Magnetic Resonance Procedures: Health Effects and Safety

The author and publisher of this book disclaim any liability for the acts of any physician, individual, group, or entity acting independently or on behalf of any organization that receives any information for any medical procedure, activity, service, or other situation through the use of this book.

The content of this book makes no representations or warranties of any kind, expressed or implied, as to the information content, materials, or products included in this book. The author assumes no responsibilities for errors or omissions that may include technical or other inaccuracies or typographical errors.

The author accepts no legal responsibility for any injury and/or damage to persons or property from any of the methods, products, instructions, or ideas contained herein.

The author will not be liable for any damages of any kind arising from the use of this book, including but not limited to direct, indirect, incidental, punitive, and consequential damages.

The information and comments provided in this book are not intended to be technical or medical recommendations or advice for individuals or patients. The information and comments provided herein are of a general nature and should not be considered specific to any individual or patient, whether or not a specific patient is referenced by the physician, technologist, individual, group, or other entity seeking information.

The author takes no responsibility for the accuracy or validity of the information contained in this book nor the claims or statements of any manufacturer. Manufacturers' product specifications are subject to change without notice. Always read the product labeling, instructions, and warning statements thoroughly before using any medical product or similar device.

Regarding the MR compatibility or MR safety for a given material, implant, device, or object that may be discussed herein, because of the ongoing research, equipment modifications, and changes in governmental regulations, no suggested product information should be used unless the reader has reviewed and evaluated the information provided with the product discussed or by reviewing the pertinent literature.

Magnetic Resonance Procedures: Health Effects and Safety

Edited by
Frank G. Shellock, Ph.D.

Foreword by—
William G. Bradley, Jr., M.D., Ph.D., FACR

CRC Press
Boca Raton   London   New York   Washington, D.C.

Library of Congress Cataloging-in-Publication Data

Magnetic resonance procedures : health effects and safety / written and edited by Frank
  G. Shellock.
      p. cm.
    Includes bibliographical references and index.
    ISBN 0-8493-1044-X (alk. paper)
    1. Magnetic resonance imaging—Safety measures. 2. Magnetic resonance
imaging—Health aspects. I. Shellock, Frank G.
    RC78.7.N83 M3478 2000
    616.07′548′0289—dc21   00-045430

Foreword

Magnetic Resonance Imaging (MRI) has revolutionized medical diagnosis over the past two decades. Even in the very beginning, however, it was clear that this wonderful new technique had a potentially significant downside. Early reports of airborne gas tanks and screwdrivers pointed to the safety precautions necessary around strong magnets. The death of a patient with a ferromagnetic aneurysm clip several years ago indicates that there is still potential for harm.

Some of the early concerns regarding oncogenesis and mutagenesis from the main magnetic field, the gradient fields, or the radiofrequency (RF) fields have been effectively eliminated. Concerns about pacemakers were raised early on but appear to be evolving — as have many of the safety areas for MRI. This evolving concern is particularly true considering the proliferation of MR systems with higher field strengths and stronger gradients. To be more specific, 3- and 4-Tesla magnets deposit considerably more RF energy and exert much more torque than the 1.5-T systems which were considered "high field" until recently. The stronger, faster gradients associated with the latest class of "cardiovascular" MRI scanners are now routinely capable of causing physiologic stimulation.

Frank Shellock, Ph.D., has done an excellent job of assembling an international, world class set of contributors for this timely and comprehensive text on health effects and safety issues in MRI. He and his contributors have put together an exhaustive analysis of these issues. The level of detail is appropriate for physicians, physicists, and MRI technologists.

This book represents the result of over 15 years of involvement in the field of MR safety by Dr. Shellock. In the 1980s, Dr. Shellock was co-chairman of the original MR Safety Committee of the Society for Magnetic Resonance Imaging (SMRI) (now merged with the SMRM to become the ISMRM). His annual pocket guides MR Procedures and Metallic Objects can be found in practically every MR center in the world. Thus, this book represents the culmination of many years of work and involvement in the area of MR safety. Dr. Shellock and his contributors are to be congratulated for having published a work that should probably be available in every MRI center in the world.

William G. Bradley, Jr., M.D., Ph.D., FACR
Professor of Radiology
University of California, Irvine
Director of MRI and Radiology Research
Long Beach Memorial Medical Center
Long Beach, CA (U.S.A.)

Preface

Magnetic resonance (MR) procedures continue to expand with regard to usage and complexity. Understandably, health effects and safety issues are important aspects of this diagnostic modality.

The last book on these topics was published in 1996. Since then, technological advances have yielded MR systems with higher static magnetic fields (up to 8.0 Tesla!), faster and higher gradient magnetic fields, and more powerful radiofrequency (RF) transmission coils. Therefore, it is necessary to reconsider, update, and revise many of the health effects and safety issues according to the changes that have occurred in MR technology.

The purpose of writing this book was to create the definitive resource of theoretical and practical information on MR health effects, safety, and patient management. While previous books on this topic were written by one or two authors, the sophisticated nature of MR now requires additional input from a wide range of experts in the field. Therefore, an international group of highly respected health effects and safety specialists representing radiologists, scientists, physicists, MR technologists, and clinicians contributed to this book. To my knowledge, this is the first authoritative textbook with multiple contributing authors devoted to the important topics of MR health effects and safety.

Because of demands by government agencies, private, and professional organizations for MR facilities to ensure patient safety, I believe that all MR healthcare workers (i.e., radiologists, physicists, MR technologists, facility managers, hospital administrators, and vendors) will find the content of this book to be particularly timely and essential.

As always, I welcome suggestions and comments that may serve to improve this book and will strive to incorporate them into the next edition. Finally, if you have a specific question or concern, please do not hesitate to visit my web site, www.MRIsafety.com, or contact me by e-mail.

Frank G. Shellock

The Editor

Frank G. Shellock, Ph.D., is a physiologist with more than 15 years of experience conducting laboratory and clinical investigations in the field of magnetic resonance imaging. He is an Adjunct Clinical Professor of Radiology at the University of Southern California, School of Medicine; the president of Shellock R & D Services, Los Angeles, CA; and a Special Employee for the U.S. Food and Drug Administration.

Dr. Shellock is a member of the Safety Committee and the Educational Committee for the International Society for Magnetic Resonance in Medicine; a former member of the Board of Directors of the Society for Magnetic Resonance Imaging; a member of the Radiological Society of North America, the American Society for Testing and Materials (subcommittee on MR Safety and Compatibility), the American College of Radiology (committee for Standards and Accreditation of the Commission on Neuroradiology and MR); and a Fellow of the American College of Sports Medicine. He is the recipient of a National Research Service Award from the National Institutes of Health, National Heart, Lung, and Blood Institute and has received numerous research grants from governmental agencies and private organizations.

Dr. Shellock has published four textbooks, over 50 book chapters, and more than 150 peer-reviewed articles. As a commitment to the field of MRI safety, Dr. Shellock developed and maintains the popular web site, www.MRIsafety.com. This web site serves as an important information resource for magnetic resonance healthcare workers and patients.

Contributors

Robert A. Bell, Ph.D.
President
R.A. Bell and Associates
Encinitas, CA

Joe D. Bourland, Ph.D.
Senior Research Engineer
Department of Computer and
  Electrical Engineering
Purdue University
West Lafayette, IN

Patrick M. Colletti, M.D.
Director, Imaging Sciences Center
Professor of Radiology
University of Southern California
  School of Medicine
Los Angeles, CA

Om P. Gandhi, Sc.D.
Professor of Electrical Engineering
University of Utah
Salt Lake City, UT

Randy L. Gollub, M.D., Ph.D.
Assistant Professor
Assistant Director of Psychiatric Neuroimaging
Department of Psychiatry
Massachusetts General Hospital
Charlestown, MA

Alexander V. Kildishev, Ph.D.
Post-Doctoral Research Associate
Department of Biomedical Engineering
Purdue University
West Lafayette, IN

Mark McJury, Ph.D.
Senior Research Scientist
Department of Radiotherapy Physics
Weston Park Hospital
Sheffield, U.K.

John A. Nyenhuis, Ph.D.
Professor of Biomedical Engineering
Department of Computer and Electrical
  Engineering
Purdue University
West Lafayette, IN

Val M. Runge, M.D.
Rosenbaum Professor of Diagnostic Radiology
Department of Diagnostic Radiology
University of Kentucky
Lexington, KY

Anne M. Sawyer-Glover, R.T. (R)(MR)
Manager, MR Whole-Body Research Systems
Richard M. Lucas Center for MRS/I
Department of Radiology
Stanford University School of Medicine
Stanford, CA

Daniel J. Schaefer, Ph.D.
Principal Engineer
General Electric Medical Systems
Milwaukee, WI

John F. Schenck, M.D., Ph.D.
Senior Scientist
General Electric Corporate Research and
  Development Center
Schenectady, NY

Frank G. Shellock, Ph.D.
Adjunct Clinical Professor of Radiology
University of Southern California and
  Shellock R & D Services, Inc.
Los Angeles, CA

Chris D. Smith, Ph.D.
Research Assistant
School of Electrical and Computer Engineering
Purdue University
West Lafayette, IN

Loren A. Zaremba, Ph.D.
Scientific Reviewer
Radiological Devices Branch
Office of Device Evaluation
Center for Devices and Radiological Health
  (CDRH)
Food and Drug Administration
Rockville, MD

Dedication

To my loving parents, Frank A. Shellock and Eleanor M. Shellock

Contents

1 Health Effects and Safety of Static Magnetic Fields*

John F. Schenck

CONTENTS

I. INTRODUCTION

The possibility that some hazard may be associated with exposure to the strong magnetic fields required to perform magnetic resonance imaging (MRI) has been of concern since the introduction of this technique in the late 1970s. Although MRI studies require patients to be exposed to strong

---

* This chapter is reprinted with modifications from the article entitled "Safety of Strong, Static Magnetic Fields." With permission from *J. Magn. Reson. Imaging*, 12, 2–19, 2000.

static magnetic fields throughout the duration of the examination, there is good reason to believe in the inherent safety of these procedures. Informal market research studies suggest that more than 150 million diagnostic MRI examinations were performed worldwide between the onset of clinical MRI in the early 1980s and the end of 1999. These studies also indicate that more than 20 million examinations are performed worldwide on a annual basis (more than 50,000 each day). Notably, the vast majority of these MRI examinations are conducted without any sign of patient injury.

Concerns for patient safety have been raised in regard to each of the three distinct fields used in MRI: the radiofrequency (RF) transmission field, B_1; the time-dependent gradient fields; and the static field, B_0. These electromagnetic fields are essential features of the operation of the magnetic resonance (MR) system, and each of them interacts with every component of the patient's body. The safety aspects of the RF and gradient fields are easier to quantify than those of the static magnetic field. The reason is that for RF and gradient fields, clear-cut physical phenomena establish upper limits for safe patient exposure (Table 1.1).

In contrast, as long as proper precautions are taken, such as assuring the absence of magnetic materials and avoiding rapid patient motion, neither theoretical nor experimental studies have demonstrated an upper limit for safe exposure to intense static magnetic fields. Therefore, at the present time, the limits on the strength of the static magnetic fields for MR systems used in MRI are set by technical, regulatory, and cost factors. The limits are not related to the ability of patients to tolerate the static magnetic fields safely.

Although there are few, if any, rigorously established magnetic field effects on human biology, this topic is the subject of vast literature that began several centuries ago and which has recently grown rapidly because of the widespread success of MRI as a clinical imaging modality. Several bibliographies of the earlier literature[1-4] and a recent historical summary[5] are available. A complete bibliography of the field at the present time is not possible, but a representative listing of books,[6-20] reviews,[21-24] and research reports[25-88] is included in the references for this chapter. As will be discussed below, the absence of harmful effects of strong, static magnetic fields can be attributed to the absence of ferromagnetic components in human tissues and to the extremely small value of the magnetic susceptibility of these tissues.

Deaths attributed to MRI procedures are extremely rare. Exact quantification is not possible because there is no uniform reporting mechanism of adverse events for this imaging modality which is heavily utilized worldwide. Furthermore, the possibility of underreporting of severe adverse events must be considered. However, a brief literature review in 1998 found reports of seven deaths attributed to the use of MRI.[89-91] These incidents included one death during examination for cerebral infarction, one death involving a ferromagnetic cerebral aneurysm clip, and five deaths related to inadvertent scanning of patients with cardiac pacemakers. Importantly, the role of the MRI examination in the fatal outcome was not certain in several of these reports. However, this small group underscores the importance of efforts to avoid performing MRI procedures in patients with ferromagnetic implants, foreign bodies, or implanted electronic devices. The large number of trouble-free studies attest to

TABLE 1.1
Comparison of the Physical Effects of the Various Fields Applied to Patients during MRI

Type of Field	Physical Limitation on Human Exposure
Switched gradient fields	Peripheral nerve stimulation[a,b]
RF B_1 fields	Tissue heating[a]
Static B_0 fields	Not known

[a] The origin of both these effects can be attributed to the electric field that accompanies all time-dependent magnetic fields and not to the magnetic field itself.

[b] Both the rate of change of the field and the duration of the change must be above threshold values for stimulation to occur.

the high level of safety that has been achieved in this modality. The much smaller number of serious complications is a reminder of the importance of continued vigilance.

This chapter will present an historical perspective of human exposure to magnetic fields, discuss information pertaining specifically to the magnetic fields of the MRI environment, and review various health effects and safety aspects related to exposure to strong, static magnetic fields.

II. HISTORICAL REVIEW OF HUMAN EXPOSURE TO MAGNETIC FIELDS

All human beings are continually exposed to the magnetic field of the Earth, which is approximately 0.5 gauss or 5×10^{-5} T. This field is weak and unobtrusive, and, except for the use of magnetic compasses, people are generally unaware of its existence. Naturally occurring magnetic minerals, such as magnetite, also known as lodestone (Fe_3O_4), have been known for several thousand years.[1] As early as the first or second century A.D., the Greek medical writer Dioscorides is said to have claimed a therapeutic role for magnetic minerals in treating arthritis and other diseases.

Mineral magnets, made from naturally occurring magnetite, are quite limited in the strength and spatial extent of the magnetic fields they can produce. For example, a fully magnetized sphere of magnetite produces a peak field of about 0.4 T, and this only occurs over a small region near its north and south poles. Using metallurgy to produce iron or steel magnets can produce fields perhaps three times stronger than this. The introduction of electromagnets in the early 19th century made it possible to produce strong fields over larger regions, but these were limited by the available power supplies and the heating of the current-carrying coils. Only after the discovery of high field (i.e., type 2) superconductors in the mid-20th century[92] did it become technically possible to achieve the intense whole-body field strengths currently used in MRI.

However, after it became possible to produce strong magnetic fields, only a relatively small number of people involved in specific professions, such as experimental high-energy physics and electromagnetic ore extraction, actually came into contact with them. Therefore, the routine use of whole-body magnets at strengths up to 1.5 T in clinical MRI, which began in the early 1980s, introduced a new degree of human exposure to magnetic fields.

Magnetotherapy is the use of magnets or coils to apply a magnetic field, usually much smaller than those used in MRI, to a patient's body for therapeutic purposes. For centuries it has been proposed in one form or another as a magical method of treating diverse conditions such as headache, seizures, and asthma. As discussed below, even though the magnetic forces on tissues are in all likelihood far too small to really produce any such effects, and no objective evidence has been provided for its effectiveness, magnetotherapy has been an impressively resilient form of folk medicine since ancient times. There has also been a fairly constant polarization of attitudes toward its effectiveness with one relatively small, but often vocal and highly popular, group of advocates opposed by a more mainstream scientific group of opponents who found the technique implausible and dismissed it as a form of quackery or self-deception. This was evident in the 16th century with the flamboyant German physician and alchemist Paracelsus (Theophrastus von Hohenheim) promoting the therapeutic powers of powdered magnetic iron oxides opposed by the famous English physician William Gilbert who ridiculed the idea of using magnets for therapeutic purposes.[5] In particular, Gilbert pointed out that grinding a magnetic lodestone into a powder for medical purposes, as recommended by Paracelsus, randomizes the magnetic effects of the individual grains and weakens the overall magnetic influence to the vanishing point.

The Viennese physician Anton Mesmer (1734 to 1815) began practicing in Paris in 1778. His therapeutic use of magnetism became sensationally successful, and by 1784 he was perhaps the most famous and controversial physician in Europe.[13] He came to believe that the curative powers did not originate in the mineral magnets themselves, but in a universal force, analogous to gravitation and called animal magnetism, which he personally was capable of concentrating and transmitting for therapeutic effect. The turbulent therapeutic sessions conducted at his upscale

Parisian clinic became controversial to the point of scandal, and a royal commission was appointed that year by Louis XVI to evaluate Mesmer's technique. This commission was composed of some of the most famous physicians and scientists of this pre-Revolutionary period including, among others, Benjamin Franklin, Antoine Lavoisier, and Joseph Guillotine.[81] They compared the results obtained using the so-called magnetized therapeutic devices with those of sham substitutes and concluded that the positive results obtained were the results of the power of suggestion acting in naive subjects, that "magnetism without imagination produces nothing," and that "this nonexistent fluid is without utility."

Mesmer was followed in the 19th century both in Europe and in North America by practicing "magnetizers" who, for the most part, were probably simple quacks. However, another line of investigation prompted by animal magnetism explored the power of suggestion. These studies led to concepts such as hypnotism, magnetic sleep, and alternate states of consciousness. Thus, these ideas have a direct ancestral relation to modern psychotherapeutic practice.[18]

In the late 19th and early 20th century, American entrepreneurs such as Dr. C. J. Thatcher, Gaylord Wilshire (for whom Wilshire Boulevard in Los Angeles is named), and Dr. Rodney Madison made heavy use of mail-order merchandising and radio advertising to promote magnet garments and devices that were claimed capable of curing an almost limitless array of diseases.[78,85] These devices, sold under names such as Theronoid and I-on-a-co, were investigated by the American Medical Association (AMA) bureau on medical fraud and the Federal Trade Commission (FTC). The Better Business Bureau and the FTC banned advertising of the Theronoid as a therapeutic device in 1933.[28]

Macklis[78] suggests that, after the American Civil War, the newly industrialized farm belts of the rural Midwest, with few well-trained physicians and a history of self-doctoring, were fertile ground for the merchandising of magnetic salves, liniments, and boot insoles. It is interesting, however, that at the beginning of the 21st century, in a well-educated country which is much less rural than it was 100 years ago, with many well-trained physicians, magnetotherapy appears to have at least as high, if not higher, a degree of popular acceptance as a mode of alternative medicine in America than at any previous time. Furthermore, although this treatment modality still lacks a convincing theoretical and experimental rationale to justify its use, there does not seem to be any organized governmental or professional effort to regulate or investigate the business practices associated with it. In this sense, the present era seems more gullible, or at least less critical, than preceding generations.

For example, widely distributed mail-order gift catalogs routinely advertise mattresses with magnetic pads sewn into them that claim to provide various health benefits and that sell for up to $1000. There are estimates that such products currently have sales in the order of $1 billion per year.[84] Additionally, a popular, physician-authored book published in 1998 claims that magnets can be used to provide relief from arthritis, menstrual cramps, carpal tunnel syndrome, and many other disorders.[20]

In the 1960s, the onset of the space program led to a series of studies concerned with possible magnetic-field-related safety problems for astronauts.[33,34] It was thought that these might arise either because the astronauts would not be exposed to the ordinarily ubiquitous magnetic field of the Earth while in space or because proposed magnetohydrodyamic propulsion and cosmic ray shielding techniques might expose them to unusually intense magnetic fields. At about the same time, additional studies were undertaken to address safety concerns about the strong magnets being utilized in high-energy physics laboratories.[38]

III. HISTORY OF MAGNETIC FIELD EXPOSURE DURING MRI

The introduction of MRI as a clinical imaging modality in the early 1980s led to the design, fabrication, and wide dissemination of new forms of large and powerful magnets and to the large increase in the level of human exposure to strong magnetic fields. MRI magnets are characterized by their large size and the highly homogeneous fields at their centers. These magnets are normally

TABLE 1.2
Historical Development of MRI Magnetic Field Strength

Field Strength (Tesla)	Date of Introduction	Institution	Type	Comments
0.05-0.10	1977	State University of New York, Brooklyn	Superconducting	This machine produced an early thoracic image
0.7	1977	University of Nottingham	Iron core electromagnet	This machine, with a 13-cm gap, produced an early wrist image
0.04	1980	Aberdeen	Air core electromagnet	This machine was used for the first clinical MRI studies
0.35	1981	Hammersmith, Diasonics	Whole body, superconducting	These machines were the first whole-body superconducting scanners
1.5	1982	General Electric	Whole body, superconducting	Whole-body magnets at 1.5 T have been in widespread clinical use since the mid-1980s
4.0	1987	Siemens, General Electric, Philips	Whole body, superconducting	During the late 1990s 3 T and 4 T scanners became widely available at research institutions
8	1998	Ohio State University	Whole body, superconducting	This is the highest field whole-body MRI scanner currently operating

Data from References 63, 65, 76, 77, and 93 to 101.

large enough to surround large adult humans, although smaller magnets designed to image only the head or limbs are sometimes used. The central field is intense and has homogeneity on the order of 10 parts per million (ppm) or better over spherical volumes approximately 50 cm in diameter. The magnets most commonly used in MRI are cylindrically symmetric superconducting devices, although resistive, permanent, and hybrid magnets are also utilized.

Table 1.2 provides information on the time of introduction of MR systems of various field strengths.[93–101] It should be noted that it is not the purpose of Table 1.2 to provide a rigorous historical record of priority, but rather to give the reader a feeling for the pace at which new levels of field strength have become available and accepted in clinical medicine and MRI research. The substantial financial and technical barriers experienced when developing whole-body machines of ever higher field strength are attested to by the 11-year period that elapsed between the introduction of the first 4.0 T whole-body scanners and the introduction of the first 8.0 T machine at Ohio State University in early 1998.[88]

Human MRI procedures have now been reported for field strengths ranging from 0.02[66] to 8.0 T. Specific advantages have been found for MR systems operating over a wide range of static magnetic field strengths. However, Bell has estimated that more than 60% of the MR systems operating in the U.S. in 2000 will be at static magnetic field strengths of 1.0, 1.5, or 2.0 T.[102] Up to the present time, MR systems operating at 3.0 T and higher have been utilized largely for research purposes. However, more widespread usage of these very high field units is likely in the next few years.

As indicated in Section I, a huge number of diagnostic clinical MRI procedures have been completed without major incidents. This strongly supports the view of earlier authors[25-27] that the magnetic interactions with normal tissues are within the bounds of safety up to the highest fields now in use for MRI. However, in the presence of ferromagnetic materials, a number of authors have noted the danger associated with ferromagnetic objects either implanted in the patient or located in the fringing field of the magnets (Figure 1.1).[47,52,53,56,73]

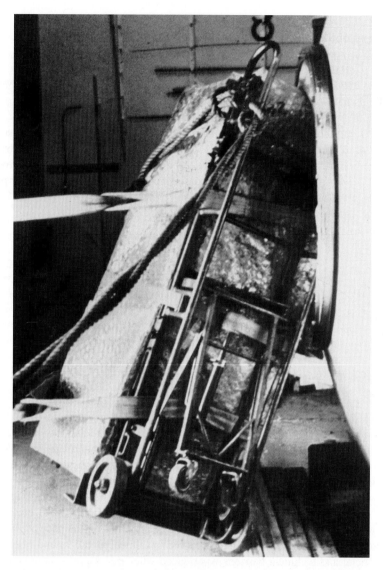

FIGURE 1.1 Magnetic field accident. The powerful and insidious nature of magnetic forces acting on ferro-magnetic materials with very large magnetic susceptibilities is demonstrated in this accident. An RF power supply was being moved in the vicinity of an unshielded 1.5-T superconducting magnet. The magnetic forces depend on the field strength and gradient and vary extremely rapidly with position. In this case, over a very short distance, the magnetic forces went from being imperceptible to a level at which the workmen moving the power supply were unable to restrain it. (Photo courtesy of Dr. W. A. Edelstein. From Schenck, J.F., *Med. Phys.*, 23, 815, 1996. With permission.)

IV. ASSESSMENT OF THE LITERATURE ON MAGNETIC FIELD EXPOSURE

A bibliographic review published in 1962,[2] well before the introduction of MRI, found 393 published reports dealing with biological effects of magnetic fields, and there have been many additional reports since that time. Of course, many of these reports do not address issues of pathological or therapeutic magnetic effects. The portion of this literature that does deal with the alleged pathological or therapeutic effects of magnetic fields is contradictory and confusing. Often, basic information such as the field strength and its variation over the organism studied is not provided. Generally, these studies do not describe the dose-response characteristics of the effect, that is the dependence on field strength and the duration of the exposure. Few, if any, have been replicated, and, in most cases, no plausible physical mechanism is put forward to explain the proposed effect. In other cases, a mechanism is proposed, but is not verified to be quantitatively large enough to explain the proposed effect. Several studies undertaken to look for harmful effects of magnetic fields have yielded negative results.[25-27,45,49,50,76,77,79]

Responding to many earlier claims for the therapeutic effectiveness of magnets, Peterson and Kennelly in 1892 collaborated on studies of magnetic field exposures at the laboratories of Thomas Edison.[26] They used the largest magnet available to them at that time (approximately 0.15 T) to carry out whole-body exposures of a dog and a young boy. They found no positive results and concluded that, "The ordinary magnets used in medicine have a purely suggestive or psychic effect and would in all probability be quite as useful if made of wood."

In 1921, Harvard physiologists Drinker and Thomson investigated possible health consequences of the exposure to magnetic fields of industrial workers.[27] They focused on the use of powerful separator magnets in the manganese industry and performed numerous experiments on nerve-muscle preparations and on living animals. Again, they found no effects of the magnetic fields and concluded that, "It seems certain that the magnetic field has no significance as a health hazard."

In many cases, efforts to reproduce positive findings have been unsuccessful. For example, in a series of publications in the 1950s, it was reported that magnetic field exposure in mice led to retardation of the overall growth rate, tumor growth rate, and white blood cell counts.[29,30] However, attempts to replicate these finding by Eiselein et al.[32] produced completely negative results. In another example, it was reported that the brainstem auditory evoked potential was delayed after exposure to a 0.35-T magnetic field.[54] Several subsequent studies failed to confirm this finding.[68,69,74]

Certainly, many factors are at work to account for the various contradictory findings in the literature. It is often difficult to isolate the effects due to the applied magnetic field from other confounding factors present. In one recent case, a finding of scientific misconduct has been made.[103–106] The power of suggestion is operative in many cases involving the subjective evaluation of magnetic field effects. It is likely that anxiety caused by the presence of a large and somewhat intimidating superconducting magnet can influence perceptions of vague discomforts. For example, Erhard et al. found that when evaluated after exposure to a 4.0-T superconducting magnet, 45% of subjects responded positively to the query, "Did you experience any unusual sensations while in the magnet?" even though the magnet was not energized.[79] Irving Langmuir suggested the term "pathological science" for situations in which experiments studying low level phenomena repeatedly fail to be replicated.[107,108]

Thus, the current situation seems to be best summarized by Budinger, who wrote in 1981[43] "From the vast literature on cell cultures, animals, and man, no experimental protocol has been found that, when repeated by other investigators, gives similar positive results." Because of the difficulty in establishing a negative conclusion, it should not be concluded that it has been proven that there are no significant biological effects of static magnetic fields. However, it does appear correct to say that the work performed to date has yet to provide a single example of a scientifically sound and rigorously verified pathological effect of such fields. The steadily increasing capability of producing ever-stronger magnets gives reason to believe that such effects will eventually be established, but probably at field strengths well above those currently used in MRI.

V. QUALITATIVE REVIEW OF POSSIBLE STATIC MAGNETIC FIELD EFFECTS ON HUMAN TISSUES

There are several physical mechanisms of interaction between tissues and static magnetic fields that could theoretically lead to pathological changes in human subjects. Quantitative analysis of each of these indicates that they are below the threshold of significance. These effects are summarized below.

A. Magnetic Forces and Torques

Tissue components that are permanently magnetized or that have magnetic susceptibilities that are positive with respect to that of water are drawn toward high field regions and vice versa.[109,110] Theoretically, this could lead to sorting of tissue components, with the more paramagnetic components moving to high field regions. However, as shown below for red blood cells, this effect is very weak in practice and not of practical significance in living tissues even in very intense static fields. Human tissues do not contain permanently magnetized components. When such materials are introduced through accident (as in shrapnel emplacement) or through surgical intervention, they represent serious hazards that must be carefully controlled and that may represent absolute contraindications for MRI procedures.

Permanently magnetized materials tend to rotate such that their magnetic moment comes into alignment with the magnetic field. Soft magnetic materials, whose magnetization is proportional to the applied field, tend to rotate such that the long axis of the object is parallel to the applied field. For magnetic foreign bodies, these effects represent an even greater potential hazard than the translational forces on such materials. Paramagnetic materials, whose susceptibilities vary with the direction of the magnetizing field (anisotropic susceptibility), tend to orient with the axis of most positive susceptibility aligned with the field. Diamagnetic materials tend to rotate such that the axis of least negative susceptibility aligns with the field. This effect can be demonstrated *in vitro,* but, as shown below, it is too weak to be operative within tissues.

B. Flow and Motion-Induced Currents in Tissues

In a truly static electric field, the electric current density, J, in tissues is determined by $J = \sigma E$, where σ is the tissue's electrical conductivity and E is the electric field. Under normal circumstances these electric fields result from processes such as the depolarization of the heart tissue. In this case, the resulting current density produces the electrocardiogram (EKG). If the tissue moves with a velocity v relative to the static field, there is an additional term in the expression for the current density, $J = \sigma(E + v \times B)$, with the term $v \times B$ acting as a motion-induced electric field.

Therefore, tissue motion, such as bulk physical movements (e.g., rapid movement into or out of the magnet or rapid head turning) or internal movements (e.g., blood flow), in strong static fields can produce additional physical effects beyond those directly associated with permanent magnetism and magnetic susceptibility. Measurement of the body surface potentials produced by blood flow in a magnetic field was long ago proposed as a form of electromagnetic flow meter.[111,112]

In the 1960s, it was shown that the EKGs of subjects (originally monkeys) located in strong magnetic fields displayed field-induced changes, particularly T-wave abnormalities.[34] It was originally suggested that this might indicate a magnetic field effect on the repolarization process in the myocardial tissues. However, a simpler effect, based on the electromotive force (emf) developed in blood flowing in a magnetic field, was subsequently shown to explain these changes.[113,114] As indicated above, when an electrically conducting fluid such as blood flows in an applied magnetic field, a transverse emf is developed. This leads to a small induced current density in the tissues. This, in turn, leads to a small electric voltage on the body surface, which, like the conventional EKG, can be detected by the use of metal electrodes on the skin. This effect is now easily demonstrated in patients in clinical MR systems and contributes to the difficulty in obtaining good EKGs during MRI procedures.

This induced emf is proportional to the velocity of blood flow and to the magnetic field strength. This effect has recently been studied in humans at field strengths as high as 8.0 T.[88] At the highest field strengths currently available, the flow-induced current densities are below the threshold levels to cause nerve or muscle stimulation effects.[115] However, at some level of magnetic field strength, it seems likely that the flow-induced currents surrounding blood vessels would reach levels capable of causing extraneous nerve or muscle excitation. Theoretically, this effect may eventually become the limiting factor in the ability of humans to tolerate extremely high static magnetic fields.[77,86]

C. Magnetic Effects on Chemical Reactions

The proper metabolic functioning of tissues requires the continual functioning of a huge number of chemical reactions. There are situations in which an applied static magnetic field might alter the rate or equilibrium positions of such reactions.[116-123] For example, if the products of a chemical reaction are more paramagnetic than the reactants, then the presence of a magnetic field could shift the reaction equilibrium to increase the concentration of the products. The dissociation of molecules consisting of oxygen bound to hemoglobin (which are diamagnetic) into separate molecules of oxygen and hemoglobin (each of which is paramagnetic) is an example of this possibility. In this case, an applied field should lower the energy barrier for the dissociation of the bound pair and favor the production of the paramagnetic products. However, calculations indicate that even in an applied field of 4.0-T, the free energy barrier to dissociation (about 64,000 J/mol) in this reaction is changed by only about 1 J/mol. This small energy shift will have less effect on the reaction equilibrium than a temperature change of 0.01°C.[77]

Although a static magnetic field, acting on small differences between the susceptibilities of the products and the reactants, does not significantly affect the equilibrium position of chemical reactions, there is another mechanism that has been shown to allow magnetic fields to alter somewhat the dynamics of certain chemical reactions. Specifically, this refers to the dissociation of a binary molecule, AB, present in some solvent, where A and B are joined by a non-magnetic electron-pair bond, into two radicals, A and B. In the bound state, the two electrons have opposite spins so that together they form a singlet state with a total spin equal to zero.

If AB spontaneously dissociates, because of thermal agitation, into separate radicals A and B, each radical can, for a short time, be considered as residing within a cage of surrounding solvent molecules that impedes the complete separation of the radicals from one another. If A and B recombine before separating from one another, the process is called geminate recombination, and the so-called cage product, AB, is formed. On the other hand, if they ultimately diffuse apart, an escape product, A and B, is formed.

If an applied magnetic field is present, and if the magnetic moments are not the same for the two radicals, the spins of the two separating radicals will precess at somewhat different rates. Geminate recombination is only possible if the two radicals are still in a singlet state (total spin of zero) when they reencounter one another. If the differing rates of spin precession have given the total spin wave function a significant portion of triplet character, the probability of bond reformation will be reduced, and the yield of escape products will be increased.

A complete discussion of this effect is beyond the scope of this chapter. However, there is experimental evidence for an effect of static magnetic fields on the yields of some photochemical and organic chemistry reactions involving free radical intermediates. In general, the effects are not large, and effects on reactions of biochemical significance have not been reported. These effects depend on field strength in a complicated way. Certain reaction paths are enhanced, then retarded as the field strength is increased.[117-123] The field effect on the yield of these reactions is small and not linearly proportional to field strength. This effect has not been demonstrated in biochemical reactions, and its relevance to magnetic field safety is uncertain. It does not appear that the cage mechanism would be relevant to enzyme-mediated reactions.

D. Possible Ferromagnetic Tissue Components

The inherent weakness of the interaction of diamagnetic tissue components with external magnetic fields is a consequence of the extremely small susceptibility values of these materials. This conclusion would need reexamination if human tissues were found to contain significant amounts of ferromagnetic or strongly paramagnetic materials.[124-129] Small amounts of some paramagnetic, but not ferromagnetic, substances are natural tissue components. For example, 70-kg adult humans have about 3.7 g of iron in their tissues. However, this iron is not present in a bulk ferromagnetic form, but is distributed in various chemical compounds such as hemoglobin, ferritin, and hemo-siderin, which are only weakly paramagnetic and do not interact strongly with applied fields. The concentrations of these paramagnetic substances are not large enough to convert the overall sus-ceptibility of any tissue (including blood) from diamagnetic to paramagnetic components.[80]

Small amounts of particulate magnetite have been found in the lungs and in other tissues of people who are occupationally exposed to rock dust, such as coal miners.[124-128] Additionally, contamination with magnetite and other iron oxides can result from tattooing.[124-128] It has also been shown that small particles such as these can spread within the body.[62] However, no evidence has been presented for a biological function of ferromagnetic particles or of a related pathology associated with their exposure to strong magnetic fields.

Electron microscopy evidence from autopsy studies[129] has been presented for the presence of extremely small magnetite particles, less than 500 Å in diameter, in human brain and other tissues. Possible functional roles for such particles were also presented. As with other such studies, addi-tional confirmation and studies to rule out an exogenous source for these particles are desirable. Such small particles do not produce MR imaging artifacts, at least by using conventional pulse sequences, and if ferromagnetic particles much larger than this were present, it is likely they could be detected in this way. Such artifacts have not been observed.

Local edema and tissue swelling as well as localized image artifacts have been noted during MRI of patients with tattooing or permanently implanted eye shadow. This effect has been attributed to an interaction of the RF field with electrically conducting components of the implanted pig-ments.[55,58,60-62] However, the B_1 field does not produce significant local heating interactions with small metallic implants such as surgical hemostasis clips and is unlikely to do so with relatively poorly conducting oxides. A more likely explanation is that the implanted pigments contain irreg-ularly shaped magnetic iron oxide particles and these particles twist such that their long axis is aligned with the applied field when the patient enters the magnet. The magnetic fields of these particles lead to the observed image artifacts, and the twisting may produce local tissue irritation causing the edema formation. Any patient motion while in the magnetic field would tend to exacerbate this tissue irritation.

E. MAGNETORESISTANCE AND THE HALL EFFECT

The motion of electrons and ions in solution is altered in the presence of a strong magnetic field, and it has been conjectured that this could lead to a field-dependent modification of the depolarizing currents which are responsible for the propagation of the nerve and muscle action potentials. If the mean free path of the current carriers and the time between collisions are sufficiently long, the effective resistivity is increased and transverse electric fields are generated (Hall effect) when a conductor is placed in a magnetic field. However, the action potentials of nerve and muscle tissue are dependent on ionic currents. These ions have extremely short mean free paths (~1 Å) and collision times (10^{-12} s), and, therefore, magnetic fields will have negligible effects on the currents associated with action potentials.[50]

F. MAGNETOHYDRODYNAMIC (MHD) FORCES AND PRESSURES

Currents flowing in tissues experience a body force, $\mathbf{J} \times \mathbf{B}$, and the resulting pressures and forces are transmitted to the tissues. These forces can be substantial in flowing liquid metals such as mercury. However, flowing physiological fluids such as blood have much lower electrical conduc-tivities than mercury, and MHD forces on flowing blood are very small compared to the naturally occurring hemodynamic forces in the vascular system. Therefore, contrary to early speculations, there is no requirement for increased heart activity to maintain the cardiac output in the presence of a strong, static magnetic field.[59,71] On the other hand, it may be that very small MHD forces operating on the endolymphatic tissues of the inner ear are the source of sensations of nausea and vertigo sometimes reported by human subjects in the presence of higher static magnetic fields.[76,77]

G. MAGNETOSTRICTION

Ferromagnetic materials change their size and shape slightly when exposed to strong magnetic fields.[130] However, these changes are very small, and human tissues do not normally contain ferromagnetic materials. Any effect in human tissue would be extremely minor compared to the naturally occurring forces of thermal expansion and mechanical stresses.

VI. QUANTITATIVE ASPECTS OF STATIC FIELD EXPOSURE

To proceed from a qualitative to a quantitative analysis of the magnetic responses of tissues, the concept of magnetic susceptibility will be introduced and its consequences explored. An important goal of this analysis is to emphasize that the quantitative differences between the magnetic properties of ferromagnetic materials and those of plant and animal tissues are so great that in many cases there is a qualitatively different character to their response to applied magnetic fields. A common error in predicting the response of tissues to applied fields is to extrapolate from familiar experiences with ferromagnetic materials, whereas tissue components will not necessarily conform to these expectations. The approach is to introduce the concept of magnetic susceptibility and then to relate this to the magnetic energy forces and torques which determine the response of tissues to applied magnetic fields.

A. MAGNETIC SUSCEPTIBILITY AND THE CLASSIFICATION OF MAGNETIC MATERIALS

Permanently magnetized materials such as bar magnets and compass needles can be extremely hazardous in the MR environment, and, in the exceptional situations in which they are required in MRI work, they must be rigorously controlled. Ordinarily, they should be excluded from these locations or environments and will not be further discussed in this chapter. All materials that are not permanently magnetized are characterized by a physical parameter called the magnetic volume susceptibility or just the susceptibility.[80] The physical basis for the apparent lack of responsiveness of biological tissues to applied magnetic fields is primarily due to the very small values of their magnetic susceptibilities.

In this chapter, SI or MKS units will be used exclusively, and boldface symbols will be used to designate vector quantities. Most material objects are not spontaneously magnetic in the sense that they do not create a magnetic field in their environment unless they are exposed to an external magnetic field. Such external fields are usually generated by permanently magnetized materials or by electric currents. The response of the materials when placed in an external field that has been generated by some means is to develop a magnetic polarization, which is measured by the magnetization or magnetic dipole moment per unit volume. The strength of the induced magnetization is proportional to the magnetic field and the susceptibility, χ. In SI units, χ is dimensionless and is defined by the equation $\mathbf{M} = \chi\mathbf{H}$, where $\mathbf{M}$ is the magnetization at the point in question and $\mathbf{H}$ is the local value of the magnetic field strength.

At each point, these fields are related to $\mathbf{B}$, the magnetic flux density by the formula $\mathbf{B} = \mu_0(\mathbf{H} + \mathbf{M})$. The magnetization of the sample becomes the source of a second, or induced, magnetic field. The interaction of the applied and the induced fields leads to interactions between the magnetized object and the permanent magnets or currents that created the originally applied field. To distinguish between the total field $\mathbf{B}$ and the applied field at a point, the symbol $\mathbf{B}_0$ for the applied field will be used.

In most materials, the induced magnetization is parallel to $\mathbf{H}$, and, in this case, $\mathbf{M}$, $\mathbf{B}$, and $\mathbf{H}$ all point in the same direction. In this common situation, the materials are referred to as isotropic and χ is a scalar quantity. In some cases, the material magnetizes in some directions more easily than in others. In this case, the magnetization is not necessarily parallel to the magnetic field, the material is anisotropic, and χ is a symmetric tensor. Except for a brief discussion of the weak torques present in certain biological crystals, this chapter will assume that the materials under discussion are isotropic. Note that the field **H** used in the definition of χ is the sum of the applied and induced fields at the point in question. Therefore, for materials with large susceptibilities, it is necessary to determine the magnetization of an object self-consistently by accounting for the effects of the induced as well as the applied field. This will be done below for ellipsoidal objects through the use of demagnetizing coefficients. On the other hand, the fields induced by the magnetization of objects, such as biological materials, with very small susceptibilities are feeble compared to the applied fields and may often be neglected. In this important case, the magnetization is determined entirely by the applied field.

If the material is isotropic, **M** will be parallel to **H** and **B**, and, as discussed below, there will be no torques attempting to align the object with the local fields. More precisely, we can say that in this situation any such torques that are present are so small as to be negligible in comparison to other biological forces acting on the tissue component.

All non-permanently magnetized materials have non-zero values of χ and are to some extent magnetic. Materials may be classified into three large groups based on their susceptibility values. Energy considerations show that χ values less than -1.0 are not possible, while any value of $\chi > -1$ is possible.[132] Materials with negative susceptibilities, that is, with $-1.0 < \chi < 0$, are called diamagnetic. They magnetize in the direction opposite to the local magnetic field and are repelled from regions of strong magnetic fields.

All materials have diamagnetic tendencies and will be in this class unless they also contain some components, such as magnetic ions of the transition elements, which provide an overriding positive contribution to χ. Materials with positive values for χ are referred to as paramagnetic and are attracted to regions of strong magnetic fields. Materials in which $|\chi|$ is less than approximately 0.01 or so are not overtly responsive to casual testing with hand-held magnets and are often considered as non-magnetic. This class includes the vast majority of common materials and, with rare exceptions such as magnetotactic bacteria, all living tissues.

The third group of materials has $|\chi| \geq 0.01$ and is referred to in this chapter as ferromagnetic or magnetic. These materials can respond very strongly to an applied magnetic field and can present real dangers if present in the vicinity of an MR system (Figure 1.1). In contrast to permanent magnets or hard magnetic materials, these materials are also referred to as soft magnetic materials as their magnetic properties are not manifested until they are exposed to an external field.

Figure 1.2 illustrates a fundamental physical fact — the enormous range of susceptibility values that occur in nature.[80] The vast majority of materials has susceptibility values much less than 0.001, and for such materials magnetic forces are quite weak and require special efforts to demonstrate them. In particular, the vast majority of biological tissues has susceptibilities in a narrow range of about ±20% from the susceptibility of water, $\chi_{H_2O} = -9.05 \times 10^{-6}$ in SI units. If it were not the case that biological tissues all have similar susceptibility values, MRI would be severely limited or impossible because of the strong local field variations and, therefore, position-dependent variations in the Larmor frequency, that would be produced by local variations in χ.

The forces involved with diamagnetic repulsion are normally so small as to be negligible. It is true that when a patient is moved into an MR system, the magnet exerts a small force to oppose this motion, but this force is so small as to be unnoticeable. The materials commonly thought of as magnetic, on the other hand, can have susceptibility values of 1000 or more and can respond forcefully to applied magnetic fields. As discussed further below, this huge quantitative variation in susceptibility values leads to qualitatively differing responses of ferromagnetic and "non-magnetic" materials to applied fields.

Geim and his associates have recently managed to use the very weak repulsive forces operating between magnets and diamagnetic materials such as living tissues to suspend small frogs and other diamagnetic objects against the pull of gravity in the space above a vertical small bore magnet operating at 16 T.[109,110] Interestingly, this dramatic exposure to strong magnetic fields did not produce any visible harm to the frogs.

SUSCEPTIBILITY SPECTRUM

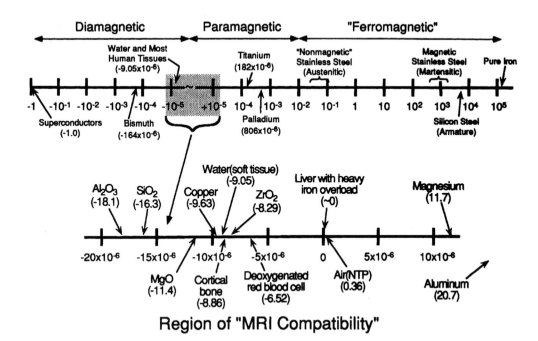

Region of "MRI Compatibility"

FIGURE 1.2 Spectrum of magnetic susceptibilities. The upper diagram uses a logarithmic scale to indicate the full range of observed magnetic susceptibility values: it extends from $\chi = -1.0$ for superconductors to $\chi > 100,000$ for soft ferromagnetic materials. The bottom diagram uses a linear scale (in ppm) to indicate the properties of some materials with $|\chi| < 20$ ppm. The susceptibilities of most human tissues range from -7.0 to -11.0 ppm. (From Schenck, J.F., *Med. Phys.*, 23, 815, 1996. With permission.)

B. MAGNETIC FIELD ENERGY

When an object such a metallic aneurysm clip is placed in a magnetic field, it experiences translational movements and torques that tend to cause it to move and rotate with respect to the direction of the field. The resulting translational forces and torques depend on the nature of the material and the strength of the magnetic field, ranging from absolutely negligible to potentially lethal values. Typically, to understand whether these forces and torques will be at a significant level in a given situation, it is necessary to have mathematical expressions that can be used to calculate them.

Once a magnetic potential energy function, U, is available to relate the magnetic energy of the object to its location, orientation, and material properties, standard techniques of physics (virtual work) can be used to generate the necessary expressions for the forces and torques. The dipole moment is the integral of the magnetization, $\mathbf{M}$, over the volume, V, of the object. If the magnetization is uniform over the object, $\mathbf{m} = \mathbf{M}V$. If a material with a permanent dipole moment $\mathbf{m}$ is brought to a point P within a magnetic field, it acquires an energy $U = \mathbf{m} \bullet \mathbf{B}_0$. If an object which has a magnetic moment that is proportional to the applied field is brought to P and thereby acquires an induced moment $\mathbf{m}$, its energy is $U = \frac{1}{2}\mathbf{m} \bullet \mathbf{B}_0$. In both cases, $\mathbf{B}_0$ is the field existing at P prior to the introduction of the material, and it is assumed that the sources of this field are kept constant when the material is introduced into the field. The factor $\frac{1}{2}$ accounts for the fact that, in the second case, as the material is brought into the magnetic field, its moment gradually increases from zero to $\mathbf{m}$, rather than being at the value $\mathbf{m}$ along the entire path. Thus, the magnetic energy is determined by the strength of the dipole moment, the strength of the magnetic field, and the angle between these two vector quantities.[131-134]

The magnetic field exerts forces and torques on the object that have the effect of increasing the magnetic energy. As shown below, the effect of the forces is to attract paramagnetic materials toward regions of stronger field strength and to push diamagnetic materials toward regions of weaker field strength. The effects of the torques are to turn the object such that $\mathbf{m}$ is brought into alignment with $\mathbf{B}_0$. Writing $\mathbf{F}$ for the force and $\mathbf{T}$ for the torque, we have the following:

$$\mathbf{F} = \nabla U \text{ and } \mathbf{T} = \frac{\partial U}{\partial \theta}\mathbf{u} = \mathbf{M} \times \mathbf{B}_0$$

where θ is the angle between $\mathbf{M}$ and $\mathbf{B}$ and $\mathbf{u}$ is the unit vector perpendicular to the plane of $\mathbf{M}$ and $\mathbf{B}$.

In many texts, such as Bleaney and Bleaney,[133] the expressions above for U, $\mathbf{F}$, and $\mathbf{T}$ all have a minus sign in front of the term on the right-hand side of the equation; that is, the definitions are $U = -\mathbf{m} \bullet \mathbf{B}_0$, $\mathbf{F} = -\nabla U$, and $\mathbf{T} = -((\partial U)/(\partial \theta))\mathbf{u}$. This sign is determined by whether or not the energy required to maintain the magnetic field at a constant level as the dipole is moved is included in the definition of the magnetic potential energy.[131-133] The choice of this convention does not affect the final formulas for the force and torque on the dipole. If an object has volume V and susceptibility χ,

$$\mathbf{m} = \mathbf{M}V = \chi V \mathbf{H}_0 = \frac{\chi}{\mu_0} V \mathbf{B}_0 \text{ and } U = \frac{1}{2}\mathbf{M} \bullet \mathbf{B}_0 = \frac{1}{2}\frac{\chi V}{\mu_0} B_0^2$$

This formula assumes that the absolute value of the susceptibility is much less than one and that the particle is sufficiently small that B_0 does not change significantly over it.

C. Demagnetizing Factors

To make use of the formulas for the translational forces and torque on materials that do not have a fixed dipole moment, but which instead have a magnetization induced by the applied field, it is necessary to determine the field-induced dipole moment. In general, this is a complicated process, but it can be simplified in the case of ellipsoids. The results for ellipsoids such as spheres, plates, and cylinders can be used in many cases to get an adequate idea of the behavior of less symmetric objects.

If a field is applied along a principal axis of an ellipsoid and the susceptibility is isotropic, the induced internal field is parallel to the applied field and is given by $\mathbf{H}_{dm} = -D\mathbf{M}$, where D, the demagnetizing factor, is a shape-dependent number with a value between zero and one.[80,130] A general ellipsoid has three distinct principal axes, and the sum of the three demagnetizing factors is always equal to one; the three principal axes of a sphere are equivalent, and, therefore, the demagnetizing factor for any direction must be one third. For cylinders transverse to the applied field, $D = 1/2$; for long cylinders parallel to this field, $D = 0$. The total internal field $\mathbf{H}$ is uniform and is the sum of the applied field, $\mathbf{H}_0 = \mathbf{B}_0/\mu_0$, and the demagnetizing field, $\mathbf{H}_{dm}$. Using $\mathbf{M} = \chi\mathbf{H}$ and $\mathbf{B} = \mu_0(\mathbf{H} + \mathbf{M})$, the total internal fields are given in terms of the applied field $\mathbf{B}_0$ by

$$\mathbf{B} = \mathbf{B}_0(1 + \chi)/(1 + D\chi),$$

$$\mu_0 \mathbf{H} = \mathbf{B}_0/(1 + D\chi),$$

$$\text{and } \mu_0 \mathbf{M} = \mathbf{B}_0\chi/(1 + D\chi).$$

Here it is assumed that $\mathbf{B}_0$ is in the direction of one of the principal axes and D is the demagnetizing factor for that axis. If $\mathbf{B}_0$ is not along a principal axis, it may be resolved into components along these axes, and the resulting fields are summed to get the total fields. An examination of these formulas shows how the shape of an object (acting through D) and the magnetic properties (acting through χ) interact with $\mathbf{B}_0$ to establish the magnetic response of the object to an applied field. A general ellipsoid has three independent principal axes and three different demagnetizing factors, but it is simpler and often sufficient to consider only ellipsoids of revolution: they have two equivalent principal axes, and, therefore, two of the demagnetizing factors are equal.

These equations show that the first order for strongly magnetic materials ($\chi \gg 1$), the internal $\mathbf{B}$ field and the magnetization are *independent of the susceptibility* and are determined only by the shape of the object. Conversely, for $|\chi| \ll 1$, $\mathbf{M}$ is parallel to the applied field, is equal to $\chi \mathbf{B}_0/\mu_0$, and is *independent of the shape of the ellipsoid*. An immediate consequence is that the forces and torques experienced by a ferromagnetic object in a magnetic field depend crucially on the object's shape, while the forces and torques on a biological object with a very small susceptibility are essentially independent of the object's shape.

D. MAGNETIC FORCES AND TORQUES

The magnetic force for an isotropic object with a field-induced magnetization in the direction x is given by

$$F_x = \frac{\partial U}{\partial x} = \frac{\chi V}{\mu_0} B \frac{\partial B}{\partial x}$$

If χ is positive, the force will be in the direction of increasing B_0 and vice versa. For a strongly magnetic object such as a ferromagnetic aneurysm clip,

$$F_z = \frac{V}{2\alpha\mu_0} B_z \frac{\partial B_z}{\partial z},$$

and for a weakly magnetic object,

$$F_z = \frac{V}{2\mu_0} \chi B_z \frac{\partial B_z}{\partial z}.$$

The torque, $\mathbf{T}$, is given by $\mathbf{T} = \mathbf{M} \times \mathbf{B}_0$ or, if the y-axis is perpendicular to $\mathbf{B}_0$ and $\mathbf{M}$,

$$T_y = \frac{\partial U}{\partial \theta} = MB_0 \sin\theta,$$

where θ is the angle between $\mathbf{M}$ and $\mathbf{B}_0$.

1. Comparison of Risks from Translational Forces and Torques

Table 1.3 provides a summary of the expressions for the magnetic energy, force, and torque which act on ellipsoids of revolution and emphasizes how the limiting forms of these expressions for large and small values of the susceptibility predict qualitatively differing behavior in these two cases. The demagnetizing factor along the axis of symmetry is D_a, and the radial demagnetizing factor is D_r. Therefore, $D_a + 2D_r = 1$. For a long, needle-like ellipsoid, $D_a \to 0$ and $D_r \to \frac{1}{2}$. For a sphere, $D_a = D_r = \frac{1}{3}$. For a flat, disk-like ellipsoid, $D_a \to 1$ and $D_r \to 0$. Expressions for demagnetizing factors for the full range of ellipsoids of revolution are given in Reference 80. The applied field and the axis of symmetry are in the x,z plane, and the angle between them is θ.

TABLE 1.3
Magnetic Properties of Ellipsoids of Revolution

	Full Expression	Soft Magnetic Materials $\chi D_a, \chi D_r \gg 1$	Non-Magnetic Materials $|\chi| \ll 1$
U	$\dfrac{\chi V B_0^2}{2\mu_0}\left[\dfrac{\cos^2\theta}{1+\chi D_a}+\dfrac{\sin^2\theta}{1+\chi D_r}\right]$	$\dfrac{V B_0^2}{2\mu_0}\left[\dfrac{\cos^2\theta}{D_a}+\dfrac{\sin^2\theta}{D_r}\right]$	$\dfrac{\chi V B_0^2}{2\mu_0}$
F_z	$\dfrac{\chi V}{\mu_0}B_0\dfrac{\partial B_0}{\partial z}\left[\dfrac{\cos^2\theta}{1+\chi D_a}+\dfrac{\sin^2\theta}{1+\chi D_r}\right]$	$\dfrac{V}{\mu_0}B_0\dfrac{\partial B_0}{\partial z}\left[\dfrac{\cos^2\theta}{D_a}+\dfrac{\sin^2\theta}{D_r}\right]$	$\dfrac{\chi V}{\mu_0}B_0\dfrac{\partial B_0}{\partial z}$
M_x	$\dfrac{\chi B_0}{\mu_0}\left[\dfrac{D_r-D_a}{(1+\chi D_a)(1+\chi D_r)}\right]\cos\theta\sin\theta$	$\dfrac{B_0}{\mu_0}\dfrac{D_r-D_a}{D_a D_r}\cos\theta\sin\theta$	$\dfrac{\chi B_0}{\mu_0}(D_r-D_a)\cos\theta\sin\theta$
M_z	$\dfrac{\chi B_0}{\mu_0}\left[\dfrac{\cos^2\theta}{1+\chi D_a}+\dfrac{\sin^2\theta}{1+\chi D_r}\right]$	$\dfrac{B_0}{\mu_0}\left[\dfrac{\cos^2\theta}{D_a}+\dfrac{\sin^2\theta}{D_r}\right]$	$\dfrac{\chi B_0}{\mu_0}$
T_y	$\dfrac{\chi^2 V B_0^2}{\mu_0}\dfrac{D_a-D_r}{(1+\chi D_a)(1+\chi D_r)}\cos\theta\sin\theta$	$\dfrac{V B_0^2}{\mu_0}\dfrac{D_a-D_r}{D_a D_r}\cos\theta\sin\theta$	$\dfrac{\chi^2 V B_0^2}{\mu_0}(D_a-D_r)\cos\theta\sin\theta$

Note: The first column gives the complete expression for the magnetic potential energy (U), force (F_z), magnetization (M_x and M_z), and torque (T_y) for an ellipsoid of revolution in a magnetic field along the z-axis. The symmetry axis is in the x-direction and θ is the angle between this axis and the magnetic field. The second column gives approximations appropriate for soft magnetic materials, and the third column gives approximations appropriate to materials such as biological tissues with very small susceptibilities. For objects inside a medium of uniform susceptibility, such as water or tissue with $\chi = \chi_{H_2O}$, χ should be replaced by $\Delta\chi = \chi - \chi_{H_2O}$. It is assumed that B_z is the only non-zero component of B_0 at the location of the object and that the spatial derivatives of the transverse components, $(\partial B_x/\partial x)$, $(\partial B_y/\partial x)$, etc., are all zero. This is the case along the central axis of the magnets commonly used in MRI. At other points in the field, there may be non-zero force components in addition to F_z, but the qualitative physical principles are unchanged.

A patient with an implanted magnetic object, such as a metallic aneurysm clip, is at risk from both the tendency of the object to move into the magnetic field as a result of translational forces and the tendency of the object to twist into alignment with the magnetic field. The relative strength of these two effects depends on the shape and susceptibility of the object and on its position in the field of the magnet. It will now be shown that in many situations the torque represents a greater hazard than the translational force.

To simplify the analysis, regions near the central axis of a cylindrical magnet are considered. If the object is spherically symmetrical, only translational forces are present, as the induced magnetization is parallel to the applied field and there is no torque and no tendency for it to rotate. However, if the object is long and slender (i.e., needle-like or thin) and flat (i.e., plate-like), very substantial torques may be encountered. Needle-shaped objects tend to turn their long axis parallel to the field direction, and plate-like objects tend to turn their flat surfaces parallel to the field lines.

For a needle-like object ($D_a \ll D_r$) located on the z-axis of the magnet, the maximum translational force will be with the needle aligned with the field ($\theta = 0$) and at the z-location it will be where the product $B_z(\partial B_z/\partial z)$ is at a maximum. Note that near the center of imaging magnets the field is constant (although large) and $(\partial B_z/\partial z) = 0$, meaning that there is no translational force, even on strongly magnetic objects, in this location. The function $B_z(\partial B_z/\partial z)$ is therefore zero both well outside the magnet and near its center. This product goes through a maximum near the opening to the bore for most magnets, and at this location the attractive translational force will be at its maximum. This maximum will tend to be stronger and more localized for unshielded than for shielded magnets. The maximum translational force for a needle-like object on the magnet's axis is

$$F_{trans}^{max} = \frac{V}{\mu_0 D_a}\left[B_z\frac{\partial B_z}{\partial z}\right]_{max}$$

We define the F_{torque} as the strength of the force couple applied to either end of the symmetry axis that would be required to prevent the ellipsoid from turning into alignment with $\mathbf{B}_0$. Along the z-axis the maximum torque will occur at the center of the magnet and for $\theta = \pi/4$. Taking the total length of the ellipsoid as $2\,L$ and using absolute values for the force,

$$F_{torque}^{max} \approx \frac{V}{2\mu_0 LD_a}B_z^2\Big|_{max}.$$

Then

$$\frac{F_{torque}^{max}}{F_{trans}^{max}} = \frac{1}{2L}B_z^2\Big|_{max}\Big/\left[B_z\frac{\partial B_z}{\partial z}\right]_{max}.$$

For one unshielded magnet where these values have been published,[76]

$$B_z^{max} = 4.0\text{T} \quad\text{and}\quad \left[B_z\frac{\partial B_z}{\partial z}\right]_{max} = 8.8\text{T}^2/m.$$

For most superconducting cylindrical magnets, whatever their field strength, it is expected that the ratio

$$B_z^2\Big|_{max}\Big/\left[B_z\frac{\partial B_z}{\partial z}\right]_{max}$$

will be approximately of the same order of magnitude, 1.8/m, as in the current case. However, this ratio will be smaller in shielded magnets. In the current example, if $L = 1$ cm $= 0.01$ m, then $(F_{\text{torque}}^{\text{max}} / F_{\text{trans}}^{\text{max}}) = 90$.

This calculation illustrates the important fact that, for non-spherical magnetic implants, the patient's tissues may be required to exert substantially more force to prevent them from twisting in place than is required to prevent them from undergoing translational motion. Therefore, an implant such as an aneurysm clip that is substantially longer than its width is much more likely to injure a patient by twisting than by undergoing translational motion.

This can be readily verified by carefully moving a paper clip or similar small magnetic test structure around in the bore of a magnet. A relatively mild attractive translational force will be found, and it will be maximum near the opening into the scanner. It will vanish well inside the magnet near the region of imaging. A much stronger force will be required to twist the paper clip out of alignment with the field. This torque will be greatest near the magnet center and for the axis of the paper clip at 45° to the z-axis. To avoid the possibility of injury, of course, care should be taken not to lose control of the paper clip, and this experiment should not be attempted with anyone inside the bore of the MR system.

An interesting result in Table 1.3 is that the torque on an object, such as a tissue component, with $|\chi| \ll 1$ is proportional to χ^2. It is sometimes thought that diamagnetic and paramagnetic materials tend to line up differently in a uniform magnetic field. This result shows that the alignment torque is independent of the sign of χ and that both types of materials tend to align with the long axis parallel to the field. More importantly, however, this also shows that for very small values of χ, this shape-dependent alignment tendency is negligibly small. This is an example of how magnetic materials and materials with very low susceptibilities can exhibit qualitatively different responses to applied fields. Thus, a flat, plate-like magnetic object, such as a washer, has a very strong tendency to align itself with its face parallel to the field. It is sometimes said that red blood cells, which also have an approximately plate-like geometry, tend to align with their flat side parallel to the applied field. However, since $\chi^2 \approx 10^{-10}$, for these cells the shape-dependent alignment torque is completely negligible.

2. Torque Caused by Anisotropic Susceptibility

It has just been shown that the shape-dependent torque on biological materials is negligible because of the presence of an χ^2 factor in the expression for the torque. However, another source of field dependence has been observed on several occasions in biological samples and can be explained by anisotropic susceptibility. This is normally observed when a large number of macromolecules or cells are bound together in a crystalline or quasi-crystalline structure so that they all present the same orientation to the applied magnetic field. In this way, the torques on individual elements are summed over all the molecules or cells in a volume V. Suppose that the susceptibility in one direction in this volume is χ_1 and that the angle between this direction and the applied field is θ. Also assume that, for simplicity, in both orthogonal directions the susceptibility is χ_2 and that $|\chi_1|, |\chi_2| \ll 1$. Then the magnetic energy is given by

$$U = \frac{1}{2} V \mathbf{M} \bullet \mathbf{B}_0 = \frac{V B_0^2}{2\mu_0}[\chi_1 \cos^2\theta + \chi_2 \sin^2\theta] \, ,$$

and the torque is given by

$$T = \frac{\partial U}{\partial \theta} = \frac{V B_0^2}{\mu_0}(\chi_2 - \chi_1)\sin\theta\cos\theta \, .$$

Normally, for biological materials, both χ_1 and χ_2 will be negative and of the order of -10^{-5}. The object will try to orient itself such that the axis with the least negative value of χ is aligned with the field. It is found that the magnitude of $\Delta\chi = \chi_1 - \chi_2$ can be on the order of $1 - 10\%$ of the average susceptibility, $(\chi_1 + 2\chi_2)/3$, or in the range of 10^{-7} to 10^{-6}.

This factor is much larger than the factor 10^{-10} calculated above for the shape-dependent torque. This is one reason why anisotropy-dependent torques have been demonstrated in biological materials, while shape-dependent torques have not. Also important in the above expression for the torque is the volume, V. This factor shows that the torque can be enhanced by aggregating more anisotropic molecules or cells together.

Some time ago, Murayama[35,36] demonstrated that the red blood cells (RBCs) of sickle cell anemia can be aligned *in vitro* by a field of 0.5 T. The explanation for this is that the hemoglobin molecules in normal RBCs are free in solution and randomly oriented, and this leads to an isotropic susceptibility for normal cells. In sickle cell RBCs, the hemoglobin S molecules tend to aggregate and polymerize to form fibers and gel-like structures with many equivalently oriented hemoglobin molecules bound together. This structure amplifies the anisotropy of the individual molecules and leads to the anisotropy-dependent orientation discovered by Murayama. Although this effect is easily demonstrated in the test tube environment, the red cells of sickle cell patients are not aligned by magnetic fields. This is because the shear forces present in flowing blood are orders of magnitude larger than is required to overwhelm the forces of magnetic orientation.[51,64,67,75]

A similar orientation effect has been observed in fibrin gels, retinal rod cell preparations, and nucleic acid solutions.[135-140] Again, these effects are observed *in vitro* and would probably be too small to affect the orientations of the equivalent structures *in vivo*. However, the equation above shows that the orienting torque is proportion to B_0^2, and going to ever-higher field strengths may lead to an observable *in vivo* effect. A step in this direction has recently been reported by a group that used a 16.0-T magnet to orient the cleavage planes of the developing frog embryo.[141] The investigators attributed this result to the anisotropy-dependent alignment of tubulin molecules.[142] If this effect is confirmed, it may become one of the first repeatable magnetic field effects on biological tissues.

a. Field-Induced Alignment of Water Molecules

One argument sometimes proposed to provide a rationale for magnetotherapy is that the application of magnetic fields can cause a local alignment of water molecules which results in significant alterations in tissue biological and physiological processes.

Therefore, it is of interest to determine how much alignment of water molecules can be produced in this way. In water the molecules have a random range of orientations and this leads to $\chi = -9.05 \times 10^{-6}$. The asymmetry of the water molecule leads to about a 1% variation in χ along the principal axes of the molecule.[143] The magnetic alignment energy of a water molecule may be estimated as follows. The susceptibility of water is $\chi = -9.05 \times 10^{-6}$, and the magnetization in an applied field of 1.0 T is $M = \chi H = (\chi/\mu_0)B = -7.2$ A/m; 3.34×10^{28} water molecules per cubic meter; this gives an average dipole moment per water molecule in a 1.0-T field of $m = -2.16 \times 10^{-28}$ J/T. Using the 1% value for the anisotropy of the molecular magnetization gives a maximum magnetic energy change as the molecular orientation changes of $\Delta E = 2.16 \times 10^{-30}$ J. At 37°C, $kT = 4.28 \times 10^{-21}$ J, and this gives $(\Delta E/kT) = 5.0 \times 10^{-10}$ for an applied field of 1.0 T.

Therefore, as the magnetic energy is proportional to the square of the applied field, it would require a field approaching 450 T to achieve a deviation of 0.01% from a random orientation. Additionally, the alignment to be expected in fields of normal strength is totally negligible. This is consistent with the lack of observation of any magnetic field-induced alignment of water molecules at the field strengths currently used in MRI.

E. FIELD-INDUCED TRANSLATIONAL FORCES IN TISSUES

In a non-uniform magnetic field, those tissue components that are less diamagnetic than the average tissue components tend to move toward the higher field regions and vice versa. It might be thought that even a very small differential force on tissue elements might disturb some delicate biological process and lead to tissue injury. It is possible to make a quantitative argument that, in the normal course of events, biological structures contend with much greater internal forces than are produced by susceptibility variations among the tissue components.[24,77] Tissue components must have mechanisms that prevent them from being disrupted by the gravitational and acceleration forces which are continually experienced during normal activity, and these same mechanisms are expected to resist the smaller magnetic forces.

The approach is to show that even under extreme conditions in a very high field magnet, the differential magnetic forces are much smaller than the differential gravitational forces, which are themselves too small to have physiological consequences. The RBCs in blood are again used as an example. These cells are slightly denser than the surrounding plasma and, therefore, continually tend to sink in plasma. This phenomenon taking place in a test tube is the basis of the erythrocyte sedimentation rate (ESR) study, which is a well-known test for blood protein abnormalities. This gravitational separation is very slow, however, and in the body this tendency for RBCs to sink is completely overwhelmed by the hemodynamic forces present in flowing blood.

The presence of iron atoms in hemoglobin makes the RBCs slightly less diamagnetic than plasma, and as a result, the RBCs have a tendency to move relative to the plasma toward regions of strong magnetic fields. From Table 1.3 this force is seen to be

$$\frac{(\chi_{rbc} - \chi_{plasma})V_{rbc}}{\mu_0}B_0\frac{\partial B_0}{\partial z}.$$

In an unusually strong (4.0 T) clinical imaging magnet, the maximum value of $B_0(\partial B_0/\partial z)$ is about 8.8 T^2/m. Accounting for the four paramagnetic iron atoms per molecule of deoxygenated hemoglobin gives an $\chi_{rbc} = -6.53 \times 10^{-6}$, and the susceptibilty of plasma is taken equal to that of water or -9.05×10^{-6}. The mass density differences that lead to the ESR are given by $\rho_{rbc} = 1.093$ g/cc and $\rho_{plasma} = 1.027$ g/cc. The ratio of the magnetic and gravitational forces is given by

$$\frac{F_m}{F_g} = \frac{1}{\mu_0 g}B\frac{\partial B}{\partial z}\frac{\chi_{rbc} - \chi_{plasma}}{\rho_{rbc} - \rho_{plasma}} = 0.027,$$

where $g = 9.8$ m/s^2 is the acceleration of gravity. Even in this case with an unusually strong magnetic field, the maximum magnetic force tending to separate the RBCs from the plasma is less than 3% of the gravitational forces, and these gravitation forces have negligible effects in living organisms. Although many magnetic effects on tissue are not precisely zero, they are very small in comparison to other familiar stresses that are easily resisted by the cohesive and stabilizing forces present in tissues.

VII. SENSORY EFFECTS AND MAGNETIC FIELDS

Mild, low level sensory effects have often been reported to be associated with motion in strong magnetic fields.[34,38,70,76] The reported effects are transient and not harmful. Care must be taken in assessing these reports because of the subjective nature and the low incidence of the observed effects. It has been shown that reports of field-induced sensory effects in the vicinity of superconducting magnets can be elicited even when the magnets are turned off.[79] However, when efforts have been made to distinguish between the responses of subjects exposed to 1.5- and 4.0-T magnets, a higher incidence of positive reports has originated from those subjected to the 4.0-T field.[76] This finding supports the concept of field-dependent sensory effects. Statistically significant ($p < 0.05$) evidence was found for sensations of nausea, vertigo, and metallic taste in association with exposure to an MR system operating with a 4.0-T static magnetic field. Notably, statistically significant evidence was not found for other effects such as headache, tinnitus, hiccuping, vomiting, and numbness which have sometimes been attributed to magnetic field exposure. At 4.0 T, evidence was also found for magnetophosphenes, which are sensations of brief flashing lights when the eyes are moved rapidly while in the presence of the magnetic field. The observation of this effect required the room to be darkened.[76]

Each of these positive effects can be plausibly ascribed to the activation of highly sensitive sensory tissues by very weak electrical currents induced in tissues by motion of the body through the magnetic fields. Sensations of nausea are likely the result of extraneous excitation of motion sensations by weak MHD forces in the semicircular canals of the inner ear and the resulting conflict between the position sensing apparatus of the vestibular and visual systems. It is also possible that these forces could arise from a diamagnetic anisotropy of the inner ear receptors. Even mild levels of extraneous sensory effects can be disconcerting. Therefore, the comfort of patients to be scanned at very high field strengths will be enhanced by moving them in and out of the magnet slowly and by minimizing their motion while they are within the magnet.

VIII. TEMPERATURE EFFECTS AND MAGNETIC FIELDS

There are conflicting statements in the literature regarding the effect of static magnetic fields on body and skin temperatures of mammals.[144-147] Research has suggested that exposure to static magnetic fields either increases or both increases and decreases temperature depending on the orientation of the organism in reference to the static magnetic fields.[144] Other studies state that static magnetic fields have virtually no effect on skin and body temperatures of mammals.[145-147]

Notably, none of the investigators that identified a static magnetic field effect on temperatures proposed a plausible mechanism for this response. In addition, studies that reported that static magnetic field-induced skin and/or body temperature changes used laboratory animals known to have labile temperatures or used instrumentation that was likely affected by the static magnetic fields recorded erroneous information.

Investigations conducted in laboratory animals and human subjects indicated that exposure to intense static magnetic fields and/or gradient magnetic fields does not alter skin and body temperatures.[145-147] It should be noted that the investigations conducted in human subjects used a special fluoroptic thermometry system known to be unperturbed by high-intensity static magnetic fields. Thus, it is generally believed that exposure to static magnetic fields does not alter temperature in human subjects.

IX. REGULATORY CONSIDERATIONS

The U.S. Food and Drug Administration (FDA) has regulated the use of MRI since the late 1970s. Similar regulatory activities have been carried out in the U.K. by the National Radiological Protection Board (NRPB) and in the European Union by the International Electrotechnical Commission (IEC). The regulatory positions of these three agencies are generally consistent, although they differ somewhat in detail.[148-158]

MRI was the first major imaging modality required to demonstrate safety and efficacy as required by the Medical Devices Act as passed by Congress in 1977. During the 1980s, several manufacturers sought approval to market MR systems in the U.S., and their applications were considered on a case-by-case basis. With the availability of substantial positive clinical experience, the FDA reclassified MR scanners operating below 2.0 T as non-significant risk devices in 1987. Further experience led the FDA in 1996 to designate all field strengths below 4.0 T as non-significant risk. Currently, in the U.S. the exposure of research subjects to fields above 4.0 T requires the informed consent of the subjects and the approval of the research protocol by an institutional review board (IRB).

A. REGULATION OF OCCUPATIONAL EXPOSURE

Some groups of workers may experience a more or less chronic exposure to strong magnetic fields in their working environment. These groups include researchers in experimental high-energy physics and hospital technologists working with MRI. Several attempts have been made to provide regulatory guidelines for the chronic exposure of people occupationally required to work near strong magnets. These guidelines customarily take the form of limits on the integrated field exposure over the course of an 8-h working day. An example is the time-weighted average field exposure of 0.2 T per 8-h day proposed by the NRPB of the U.K. The use of this guideline would mean that a worker could be in a 2000-gauss (0.2 T) field for the entire working day or in a field of 1.6 T for 1 h. In common with several other guidelines, the NRPB exposure guidelines permit a substantially higher average field (2.0 T per 8-h day) if the extremities only, but not the head or trunk, are exposed to the field.

Other than injuries related to ferromagnetic forces, the literature does not contain any scientifically confirmed harmful effect of static field exposure, and therefore, it does not provide a scientific rationale to serve as a basis for designating a particular magnetic field strength as unsafe. In particular, it follows that there is no confirmed experimental evidence for any cumulative harmful effect of magnetic field exposure. A related difficulty is the rapid spatial variation of the magnetic fields typically found in workplace environments. A magnet is rated typically by the magnetic field strength at its center. However, the field falls off rapidly with distance away from the magnet, and, except in unusual circumstances, the exposure of workers to environmental magnetic fields as they move about performing their responsibilities is not characterized by a single value that can be readily averaged over a period of time.

Although there are experiments and theoretical analyses to support the belief that the proposed mechanisms of tissue injury are not harmful at the field strengths currently available, the literature also does not contain extensive controlled studies demonstrating the absolute safety of prolonged magnetic field exposure. It is therefore prudent and logical to take reasonable precautions against casual and readily avoidable exposure to intense fields and to provide guidelines based on the best available information for the exposure of workers whose duties require working in the vicinity of magnetic fields. Furthermore, it is important and desirable that additional data be collected and analyzed to provide improved confidence in the safety of magnetic field exposure.

X. SUMMARY AND CONCLUSIONS

For the vast majority of the more than 100 million clinical MRI studies performed since the early 1980s, there has not been any evidence of harm to the patients from the static magnetic field. The relatively few injuries that have occurred have been attributed to the inadvertent presence of ferromagnetic materials or cardiac pacemakers. Results on investigations conducted in human subjects in fields up to 8.0 T and on laboratory animals up to 16.0 T indicate that there is a substantial margin of safety remaining above the highest static magnetic fields currently in clinical use (i.e., in the range of 3.0 to 4.0 T). This safety margin, of course, is no indication that efforts should not continue to energetically search for signs of unexpected field-related health issues. In particular, there is a need for improved techniques for protecting patients from injuries caused by the occult presence of ferromagnetic foreign bodies. It may be some time before whole-body MRI magnets operating above 8.0 T become available to study the ability of human subjects to withstand even stronger fields. However, small bore magnets designed to permit nuclear magnetic resonance (NMR) chemistry studies at frequencies approaching 1 GHz may soon be available in the range of 20.0 to 25.0 T, and these will undoubtedly be used to determine if small animals can tolerate fields of this strength.[159,160]

Although there have been many reports of potentially harmful biological effects of magnetic fields on cells, tissues, or organisms, none of these has been thoroughly verified and firmly established as a scientific fact. Given this experience, it seems reasonable to require the replication of any experiment claiming to demonstrate a biological effect of static fields before it is accepted as the basis of a regulatory standard. Also, many physical mechanisms have been suggested as possible sources of magnetic field effects on biological processes. However, it is often the case that relatively simple calculations that would indicate that the proposed effect is of an insignificant order of magnitude at the static magnetic field strengths used in MRI are not provided. Again, before any such mechanisms are used as the basis of a regulatory standard, serious efforts should be made to calculate the size of the magnetic forces involved and compare them with other comparable forces of which tissues are known to withstand without injury.

The lack of serious effects of the magnetic fields in current use on tissues is attributed to the very weak diamagnetic susceptibility of these tissues. At very high static magnetic field strengths, there is considerable evidence for mild sensory effects such as vertigo, metallic taste, and magnetophosphenes, but there is no evidence that these effects are at all harmful. These effects, vertigo in particular, can be reduced by moving patients slowly while they are in regions of very strong magnetic fields.

There is a need for additional studies to support the belief that extended exposure to magnetic fields during interventional MRI and related activities is not harmful. Although there is no evidence for a cumulative effect of magnetic field exposure on health, further studies of the exposed populations will be helpful in establishing rational guidelines for occupational exposure to magnetic fields.

It is of interest to speculate on the physical process that will provide the ultimate upper limit on the ability of humans to withstand intense magnetic fields. Some effects, such as the field-induced alignment of water molecules, are so ineffective that they are unlikely to ever be observed. On the other hand, as ever-higher field strengths become available, it is likely that either flow-induced EMFs or diamagnetic anisotropy will eventually become a truly limiting factor. However, it appears that substantial safety margins still exist and high field MRI will remain a fertile area for research and clinical applications. With proper precautions, it is likely that human subjects will safely tolerate whole-body fields considerably higher than any that have yet been experienced.

REFERENCES

1. Mottelay, P.F., *Bibliographical History of Electricity and Magnetism Chronologically Arranged*, Charles Griffin & Co, London, 1922.
2. Davis, L.D., Pappajohn, K., Plavnieks, I.M., Spiegler, P.E., and Jacobius, A.J., Bibliography of the biological effects of magnetic fields, *Fed. Proc. Suppl.*, 12, 1-38, 1962.
3. Gross, L., Bibliography of the biological effects of static magnetic fields, in *Biological Effects of Magnetic Fields*, Barnothy, M.F., Ed., Plenum Press, New York, 1964, 297-311.
4. Gartrell, R.G., *Electricity, Magnetism, and Animal Magnetism: A Checklist of Printed Sources 1600–1850*, Scholarly Resources, Inc., Wilmington, DE, 1975.
5. Mourino, M.R., From Thales to Lauterbur, or from the lodestone to MR imaging: magnetism and medicine, *Radiology*, 180, 593-612, 1991.
6. Binet, A. and Féré, C., *Animal Magnetism*, Kegan Paul, London, 1887; Reprinted, Gryphon Editions, New York, 1993.
7. Barnothy, M.F., Ed., *Biological Effects of Magnetic Fields*, Plenum Press, New York, 1964.
8. Kholodov, Y.A., *The Effect of Electromagnetic and Magnetic Fields on the Central Nervous System*, NASA Technical Translation F-465, Clearing House for Federal Scientific and Technical Information, Springfield, VA, 1967.

9. Barnothy, M.F., Ed., *Biological Effects of Magnetic Fields, Volume 2*, Plenum Press, New York, 1969.

10. Pressman, A.S., *Electromagnetic Fields and Life*, Sinclair, F.L. and Brown, F.A., Jr., translators, Plenum Press, New York, 1970.

11. Kholodov, Y.A., Ed., *Influence of Magnetic Fields on Biological Objects*, JPRS 63038, National Technical Information Service, Springfield, VA, 1974.

12. Llaurado, J.G., Sances, A., and Battocletti, A.J.H., Eds., *Biologic and Clinical Effects of Low-Frequency Magnetic and Electric Fields*, Charles C Thomas, Springfield, IL, 1974.

13. Buranelli, V., *The Wizard from Vienna: Franz Anton Mesmer*, Coward, McCann and Geohagen, New York, 1975.

14. Tenforde, T.S., Ed., *Magnetic Field Effect on Biological Systems*, Plenum Press, New York, 1979.

15. Herlach, F., Ed., *Strong and Ultrastrong Magnetic Fields and Their Applications*, Springer-Verlag, Berlin, 1985.

16. Maret, G., Boccara, N., and Kiepenheuer, J., Eds., *Biophysical Effects of Steady Magnetic Fields*, Springer-Verlag, Berlin, 1986.

17. Polk, C. and Postow, E., *Handbook of Biological Effects of Electromagnetic Fields*, CRC Press, Boca Raton, FL, 1986.

18. Crabtree, A., *From Mesmer to Freud: Magnetic Sleep and the Roots of Psychological Healing*, Yale University Press, New Haven, CT, 1993.

19. Shellock, F.G. and Kanal, E., *Magnetic Resonance: Bioeffects, Patient Safety, and Patient Management, 2nd Edition*, Lippincott-Raven, Philadelphia, 1996.

20. Whitaker, J. and Adderly, B., *The Pain Relief Breakthrough: The Power of Magnets to Relieve Backaches, Arthritis, Menstrual Cramps, Carpal Tunnel Syndrome, Sports Injuries and More*, Little, Brown, Boston, 1998.

21. Quinan, J.R., The use of the magnet in medicine: a historical study, *Md. Med. J.*, 14, 460–465, 1886.

22. Schaefer, D.J., Safety aspects of magnetic resonance imaging, in *Biomedical Magnetic Resonance Imaging: Principles, Methodology and Applications*, Wehrli, F.W., Shaw, D., and Kneeland, J.B., Eds., VCH Verlagsgesellschaft, Weinheim, 1988, 553-578.

23. Shellock, F.G., Kanal, E., and Moscatel, M., Bioeffects and safety considerations, in *Magnetic Resonance Imaging of the Brain and Spine, 2nd Edition*, Atlas, S.W., Ed., Lippincott-Raven, Philadelphia, 1996, 109-148.

24. Schenck, J.F., MR safety at high magnetic field strengths, in *Magnetic Resonance Imaging Clinics of North America: MR Safety, Volume 6(4)*, Kanal, E., Ed., W. B. Saunders, Philadelphia, 1998, 715-730.

25. Hermann, L., Hat das magnetische Feld directe physiologische Wirkungen?, Pflügers Arch. *Gesammte Physiol. Menschen Thiere*, 43, 217-234, 1888.

26. Peterson, F. and Kennelly, A.E., Some physiological experiments with magnets at the Edison Laboratory, *N.Y. Med. J.*, 56, 729-734, 1892.

27. Drinker, C.K. and Thomson, R.M., Does the magnetic field constitute an industrial hazard?, *J. Ind. Hyg.*, 3, 117-129, 1921.

28. American Medical Association, Theronoid and vitrona: the magic horse collar campaign continues, *J. Am. Med. Assoc.*, 96, 1718-1719, 1931.

29. Barnothy, M.F., Barnothy, J.M., and Boszormenyi-Nagy, I., Influence of magnetic field upon the leucocytes of the mouse, *Nature*, 177, 577-578, 1956.

30. Barnothy, M.F. and Barnothy, J.M., Biological effect of a magnetic field and the radiation syndrome, *Nature*, 181, 1785-1786, 1958.

31. Freeman, M.W., Arrott, A., and Watson, J.H.L., Magnetism in medicine, *J. Appl. Phys.*, 31, 404S-405S, 1960.

32. Eiselein, T.E., Boutell, H.M., and Biggs, M.W., Biological effects of magnetic fields — negative results, *Aerosp. Med.*, 32, 383-386, 1961.

33. Beischer, D.E., Human tolerance to magnetic fields, *Astronautics*, 7, 24-25, 46, 48, 1962.

34. Beischer, D.E. and Knepton, J.C., Jr., Influence of strong magnetic fields on the electrocardiogram of squirrel monkeys (*Saimiri sciureus*), *Aerosp. Med.*, 35, 939-944, 1964.

35. Murayama, M., Orientation of sickled erythrocytes in a magnetic field, *Nature*, 206, 420-422, 1965.

36. Murayama, M., Molecular mechanism of red cell "sickling," *Science*, 153, 145-149, 1966.

37. Malinin, G.I., Gregory, W.D., Morelli, L., Sharma, V.K., and Houck, J.C., Evidence of morphological and physiological transformation of mammalian cells by strong magnetic fields, *Science*, 194, 844-846, 1976.

38. St. Lorant, S.J., Biomagnetism: a review, in *SLAC Publication 1984*, Stanford Linear Accelerator, Stanford, CA, 1977, 1-9.

39. Ketchen, E.E., Porter, W.E., and Bolton, N.E., The biological effects of magnetic fields on man, *Am. Ind. Hyg. Assoc. J.*, 39, 1-11, 1978.

40. Budinger, T.F., Threshold for physiological effects due to rf and magnetic fields used in NMR imaging, *IEEE Trans. Nucl. Sci.*, NS-26, 2821-2825, 1979.

41. Saunders, R.D., Biological hazards of NMR, in *Proceedings of an International Symposium on Nuclear Magnetic Resonance Imaging*, Witcofski, R.L., Karstaedt, N., and Partain, C.L., Eds., Bowman Gray School of Medicine, Winston-Salem, NC, 1981, 65-71.

42. Battocletti, J.H., Salles-Cunha, S., Halbach, R.E., Nelson, J., Sances, J.R., and Antonich, F.J., Exposure of rhesus monkeys to 20000 G steady magnetic field: effect on blood parameters, *Med. Phys.*, 8, 115-118, 1981.

43. Budinger, T.F., Nuclear magnetic resonance (NMR) *in vitro* studies: known thresholds for health effects, *J. Comput. Assist. Tomogr.*, 5, 800-811, 1981.

44. Hong, C.-Z., Lin, J.C., Bender, L.F., Schaeffer, J.N., Meltzer, R.J., and Causin, P., Magnetic necklace: its therapeutic effectiveness on neck and shoulder pain, *Arch. Phys. Med. Rehabil.*, 63, 462-466, 1982.

45. Budinger, T.F., Hazards from d.c. and a.c. magnetic fields, in *Book of Abstracts*, Society of Magnetic Resonance in Medicine, Berkeley, CA, 1982, 29-30.

46. Milham, S., Mortality from leukemia in workers exposed to electrical and magnetic fields [Letter], *N. Engl. J. Med.*, 307, 249, 1982.

47. New, P.F.J., Rosen, B.R., Brady, T.J., et al., Potential hazards and artifacts of ferromagnetic and nonferromagnetic surgical and dental materials and devices in nuclear magnetic resonance imaging, *Radiology*, 1983, 139-148, 1983.

48. Saunders, R.D. and Smith, H., Safety aspects of NMR clinical imaging, *Br. Med. Bull.*, 40, 148-154, 1984.

49. Budinger, T.F., Bristol, K.S., Yen, C.K., and Wong, P., Biological effects of static magnetic fields, in *Book of Abstracts*, Society of Magnetic Resonance in Medicine, Berkeley, CA, 1984, 113-114.

50. Budinger, T.F. and Cullander, C., Health effects of *in vivo* nuclear magnetic resonance, in *Biomedical Magnetic Resonance*, James, C.E. and Margulis, A., Eds., Radiology Research and Education Foundation, San Francisco, 1984, 421-441.

51. Brody, A.S., Sorette, M.P., Gooding, C.A., Listerud, J., Clark, M.R., Mentzer, W.C., Brasch, R.C., and James, T.L., Induced alignment of flowing sickle erythrocytes in a magnetic field: a preliminary report, *Invest. Radiol.*, 20, 560-566, 1985.

52. Kelly, W.M., Paglen, P.G., Pearson, J.A., San Diego, A.G., and Soloman, M.A., Ferromagnetism of intraocular foreign body causes unilateral blindness after MR study, *Am. J. Neuroradiol.*, 7, 243-245, 1986.

53. Gleick, J., Man hurt as medical magnet attracts forklift, *New York Times*, p. A21, June 5, 1986.

54. von Klitzing, L., Do static magnetic fields of NMR influence biological signals?, *Clin. Phys. Physiol. Meas.*, 7, 157-160, 1986.

55. Lund, G., Nelson, J.D., Wirtschafter, J.D., et al., Tattooing of eyelids: magnetic resonance imaging artifacts, *Ophthalmic Surg.*, 17, 550-553, 1986.

56. Fowler, J.R., Ter Penning, B., Syverud, S.A., and Levy, R.C., Magnetic field hazard [Letter], *N. Engl. J. Med.*, 314, 1517, 1986.

57. Miller, G., Exposure guidelines for magnetic fields, *Am. Ind. Hyg. Assoc. J.*, 48, 957-968, 1987.

58. Jackson, J.G. and Acker, J.D., Permanent eyeliner and MR imaging [Letter], *Am. J. Roentgenol.*, 149, 1080, 1987.

59. Budinger, T.F., Magnetohydrodynamic retarding effect on blood flow velocity at 4.7 tesla found to be insignificant, in *Book of Abstracts*, Society of Magnetic Resonance in Medicine, Berkeley, CA, 1987, 183.

60. Jackson, J.G. and Acker, J.D., Permanent eyeliner and MR imaging [Letter], *Am. J. Roentgenol.*, 149, 1080, 1987.

61. Sacco, D.C., Steiger, D.A., Bellon, E.M., et al., Artifacts caused by cosmetics in MR imaging of the head, *Am. J. Roentgenol.*, 148, 1001-1004, 1987.

62. Wolfley, D.E., Flynn, K.J., and Cartwright, J., Eyelid pigment implantation: early and late histopathology, *Plast. Reconstr. Surg.*, 82, 770-774, 1988.

63. Schenck, J.F., Dumoulin, C.L., Mueller, O.M., et al., Proton imaging of humans at 4.0 tesla, in *Book of Abstracts*, Society of Magnetic Resonance in Medicine, Berkeley, CA, 1988, 153.

64. Brody, A.S., Embury, S.H., Mentzer, W.C., Winkler, M.L., and Gooding, C.A., Preservation of sickle cell bloodflow patterns during MR imaging: an *in vivo* study, *Am. J. Roentgenol.*, 151, 139-141, 1988.

65. Redington, R.W., Dumoulin, C.L., Schenck, J.F., et al., MR imaging and bio-effects in a whole-body 4.0 tesla imaging system, in *Book of Abstracts*, Society of Magnetic Resonance in Medicine, Berkeley, CA, 1988, 20.

66. Wahlund, L.-O., Agartz, I., Almqvist, O., et al., The brain in healthy aged individuals, *Radiology*, 174, 674-679, 1990.

67. Mankad, V.N., Williams, J.P., Harpen, M.D., Manci, E., Longenecker, G., Moore, R.B., Shah, A., Yang, Y.M., and Brogdon, B.G., Magnetic resonance imaging of bone marrow in sickle cell disease: clinical, hematological, and pathologic correlations, *Blood*, 75, 274-283, 1990.

68. Hong, C.-Z. and Shellock, F., Short term exposure to a 1.5 tesla static magnetic field does not affect somato-sensory-evoked potentials in man, *Magn. Reson. Imaging*, 8, 65-69, 1990.

69. Muller, S. and Hotz, M., Human brainstem auditory evoked potentials (BAEP) before and after MR examinations, *Magn. Reson. Med.*, 16, 476-480, 1990.

70. Schenck, J.F., Dumoulin, C.L., and Souza, S.P., Health and physiological effects of human exposure to whole-body 4 tesla magnetic fields during magnetic resonance scanning, in *Book of Abstracts*, Society of Magnetic Resonance in Medicine, Berkeley, CA, 1990, 277.

71. Keltner, J.R., Roos, M.S., Brakeman, P.R., and Budinger, T.F., Magnetohydrodynamics of blood flow, *Magn. Reson. Med.*, 16, 139-149, 1990.

72. Phillips, M.E., Industrial hygiene investigation of static magnetic fields in nuclear magnetic resonance facilities, *Appl. Occup. Environ. Hyg.*, 5, 353-358, 1990.

73. Kelsey, C.A., King, J.N., Keck, G.M., Chiu, M.T., Wolfe, D.M., and Orrison, W.W., Ocular hazard of metallic fragments during MR imaging at 0.06 T, *Radiology*, 180, 282-283, 1991.

74. Buettner, U.W., Human interactions with ultra high fields, in *Biological and Safety Aspects of Nuclear Magnetic Resonance Imaging and Spectroscopy,* Magin, R.L., Liburdy, R.P., and Persson, B., Eds., New York Academy of Sciences, New York, 1992, 59-66.

75. Schenck, J.F., Quantitative assessment of the magnetic forces and torques in red blood cells: implications for patients with sickle cell anemia, in *Book of Abstracts*, Society of Magnetic Resonance in Medicine, Berkeley, CA, 1992, 3405.

76. Schenck, J.F., Dumoulin, C.L., Redington, R.W., Kressel, H.Y., Elliott, R.T., and McDougall, I.L., Human exposure to 4.0-tesla magnetic fields in a whole-body scanner, *Med. Phys.*, 19, 1089-1098, 1992.

77. Schenck, J.F., Health and physiological effects of human exposure to whole-body four-tesla magnetic fields during MRI, in *Biological and Safety Aspects of Nuclear Magnetic Resonance Imaging and Spectroscopy,* Magin, R.L., Liburdy, R.P., and Persson, B., Eds., New York Academy of Sciences, New York, 1992, 285-301.

78. Macklis, R.M., Magnetic healing, quackery, and the debate about the health effects of electromagnetic fields, *Ann. Intern. Med.*, 118, 376-383, 1993.

79. Erhard, P., Chen, W., Lee, J.-H., and Ugurbil, K., A study of effects reported by subjects at high magnetic fields, in *Book of Abstracts*, Society of Magnetic Resonance, Berkeley, CA, 1995, 1219.

80. Schenck, J.F., The role of magnetic susceptibility in magnetic resonance imaging: magnetic field compatibility of the first and second kinds, *Med. Phys.*, 23, 815-850, 1996.

81. Shermer, M., Salas, C., and Salas, D., Testing the claims of Mesmerism: commissioned by King Louis XVI; designed, conducted and written by Benjamin Franklin, Antoine Lavoisier and others [translation of the 1784 report of the commissioners charged by the king to examine animal magnetism], *Skeptic*, 4, 66-83, 1996.

82. Minczykowski, A., Wlodzimierz, P., Smielecki, J., Sosnowski, P., Szczepanik, A., Eder, M., and Wysocki, H., Effects of magnetic resonance imaging on polymorphonuclear neutrophil functions, *Acad. Radiol.*, 3, 97-102, 1996.

83. Vallbona, C., Hazlewood, C.F., and Jurida, G., Response of pain to static magnetic fields in postpolio patients: a double-blind pilot study, *Arch. Phys. Med. Rehabil.*, 78, 1200–1203, 1997.

84. Horstman, J., Explorations: magnets, *Arthritis Today*, 12, 48-51, 1998.

85. Ramey, D.W., Magnetic and electromagnetic therapy, *Sci. Rev. Alt. Med.*, 2, 13–19, 1998.

86. Kinouchi, Y., Yamaguchi, H., and Tenforde, T.S., Theoretical analysis of magnetic field interactions with aortic blood flow, *Bioelectromagnetics*, 17, 21-32, 1996.

87. Feingold, L., Magnet therapy, *Sci. Rev. Alt. Med.*, 3, 26-33, 1999.

88. Kangarlu, A., Burgess, R.E., Zhu, H., Nakayama, T., Hamlin, R.L., Abduljahl, A.M., and Robitaille, P.M.L., Cognitive, cardiac, and physiological safety studies in ultra high field magnetic resonance imaging, *Magn. Reson. Imaging*, 17, 1407-1416, 1999.

89. Klucznik, R.P., Carrier, D.A., Pyka, R., et al., Placement of a ferromagnetic intracerebral aneurysm clip with a fatal outcome, *Radiology*, 187, 587-599, 1993.

90. Kanal, E. and Shellock, F., MR imaging of patients with intracranial aneurysm clips, *Radiology*, 187, 612-614, 1993.

91. Gimbel, J.R., Johnson, D., Levine, P.A., et al., Safe performance of magnetic resonance imaging on five patients with permanent cardiac pacemakers, *PACE (Pacing and Clinical Electrophysiology)*, 19, 913-919, 1996.

92. Wilson, M.N., *Superconducting Magnets*, Clarendon Press, Oxford, 1983.

93. Hinshaw, W.S., Bottomley, P.A., and Holland, G.N., Radiographic thin-section image of the human wrist by nuclear magnetic resonance, *Nature*, 270, 722-723, 1977.

94. Hinshaw, W.S., Andrew, E.R., Bottomley, P.A., et al., Display of cross sectional anatomy by nuclear magnetic resonance imaging, *Br. J. Radiol.*, 51, 273-280, 1978.

95. Damadian, R., Minkoff, L., and Goldsmith, M., Field-focusing nuclear magnetic resonance (FONAR), *Naturwissenschaften*, 65, 250–252, 1978.

96. Edelstein, W.A., Hutchison, J.M.S., Johnson, G., et al., Spin warp NMR imaging and applications to human whole-body imaging, *Phys. Med. Biol.*, 25, 751-756, 1980.

97. Vetter, J., Siebold, H., and Söldner, L., A 4 T superconducting whole-body magnet for MR-imaging and spectroscopy, in *Book of Abstracts*, Society of Magnetic Resonance in Medicine, Berkeley, CA, 1987, 181.

98. Vetter, J., Ries, G., and Reichert, T., A 4-tesla superconducting whole-body magnet for MR imaging and spectroscopy, *IEEE Trans. Magn.*, 24, 1285-1287, 1988.

99. Barfuss, H., Fischer, H., Hentschel, D., et al., Whole-body MR imaging and spectroscopy with a 4-T system, *Radiology*, 169, 811-816, 1988.

100. Barfuss, H., Fischer, H., Hentschel, D., et al., *In vivo* magnetic resonance imaging and spectroscopy of humans with a 4T whole-body magnet, *Nucl. Magn. Reson. Biomed.*, 3, 31-45, 1990.

101. Chu, S.C., The development of a 4T whole body system for clinical research, *Jpn. J. Magn. Reson. Med.*, 10 S1, 63-64, 1990.

102. Bell, R.A., Economics of MRI technology, *J. Magn. Reson. Imaging*, 6, 10-25, 1996.

103. Liburdy, R.P., Biological interactions of cellular systems with time-varying magnetic fields, in *Biological and Safety Aspects of Nuclear Magnetic Resonance Imaging and Spectroscopy*, Magin, R.L., Liburdy, R.P., and Persson, B., Eds., New York Academy of Sciences, New York, 1992, 74-95.

104. Vergano, D., EMF researcher made up data, ORI says, *Science*, 285, 23, 25, 1999.

105. Broad, W.J., Data tying cancer to electric power found to be false, *New York Times*, p. 1, July 24, 1999.

106. Liburdy, R.P., Calcium and EMFs: graphing the data [Letter], *Science*, 285, 337, 1999.

107. Hall, R.N., Pathological science, *Speculations Sci. Technol.*, 8, 77, 1985.

108. Langmuir, I., Pathological science [transcribed and edited by Hall, R.N.], *Phys. Today*, 10, 36-48, 1989.

109. Berry, M.V. and Geim, A.K., Of flying frogs and levitrons, *Eur. J. Phys.*, 18, 307-313, 1997.

110. Geim, A.K., Simon, M.D., Boamfa, M.I., and Heflinger, L.O., Magnet levitation at your fingertips, *Nature*, 400, 323-324, 1999; Correction, *Nature*, 402, 604, 1999.

111. Kolin, A., Improved apparatus and technique for electromagnetic determination of blood flow, *Rev. Sci. Instr.*, 23, 235-242, 1952.

112. Kanai, H., Yamano, E., Nakayama, K., Kawamura, N., and Furuhata, H., Transcutaneous blood flow measurement by electromagnetic induction, *IEEE Trans. Biomed. Eng.*, BME-21, 144-151, 1974.

113. Togawa, T., Okai, O., and Ohima, M., Observation of blood flow e.m.f. in externally applied strong magnetic fields by surface electrodes, *Med. Biol. Eng.*, 5, 169-170, 1967.

114. Tenforde, T.S., Gaffey, C.T., Moyer, B.R., and Budinger, T.F., Cardiovascular alterations in Macaca monkeys exposed to stationary magnetic fields: experimental observations and theoretical analysis, *Bioelectromagnetics*, 4, 1-9, 1983.

115. Winfrey, A.T., The electrical thresholds of ventricular myocardium, *J. Cardiovasc. Physiol.*, 1, 393-410, 1990.

116. Haberditzl, W., Enzyme activity in high magnetic fields, *Nature*, 213, 72-73, 1967.

117. Atkins, P.W., Magnetic field effects, *Chem. Br.*, 12, 214-218, 1976.

118. Atkins, P.W. and Lambert, T.P., The effect of a magnetic field on chemical reactions, *Ann. Rep. Prog. Chem.*, A72, 67-88, 1976.

119. Brocklehurst, B., Spin correlation in the geminate recombination of radical ions in hydrocarbons. I. Theory of the magnetic field effect, *J. Chem. Soc. Faraday Trans.*, 2, 72, 1869-1864, 1976.

120. McLauchlan, K.A., The effects of magnetic fields on chemical reactions, *Sci. Prog. (Oxford)*, 67, 509-529, 1981.

121. Turro, N.J., Influence of nuclear spin on chemical reactions: magnetic isotope and magnetic field effects (a review), *Proc. Natl. Acad. Sci. U.S.A.*, 80, 609-621, 1983.

122. Gould, I.R., Turro, N.J., and Zimmt, M.B., Magnetic field and magnetic isotope effects on the products of organic reactions, in *Advances in Physical Organic Chemistry, Volume 20*, Gold, V. and Bethel, D., Eds., Academic Press, New York, 1984.

123. Steiner, U.E. and Ulrich, T., Magnetic field effects in chemical kinetics and related phenomena, *Chem. Rev.*, 89, 51-147, 1989.

124. Cohen, C., Ferromagnetic contamination in the lungs and other organs of the body, *Science*, 180, 745-748, 1973.

125. Freedman, A.P., Robinson, S.E., and Johnston, R.J., Non-invasive magnetopneumographic estimation of lung dust loads and distribution in bituminous coal workers, *J. Occup. Med.*, 22, 613-618, 1980.

126. Cohen, D. and Nemoto, I., Ferrimagnetic particles in the lung. I. The magnetizing process, *IEEE Trans. Biomed. Eng.*, 31, 261-273, 1984.

127. Cohen, D., Nemoto, I., Kaufman, L., et al., Ferrimagnetic particles in the lung. II. The relaxation process, *IEEE Trans. Biomed. Eng.*, 31, 274-284, 1984.

128. Moatamed, F. and Johnson, F.B., Identification and significance of magnetite in human tissues, *Arch. Pathol. Lab. Med.*, 110, 618-621, 1986.

129. Kirschvink, J.L., Kobayishi-Kirschvink, A., and Woodford, B.J., Magnetite biomineralization in the human brain, *Proc. Natl. Acad. Sci. U.S.A.*, 89, 7683-7687, 1992.

130. Bozorth, R.M., *Ferromagnetism*, Van Nostrand, New York, 1951; Reprinted, IEEE, Piscataway, NJ, 1993, 627-699.

131. Scott, W.T., *The Physics of Electricity and Magnetism, 2nd Edition*, Wiley, New York, 1966, 323-368.

132. Landau, L.D., Lifshitz, E.M., and Pitaevskii, L.P., *Electrodynamics of Continuous Media, 2nd Edition*, Pergamon Press, Oxford, 1984, 105-128 and 217-222.

133. Bleaney, B.I. and Bleaney, B., *Electricity and Magnetism, 3rd Edition*, Oxford University Press, Oxford, 1976, 101-107.

134. Jackson, J.D., *Classical Electrodynamics, 3rd Edition*, Wiley, New York, 1999, 214.

135. Torbet, J., Freyssinet, J.-M., and Hudry-Clergeon, G., Oriented fibrin gels formed by polymerization in strong magnetic fields, *Nature*, 289, 91-93, 1981.

136. Maret, G., von Schickfus, M., Mayer, A., and Dransfeld, K., Orientation of nucleic acids in high magnetic fields, *Phys. Rev. Lett.*, 35, 397-400, 1975.

137. Worcester, D.L., Structural origins of diamagnetic anisotropy in proteins, *Proc. Natl. Acad. Sci. U.S.A.*, 75, 5475-5477, 1978.

138. Hong, F.T., Photoelectric and magneto-orientation effects in pigmented biological membranes, *J. Colloid Interface Sci.*, 58, 471-497, 1977.

139. Geacintov, N.E., Van Nostrand, F., Becker, J.F., and Tinkel, J.B., Magnetic field orientation of photosynthetic systems, *Biochim. Biophys. Acta*, 267, 65-79, 1972.

140. Hong, F.T., Mauzerall, D., and Mauro, A., Magnetic anisotropy and the orientation of retinal rods in a homogeneous magnetic field, *Proc. Natl. Acad. Sci. U.S.A.*, 68, 1283–1285, 1971.

141. Denegre, J.M., Valles, J.M., Jr., Lin, K., Jordan, W.B., and Mowry, K.L., Cleavage planes in frog eggs altered by strong magnetic fields, *Proc. Natl. Acad. Sci. U.S.A.*, 95, 14729-14732, 1998.

142. Bras, W., Diakun, G.P., Diaz, J.F., Maret, G., Kramer, H., Bordas, J., and Medrano, F.J., The susceptibility of pure tubulin to high magnetic fields: a magnetic birefringence and x-ray fiber diffraction study, *Biophys. J.*, 74, 1509-1521, 1998.
143. Kern, C.W. and Karplus, M., The water molecule, in *Water: A Comprehensive Treatise, Volume 1, The Physics and Physical Chemistry of Water*, Franks, F., Ed., Plenum Press, New York, 1972, 21-91.
144. Gemmel, H., Wendhausen, H., and Wunsch, F., Biologische Effekte statischer Magnetfelder bei NMR-tomographie am Menschen, *Radiologische Klinik*, Wiss. Mitt. Univ. Kiel., 1983.
145. Shellock, F., Schaefer, D., and Crues, J., Exposure to a 1.5 T static magnetic fields does not alter body and skin temperatures in man, *Magn. Reson. Med.*, 11, 371, 1989.
146. Shellock, F., Schaefer, D., and Gordon, C., Effect of a 1.5 T static magnetic field on body temperature of man, *Magn. Reson. Med.*, 3, 644, 1986.
147. Tenforde, T. and Levy, L., Thermoregulation in rodents exposed to homogeneous (7.55 Tesla and gradient (60 Tesla/per second) DC magnetic fields, in Proceedings of the Bioelectromagnetics Society, 7th Annual Meeting Abstracts, 1985, 7.
148. Goyan, J.E., Medical devices: procedures for investigational device exemptions, *Fed. Regist.*, 45, 3732-3759, 1980.
149. National Radiological Protection Board (NRPB), Exposure to nuclear magnetic resonance clinical imaging, *Radiography*, 47, 258-260, 1980.
150. Gundaker, W.E., Guidelines for Evaluating Electromagnetic Risk for Trials of Clinical NMR Systems, U.S. Food and Drug Administration, Rockville, MD, 1982.
151. National Radiological Protection Board (NRPB), Revised guidance on acceptable limits of exposure during nuclear magnetic resonance clinical imaging, *Br. J. Radiol.*, 56, 974-977, 1982.
152. Villforth, J.C., Guidelines for Evaluating Electromagnetic Exposure Risk for Trials of Clinical NMR Systems, U.S. Food and Drug Administration, Rockville, MD, 1982.
153. U.S. FDA, Guidance for Content and Review of a Magnetic Resonance Diagnostic Device 510(k) Application, U.S. Food and Drug Administration, Silver Spring, MD, 1988.
154. U.S. Food and Drug Administration, Magnetic resonance diagnostic device: panel recommendation and report on petitions for MR reclassification, *Fed. Regist.*, 53, 7575-7579, 1988.
155. Young, F.E., Magnetic resonance diagnostic device: panel recommendation and report on petitions for MR reclassification, *Fed. Regist.*, 53, 7575-7579, 1988.
156. Department of Health and Human Services, Guidance for Content and Review of a Magnetic Resonance Diagnostic Device 510(k) Application, U.S. Food and Drug Administration, Silver Spring, MD, 1988.
157. National Health and Medical Research Council, *Safety Guidelines for Magnetic Resonance Diagnostic Facilities: Radiation Health Series, Number 34*, Australian Government Publishing Service, Canberra, 1991.
158. International Electrotechnical Commission, International Standard: Part 2 — Particular Requirements for the Safety of Magnetic Resonance Equipment for Medical Diagnosis, CEI/IEC 601-2-33, International Electrotechnical Commission, Geneva, Switzerland, 1995.
159. Normile, D., Race for stronger magnets turns into marathon, *Science*, 281, 164-165, 1998.
160. Service, R.F., NMR researchers look to next generation of machines, *Science*, 1998, 279, 1127-1128, 1998.

2 Health Effects and Safety of Intense Gradient Fields

John A. Nyenhuis, Joe D. Bourland, Alexander V. Kildishev, and Daniel J. Schaefer

CONTENTS

I. INTRODUCTION

The pulsed gradient fields that occur in association with magnetic resonance imaging (MRI) expose the patient to a time-varying magnetic field. This field, *dB/dt*, induces an electric field and, hence, an electric current in the patient. For early magnetic resonance (MR) systems, the induced currents were not of sufficient intensity to be perceived by the patient. In echo planar and other modern imaging modalities, it is desirable to have more rapidly switched gradient fields in order to improve image quality and the speed of image acquisition. It was observed experimentally and predicted theoretically that modern gradient coil hardware may produce time-varying magnetic fields with intensity sufficient to produce a physiologic response.

The potential health effects of intense gradient fields include the onset of peripheral nerve stimulation, muscle movement, and discomfort. Fortunately, cardiac stimulation is unlikely to occur with practical levels of gradient fields used for MR procedures. Another possible health effect is the acoustic noise that results from vibrations induced by the force from the static field when the audio-frequency currents pass through the gradient coils (see Chapter 7, "Acoustic Noise and Magnetic Resonance Procedures").

This chapter reviews reports on physiologic effects of intense gradient fields and includes results from the literature. Additionally, results are presented from a study conducted at Purdue University in West Lafayette, IN that was performed on human subjects, in which the *dB/dt* intensity required to induce physiologic responses was measured. Also, presented for the first time is the distribution of *dB/dt* across the population required to induce these responses. The induced electric fields that result from the measured values of *dB/dt* are calculated in a morphologically realistic human model. Notably, the computational method along with the electric fields calculated from the Purdue University study and other measurements can be used to predict the level of *dB/dt* as a function of pulse duration that may be safely applied with a given gradient coil assembly.

II. GRADIENT COILS AND INDUCED ELECTRIC FIELDS

A patient in an MR system is exposed to static, radiofrequency (RF), and gradient magnetic fields (Figure 2.1). The gradient fields are used to produce a spatial variation in the static field, B_0, that is assumed to be in the z-direction. The signal from the precessing protons is thus a function of position and frequency content in the signal from the receiver coil and is used to construct the MR image. Since the gradient fields are pulsed or switched in time, there will be a time-varying magnetic field, *dB/dt*.

The magnetic field gradient dB_z/dx, dB_z/dy, or dB_z/dz is proportional to the current in each coil, and *dB/dt* is proportional to the time rate of change of the current. Figure 2.2 illustrates coil current and *dB/dt* waveforms for a rectangular pulse train. Note that the magnitude and direction of *dB/dt* is a function of position within the gradient coil assembly. Sinusoidal and other shapes of gradient waveforms are also used.

In a significantly simplified model, which nonetheless describes the basic features of the mechanism for inducing currents, the trunk of the patient is modeled as a conducting cylinder with the time-varying magnetic field from the z-gradient, dB_z/dt, along the length of the patient. The induced currents, the density of which is equal to the proof the conductivity and the electric field, then flows in a circular path with zero intensity at the center and maximal intensity at the surface. The intensity of the induced electric field E as a function of radial distance R from patient center is

$$E = (R/2)\, dB_z/dt \tag{2.1}$$

In a cylindrical MR system, the induced currents from the transverse x- and y-gradients are primarily due to the component of the time-varying magnetic field which is perpendicular to the

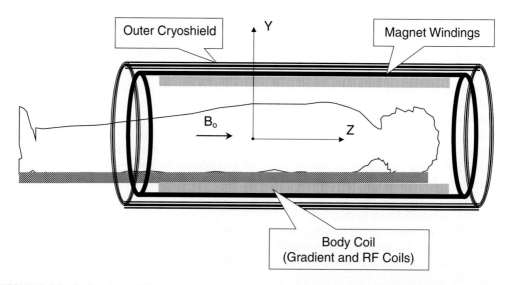

FIGURE 2.1 Patient in an MR system and coils that produce the static, RF, and gradient magnetic fields.

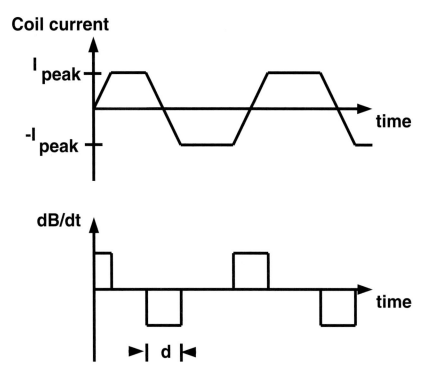

FIGURE 2.2 Waveforms for coil current and *dB/dt* for a rectangular pulse train. The ramp time *d* is the duration of the pulse of current that is induced in the patient.

axis of the bore. The currents will mostly be in the plane perpendicular to the direction of *dB/dt* and will have the greatest intensity near the patient surface. An improved calculation of induced eddy currents can be made using an ellipsoidal human model.[1] An accurate calculation requires the incorporation of the various tissue conductivities and can be done with finite elements.[2,3]

III. STIMULATION BY INTENSE MRI GRADIENT FIELDS

Early regulatory standards[4] limited pulsed gradient intensities *dB/dt* to 20 T/s in order to avoid nerve stimulation.[5,6] It was observed experimentally and predicted theoretically that modern gradient coil hardware may produce *dB/dt* intensity sufficient to produce a physiological response. The lowest level of response will be peripheral nerve stimulation (PNS), the lowest level sensation that can be felt by the patient.

The first report of physiological response was by Cohen's et al.,[7] who reported sensations in the noses of subjects exposed to transverse gradients in a prototype fast-scan or "hyperscan" MR system. Another early report was by Budinger et al.,[8] who reported neuromuscular stimulation by rapidly oscillating gradient fields created by an experimental echo planar gradient coil. A stimulus of about twice the sensation induced pain. Ueno et al.[9] made a coil to fit over the human head and applied a train of 64 trapezoidal pulsed currents which produced rectangular *dB/dt* pulses with a duration of 200 μs. (See Figure 2.2 for definition of pulse duration *d* for a trapezoidal train of gradient pulses.) A threshold of 80 to 100 T/s was observed for sensation in the middle of the forehead.

Early in the development of fast-scan MR techniques, there was concern that the heart could be at risk with respect to stimulation by pulsed gradients. Reilly[10] used literature results and a theoretical model to estimate that for long duration *dB/dt* pulses, the induced electric fields for peripheral nerve and cardiac stimulation are similar. Fortunately, for pulse durations of interest in MRI, the threshold for cardiac stimulation is much greater than for PNS.

Bourland and collaborators[11-14] measured thresholds for cardiac stimulation (induction of ectopic beats) by pulsed magnetic fields in anesthetized dogs. The coils they used induced eddy currents similar to what would be induced by an MRI z-gradient coil. The projected median cardiac threshold for a pulse duration of 530 μs was 2700 T/s. These values resulted in a ramp in the magnetic field of 1.43 T. The thresholds were found to not depend on whether or not a static magnetic field $B_0 = 1.5$ T was present. Furthermore, when near-cardiac-threshold pulses were delivered at various times during the cardiac cycle, no malignant rhythms were observed.[15] Assuming a chronaxie of 3 ms and scaling the numbers to typical human geometry result in an estimate[16] of 0.43 T for the minimal ramp in the magnetic field required to achieve cardiac stimulation in the healthy human subject.

Reilly[1,17] estimated that the threshold for the 1-percentile level is half the median stimulation threshold. Thus, for the results of Bourland et al.,[13,15,16] the 1-percentile level is projected to be 0.215 T, which is close to a value of 0.19 T extrapolated from Reilly's work. A z-gradient ramp of 0.2 T in a whole-body MR system is more than a factor of 5 greater than a ramp that will cause significant discomfort to the patient. Cardiac stimulation can be avoided by a wide margin of safety in a standard or conventional MR system.

The establishment of essentially "zero risk" of cardiac stimulation by the MRI gradient fields is reassuring. The practical physiological limit of the pulsed gradient fields is the induction of undesirable sensations, and perhaps motion, in the patient. In order to devise MRI hardware with the best possible image quality and speed of acquisition, but which does not disturb the patient, it is important to know accurately the *dB/dt* levels for physiological responses. Accordingly, several experimental studies have been undertaken in recent years to quantify the health effects of pulsed gradient fields.

Schaefer et al. measured PNS thresholds for trapezoidal pulse trains in a whole-body coil for gradients applied to a single axis[18] and simultaneously[19] to multiple axes. The thresholds for a *dB/dt* pulse duration of 200 μs ranged from 58 to 100 T/s. Stimulation sites included the scapula and other sites on the back, bridge of the nose, upper arms, legs, hands, buttocks, head, and xyphoid. For the y-axis (anterior-posterior) gradient, the stimulation threshold was reduced by about 30% when the hands were clasped, and the site of stimulation was between the fingers.

Ham et al.[20] measured PNS thresholds in a whole-body MR system for pulse durations of 400 μs. The amplitude of *dB/dt* required for stimulation ranged from 43 to 51 T/s for the three gradient directions. Abart et al.[21] studied PNS with the y-gradient in 113 human subjects with a sinusoidally ramped gradient with a period of 1200 μs and an effective ramp time of 300 μs. The sensation thresholds were expressed in milliTesla per meter (mT/m) units, but the mean threshold was inferred to be about 45 T/s. Studies of stimulation thresholds were also undertaken by Ehrhardt et al.[22] and by Frese et al.[23]

Hebrank et al.[24] measured PNS thresholds for a y-coil in 65 volunteer subjects at eight pulse durations from 200 to 1000 μs. Thresholds ranged from 24.3 at 1000 μs to 57.6 T/s at 200 μs. Jagannathan[25] described areas of health concern for the gradient and other fields in MRI. Schaefer et al.[26] recently presented a detailed review of the present understanding of patient safety in time-varying gradient fields in MRI.

Bourland et al.[16] performed an extended study of stimulation by MRI pulsed gradient fields in 84 human subjects. Trains of rectangular magnetic field pulses were applied by coils that simulated the eddy currents that are induced by the y- and z-gradient coils in a whole-body MR system with a longitudinal bore. The amplitude of *dB/dt* vs. pulse width was measured for the physiological endpoints of sensation, discomfort, and intolerance. The experimental data were fitted to the Lapicque[27,28] (hyperbolic) form of the strength duration relationship to determine the population average and standard deviation for physiologic response:

$$dB/dt = b \cdot \left(1 + \frac{c}{d}\right) \tag{2.2}$$

where b is the rheobase, the asymptotic dB/dt for long duration pulses, and c is chronaxie, the pulse duration at which dB/dt is twice the rheobase. The population average rheobase and chronaxie for the sensation threshold were 14.91 T/s and 365 μs for the y-coil and 26.17 T/s and 378 μs for the z-coil. The dB/dt values were maximal values on the axis of the coil. Significant motor contraction of either abdominal or thoracic skeletal muscles was observed for gradient field strengths approximately 50% greater than the sensation threshold. Weak muscle contractions were observed in several subjects, even though they reported no sensations. A dB/dt intensity of approximately twice the sensation threshold was described by the subjects involved in this study as "intolerable."

Robust models for prediction of the response of a neuron to an electrical stimulus have been developed by a number of investigators.[1] It appears that empirical models combined with experimental input can accurately predict the threshold for dB/dt waveforms representative of those used in MRI procedures. Havel et al.[29] demonstrated an equivalent electrical circuit for the cell membrane based upon Equation 2.2. The model was applied to stimulation by single rectangular and sinusoidal dB/dt pulses applied to the arm and yielded similar b and c for the two waveforms.

den Boer et al.[30] developed a generalization of Equation 2.2 which involved convolution of the time-dependent stimulus. This model was applied to dB/dt waveforms used in MRI and did explain correctly a number of experimental results. A more involved, yet relatively simple, model was presented by Hebrank et al.[24] Their SAFE (Stimulation Approximation by Filtering and Evaluation) model applies three temporal filters to the gradient waveform and sums the output. The filters model the generation of action potentials within nerve cells and the spread of the signal via synapses. While the model does not claim to describe the physiological behavior, it does predict all dependencies of the stimulation threshold on pulse duration, sinusoidal vs. trapezoidal, and number of gradient pulses.

When comparing peripheral nerve thresholds by different investigators, it is extremely important to consider the experimental conditions and how the data are reported. It is particularly important to note the spatial location at which the dB/dt intensity is evaluated.[31] The International Electrotechnology Commission (IEC)[32] and National Electrical Manufacturers Association (NEMA)[33] standards specify that reported dB/dt be the maximal value measured on a radius of 0.2 m from the axis for cylindrical bore magnets. For representative whole-body coils used for MRI procedures, values of dB/dt evaluated on the axis of the bore will be about 20% less for the z-gradient and about 30% less for the transverse x- and y-gradients.

Bourland et al.[16] used literature data to estimate that a dB/dt of 5500 T/s uniformly applied to the head would be required to achieve brain stimulation. This is well above the threshold for induction of intense pain, and thus, stimulation of the brain by the MRI pulsed gradients is unlikely.

Present and future regulations permit higher levels of dB/dt than previously allowed. The U.S. Food and Drug Administration (FDA) specifies that an investigational device exemption (IDE) is required if the dB/dt intensity is sufficient to produce severe discomfort or painful nerve stimulation.[34] The upcoming IEC standard will probably allow dB/dt of 80% of the mean sensation threshold for normal operation and 100% of the mean for level 1 controlled operation. These new regulations protect the safety of the patient, while permitting the maximal therapeutic benefit of the new MRI techniques.

IV. HUMAN PHYSIOLOGIC RESPONSE TO INTENSE MRI GRADIENT MAGNETIC FIELDS

Given that the regulatory standards for pulsed gradient intensity are now specified in terms of physiologic response, rather than absolute values of dB/dt, an understanding of the statistical distribution of the bioeffects of the pulsed gradients is important. In this section, previously unpublished data from the Purdue University study on the statistical distribution of pulsed gradient intensities required for physiologic response are presented. A computer model is used to calculate the intensity of induced electric fields for *dB/dt* at the sensation threshold. Notably, the information and methods in this section can be used to predict the *dB/dt* thresholds for physiologic response for various types of MRI gradient coils.

A. MEASUREMENT TECHNIQUES TO ASSESS PHYSIOLOGIC RESPONSES

This experimental procedure has previously been described.[16] Figures 2.3 and 2.4 depict the coils that were used in the study. The coils are designed to reproduce the stimulating effects of gradient coils in a whole-body, cylindrical-bore MR system. The coils were wound on cylindrical forms with a diameter of 65 cm. The y-coil is illustrated in Figure 2.3. It closely resembles an actual MRI gradient coil. It consists of 4 spiral windings of 24 turns. Each spiral winding sub-tends an angle of nearly 180° on the cylindrical form and has a length equal to the diameter of the form. Note that the y-component of the magnetic field is the one likely to yield the greatest intensity of eddy currents. The z-coil, illustrated in Figure 2.4, consists of a single winding with a length of half of the diameter. This simulates the windings on either end of an actual gradient coil. The single winding was used to generate the largest possible amplitude of dB_z/dt. Two z-coils, one with 30 turns and the other with 75 turns, were used to achieve a wide range of ramp times *d* with the available generator.

A modified General Electric Ramp Accelerator Module (GRAM)[35] and linear amplifier were used to generate current trains with linear ramps, depicted in Figure 2.2, producing 127 rectangular *dB/dt* pulses. The peak output voltage of the generator was ±3750 V and maximal currents were ±325 A. For the coils used, the achievable *dB/dt* pulse widths ranged from 50 to 1000 μs. The

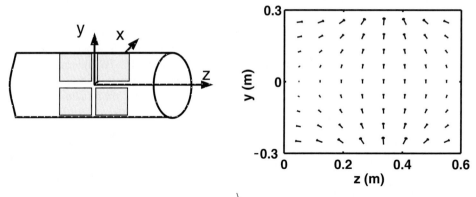

FIGURE 2.3 Layout of the coil for generation of the y-gradient and the field pattern in the y,z plane.

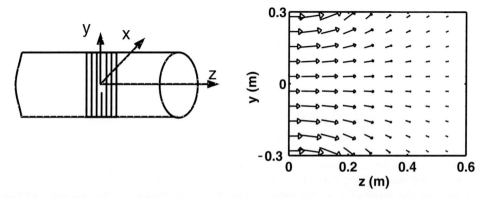

FIGURE 2.4 Layout of the coil producing a magnetic field pattern simulating the stimulating characteristics of the MRI z-gradient coil and field pattern in the y,z plane.

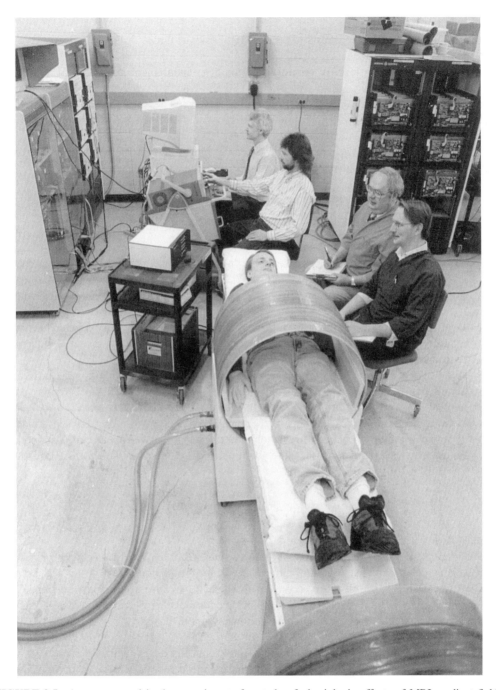

FIGURE 2.5 Apparatus used in the experiments for study of physiologic effects of MRI gradient fields. The subject is lying in a coil which simulates the stimulating effects of the MRI z-gradient coil.

plateau time between pulses was 300 μs. Figure 2.5 shows the overall apparatus and a subject in the z-coil. The subject lies supine, and the axial position of the subject umbilicus relative to the coil center is adjusted to yield the lowest thresholds. Rectangular *dB/dt* pulses with nine different durations as defined in Figure 2.2 — of 50, 70, 100, 150, 200, 300, 500, 700, and 1000 μs — were applied to the coil. The subjects were asked to rate the response induced by a pulse train according to the following scale:

0: not felt

1: no discomfort (sensation threshold for PNS)

3: slightly uncomfortable

5: uncomfortable, but a level of comfort that could be endured for the length of a scan if medically necessary

7: very uncomfortable

10: intolerable (it would not be possible to undergo a scan at this level of discomfort)

The amplitude of the *dB/dt* pulses in the train was increased in 10% increments until one of the following conditions was met:

1. The subject reported a 10 or requested that no stronger field be applied.
2. A *dB/dt* intensity twice the sensation threshold was achieved.
3. A system limit was encountered.

The data points presented here are essentially "measured data" and were obtained as follows:

1. For the applied train of current pulses, the peak current amplitude and *dB/dt* pulse width *d* were measured.
2. From knowledge of the coil constant (magnetic field per unit current), a value of *dB/dt* intensity is obtained. *dB/dt* intensities reported in this section are the maximal values at a distance 0.2 m from the center of the bore.*
3. If the subject assigned the same score to *dB/dt* pulses of the same duration but different amplitudes (in a typical experimental session, approximately 250 pulse trains were applied), the lowest *dB/dt* intensity would be taken to be the correct one.
4. If the subject did not describe any of the applied pulse trains to produce a sensation of 1, 5, or 10, a fitting procedure was attempted to extrapolate the "measured" data point. For each coil and ramp duration, a three-parameter power function of the form in Equation 2.3 is used.

$$\text{Score} = \alpha + \beta \cdot (dB/dt)^{\gamma} \tag{2.3}$$

where α, β, and γ are the fitting parameters.

The dependence on pulse duration of time-varying *dB/dt* required to achieve physiologic response is modeled by the strength-duration relationship in Equation 2.2.

The extrapolation was felt to be a conservative one. It was used only if experimental *dB/dt* values were available for the same coil type and pulse duration at a response level near the missing datum. The extrapolation was used under the following circumstances:

1. There is no response datum available at score 1, but there is a datum for score 2.
2. There is no datum available at score 5, but there are data available for response scores of 4 or 6.
3. There is no datum available at score 10, but there are data available for a response scores of 8 or 9.

---

* The Purdue University group reported *dB/dt* measured on the axis of the bore.[16] For the coils in Figure 2.3 and 2.4, the ratio of maximal field at a radius of 0.2 m compared to the axis is 1.44 for the y-coil and 1.21 for the z-coil. Results presented here incorporate correction of a systematic error and an improved method of data analysis, which would lower the previously reported *dB/dt* values by abut 10%.

It was necessary to limit the amount of data accrued to maintain the experiment time under 2 h to avoid subject fatigue. Thus, measurements were made with only one transverse coil. Because the x-coil has the greatest thresholds, measurements were made with the y-coil only because knowledge of the lower thresholds is more clinically relevant.

This study was conducted with the consent and under the advice of the Purdue University Committee for the Use of Human Research Subjects, the university's equivalent of an institutional review board. As a safety precaution, test train pulses were synchronized to the R-wave of the electrocardiogram (ECG), and the ECG was continuously monitored by a team member. The subjects wore surgical gloves to prevent stimulation in the hands.

B. Measured *dB/dt* Intensities for Physiologic Responses

Experimental results for a single subject are shown in Figure 2.6. These results are representative of those obtained for each of the 84 subjects in the study. The points are measurements for intensity levels of 1 (PNS sensation threshold), 5 (uncomfortable), and 10 (intolerable). The symbols in the graphs indicate whether the points are measured data or extrapolated from measurements at nearby scores according to the procedure described above. The solid lines in Figure 2.6 are best fit for the hyperbolic form of the strength-duration relationship in Equation 2.2.

Visual inspection of Figure 2.6 shows that measured data and extrapolated data together are well fit by the same rheobase *b* and chronaxie *c* parameters. Figure 2.6 shows that the intensity of the *dB/dt* pulse required to achieve physiologic response increases as the pulse duration decreases. The intensity required to achieve a response score of 5 is approximately 50% above the threshold and a score of 10 requires *dB/dt* approximately twice that of the threshold.

Figure 2.7 is a histogram of the axial positions of subjects that resulted in the lowest sensation thresholds. For the y-coil, the lowest thresholds occurred when the subject was positioned so that the umbilicus was approximately 10 cm from the coil center (the typical subject was initially placed with the umbilicus at the coil center, and the lowest threshold was observed when the subject was moved in the cranial direction 10 cm of the coil).

This situation corresponds to the peak of the y-component of the magnetic field of the coil pair in Figure 2.3 proximal to the head being approximately centered over the thorax. A few subjects reported the lowest thresholds at a position of about –40 cm; this corresponds to the coil pair distal to the head being centered over the thorax. For the z-coil, the lowest thresholds occur for a subject position of about –20 cm. This corresponds to the single coil of Figure 2.4 being approximately centered over the thorax.

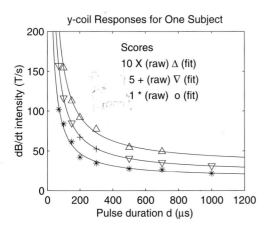 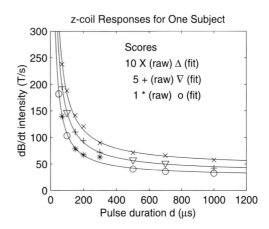

FIGURE 2.6 Plots of field intensity *dB/dt* vs. pulse duration for a single subject for physiologic response levels of 1 (PNS threshold), 5 (uncomfortable), and 10 (intolerable) for the y- and z-coils. The points are measured as explained in the text, and the lines are fit to the strength-duration relationship in Equation 2.2.

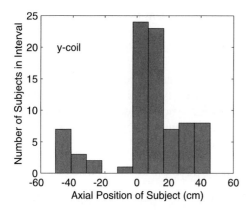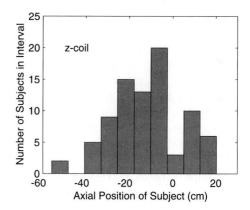

FIGURE 2.7 Histogram of subject positions which produced the lowest thresholds for the y- and z-coils. A zero position means that the umbilicus is at the coil center, and a positive position means the head of the subject is moved away from the coil center.

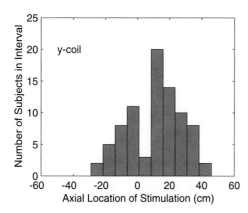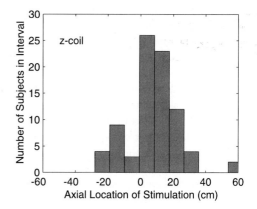

FIGURE 2.8 Histogram of axial locations where the subjects reported sensation (score = 1). Zero locations mean stimulation occurred at the level of the umbilicus. A positive location means stimulation occurred cranial of the umbilicus, and a negative location means stimulation was caudal of the umbilicus.

Figure 2.8 is a histogram of locations where subjects felt the sensation for the lowest level of stimulus (score = 1). For the y-coil, the majority of stimulations occurred some 20 cm cranial of the umbilicus, which is at the approximate level of the xiphoid. The few instances of negative location are due to stimulation occurring somewhere in the hip region. For the z-coil, a representative location is also somewhere in the thorax, with just a few subjects reporting sensation in the hip region.

Pulse field intensities for the subject population for three levels of response are shown in rank order in Figure 2.9 for *dB/dt* pulse duration of 200 µs for the y- and z-coils. Similarly, Figure 2.10 shows measured thresholds for a pulse duration of 500 µs. In these graphs, each point represents an experimental datum, either one that is directly measured or extrapolated as described above. For the sensation threshold (response of 1), most of the *dB/dt* data are direct measurements (* symbol) and only a few are projected (o symbol). On the other hand, a larger fraction of the data is projected for the scores of 5 and 10.

Even with the selective fitting scheme, a *dB/dt* intensity was not obtained for all of the subjects for the scores of 5 and 10. For instance, for a score of 10 at duration 200 µs, *dB/dt* intensity was not obtained for 31 subjects with the y-coil and for 35 subjects with the z-coil. This is because of equipment limitations and the experimental protocol stipulation that the subject not be exposed to

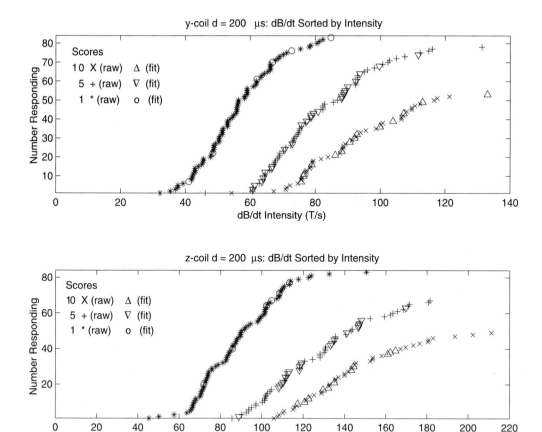

FIGURE 2.9 Rank ordered *dB/dt* intensities for the 84-subject population at a pulse duration of 200 μs for the y- and z-coils. Each symbol represents a data point for an individual subject. The points are either direct measurements or extracted from measurements as explained in the text.

dB/dt intensity in excess of twice the sensation threshold. It is not surprising given the subjective nature of pain (and the stoicism of Purdue University students!) that some subjects had a high criterion of what they would describe as tolerable.

We use the median *dB/dt* intensity to characterize the overall population response. This is the 42nd highest intensity in the 84-subject population. Use of the median intensity to determine the actual population average is useful because the missing *dB/dt* values are generally at the higher intensities. With missing data, taking the average of the available *dB/dt* values will underestimate the actual average intensity.

Table 2.1 shows median *dB/dt* intensities for the overall population. A null entry means that a *dB/dt* intensity is available for fewer than 42 of the 84 subjects. The null entries are generally for scores of 5 and 10 at the short and long pulse durations, where hardware limitations made difficult the application of sufficiently intense pulses.

For response scores of 1, for which there is a *dB/dt* datum for most subjects, the mean and median *dB/dt* intensities are nearly the same. For $d = 200$ μs, means for the y- and z-coils are 55.8 and 88.3 T/s, respectively. At $d = 500$ μs, the respective means are 33.8 and 52.6 T/s.

A fitting procedure for the score = 1 median *dB/dt* data in Table 2.1 indicates that a chronaxie of approximately 380 μs is the best fit for the score of 1 and will also fit the data for scores of 5 and 10. A relative least square error criterion was used to determine values of the rheobase for the two coils and three intensity levels that best fit the strength-duration relationship in Equation 2.2.

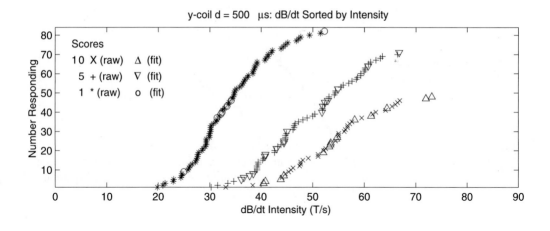

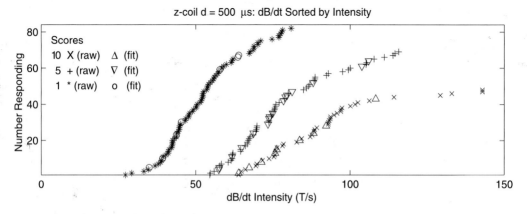

FIGURE 2.10 Same as Figure 2.9, except at a *dB/dt* pulse duration of 500 μs.

TABLE 2.1
Median *dB/dt* Intensities for Physiologic Response for the 84-Subject Population

$d(\mu s)$	y-Coil *dB/dt*			Z-Coil *dB/dt*		
	Score = 1	5	10	Score = 1	5	10
50	—	—	—	232	367	—
70	113	178	—	180	279	380
100	91	135	—	137	215	271
150	68	104	133	102	160	217
200	55	79	107	86	133	173
300	42	61	83	66	93	124
500	33	52	64	52	78	106
700	28	44	—	45	67	100
1000	27	—	—	40	61	—

Let dB/dt_i represent a median datum for a given coil and score in Table 2.1. The relative mean square error ε_r^2 is

$$\varepsilon_r^2 = \sum_i \left(\frac{dB/dt_i - b(1 + c/d_i)^2}{b(1 + c/d_i)} \right) \tag{2.4}$$

where the sum includes up to nine durations. Taking the derivative of ε_r^2 with respect to b and setting to 0 results in the best fit for b:

$$b = \frac{\sum_i \left(\frac{dB/dt_i}{1 + c/d_i}\right)^2}{\sum_i \left(\frac{dB/dt_i}{1 + c/d_i}\right)} \tag{2.5}$$

Applying Equation 2.5 to the results in Table 2.1 yields the rheobases in Table 2.2.

Figure 2.11 plots the median thresholds from Table 2.2 as a function of the pulse duration d. Superimposed on the data points are the strength duration curves calculated from Equation 2.2 using a chronaxie of 380 μs and the rheobases from Table 2.2.

The rheobases in Table 2.2 combined with a chronaxie of 380 μs describe the overall median response to the pulsed groove fields. The ratio of the z to y rheobases for the same score falls in the narrow range of 1.56 to 1.62. Noteworthy are the relative values of rheobases for the different response levels. The ratio of rheobase of score 5 relative to threshold is 1.51 and 1.57 for the y- and z-coils, respectively. For a score of 10, the ratios relative to the rheobase are 1.96 and 2.08 for the y- and z-coils, respectively.

For comparison, the fitting procedure was applied to y-gradient thresholds for eight durations from 200 to 1000 μs recently presented by Hebrank et al.[24,25] Applying a chronaxie of 380 μs results in a rheobase of 19.0 T/s, an excellent agreement with the value of 18.8 T/s in the Purdue University study.

An important result of the Purdue University experiments is the distribution of thresholds across the population. For example, it would be highly desirable to provide the answer to the following question from these data: If the gradient field were limited such that a small percentage of the

TABLE 2.2
**Population Median Rheobases Calculated from the *dB/dt*
Intensity in Table 2.1 Assuming Chronaxie *c* = 380 μs**

y-Coil Rheobases (T/s)			z-Coil Rheobases (T/s)		
Score = 1	5	10	Score = 1	5	10
18.8	28.3	36.9	28.8	44.0	59.8

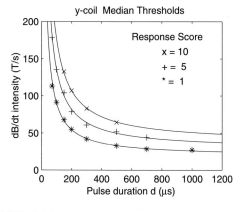
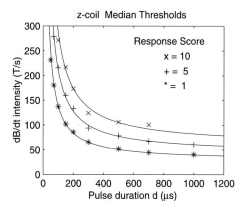

FIGURE 2.11 Median *dB/dt* intensities vs. pulse duration for the 84 subjects. The points are the calculated medians from Table 2.1 and the curves are from the strength-duration relationship in Equation 2.2 with chronaxie *c* = 380 μs and rheobase *b* from Table 2.2.

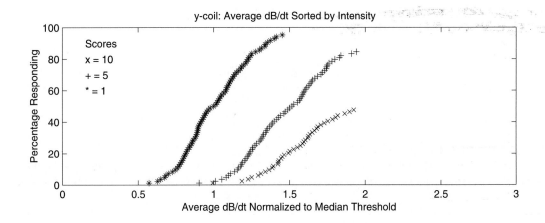

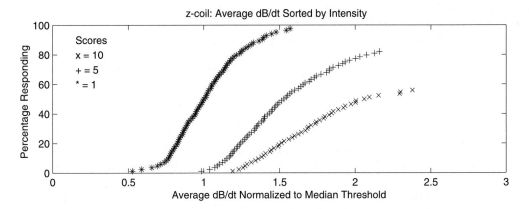

FIGURE 2.12 Combined sorted *dB/dt* intensities for the 84-subject population. The thresholds are normalized to the median value of *dB/dt* for the sensation threshold (score = 1).

population could just sense the field, what (smaller) percentage would find the sensation as uncomfortable and what (yet smaller) percentage would find the sensation as intolerable?

An indication of threshold distribution can be appreciated from examination of Figures 2.9 and 2.10. In Figure 2.12, a summary of the overall population thresholds is presented. The thresholds are normalized to the median sensation threshold. Each point in Figure 2.12 is calculated by averaging the *dB/dt* intensities over the nine durations in the following manner:

1. Measured *dB/dt* intensities for a given score, coil type, and duration are sorted in rank order (1 to 84) of increasing intensity over the 84 subjects, for example, as is done in Figures 2.9 and 2.10 for *d* = 200 and 500 μs. The *dB/dt* values are normalized with a relative *dB/dt* of 1 corresponding to the median sensation threshold.
2. The average relative *dB/dt* values for a given rank (1 to 84) are calculated by averaging over the nine durations. This value is plotted in Figure 2.12 if *dB/dt* intensities were obtained for at least four durations at a given rank.

Key features to note in Figure 2.12 are

1. For the sensation threshold (score = 1), the lowest 1-percentile is slightly more than half of the median.

2. The lowest 1-percentile of uncomfortable (score = 5) is approximately equal to the median of the sensation threshold.
3. The lowest 1-percentile of intolerable (score = 10) is approximately 20% above the median sensation threshold.
4. At 20% above the median sensation threshold, approximately 80% of the subjects report stimulation.

It is interesting to explore a possible relationship between *dB/dt* thresholds and morphological and other characteristics of the subjects. For instance, one might expect larger subjects to have lower thresholds because of the larger eddy current loops.

Figure 2.13 shows *dB/dt* required for the threshold of sensation (score = 1) vs. the girth at the level of the umbilicus of the subjects. There is no evidence for a correlation for the y-coil thresholds. On the other hand, there is some, but not dramatic, evidence for slight decrease in z-coil thresholds with increasing girth. Plots of thresholds vs. subject weight which are shown in Figure 2.14 for the y- and z-coils indicate little if any correlation with weight. Sensation thresholds as a function of subject age are shown in Figure 2.15, and there is no indication of a correlation. Subject gender is indicated by the symbol type in Figures 2.13 to 2.15, and there is no indication that the thresholds depend on gender.

These results are in agreement with the observations of Abart et al.[21] who found no correlation in their study of the dependence of stimulation thresholds on the parameters of age, body surface,

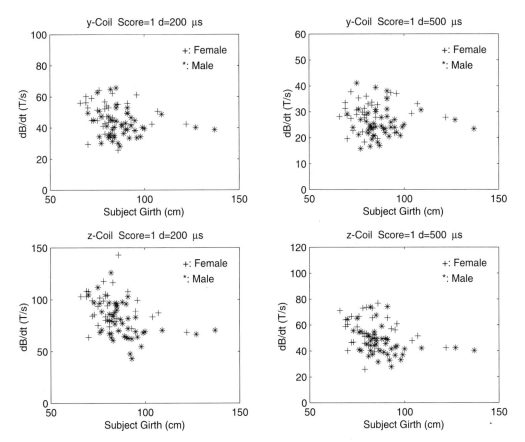

FIGURE 2.13 *dB/dt* intensity for sensation (score = 1) vs. subject girth (waist size) at the level of the umbilicus for the y- and z-coils for pulse durations of 200 and 500 μs.

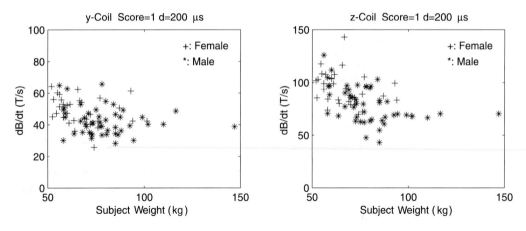

FIGURE 2.14 Thresholds for sensation (score = 1) vs. subject weight for the y- and z-coils at a pulse duration of 200 μs.

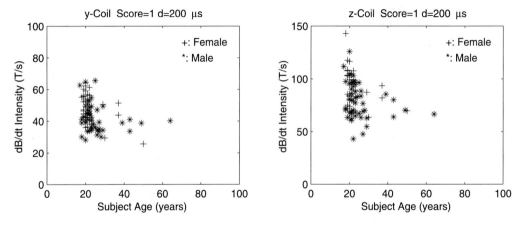

FIGURE 2.15 Thresholds for sensation (score = 1) vs. subject age for the y- and z-coils at a pulse duration of 200 μs.

and gender. On the other hand, women exhibited lower thresholds than men for perception and annoyance when stimuli were applied via electrodes to the forearm and fingertip.[36]

Reilly[37] has calculated that thresholds for biphasic pulses separated by greater than 50% of chronaxie will be nearly the same as for isolated pulses. Thus, the pulse separation of 300 μs in the Purdue University experiments was sufficiently large to avoid the increase in threshold that occurred for closely spaced biphasic pulses.

V. FINITE ELEMENT CALCULATION OF INDUCED CURRENTS

Calculations were undertaken on the Purdue University data with the principal objective of obtaining a statistical characterization of the electric field induced in the body for a given dB/dt. This information can then be applied to the measured dB/dt thresholds to determine the peak-induced electric field that was required to achieve a given physiologic response in the subjects. Once the electric field required for stimulation is known, the computer model can be used to predict the amount of time-varying current, dI/dt, that will be required to achieve a physiologic response for an arbitrary gradient coil assembly.

A. CALCULATION METHOD

The eddy current density induced by the coils of Figures 2.3 and 2.4 was calculated in a model with a human shape and uniform conductivity. The calculations were made with the commercial ANSYS v. 5.4. finite element program. The human model was created at the Biomedical Institute at Karlsruhe University, Germany (http://www-ibt.etec.uni-karlsruhe.de/MEETMan_eng.html) as a MEET project (Models for Simulation of Electromagnetic, Elastomechanic and Thermal Behavior of Man). Meet Man originated from the Visible Human Project of the National Library of Medicine in Bethesda, MD.

The voxels in the Meet Man model are 8 mm on a side. The voxels were scaled by a factor of 0.95 so that the model would fit into the coils. To not exceed the 64,000 node limit of the Ansys license, eight smaller voxels, 7.6 mm on a side, were combined to create larger voxels, 15.2 mm on a side. Voxels in the uniform conductivity model consist either of tissue or air. For example, there is air in the lungs and sinuses. A simple "voting" procedure in each assembly of eight initial voxels was used to decide the conductivity of the larger voxel. If four or more of the initial voxels are tissue, then the conductivity of the larger voxel will be that of tissue. The same electrical conductivity of 0.25 S/m was assumed for all tissues. The assumption of uniform conductivity allowed the model to be symmetric about the sagittal plane. Furthermore, the legs and arms were not included in the calculations.

The ANSYS model consisted of 10,737 tissue elements, and the total number of element was 42,120. The element type was SOLID97. This element has eight nodes and up to five degrees of freedom (DOFs), including magnetic vector potential (Ax, Ay, Az) and the electric scalar potential (VOLT).

Direct node/element generation was used to simplify the meshing. An initial grid was generated in a rectangular block with 36 elements in the x-direction, 40 elements in the y-direction, and 144 elements in the z-direction. An additional outer layer of free air was enclosed in an external boundary.

The magnetic vector potential produced by the gradient coil was the load applied to the boundary. A harmonic solution was used, and the frequency was 1 kHz, a frequency consistent with those used in MRI procedures. For the y- and z-coils, a flux-parallel (magnetic) boundary condition was applied to all nodes on the plane of symmetry (z,y plane).

Figure 2.16 shows the arrow plot of the induced eddy currents for the y-coil in the x,z plane, the center coronal plane of the patient model. Since the calculation assumes symmetry about the sagittal mid-plane, the eddy currents were only calculated for the left half. The currents in the right

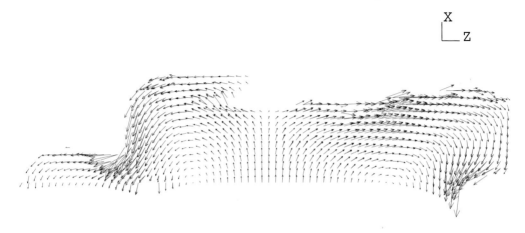

FIGURE 2.16 Pattern of calculated induced currents in the center coronal plane of the patient model for the y-coil of Figure 2.3.

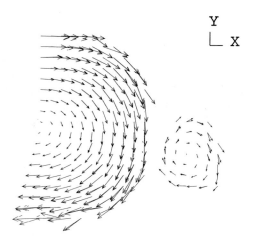

FIGURE 2.17 Pattern of calculated induced currents in the center axial plane of the patient model for the z-coil of Figure 2.4.

half are extrapolated by symmetry. There are two approximately circular patterns of induced currents with lowest intensity at patient center and greatest intensity at patient periphery.

Figure 2.17 shows the arrow plot of induced currents for the z-coil in an axial plane near the umbilicus. Again, because of the plane symmetry, currents are displayed for only half of the model. The larger semicircle at the left is the trunk, and the smaller circle at the right is the left arm. As expected, the time-varying magnetic field in the z-direction produces a circumferential eddy current pattern. Consistent with predictions for a conducting cylinder in Section II, the induced current intensity is near zero at the center of the trunk and arm and greatest at the periphery. The induced electric intensity at the periphery of the trunk is about twice that of the electric field at the periphery of the arm, a consequence of the larger trunk radius.

B. CALCULATION OF ELECTRIC FIELDS FOR STIMULATION

In this section, the electric field for physiologic response is calculated by making use of the computer model and the *dB/dt* thresholds presented here for the y- and z-coils. The experimental results are presented in terms of *dB/dt* for a specific coil. The electric field induced in the tissue (which is proportional to the induced currents) is the probable mechanism for stimulation. The intensity of electric field for a given *dB/dt* will depend on the geometry of the gradient coils and the patient position relative to the coils. The objective here is to take the *dB/dt* thresholds from the experimental study and to apply them to the numerical model to determine the induced electric fields that result in a physiologic response in the subject. Then knowing the required electric field, it will be possible to predict how much time-varying current, *dI/dt,* is required to produce sensation or other physiologic response for other gradient coils.

An overview of the calculation is as follows.

1. The geometry of the y- and z-coils is used to calculate the magnetic vector potential, which is applied to the boundary nodes for the ANSYS calculation. Also calculated is the maximal magnetic field on the axis at a radial distance of 0.2 m from the coil axis. The maximal field is 49.1 µT/A for the y-coil and 61.9 µT/A for the 30-turn z-coil.
2. The induced electric field is calculated in the 10,737 voxels of the half-body model. The calculation assumes that the time-varying current is 10^9 A/s. Using the symmetry, the induced field is calculated for the 21,474 voxels in the whole-body model.

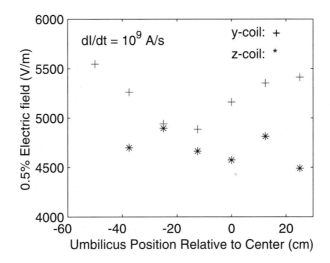

FIGURE 2.18 Calculated electric field for the human model as a function of the umbilicus location relative to the coil center. A positive position means the subject is moved cranial. A current of 10^9 A/s is applied to the coils of Figures 2.3 and 2.4.

The induced electric fields are sorted to determine the upper half percentile of the electric field. That is, 99.5% of the voxels will have a lower induced field. It was found that taking the upper half percentile of the electric field is a good means for estimating the maximal electric field; evaluating the electric field at a lower percentile may result in a value that is affected by computational artifacts at a few nodes. The value of the 0.5-percentile electric field was calculated as a function of position of subject umbilicus relative to the coil center; results are shown in Figure 2.18. A negative position means that more of the thorax is inside the coil. The range of position plotted in Figure 2.18 is approximately the same as the range of positions in the experiments at which the subjects exhibited the lowest thresholds. For the y-coil, the greatest induced field occurs at the approximate positions of 20 and –50 cm; these positions are consistent with the axial positions of lowest threshold in Figure 2.7. For the z-coil, the maximal electric field occurs at position of about –20 cm, and the induced electric field is a less strong function of position that is the induced field from the y-coil. These observations are consistent with experimental results in Figure 2.8 for the z-coil, which shows a relatively broad range of positions for lowest threshold.

From the data in Figure 2.18, 5400 V/m is seen to be a good representation of the electric field for the y-coil for $dI/dt = 10^9$ A/s, and 4900 V/m is a good representation for the z-coil. The induced electric field E_1 per unit dB/dt for the two coils then is

$$E_1(\text{y-coil}) = \frac{(5400 \text{ V/m})/(10^9 \text{ A/s})}{49.1 \text{ } \mu\text{T/A}} = 0.11 \text{ } (V/m)/(T/s) \qquad (2.6)$$

$$E_1(\text{z-coil}) = \frac{(4900 \text{ V/m})/(10^9 \text{ A/s})}{61.9 \text{ } \mu\text{T/A}} = 0.080 \text{ } (V/m)/(T/s) \qquad (2.7)$$

The rheobase electric fields b_{Ey} and b_{Ez} for onset of sensation can now be determined.

$$b_{Ey} = (18.8 \text{ T/s})(0.11 \text{ } (V/m)/(T/s)) = 2.07 \text{ V/m} \qquad (2.8)$$

$$b_{Ez} = (28.8 \text{ T/s})(0.080 \text{ } (V/m)/(T/s)) = 2.30 \text{ V/m} \qquad (2.9)$$

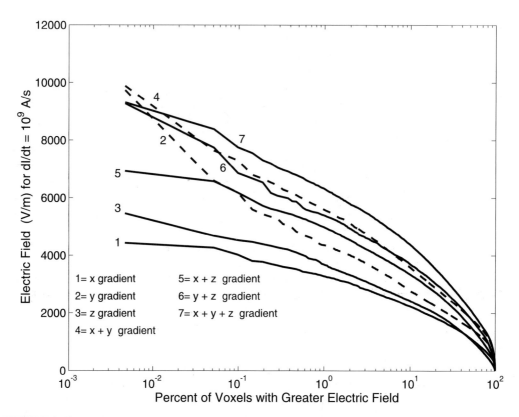

FIGURE 2.19 Induced electric field intensity vs. percent of voxels for simultaneous application of switched gradients.

The similarity of the electric field rheobases for the y- and z-coils suggests that stimulation occurs when the induced electric field has reached a suitably high level. The electric field appears to be a reliable predictor of whether a given pulse sequence will be of sufficient intensity to cause stimulation in other MR system geometries, such as open gradient.

The stimulating potential of simultaneous gradient combinations can be predicted with the method described here. Figure 2.19 illustrates some examples of the effect of combined gradients on the magnitude of the electric field. Shown is the electric field vs. percent of voxels stimulated for actual whole-body gradient coils for a constant dI/dt. Key features to note include that the 0.5-percentile electric field induced by the y-gradient coil is approximately 40% greater than that of x-gradient coil and that simultaneous application of the x- and z-gradients with the y-gradient does not result in a significant increase of electric field over that produced by the y-gradient alone.

C. Discussion of Electric Field Calculations

The calculated rheobase electric fields (2.07 V/m for the y-coil and 2.30 V/m for the z-coil) are less than some previous literature reports. A chronaxie of 402 μs and an electric field rheobase of 4.19 V/m were reported by Havel et al.[29] for stimulation of the forearm with the equivalent of a single rectangular pulse of magnetic field. Reilly[37] has predicted a rheobase electric field of 6.2 V/m for excitation of 20-μm diameter fibers. On the other hand, Reilly estimated a characteristic time for excitation of about 130 μs, about a factor of 3 less than reported here.

There are several possible reasons for the seemingly low electric field rheobase for whole-body stimulation with pulsed magnetic fields. There will be a local enhancement of the electric field in the body due to concentration of eddy currents by non-conducting structures such as bone. This would result in a greater maximal electric field than is calculated with a uniform conductivity human model. It seems reasonable that the electric field enhancement in the trunk of the body, where many bones are relatively close to the skin, will be greater than in the forearm. Another contributing factor may be physiologic summation by the subject of the *dB/dt* pulses in a train, resulting in a lower threshold than for single pulses. Differences in anatomy between nerves in the thorax and the forearm may also be a factor. Calculation of the electric fields for a non-uniform conductivity human model may be desirable and would be a relatively straightforward extension of this work.

Heating of tissue by the pulsed gradients will be insignificant. Consider an extreme case of a pulse duration of 50 μs. With chronaxie of 380 μs and an electric field rheobase of 2.3 V/m, the sensation threshold will be 19.8 V/m. Assuming a conductivity of 0.5 S/m, the peak power deposition will be 0.20 W/kg. This is more than an order of magnitude less than the allowable specific absorption ratio (SAR) which may be applied with the RF field.[28] The partial duty cycle of the gradients further reduces the heating.

VI. ACOUSTIC NOISE

The static field will result in torques and forces on the gradient coils when currents are applied. The gradient currents are in the audio-frequency range, and thus, the MR system produces an acoustic noise that is manifested as a "banging" or "beeping" sound, depending upon the pulse sequence as well as other factors.[38] The actual noise levels will depend on the selected scan protocol,[39] and one expects that the noise will be greater for larger static field and higher amplitudes of gradients. Temporary hearing loss can be caused by the intense sounds in MRI, even those that fall within recommended levels.[40] Earplugs that, when properly used, will reduce noise by 10 to 20 dB prevented the hearing loss.[40] The FDA specifies that noise levels must meet the requirements of local regulatory bodies, such as the U.S. Occupational Safety and Health Administration.[41] A thorough discussion of this topic is presented by Dr. Mark McJury in Chapter 6.

VII. SUMMARY AND CONCLUSIONS

The principal health effect of concern for the pulsed gradient fields is the potential for PNS. The practical health effect that patients will experience most is the loud noise due to the gradient magnetic fields. Present and upcoming regulatory standards will permit *dB/dt* intensities that will result in PNS in some patients. However, painful stimulation is to be avoided. Cardiac stimulation by the pulsed gradients is essentially impossible.

Notably, the most important new results in this chapter are shown in Figure 2.12. The 1-percentile for uncomfortable stimulation is approximately equal to the medium threshold for onset of sensation. The PNS threshold measurements in human subjects yield a chronaxie of 380 μs, and a computation using data from the measurements yields a rheobase electric field of about 2.2 V/m. Using these values for rheobase and chronaxie, it would be possible to predict the stimulation thresholds for combinations of current for an arbitrary MR system geometry, such as open gradient. Recently presented models offer a simple means of predicting the stimulating potential for non-rectangular *dB/dt* waveforms.

ACKNOWLEDGMENTS

Sponsors of research at Purdue University on MRI safety include General Electrical Corporation, the Magnetic Health Science Foundation of Japan, the National Institutes of Health (Grant CA 62224), and the National Science Foundation (NATO-NSF Grant DGE 9804545).

We thank W.A. Tacker, C.F. Babbs, K.S. Foster, G.P. Graber, J. Jones, R. Hendricks, L.A. Geddes, and W. Schoenlein for their considerable medical and technical assistance.

REFERENCES

1. Reilly, J.P., Principles of nerve and heart excitation by time-varying magnetic fields, *Ann. N.Y. Acad. Sci.,* 649, 96, 1992.
2. Mouchawar, G.A., Nyenhuis, J.A., Bourland, J.D., et al., Magnetic stimulation of excitable tissue: calculation of induced eddy-currents with a three-dimensional finite-element model, *IEEE Trans. Magn.,* 29, 3355, 1993.
3. Ragan, P.M., Wang, W., and Eisenberg, S.R., Magnetically induced currents in the canine heart: a finite element study, *IEEE Trans. Biomed. Eng.,* 42, 1110, 1995.
4. Athey, T.W., Current FDA guidance for MR patient exposure and considerations for the future, *Ann. N.Y. Acad. Sci.,* 649, 242, 1992.
5. Barker, A.T., An introduction to the basic principles of magnetic nerve stimulation, *J. Clin. Neurophysiol.,* 8, 26, 1991.
6. Ueno, S. and Iwasaka, M., Magnetic nerve stimulation and effects of magnetic fields on biological, physical and chemical processes, in *Biological Effects of Magnetic and Electromagnetic Fields,* S. Ueno, Ed., Plenum Press, New York, 1996, 1.
7. Cohen, M.S., Weisskopf, M.R., Rzedian, R.R., et al., Sensory stimulation by time varying magnetic fields, *Magn. Reson. Med.,* 14, 409, 1990.
8. Budinger, T.F., Fischer, H., Hentshel, D., et al. Physiological effects of fast oscillating magnetic field gradients, *J. Comput. Assist. Tomogr.,* 15, 609, 1991.
9. Ueno, S., Hiwaki, O., Matsuda, T., et al., Safety problems of dB/dt associated with echo planar imaging, *Ann. N.Y. Acad. Sci.,* 649, 396, 1992.
10. Reilly, J.P., Magnetic field excitation of peripheral nerves and the heart: a comparison of thresholds, *Med. Biol. Eng. Comput.,* 29, 571, 1991.
11. Mouchawar, G.A., Bourland, J.D., Nyenhuis, J.A., et al., Closed-chest cardiac stimulation with a pulsed magnetic field, *Med. Biol. Eng. Comput.,* 30, 162, 1992.
12. Nyenhuis, J.A., Bourland, J.D., Mouchawar, G.A., et al., Magnetic stimulation of the heart and safety issues in magnetic resonance imaging, in *Biomagnetic Stimulation,* S. Ueno, Ed., Plenum Press, New York, 1994, 75.
13. Bourland, J.D., Nyenhuis, J.A., Mouchawar, G.A., et al., Z-gradient coil eddy-current stimulation of skeletal and cardiac muscle in the dog, *Soc. Magn. Reson. Med. Proc. 10th Ann. Meet.,* 969, 1991.
14. Nyenhuis, J.A., Bourland, J.D., Schaefer, D.J., et al., Measurement of cardiac stimulation thresholds for pulsed Z-gradient fields in a 1.5 T magnet, *Soc. Magn. Reson. Med. Proc. 11th Ann. Meet.,* 586, 1992.
15. Bourland, J.D., Nyenhuis, J.A., Schaefer, D.J., et al., Gated, gradient-induced cardiac stimulation in the dog: absence of ventricular fibrillation, *Soc. Magn. Reson. Med. Proc. 11th Ann. Meet.,* 4804, 1992.
16. Bourland, J.D., Nyenhuis, J.A., and Schaefer, D.J., Physiologic effects of intense MRI gradient fields, *Neuroimaging Clin. North Am.,* 9, 363, 1999.
17. Reilly, J.P., *Electrical Stimulation and Electropathology,* Cambridge University Press, Cambridge, U.K., 1992, 180.
18. Schaefer, D.J., Bourland, J.D., Nyenhuis, J.A., et al., Determination of gradient-induced, human peripheral nerve stimulation thresholds for trapezoidal pulse trains, *Proc. Int. Soc. Magn. Reson. Med.,* 2, 101, 1994.
19. Schaefer, D.J., Bourland, J.D., Nyenhuis, J.A., et al., Effects of simultaneous gradient combinations on human peripheral nerve stimulation thresholds, *Soc. Magn. Reson. Med. Proc. 11th Ann. Meet.,* 1220, 1995.
20. Ham, C.L.G., Engels, J.M.L., van de Weil, G.T., and Machielsen, A., Peripheral nerve stimulation during MRI: effects of high gradient amplitudes and switching rates, *J. Magn. Res. Imaging,* 7, 933, 1997.
21. Abart, J., Eberhardt, K., Fischer, H., et al., Peripheral nerve stimulation by time-varying magnetic fields, *J. Comput. Assist. Tomogr.,* 21, 532, 1997.
22. Ehrhardt, J.C., Lin, C.S., Magnotta, V.A., Fisher, D.J., and Yuh, W.T.C., Peripheral nerve stimulation in a whole-body echo-planar imaging system, *J. Magn. Reson. Imaging,* 7, 405, 1997.
23. Frese, G., Hebrank, F.X., Renz, W., and Storch, T., Physikalische Parameter bei der Anwendung der MRT, *Radiologe,* 38, 750, 1998.

24. Hebrank, F.X. and Gebhardt, M., SAFE-Model — a new model for predicting peripheral nerve stimulations in MRI, *Proc. Int. Soc. Magn. Reson. Med.,* 8, 2007, 2000.

25. Jagannathan, N. R., Magnetic resonance imaging: bioeffects and safety concerns, *Indian J. Biochem. & Biophysics*, 36, 341, 1999.

26. Schaefer, D.J., Bourland, J.D., and Nyenhuis, J.A., Review of patient safety in time-varying gradient fields, *J. Magn. Reson. Imaging,* 12, 20, 2000.

27. Lapicque, L., Definition experimental de l'excitation, *C. R. Acad. Sci.,* 67, 280, 1909.

28. Irnich, W. and Schmitt, F., Magnetostimulation in MRI, *Magn. Reson. Med.,* 33, 619, 1995.

29. Havel, W.J., Nyenhuis, J.A., Bourland, J.D., et al., Comparison of rectangular and damped sinusoidal dB/dt waveforms in magnetic stimulation, *IEEE Tran. Magn.,* 33, 4269, 1997.

30. den Boer, J.A., Bakker, R.M., Ham, C., and Smink, J., Generalization to complex stimulus shape of the nerve stimulation threshold based on existing knowledge of it relation to stimulus duration for rectangular stimuli, *Proc. Int. Soc. Magn. Reson. Med.,* 7, 108, 1999.

31. Nyenhuis, J.A., Bourland, J.D., and Schaefer, D.J., Analysis from a stimulation perspective of the field patterns of magnetic resonance imaging coils, *J. Appl. Phys.,* 81, 4313, 1997.

32. International Electrotechnology Commission, Particular requirements for the safety of magnetic resonance equipment for medical diagnosis, in Diagnostic Imaging Equipment, Publication IEC 60601-2-33, Medical Electrical Equipment, Part 2, International Electrotechnology Commission International Electrotechnical Commission (IEC), Geneva, Switzerland.

33. National Electrical Manufacturers Associations, Measurement Procedure for Time-Varying Gradient Fields (dB/dt) for Magnetic Resonance Imaging Systems, NEMA Standards Publication No. MS 7-1993, National Electrical Manufacturers Association, Washington, D.C., 1994.

34. United States Food and Drug Administration, Magnetic Resonance Diagnostic Devices Criteria for Significant Risk Investigations, at URL http://www.fda.gov/cdrh/ode/magdev.html, 1997.

35. Mueller, O.M., Roemer, P.B., Park, J.N., et al., A general purpose non-resonant gradient power system, *Soc. Magn. Reson. Med. Proc. 10th Ann. Meet.,* 130, 1991.

36. Larkin, W.D., Reilly, J.P., and Kittler, L.B., Individual differences in sensitivity to transient electrocutaneous stimulation, *IEEE Trans. Biomed. Eng.,* BME-33, 494, 1986.

37. Reilly, J.P., Peripheral nerve stimulation by induced electric current: exposure to time-varying magnetic fields, *Med. Biol. Eng. Comput.,* 27, 101, 1989.

38. Savoy, R.L., Ravicz, R.E., and Gollub, R., *The Psychophysical Laboratory in the Magnet: Stimulus Delivery, Response Recording, and Safety, Functional MRI,* C. Moonen and P. Bandettini, Eds., Springer-Verlag, New York, 1999.

39. Hedeen, R.A. and Edelstein, W.A., Characterization and prediction of gradient acoustic noise in MR imagers, *Magn. Res. Med.,* 37, 7, 1997.

40. Brummett, R.E., Talbott, J.M., and Charuhas, P., Potential hearing loss resulting from MR imaging, *Radiology,* 169, 539, 1988.

41. United States Occupational Safety and Health Administration Standard for Occupational Noise Exposure, at URL http://www.osha-slc.gov/OshStd_data/1910_0095.html.

3 Health Effects and Safety of Radiofrequency Power Deposition Associated with Magnetic Resonance Procedures

Daniel J. Schaefer

I. INTRODUCTION

Radiofrequency (RF) energy is defined as non-ionizing electromagnetic radiation in the frequency range of 0 to 3000 GHz, as distinguished from the very high photon energies and frequencies associated with ionizing electromagnetic radiation (e.g., gamma and X-rays). The RF spectrum includes radar, ultra high frequency (UHF) and very high frequency (VHF) television, AM and FM radio, and microwave communication frequencies. Resonant RF magnetic fields are used in magnetic resonance (MR) for imaging and spectroscopy procedures.[1]

This chapter will present and discuss various important aspects of RF power deposition associated with MR procedures with an emphasis on non-clinical physical factors, calculations, and measurements used to characterize this electromagnetic field.

II. RF MAGNETIC FIELDS AND MR PROCEDURES

During an MR procedure, the patient absorbs a portion of the transmitted RF energy, which may result in tissue heating.[2-16] Thus, whole-body and localized heating are the primary safety concerns associated with the absorption of RF energy. Notably, the elevation of core body temperatures to sufficiently high levels may be life-threatening.[2,17,18] With local transmit coils, the primary safety concern is to prevent burns by limiting localized heating.

The specific absorption ratio (SAR) is the RF power absorbed per unit mass of tissue and is the dosimetric means by which RF energy is characterized. SAR serves as a crude measure of heating potential. It is essential for patient safety to limit whole-body and localized temperatures to appropriate SAR levels.[2,18-22] Therefore, national and international safety standards[2,19-21] appropriately limit SAR for clinical MR procedures. Heating experienced by the patient during an MR procedure depends on the RF power deposited per unit mass (or SAR), ambient temperature, relative humidity, airflow rate, blood flow, and patient insulation.

Resonant frequency scales with static field strength and nuclei of interest. For protons, the resonant RF frequency is 42.57 MHz/T.[1] The tip angle is proportional to the area under the envelope of the RF waveform. Typically, the amplitude of the RF pulse (i.e., the tip angle) is adjusted to maximize the received signal. For a given waveform, RF energy is proportional to the square of the tip angle. Only the magnetic component of the RF field is useful in MR. Designs usually reduce electric field coupling to patients. Since power deposition is mostly through magnetic induction, the distribution of RF power deposition associated with the MR procedure tends to be mostly peripheral or on the surface of the subject's body.[9-11] Plane wave exposures (in non-MR applications) may lead to greater heating at depth.[18,24]

The average RF power (and SAR) is proportional to the number of images per unit time and peak RF power. Peak RF power depends on patient dimensions, RF waveform, tip angle, and whether the system's RF coil is operating in a linear or quadrature (i.e., has a circularly polarized magnetic field vector) mode during transmission of RF energy. It should be noted that quadrature excitation lowers RF peak power requirements and SAR by a factor of two and stirs any field inhomogeneities.[10] For a given field strength and RF waveform, SAR is independent of the type of nucleus.

III. MR SAFETY STANDARDS

The U.S. Food and Drug Administration (FDA) has published "Non-Significant Risk Criteria" for MR devices.[22] These criteria state that clinical MR examinations need an investigational device exemption (IDE) if the SAR exceeds the following levels:

1. 4 W/kg (averaged over the whole body over any 15-min period)
2. 3 W/kg (averaged over the head over any 10-min period)
3. 8 W/kg in any gram (head or torso, averaged over any 5-min period)
4. 12 W/kg in any gram (extremities, averaged over any 5-min period)

The International Electrotechnical Commission (IEC)[23] has also developed a widely used MR safety standard. The IEC MR safety standard is three tiered. The first tier is referred to as the NORMAL OPERATING MODE and is for routine scanning of patients. The second tier is designated as the FIRST LEVEL CONTROLLED OPERATING MODE. The MR system operator must take a deliberate action (usually using an ACCEPT button on the MR system console) to enter the FIRST CONTROLLED OPERATING MODE. This mode provides higher MR system performance, but requires the MR healthcare worker to closely monitor the patient during the MR procedure. Finally, the third tier is the SECOND CONTROLLED OPERATING MODE, which is used only for research purposes under limits controlled by an investigational review board (IRB).

When the environmental temperature is ≤24°C and the relative humidity is ≤60%, the current IEC MR safety standard for RF energy during an MR procedure permits (assuming SAR averaged over any 10-s period ≤ five times the average SAR limit) the following:

1. Whole-body SAR (averaged over any 15-min period)
   a. the NORMAL OPERATING MODE — SAR ≤ 1.5 W/kg
   b. the FIRST LEVEL CONTROLLED OPERATING MODE — SAR ≤ 4 W/kg
   c. the SECOND LEVEL CONTROLLED OPERATING MODE — SAR > 4 W/kg
2. Head SAR (averaged over any 10-min period)
   a. the NORMAL OPERATING MODE — SAR ≤ 3 W/kg
   b. the SECOND CONTROLLED OPERATING MODE — SAR > 3 W/kg
3. Local tissue SAR (averaged over any 5-min period)
   a. the NORMAL OPERATING MODE
      • SAR ≤ 8 W/kg in the head or torso
      • SAR ≤ 12 W/kg in the extremities
   b. the SECOND CONTROLLED OPERATING MODE — SAR > NORMAL MODE

Note that a new, second edition of the IEC MR safety standard with updated limits may be approved by the summer of 2001.

Another IEC safety standard[25] also establishes safety criteria for electrical safety and limits surface contact temperatures to 41°C. Note that during an MR procedure using a high SAR, the average skin temperature of a human subject approaches 37°C (a 4°C margin for temperature rise). During an MR procedure using a very low SAR, the average skin temperature is typically 33°C (an 8.0°C margin for temperature rise).

IV. MAGNETIC AND ELECTRIC FIELDS: SAR CALCULATIONS

The patient's RF power absorption during an MR procedure can be approximated from quasi-static analysis, assuming that the electric field coupling to the patient can be neglected[26,27] as well as the RF phase. In practice, quasi-static approximations for these calculations appear to be accurate for MR systems operating with static magnetic fields up to about 1.5 T. Calculation of actual SAR levels at very high static magnetic field strengths may require numerical techniques. Quasi-static methods will usually overestimate whole-body and local SARs when conductor dimensions approach a wavelength.

Assume a line segment of length dl carries current I and is located at vector r' from the origin, O (see Figure 3.1). The magnetic vector potential A at a point located at vector $r(x_2, y_2, z_2)$ from the origin may be expressed as[24,27,28]

$$\bar{A}(\bar{r}) = \frac{\mu I(\bar{r}') \cdot dl'}{4\pi|r - r'|} \tag{3.1}$$

The RF magnetic field, B_1, may then be found from the magnetic vector potential:

$$B_1 = \nabla \times \bar{A} \Rightarrow B_{1x} = \frac{\partial A_z}{\partial y} - \frac{\partial A_y}{\partial z}, B_{1y} = \frac{\partial A_x}{\partial z} - \frac{\partial A_z}{\partial x}, \text{ and } B_{1z} = \frac{\partial A_y}{\partial x} - \frac{\partial A_x}{\partial y} \tag{3.2}$$

Note that B_1 scales with current. Coil current is scaled until the desired B_1 is produced at the appropriate site. Usually, the 180-degree pulse centers on the site resulting in the greatest total return signal. The signal distribution, $S(x, y, z)$, might be approximated as

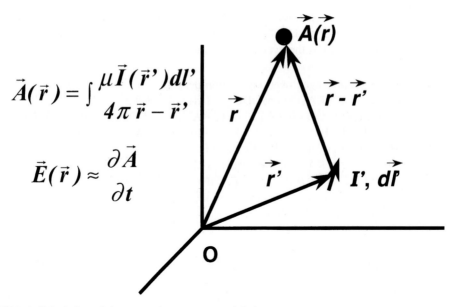

$$\vec{A}(\vec{r}) = \int \frac{\mu \vec{I}(\vec{r}')dl'}{4\pi \, \vec{r} - \vec{r}'}$$

$$\vec{E}(\vec{r}) \approx \frac{\partial \vec{A}}{\partial t}$$

FIGURE 3.1 Calculation of the magnetic vector potential, A.

$$S(x, y, z) = \sin\left(\frac{\pi B_1(x, y, z)}{2B_{1\,\mathrm{max}}}\right)^3. \qquad (3.3)$$

The total signal is the sum of the signal from all locations. Magnetic vector components are scaled by the coil current required to produce the 180° (or whatever is desired) tip angle.

Let ω be the radian frequency. Without significant capacitive coupling, the electric field, E, may be expressed as

$$E \approx \frac{\partial A}{\partial t} = -\omega A. \qquad (3.4)$$

V. THEORETICAL ESTIMATION OF WHOLE-BODY SAR

The SAR was defined above as the power absorbed per unit mass. Let DC be the ratio of average to peak power over the pulse repetition period; let σ be the electrical conductivity; and let ρ be the density of the surrounding tissue. SAR (at a point) may be expressed as

$$\mathrm{SAR} = \frac{\sigma DC|E|^2}{2\rho} = \frac{\sigma DC|\omega A|^2}{2\rho}. \qquad (3.5)$$

For RF coils that produce homogeneous B_1 fields, it is possible to investigate the whole-body average and peak SARs theoretically for certain object shapes. The patient's power absorption during an MR procedure can be approximated from quasi-static analysis, assuming that electric field coupling to patients can be neglected.[15,27] Consider a homogeneous tissue sphere of radius R. Assume that this sphere is placed in a uniform RF magnetic field of strength B_1. The total average RF power, P_{total}, deposited in the sphere may be expressed as

$$P_{\mathrm{total}} = \frac{\sigma DC\pi\omega^2 B_1^2 R^5}{15} \qquad (3.6)$$

The average SAR, SAR_{ave}, may be expressed as

$$SAR = \frac{P_{total}}{\rho\left(-\frac{4}{3}\pi R^3\right)} = \frac{\sigma DC \omega^2 B_1^2 R^2}{20\rho} \tag{3.7}$$

The highest spatial peak SAR, SAR_{peak}, for a homogeneous sphere may be found:

$$SAR_{peak} = \frac{\sigma DC \omega^2 B_1^2 R^2}{8\rho} = 2.5 SAR_{ave}. \tag{3.8}$$

RF energy-induced heating during the MR procedure is by magnetic induction. Power deposition in homogeneous spheres immersed in uniform RF magnetic fields increases with the fifth power of the radius R (see Equation 3.6). Because heating is largely peripheral and little deep body heating occurs in a human subject, the body may more easily dissipate the additional heat load. The RF power, P, deposited between a smaller radius, $r = \alpha * R$ (where $\alpha < 1$), and the outer radius, R, normalized to the total power deposited is n[9]:

$$n = \frac{P(R) - P(r)}{P(R)} = \frac{R^5 - r^5}{R^5} = 1 - \alpha^5. \tag{3.9}$$

Equation 3.8 shows that peak power deposition for homogeneous spheres is 2.5 times the average,[15] consistent with the peripheral nature of RF deposition during the MR procedure. From Equation 3.9, it is clear that, at least for homogeneous spheres, 87% of the total RF power deposition is in the outer third of the sphere.

RF pulses are used in MR examinations to flip the macroscopic magnetization vectors through desired angles. Recall that the nuclei precess about the static magnetic field vector in accordance to the right-hand rule. Linearly polarized waves may be treated as the superposition of left- and right-handed circularly polarized waves. Only that portion of the RF that is circularly polarized in the same sense as the nuclear precession influences the nuclei (see Figure 3.2). The other RF component contributes noise and increases RF power requirements. During the MR procedure, RF coils may be driven linearly (linearly polarized RF magnetic vector) or they may be driven in quadrature (circularly polarized RF magnetic vector). Quadrature RF transmit systems reduce patient heating during the MR procedure by a factor of two and spatially stir any RF "hot spots."[9]

Let γ be the magnetogyric ratio for a given type of nucleus. Note that the energy, W, deposited per pulse depends on the square of the RF tip angle, θ, the square of the static field strength, B_0, and inversely on RF pulse width, τ, and a waveform factor, η:

$$\theta = \int \omega dt = \eta \gamma B_{1p} \tau \Rightarrow SAR \propto W \propto \tau \omega^2 B_{1p}^2 = \frac{\gamma^2 B_0^2 \theta^2 \tau}{(\eta \gamma \tau)^2} = \frac{B_0^2 \theta^2}{\eta^2 \tau} \tag{3.10}$$

It is important to note that, for a given field strength and RF waveform, SAR is *independent* of nuclear species.

VI. RF ENERGY-INDUCED HOT SPOTS

Next, consider localized regions of RF power deposition or heating, commonly referred to as hot spots. Inhomogeneities in the electrical properties of tissue may result in high local SAR levels.

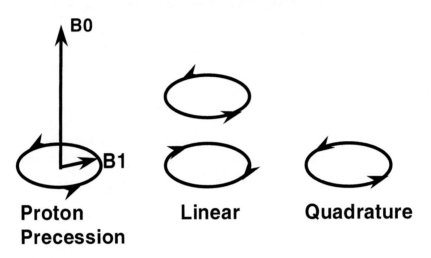

Linear: $\Big\{$ − 1/ 2 Power with Precession
− 1/ 2 power opposite precession

Quad: - power all in direction of precession
=> Power Requirements 1/2 of Linear

FIGURE 3.2 Comparison of quadrature and linear RF excitation of spins. Note that linear excitation wastes half the applied power.

Recall that RF-induced biological effects appear to depend upon temperature rather than on power deposition. A region of high local SAR may not be a region of high temperature due to blood flow or diffusion or other cooling mechanisms. The distinction between temperature hot spots and SAR hot-spots is often forgotten or misunderstood.

What effect do inhomogeneities have on the distribution of RF power deposition? Using spherical models, Schenck and Hussain[29] demonstrated that production of power deposition hot spots depends upon both the dielectric constants and the conductivities of the media. The model was later reformulated and used to investigate several problems involving worst-case conditions and magnitudes of local power deposition.[10] Assume that there is a small, homogeneous sphere (sphere 1) with permittivity ε_1 and conductivity σ_1 (Figure 3.3). Let sphere 2 be a much larger, homogeneous sphere of "standard tissue" representing the body. Sphere 2 has a permittivity ε_2 and conductivity σ_2. Sphere 1 may be placed outside sphere 2 at the pole (tangential electric field location) or at the equator (normal electric field location). In addition, sphere 1 may be placed inside sphere 2. When sphere 1 is placed near the pole of sphere 2, the local power deposition is amplified by a factor, A_p, which may be expressed as

$$A_p = \frac{9(\sigma_1^2 + \omega^2 \varepsilon_1^2)}{(\sigma_1 + 2\sigma_2)^2 + \omega^2(\varepsilon_1 + 2\varepsilon_2)^2}.$$ (3.11)

When sphere 1 is placed near the equator of sphere 2, the local power deposition amplification factor, A_e, may be expressed as

$$A_e = \frac{9(\sigma_2^2 + \omega^2 \varepsilon_2^2)}{(\sigma_1 + 2\sigma_2)^2 + \omega^2(\varepsilon_1 + 2\varepsilon_2)^2}.$$ (3.12)

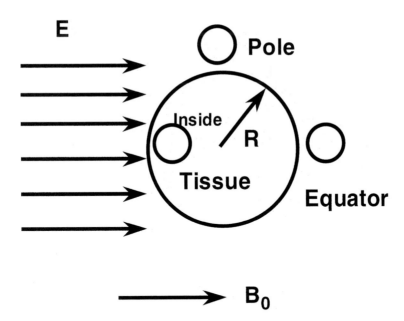

FIGURE 3.3 Effect of inhomogeneities on RF power deposition. To model the effect, a small, homogeneous sphere is placed either inside a larger tissue sphere or at the pole or equator of the larger tissue sphere (with respect to the RF electric field vector).

Finally, if sphere 1 is placed inside sphere 2, the local power deposition amplification factor, A_s, may be represented as

$$A_s = \frac{9\sigma_1(\sigma_2^2 + \omega^2\varepsilon_2^2)}{\sigma_2((\sigma_1 + 2\sigma_2)^2 + \omega^2(\varepsilon_1 + 2\varepsilon_2)^2)} = \left(\frac{\sigma_1}{\sigma_2}\right)A_e. \tag{3.13}$$

All the terms in Equations 13.11 to 13.13 are positive. The electrical properties of sphere 1 are treated as variables so that conditions for maximum amplification of local power deposition may be determined.

When sphere 1 is near the pole, amplification of local power deposition, A_p, is greatest when sphere 1 is a perfect conductor ($\sigma_1 \approx \infty$). A perfectly conducting small sphere at the pole will result in a local amplification factor of $A_p = 9$. Recall that the spatial peak SAR in a homogeneous sphere is already 2.5 times the average SAR for the sphere. Combining these results, the peak SAR at the pole is 22.5 times the SAR averaged over sphere 2. Conductive leads (e.g., monitoring equipment) placed in contact with the skin of patients may simulate this situation. Note that there is almost no amplification of local power deposition if sphere 1 is a radius or more from sphere 2. Spacing conductors well away from patients can dramatically reduce local heating potential.

Assume sphere 1 is placed near the equator of sphere 2. Then the greatest amplification of local power deposition takes place when sphere 1 electrical properties are minimal; i.e., $\sigma_1 = 0$ and $\varepsilon_1 = \varepsilon_0$ (free space value). So, for a void such as an air bubble, $A_e = 2.25$. Fat or bone at the equator produces slightly smaller amplifications.[40] When a low conductivity sphere is located near the outer edge of the equator of a larger (conductive) sphere, the local SAR is highest and is limited to 5.625 times the average SAR.

Finally, assume sphere 1 is placed inside the large sphere. This situation may simulate implanted prostheses. While local SAR is amplified the most when $\sigma_1 = 2\sigma_2$ and $\varepsilon_1 = 2\varepsilon_2$ (not a likely situation), the amplification factor is only $A_s = 1.125$. The highest local SAR works out to 2.8125 times the local average SAR.

The analyses above assume linearly polarized RF magnetic fields. Notably, if the RF coil produces quadrature excitation, then the amplification of local power deposition is reduced. The reduction in local power deposition results from rotating eddy current loops during quadrature excitation. Sphere 1 alternates between the equator and the pole of the larger sphere during quadrature excitation. So, worst-case quadrature local SAR amplification (assuming inhomogeneous biology) is 0.5 * (2.5 + 2.8125) = 2.66. For maximum SAR amplification at the equator, the electrical properties of sphere 1 approach those of a void.

Similarly, for an infinitely conducting sphere 1, during quadrature RF excitation, the worst-case local power deposition amplification would be 0.5 * (2.5 + 22.5) = 12.5. However, the presence of a conductor may complicate the production of a perfect quadrature RF field by setting up difficult boundary conditions.

RF body coils induce electric fields in patients during MR procedures. RF-induced electric fields are largest near RF coil conductors (Figure 3.4). RF coils may have high electric fields near capacitors on the coil as well. During high SAR MR examinations, placing patients well away from RF body coil conductors may reduce local power deposition and heating. The axis of birdcage RF coils is nearly a virtual ground. Conductors that must be introduced into the bore will minimally affect local SAR if they are placed along this virtual ground.

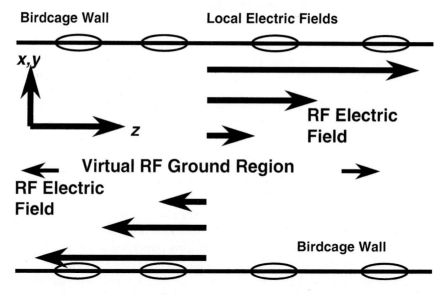

FIGURE 3.4 Electric fields inside a low pass, RF birdcage coil. Note that electric fields reach their maximum magnitude at the coil and fall to zero along the coil axis. Capacitors along the coil wall may also give rise to locally high electric fields. Any conductors should be routed along regions of low electric field or orthogonal to the electric field.

Receive-only RF coils, including most surface coils, typically use RF body coils to transmit RF excitation pulses. Receive-only coils are resonant during RF reception. However, if these RF coils were resonant during transmission of RF energy, then large currents may be produced in the receive coils. These large currents would, by Lenz's law, induce opposing RF magnetic fields. Flip angle profiles could be altered by the opposing RF magnetic fields, degrading image quality. The opposing RF magnetic fields may induce large electric fields in the body, leading to large local SAR levels. Boesigner[44] has shown conditions where the surface coil amplified normal body coil heating 47-fold. Manufacturers use high impedance blocking networks to detune surface coils and limit surface coil current during body coil excitation (Figure 3.5).

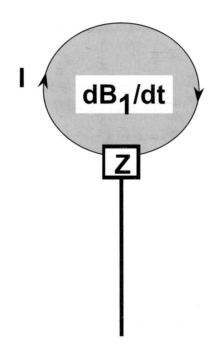

FIGURE 3.5 Receive-only surface coil with blocking network. During body coil transmit, the blocking network, Z, becomes a high impedance to prevent high induced currents from flowing on the coil. Such currents could lead to very high local SAR levels. During surface coil receive, the blocking network becomes a very low impedance to improve the image signal-to-noise ratio.

If conductive loops (e.g., associated with the use of monitoring equipment or even a coiled transmission line) are introduced into the MR system, high local SAR levels may result[30,31] (Figure 3.6). Even straight conductors may increase local SAR significantly[32-35] (Figure 3.7). Therefore, for patient safety, fiber optic devices should be used instead of conductors when possible.

Local temperature rise typically does not correlate well with local power deposition in a human subject. Thermal diffusion, blood flow, thermal radiation, sweating, and air flow may influence local temperature rise. Consider a region with a small mass, m, cooled by blood flowing from a cooler, more massive region. Under steady-state conditions, the SAR that is dumped to the more

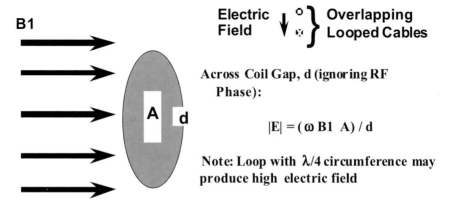

FIGURE 3.6 Any loop whose axis is parallel to the RF magnetic field may produce high currents and voltages by Faraday induction. Conductive loops should be avoided in the scanner.

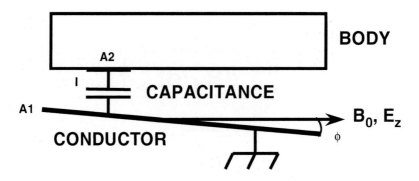

FIGURE 3.7 Even straight conductors may act as antennas and couple to the RF electric field (which is highest near the wall of the RF body coil). Loops may also short out a mode of quadrature coils, resulting in linear excitation.

massive region depends upon an energy constant, K, the specific heat, C, the temperature difference between the massive and small region, ΔT, and the mass rate of blood flow, dM/dt, and may be expressed as[11]

$$SAR = \frac{KC\Delta T}{m}\left(\frac{dM}{dt}\right). \tag{3.14}$$

The SAR required for a 1°C temperature rise in various organs may be estimated using Equation 3.14. Blood flow rates per unit mass vary from 128 ml/kg/min for normal skin to 4200 ml/kg/min for the kidneys. Table 3.1 lists local SAR levels required to produce a local temperature rise of 1°C for various organs.[23] Table 3.1 demonstrates the homogenizing property of blood flow to limit temperature hot-spots in the body. Resulting steady-state (maximum) temperature rises for each organ exposed locally to 4 W/kg are also presented in Table 3.1. Athey[36] has shown similar theoretical results demonstrating that significant thermal hot spots are not probable for typical head exposures.

TABLE 3.1
Maximum Local SAR Level for Local Temperature Rise of 1°Celsius for Various Perfused Organs[a]

Organ	Mass (kg)	Blood Flow (ml/kg/min)	Maximum SAR (W/kg)[b]	Maximum ΔT (°C)[c]
Brain	1.4	540	31	0.13
Heart (muscle)	0.3	840	48.3	0.08
Liver	2.6	577	33.4	0.12
Kidneys	0.3	4200	243.2	0.02
Skin (normal)	3.6	128	7.4	0.54
Skin (vasodilation)	3.6	1500	86.9	0.05

[a] Data calculated from Ganong.[51]
[b] Maximum local SAR level which would cause a local temperature rise of 1°C, ignoring vasodilatation and changes in cardiac output.
[c] Maximum local temperature rise for local SAR exposures of 4 W/Kg, assuming no vasodilatation and no change in cardiac output.

VII. SAR IN BIRDCAGE COILS AND CONDUCTORS NEAR PATIENTS

Ideally, birdcage coils would produce uniform B_1 fields. Perfectly uniform B_1 requires an infinitely long birdcage coil (or a spherical current density). Components of A (and thus E) must be parallel to the current density on the conductors that produced them. The B_1 field is related to magnetic vector potential:

$$\bar{B}_1 = \nabla \times \bar{A} = \hat{a}_x \left[\left(\frac{\partial A_x}{\partial y} \right) - \left(\frac{\partial A_y}{\partial x} \right) \right] + \hat{a}_y \left[\left(\frac{\partial A_x}{\partial z} \right) - \left(\frac{\partial A_z}{\partial x} \right) \right] + \hat{a}_z \left[\left(\frac{\partial A_y}{\partial x} \right) - \left(\frac{\partial A_x}{\partial y} \right) \right]. \quad (3.15)$$

Assume that (at the moment of time we look) $B_1 = B_{1x}$ ($B_{1y} = B_{1z} = 0$). Assume that RF coil conductors lie only along the z direction, then $A_y = A_x = 0$ (remember that B_1 is constant):

$$\bar{B}_1 = B_{1x} = \frac{\partial A_z}{\partial y}; \Rightarrow A_z = yB_1; \Rightarrow E_z = -\omega y B_1. \quad (3.16)$$

Let "a" be the radius of the birdcage coil. Without significant coupling, Equation 3.16 becomes

$$E_{max} = -\omega B_1 a \qquad (at(0, a, 0)). \quad (3.17)$$

Note that the z-component of the RF electric field inside an ideal birdcage coil depends linearly on the radial position. Suppose, for example, that at $\omega = 2\pi$ (63.86 MHz), $a = 0.3$ m, and $B_1 = 14.7$ µT, then $E_z = (-5898 \text{ v/m}^2)$ y and $E_{max} = 1769$ v/m.

Equation 3.16 predicts that the electric fields (and currents) in a birdcage coil of radius a need to be sinusoidal to produce a uniform magnetic field:

$$E_z(\theta) = -\omega a B_1 \sin(\theta). \quad (3.18)$$

Assume that the "duty cycle" (ratio of average to peak radio frequency power), DC, is 5%. Assume the RF coil length, h, is 0.6 m. Then a conductor of length, L (where $L \leq h$), making an angle ϕ with the z-axis, will (ignoring RF electrical length and matching issues) see a voltage, V, induced on it in the birdcage coil:

$$V = -\omega B_1 y L \cos(\phi). \quad (3.19)$$

If the conductor, whose impedance is Z, contacts a patient through a cross section of area α, the current density, J, may be expressed as

$$J = \frac{V}{\alpha Z} = \frac{-\omega B_1 L \cos(\phi)}{\alpha Z}. \quad (3.20)$$

If the patient conductivity is σ, then the local electric field, E', in the patient (at the point of conductor contact) is $E' = J/\sigma$. If the patient density is ρ, the local SAR at the point of contact may be written as

$$SAR = \frac{\sigma DC |E'|^2}{2\rho} = \frac{DC |\omega B_1 L \cos(\phi)|}{2\sigma \rho \alpha^2 Z^2}. \quad (3.21)$$

So, the SAR from conductors in the bore may be limited by making the impedance to the body large ($Z = \infty$). SAR from conductors may also be limited by keeping conductors very short ($L = 0$). Additionally, the SAR from conductors may be minimized by routing the conductors down the center of the bore ($y = 0$) or by routing them along $\phi = \pi/2$. Note that the analysis above was for a linear coil in the homogeneous region (away from coil conductors) for simplicity.

VIII. EXPERIMENTAL MEASUREMENTS OF WHOLE-BODY SAR

By measuring the RF peak forward, reflected, and (possibly) dummy load power levels required for 180° pulses (see Figure 3.8) with a known waveform, it is possible to measure the energy absorbed per pulse by the patient. Note that these measurements may be made while exposing human subjects to very low SAR levels. This information may be used to calculate whole-body SAR for any pulse with that patient in the same location. Details are in a National Electrical Manufacturers Association (NEMA) standard.[37]

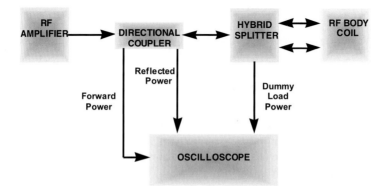

FIGURE 3.8 Experimental measurement of whole-body SAR.

IX. LOCAL SAR FROM TRANSMIT/RECEIVE RF SURFACE COILS

Planar, transmit surface RF coils are often used in MR spectroscopy studies. The primary safety concern with transmit/receive surface coils involves local SAR. While it is straightforward to calculate local RF power deposition in volume transmit coils, estimation of spatial peak SAR for planar transmit surface coils is complex. To prevent excessive local RF power deposition, it is imperative to at least estimate an upper bound for the local SAR. The local SAR is highest near the coil conductors. For such cases, simplifying assumptions may be made to calculate appropriate design limits.[38] Assume there is an anti-parallel pair of infinitely long conductors of width d, with a return distance $2 * a_1$ apart. Schenck et al.[39] showed that the inplane magnetic vector potential at a distance r from one conductor for the case where $d \ll a_1$ (and where quasi-static conditions apply) may be expressed as

$$A_z = \frac{\mu_0 I}{4\pi d} \tag{3.22}$$

$$\left[4\pi(a_1 - r) + 4r\tan^{-1}\left(\frac{2r}{d}\right) - 4(2a_1 - r)\tan^{-1}\left(\frac{2(2a_1 - r)}{d}\right) + d\ln\left(\frac{4(2a_1 - r)^2 + d^2}{4r^2 + d^2}\right) \right]$$

The local SAR may be calculated by inserting A_z from Equation 3.22 into Equation 3.5. It is necessary to scale current to levels that produce the desired B_1 at the desired location. Equations 3.2 and 3.22 may be used to find B_1:

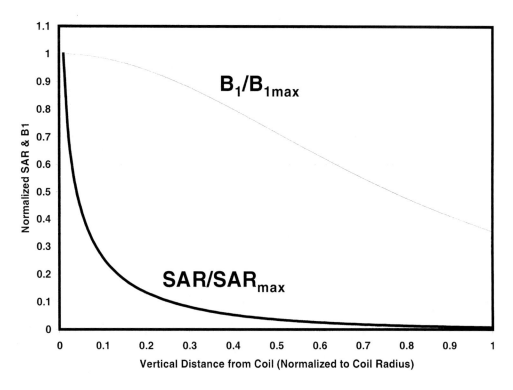

FIGURE 3.9 Normalized local SAR and B_1 vs. distance for a circular RF coil. B_1 is calculated along the coil axis. Local SAR is calculated from under the coil conductor.

$$B_1 = \frac{-\mu I}{\pi d}\left[\tan^{-1}\frac{-2(dr + 2a_1 - r)}{r^2 + d^2 - 2a_1 r} - \pi\right] \tag{3.23}$$

Note that the local SAR falls off much faster than B_1 (or signal) with distance to the patient. In Figure 3.9, normalized B_1 and normalized local SAR are plotted against the normalized distance from a planar, circular coil. A sevenfold reduction in local SAR may be achieved at the expense of a 5% reduction in B_1. Equations 3.5, 3.22, and 3.23 should permit coil designers to theoretically estimate the local SAR. Quasi-static calculations could also be done using Equations 3.1 through 3.5.

X. EXPERIMENTAL DETERMINATION OF LOCAL SAR

It is possible to experimentally measure local SAR in phantoms using materials with electrical properties and density similar to muscle.[24,40–42] To accomplish this, the temperature probe from the Luxtron Fluoroptic Thermometry System (Luxtron, Santa Clara, CA) or another nonconductive temperature probe is placed under the transmit coil conductors in contact with the tissue/phantom and thermally isolated from the coil. The local SAR may be calculated from the early (linear) portion of the heating curve:

$$SAR = 4186 C \frac{dT}{dt}. \tag{3.24}$$

In Equation 3.24, C is the specific heat of the tissue and T is the temperature. Equation 3.24 is expressed in MKS units. Other loss mechanisms (convection, radiation, and conduction) must be minimized during the experiment. Convection may be limited by using a gel phantom.[40] Conduction losses may be minimized by keeping materials insulated and by starting with the coil and the "tissue/phantom" at room temperature.

XI. SAFETY CONSIDERATIONS FOR RECEIVE-ONLY RF SURFACE COILS

Very large surface coil currents may flow[42,43] if receive-only surface coils are resonant, while RF excitation pulses are played out on the RF body coil. These currents may result in extremely high local SAR levels near the surface coil. In addition, the surface coil reaction currents would destroy B_1 homogeneity by generating opposing magnetic fields. To prevent such problems, a blocking network in the surface coil presents a high impedance to limit surface coil currents during RF excitation (see Figure 3.5). The blocking impedance required depends on coil area, magnet frequency, and how large an opposing field is to be allowed. Typical blocking impedances are a few hundred ohms. Note that in the case of phased-array receive coils, special care must be exercised to avoid the development of high local electric fields from differential voltages on adjacent conductors.

Unfortunately, surface coil blocking networks may become warm. IEC 60601-1[25] sets a surface temperature limit ($T_{limit} = 41°C$) for objects that may touch human subjects. Skin temperature under normal, non-MR, or low SAR conditions is approximately 33°C. However, during an MR procedure involving a high SAR, skin blood vessels dilate and skin temperature approaches the core temperature of approximately 37°C. In tests with phantoms initially at ambient temperature, a 4°C rise should be the limit for systems capable of high SAR. For low SAR systems, the surface coil temperature rise may be limited to 8°C above the ambient temperature.

XII. POSSIBLE MECHANISMS FOR RF BIOEFFECTS

Thermal effects arise from the temperature dependence of most biological functions. Chemical reaction rates approximately double with each 10°C rise in temperature.[45] Protein denaturation takes place at temperatures of about 45°C.[18] The fluidity of cell membranes is also affected by temperature. Thermal effects may be caused by whole-body heating of the organism or by localized heating of tissues. During an MR procedure, while only body parts in the RF transmit coil are exposed to RF magnetic fields, the entire body may be affected by thermal reactions.

The mechanisms behind non-thermal effects are not clear. The energy of a single photon at 85 MHz or 2.0 T is 5.304×10^{-26} J.[46] The energy of chemical bonds is much larger. In fact, even relatively weak hydrogen bonds between groups in protein structures have energies of 3.125×10^{-20} J.[45] Notably, thermal energy at body temperature is 4.28×10^{-21} J, five orders of magnitude greater than the energy of RF photons at 2.0 T (85 MHz).

XIII. THERMAL PHYSICS AND PHYSIOLOGY LITERATURE

RF fields are too high in frequency to stimulate excitable tissue electrically.[47] Thus, as previously mentioned, the only well-established mechanism for RF energy-related bioeffects is heating.[18] Proteins denature at roughly 45°C.[18] Guy et al.[48] showed that the SAR threshold for cataractogenesis is 100 W/kg. The highest safe core temperature for workers is considered to be 39.4°C.[24,49,50] The threshold core temperature for teratogenic effects in pregnant women is 38.9°C.[50] During a day, core temperature fluctuates 1°C.[17,51] Skin temperature fluctuates over a range of 15°C.[17] The skin pain threshold is 43°C.[52] Finally, the resting metabolic rate is 1.3 W/kg, while during vigorous exercise, in highly trained athletes, it may be as high as 18 W/kg.[24]

Consider an insulated tissue section. In 1 h, the insulated tissue will, when exposed to an SAR of 1.0 W/kg, rise approximately 1°C. Insulated tissue would rise to infinite temperature in infinite time at any finite SAR. In use, physiologic heat dissipation mechanisms of the human body limit temperature rise to a steady-state value. A body whose outer surface temperature, T_{sk}, is warmer than the ambient temperature, T_a, will radiate to the surroundings.[17] When exposed to RF power deposition, the body temperature will increase until steady-state conditions prevail. In a steady state, the body dissipates energy to the environment at the same rate that it gains energy from RF power deposition. Temperature increases initially and then asymptotically approaches the final steady-state value. The temperature time course may be expressed as

$$\Delta T = \Delta T_0\left(1 - \exp\left(\frac{-t}{\tau}\right)\right). \tag{3.25}$$

In Equation 3.25, τ is a constant, ΔT is the temperature rise at any time t, and ΔT_0 is the steady-state temperature rise. Note that an infinite duration RF exposure results in a finite, non-linear temperature rise. If σ_s is taken as the Stefan-Boltzmann constant and A is the surface area of the body, then the radiated power, P, may be expressed as

$$P = \sigma_s A(T_{sk}^4 - T_a^4) \approx 4\sigma_s A T_a^3 \Delta T. \tag{3.26}$$

Consider a hypothetical, uninsulated human subject (70 kg) who is constrained to lose energy to the environment only by radiation. Assume that the ambient temperature is 25°C and the thermal neutral (steady-state) temperature of the skin is 33°C. In a steady state, the hypothetical human would radiate about 1.4 W/kg, which is replaced by his own metabolic energy at the same rate. The result is no change in deep body or core temperature.

Next consider the same hypothetical human, but this time the skin temperature has risen to 38°C (vasodilatation of skin blood vessels may permit the skin to reach core temperature). Now the hypothetical human radiates energy at a rate of 2.4 W/kg, 1 W/kg above his metabolic rate. This hypothetical human might experience a 1°C rise in temperature in 1 h when exposed to 2 W/kg, demonstrating the importance of ambient temperature to the core temperature rise.

Adair and Berglund[53,54] utilized a mathematical thermal model of the body, based on the Gagge model,[55] to predict the effects of SAR, ambient temperature, impairment of blood flow, relative humidity, clothing, and scan time on core temperature rise. Their summarized results can be approximated with a simple program.[54] The Adair program was used to predict the effect of ambient temperature on core temperature rise[10] (Figure 3.10). For the plot, it was assumed that clothing = 0.2 clo, relative humidity was 50%, blood flow impairment was 40%, and the scan duration was 60 min. A 40% reduction in cardiac output is life-threatening.[56] From the plot, it is evident that an exposure to 4 W/kg for 1 h should result in only a 1°C core temperature rise when $T_a = 19°C$. However, if $T_a = 25°C$, then 3 W/kg is needed. A 1 h exposure to 1 W/kg even at $T_a = 27°C$ should result in no temperature rise. Ambient temperature plays an important role in core temperature rise.

XIV. SUMMARY AND CONCLUSIONS

A variety of physical factors affect the manner in which the RF fields used for MR procedures impact patients. Both whole-body and localized depositions of RF energy may result in tissue heating. In consideration of this primary safety concern of RF fields, regulatory agencies have provided guidelines based on whole-body-averaged and/or peak SARs to ensure the safe operation of MR systems. In this chapter, various techniques of calculating and estimating SARs associated with MR procedures have been described. Additionally, there has been a discussion of the possible mechanisms responsible for observed RF bioeffects and a review of the thermal physics and mathematical models used to predict human thermal responses to absorption of RF energy. This

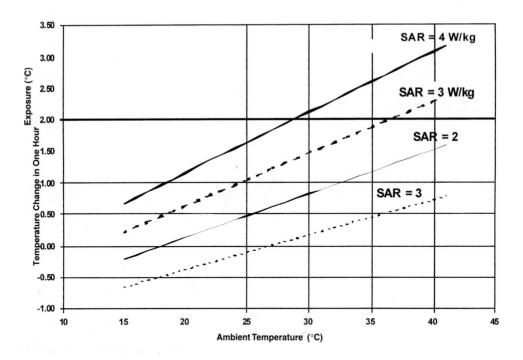

FIGURE 3.10 Effects of SAR (W/kg) and ambient temperature on human core temperature during 60-min MR scans. The polot is based on the Adair thermal model assuming a relative humidity of 50%, clothing = 0.2 clo, and a 40% impairment of blood flow at various SAR levels and ambient temperatures.

work has served as the basis for characterizing the RF fields used during MR procedures and has helped estimate the thermophysiologic alterations in patients. In this book, other chapters further explore these topics (see Chapter 4, Radiofrequency Energy-Induced Heating during Magnetic Resonance Procedures: Laboratory and Clinical Experiences; and Chapter 5, Specific Absorption Rates and Induced Current Density Distributions for Radiofrequency and Gradient Magnetic Fields Used for Magnetic Resonance Procedures).

REFERENCES

1. Mansfield, P. and P.G. Morris, NMR imaging in biomedicine, in *Advances in Magnetic Resonance*, Suppl. 2, J.S. Waugh, Ed., Academic Press, New York, 1982, pp. 310-314.
2. Athey, T.W., Current FDA guidance for MR patient exposure and considerations for the future, *Ann. N.Y. Acad. Sci.*, 649, 242-257, 1992.
3. Bernhardt, J.H., Non-ionizing radiation safety: radio-frequency radiation, electric and magnetic fields, *Phys. Med. Biol.*, 4, 807-844, 1992.
4. Budinger, T.F. and C. Cullander, Health effects of in-vivo nuclear magnetic resonance, in *Clinical Magnetic Resonance Imaging*, A.R. Margulis, C.B. Higgins, L. Kaufman, and L.E. Crooks, Eds., Radiology Research and Education Foundation, San Francisco, CA, 1984, chap. 27.
5. Budinger, T.F., Nuclear magnetic resonance technologies: health and safety, *Ann. N.Y. Acad. Sci.*, 649, 1-19, 1992.
6. Kanal, E., An overview of electromagnetic safety considerations associated with magnetic resonance imaging, *Ann. N.Y. Acad. Sci.*, 649, 204-224, 1992.
7. Persson, B.R.R. and F. Stahlberg, Potential health hazards and safety aspects of clinical NMR examinations, in *Seminars on Biomedical Applications of Nuclear Magnetic Resonance*, B.R.R. Bertil, Ed., Radiation Physics Department, Lasarettet, Lund, Sweden, 1984.

8. Saunders, R.D. and H. Smith, Safety aspects of NMR clinical imaging, *Br. Med. Bull.,* 40(2), 148-154, 1984.

9. Schaefer, D.J., Safety aspects of magnetic resonance imaging, in *Biomedical Magnetic Resonance Imaging: Principles, Methodology and Applications,* F. W. Wehrli, D. Shaw, and J. B. Kneeland, Eds., VCH Publishers, New York, 1988, chap. 13, pp. 553-578.

10. Schaefer, D.J., Dosimetry and effects of MR exposure to RF and switched magnetic fields, *Ann. N.Y. Acad. Sci.,* 649, 225-236, 1992.

11. Schaefer, D.J., Bioeffects of MRI and patient safety, in *The Physics of MRI,* Monograph No. 21, P. Sprawls and M. Bronskill, Eds., American Association of Physicists in Medicine (AAPM), American Institute of Physics, New York, 1993, pp. 607-647.

12. Shellock, F.G., Biological effects and safety aspects of magnetic resonance imaging, *Magn. Reson. Q.,* 5, 243-261, 1989.

13. Tenforde, T.S. and T.F. Budinger, Biological effects and physical safety aspects of NMR imaging and in-vivo spectroscopy, in *NMR in Medicine: Instrumentation and Clinical Applications,* Medical Monograph No. 14, S.R. Thomas and R.L. Dixon, Eds., American Association of Physicists in Medicine (AAPM), American Institute of Physics, New York, 1986, pp. 493-548.

14. Schaefer, D.J., Safety aspects of radio frequency power deposition in magnetic resonance, *MRI Clin. North Am.,* 6, 775-789, 1998.

15. Bottomley, P.A. and E.R. Andrew, RF magnetic field penetration, phase shift and power dissipation in biological tissue: implications for NMR imaging, *Phys. Med. Biol.,* 23, 630, 1978.

16. Shellock, F.G. and E. Kanal, *Bioeffects of Radiofrequency Electromagnetic Fields, Magnetic Resonance: Bioeffects, Safety, and Patient Management,* Lippincott/Raven Press, New York, 1996, pp. 25-49.

17. Carlson, L.D. and A.C.L. Hsieh, *Control of Energy Exchange,* Macmillan, London, 1982, p. 85.

18. Elder, J.E., Special senses, in *Biological Effects of Radio-Frequency Radiation,* J.E. Elder and D.F. Cahill, Eds., EPA-600/8-83-026F, U.S. Environmental Protectection Agency, Research Triangle Park, NC, Sec. 5, 1984, pp. 64-78.

19. U.S. Department of Health and Human Services, Food and Drug Administration, Magnetic resonance diagnostic device. Panel recommendation and report on petitions for MR reclassification, docket nos. 87P0214/CP through 87P-0214/CP0013, *Fed. Regist.,* 53, 7575-7579, 1988.

20. U.S. Department of Health and Human Services, Food and Drug Administration, Recommendation and report on petitions for magnetic resonance reclassification and codification of reclassification, final rule, 21 CFR part 892, *Fed. Regist.,* 54, 5077-5088, 1989.

21. U.S. Food and Drug Administration, Guidance for Content and Review of a Magnetic Resonance Diagnostic Device 510(k) Application: Safety Parameter Action Levels, Center for Devices and Radiological Health Report, Rockville, MD, 1988.

22. U.S. Food and Drug Administration, Magnetic Resonance Diagnostic Devices Criteria for Significant Risk Investigations at http://www.fda.gov/cdrh/ode/magdev.html, 1997.

23. International Electrotechnical Administration, Medical Electrical Equipment — Part 2: Particular Requirements for The Safety of Magnetic Resonance Equipment for Medical Diagnosis, IEC 60601-2-33 International Electrotechnical Commission (IEC), Geneva, Switzerland (in the U.S., copies of this standard can be obtained from the American National Standards Institute (ANSI), New York, 1995.

24. Durney, C.H., C.C. Johnson, P.W. Barber, et al., Radiofrequency Radiation Dosimetry Handbook, 2nd ed., Report SAM-TR- 78-22, USAF School of Aerospace Medicine, Brooks Air Force Base, TX, 1978, pp. 8-126.

25. International Electrotechnical Commission, Medical Electrical Equipment - Part 1: General Requirements for Safety; Safety Requirements for Medical Electrical Systems, 1992-06, Amendment 1, 1995-11 (General), IEC 60601-1-1, International Electrotechnical Commission (IEC), Geneva, Switzerland (in the U.S., copies of this standard can be obtained from the American National Standards Institute (ANSI), New York, 1995.

26. Bottomley, P.A. and E.R. Andrew, RF magnetic field penetration, phase shift and power dissipation in biological tissue: implications for NMR imaging, *Phys. Med. Biol.,* 2, 630, 1978.

27. Ramo, S., J.R. Whinnery, and T. Van Duzer, *Fields and Waves in Communication Electronics,* John Wiley & Sons, New York, 1965, pp. 108-111, 119-124.

28. Plonus, M.A., *Applied Electromagnetics,* McGraw-Hill, New York, 1978, pp. 208, 290–299, 453.

29. Schenck, J.F. and M.A. Hussain, Power Deposition During Magnetic Resonance: The Effects of Local Electrical Inhomogeneities and Field Exclusion, NMR Project Memo #84-199, General Electric Corporate Research and Development Labs, 1984.

30. Davis, P. L., L. Crooks, M. Arakawa, R. McRee, L. Kaufman, and A. R. Margulis, Potential hazards in NMR imaging: heating effects of changing magnetic fields and RF fields on small metallic implants, *Am. J. Roentgenol.,* 137, 857-860, 1981.

31. Chou, C. K., J. A. McDougall, and K. W. Chan, RF heating of implanted spinal fusion stimulator during magnetic resonance imaging, *IEEE Trans. Biomed. Eng.,* 44, 367-373, 1997.

32. Lemieux, L., P. J. Allen, F. Franconi, M. R. Symms, and D. R. Fish, Recording of EEG during fMRI experiments: patient safety, *Magn. Reson. Med.,* 38, 943-52, 1997.

33. Hofman, M.B., C. C. de Cock, J. C. van der Linden, A. C. van Rossum, F. C. Visser, M. Sprenger, and N. Westerhof, Transesophageal cardiac pacing during magnetic resonance imaging: feasibility and safety considerations, *Magn. Reson. Med.,* 35, 413-422, 1996.

34. Hess, T., B. Stepanow, and M. V. Knopp, Safety of intrauterine contraceptive devices during MR imaging, *Eur. Radiol.,* 6, 66-68, 1996.

35. Shellock, F.G., *Pocket Guide to MR Procedures and Metallic Objects: Update 2000,* Lippincott, Williams & Wilkins, New York, 2000, pp. 27-29.

36. Athey, T.W., A model of the temperature rise in the head due to magnetic resonance imaging procedures, *Magn. Reson. Med.,* 9, 177-184, 1989.

37. National Electrical Manufacturers Association, Characterization of the Specific Absorption Rate for Magnetic Resonance Imaging Systems (Radiology), NEMA MS 8-1993, National Electrical Manufacturers Association, Rosslyn, VA, 1993.

38. Schaefer, D.J., Estimation of Current Limits for RF Power Deposition from Planar, Transmit Surface Coils, Abstracts of the Society of Magnetic Resonance, Fourth Meeting, New York City, 1996, p. 1446.

39. Schenck, J. F., E. B. Boskamp, D. J. Schaefer, W. D. Barber, and R. H. Vander Heiden, Estimating Local SAR Produced by RF Transmitter Coils: Examples Using the Birdcage Coil, Abstracts of the International Society of Magnetic Resonance in Medicine, Sixth Meeting, Berkeley, CA, 1998, p. 649.

40. Chou, C. K., G. W. Chen, A. W. Guy, and K. H. Luk, Formulas for preparing phantom muscle tissue at various radiofrequencies, *Bioelectromagnetics,* 5, 435-441, 1984.

41. Gandhi, O. P. and J. Y. Chien, Absorption and distribution patterns of RF fields, *Ann. N.Y. Acad. Sci.,* 649, 132, 1992.

42. Grandolfo, M., A. Polichetti, P. Vecchia, and O. P. Gandhi, Spatial distribution of RF power in critical organs during magnetic resonance imaging, *Ann. N.Y. Acad. Sci.,* 649, 178, 1992.

43. Buchli, R., M. Saner, D. Meier, E. B. Boskamp, and P. Boesiger, Increased RF power absorption in MR imaging due to RF coupling between body coil and surface coil, *Magn. Reson. Med.,* 9, 105-112, 1989.

44. Boesinger, P., R. Buchli, M. Saner, and D. Meier, An overview of electromagnetic safety considerations associated with magnetic resonance imaging, *Ann. N.Y. Acad. Sci.,* 649, 160–165, 1992.

45. Lehninger, A.L., *Biochemistry,* Worth, New York, 1972, p. 153.

46. Halliday, D. and R. Resnick, *Physics,* John Wiley & Sons, New York, 1966, p. 873.

47. Kennelly, A. E. and E. F. W. Alexanderson, The physiological tolerance of alternating-current strengths up to frequencies of 100,000 cycles per second, *Electric. World,* 56, 154-156, 1910.

48. Guy, A.W., J.C. Lin, P.O. Kramer, and A.F. Emery, Effect of 2450 MHz radiation on the rabbit eye, *IEEE Trans. Microwave Theory Tech.,* MTT-23, 492-498, 1975.

49. Goldman, R.F., E.B. Green, and P.F. Iampietro, Tolerance of hot wet environments by resting men, *J. Appl. Physiol.,* 20, 271-277, 1965.

50. Smith, D.A., S.K. Clarren, and M.A.S. Harvey, Hyperthermia as a possible teratogenic agent, *Pediatrics,* 92, 878-883, 1978.

51. Ganong, W.F., *Review of Medical Physiology,* 6th Edition, Lange Medical Publ., Los Altos, CA, 1973, pp. 193-197, 474-476.

52. Benjamin, F.B., Pain reaction to locally applied heat, *J. Appl. Physiol.,* 52, 250-263, 1952.

53. Adair, E.R. and L.G. Berglund, On the thermoregulatory consequences of NMR imaging, *Magn. Reson. Imaging,* 4, 321-333, 1986.

54. Adair, E.R. and L.G. Berglund, Thermoregulatory consequences of cardiovascular impairment during NMR imaging in warm/humid environments, *Magn. Reson. Imaging,* 7, 25, 1989.

55. Gagge, A.P., The new effective temperature (ET) — an index of human adaptation to warm environments, in *Environmental Physiology: Aging, Heat, and Altitude*, S. Horvath and M. Yousef, Eds., Elsevier/North-Holland, Amsterdam, 1980, chap. 5, pp. 59-77.
56. Hurst, J. W., Ed., *The Heart*, McGraw-Hill, New York, 1978.

4 Radiofrequency Energy-Induced Heating during Magnetic Resonance Procedures: Laboratory and Clinical Experiences

Frank G. Shellock and Daniel J. Schaefer

I. INTRODUCTION

During a clinical magnetic resonance (MR) procedure, most of the transmitted radiofrequency (RF) power is transformed into heat within the patient's tissue as a result of resistive losses.[1] Not surprisingly, the primary health effects and safety concerns associated with the RF energy-induced heating are directly related to the thermogenic qualities of this electromagnetic field.[1-30]

Research studies conducted over the past 65 years have indicated that exposure to RF radiation may produce various physiologic effects, including those associated with alterations in visual, auditory, endocrine, neural, cardiovascular, immune, reproductive, and developmental functions.[1-30] In general, these biological changes are believed to occur due to RF energy-induced heating of tissues.

Exposure to RF energy may also cause athermal, field-specific changes in biological systems that are produced without an increase in temperature.[2,5,6,22] However, athermal effects associated with RF radiation are not well understood and have not been studied in association with the use of MR procedures. Those interested in thorough discussions of this topic are referred to the extensive reviews written by Adey[6] and Beers.[22]

Prior to 1985, there were no published reports pertaining to the effects of exposing human subjects to RF energy during MR procedures. In fact, there was a general lack of quantitative data on thermal and other physiological responses of human subjects exposed to RF radiation from any source.

The previous studies that were conducted on this topic typically examined responses to therapeutic applications of diathermy or thermal sensations related to exposure to RF radiation.[2-5,23,24] Unfortunately, these localized or limited exposures to RF energy do not relate to the exposure conditions that occur during MR procedures.

Therefore, in order to characterize the thermophysiological aspects of RF energy, several investigations have been conducted using laboratory animals, volunteer subjects, and patients. This research has yielded extremely useful and important data with regard to thermoregulatory responses to RF radiation-induced heating during MR procedures.

This chapter will the review and discuss the various aspects of RF energy-induced heating associated with MR procedures, with emphasis on the studies performed to assess thermal and other physiologic responses observed in human subjects.

II. MR PROCEDURES AND SPECIFIC ABSORPTION RATE

The thermoregulatory and other physiologic changes that a laboratory animal or human subject displays in response to exposure to RF radiation are dependent on the amount of energy that is absorbed.[3] The dosimetric term used to describe the absorption of RF radiation is the specific absorption rate (SAR).[2,3,5,19,20] The SAR is the mass normalized rate at which RF power is coupled to biologic tissue and is typically indicated in units of watts per kilogram (W/kg).

The relative amount of RF radiation that an organism encounters during an MR procedure is usually characterized with respect to the whole-body averaged and peak SAR levels (i.e., the SAR averaged in 1 g of tissue). As previously described in Chapter 3, SAR information is used by regulatory agencies with regard to safety guidelines for exposure to RF energy during MR procedures.

It should be noted that measurements or estimates of SAR are not trivial, particularly in human subjects. There are several methods of determining this parameter for the purpose of RF energy dosimetry in association with MR procedures. The SAR that is produced during an MR procedure is a complex function of numerous variables including the frequency (i.e., determined by the strength of the static magnetic field of the MR system, with resonant frequencies producing the greatest effects), the type of RF pulse used (e.g., 90° vs. 180° pulse), the repetition time, the type of RF coil used (e.g., linear vs. quadrature transmission, whole-body vs. local RF coil, receive only vs. send/receive), the volume of tissue contained within the coil, the configuration of the anatomical region exposed, the orientation of the body to the field vectors, as well as other factors.[1,19,20] Therefore, SAR, being an important parameter used to help ensure safety aspects of exposure to RF energy, may be difficult to calculate or estimate precisely for MR procedures.

III. RF ENERGY-INDUCED HEATING AND MR PROCEDURES: EVALUATION OF LABORATORY ANIMALS

Although there have been several studies performed using laboratory animals to assess thermoregulatory reactions to tissue heating associated with exposure to RF radiation, these experiments do not directly apply to the specific conditions that occur with MR procedures. Furthermore, the results of these investigations cannot be easily extrapolated to provide useful information for human subjects.[2-5,7,8,25] For example, the pattern of RF coupling and resulting absorption of RF energy to biological tissues is primarily dependent on the organism's size, anatomical features, the duration of exposure, the sensitivity of the involved tissues, and a myriad of other variables.[2-5,7,8,25] Importantly, there is no laboratory animal that sufficiently mimics or simulates the thermoregulatory responses of an organism with the dimensions and specific responses to that of a human subject. Therefore, experimental results obtained in laboratory animals cannot be simply "scaled" or extrapolated to predict thermoregulatory or other physiologic changes in human subjects exposed to RF radiation-induced heating during MR procedures. Nevertheless, experiments have been conducted in the MR environment using laboratory animals as an initial step to determine the effects of RF energy-induced heating associated with exposure to high SAR levels.

Shuman et al.[29] studied laboratory dogs undergoing MR procedures using relatively high levels of RF energy. Superficial- and deep-tissue temperatures were measured in five laboratory dogs before, during, and after exposure to RF energy to determine whether significant temperature changes could be produced in association with operation of a 1.5-T MR system.[29] The RF power output employed was 6.3 times that required for routine MR procedures, with calculated SARs that averaged 7.9 W/kg for the five dogs.

Shuman et al.[29] reported that there was a linear temperature increase of several degrees during RF exposure, with a maximal average change of 4.6°C that occurred in the urinary bladder. Overall, the temperature elevations were slightly greater in deep tissues than in superficial tissues. Shuman et al.[29] stated that these findings argue for continued caution in the design and operation of MR systems that are capable of high SARs, particularly when they are used for imaging infants or patients with altered thermoregulatory capabilities.

While the results of Shuman et al.[29] are intriguing, it should be noted that this study was conducted using anesthetized laboratory animals. As such, the findings are unlikely to pertain to conscious, adult human subjects because of the previously discussed factors related to the physical dimensions of the animals and the fact that an anesthetic agent was used that may substantially affect thermoregulation. Additionally, the thermoregulatory systems of these two species is quite dissimilar (e.g., the dogs pant to dissipate heat, while human subjects sweat).

Nevertheless, data obtained by Shuman et al.[29] may have important implications for the use of MR procedures in pediatric patients because this patient population is typically sedated or anesthetized for MR examinations and the physical dimensions of the laboratory dog are comparable to those of the pediatric population. Obviously, additional research is required to further examine this issue.

Barber et al.[30] also conducted a study to determine the effects of heating related to MR imaging. The objective of this investigation was to provide a worst-case estimate of thermal effects of MR imaging by subjecting anesthetized, unshorn sheep to RF power deposition at SARs well above approved standards for periods of time in excess of normal clinical imaging protocols.[30] The sheep underwent MR procedures using a 1.5-T, 64-MHz MR system. A control period with no RF power was followed by 20 to 105 min of RF power application. Afterward, there was a 20 min or longer recovery period with no RF power applied to the sheep. Eight sheep were given whole-body RF exposures at SARs that ranged from 1.5 to 4.0 W/kg while rectal and skin temperatures were monitored.

In addition, to determine the effects of RF energy-induced heating associated with MR imaging of the brain, Barber et al.[30] subjected four sheep to magnetic resonance imaging (MRI) procedures involving the head. The average scan time was 75 min and temperatures of the cornea, vitreous humor, head skin, jugular vein, and rectum were measured during this experiment.

In the whole-body exposure experiments, elevation of the rectal temperature was correlated with energy input. Deep-body temperature rises in excess of 2°C were attained for the whole-body averaged SAR level of 4.0 W/kg during exposure periods greater than 82 min.

In the head scanning experiments, skin and eye temperatures increased approximately 1.5°C. Additionally, the jugular vein temperature rose a maximum of 0.4°C after an average exposure time of 75 min. Animals exposed for 40 min to an SAR of 4.0 W/kg in either the body RF coil (three sheep) or the head RF coil (two sheep) were recovered and observed to be in good health for 10 weeks. Importantly, no cataracts were found in these sheep.[30]

Thus, using this animal model, Barber et al.[30] concluded that RF power deposition at SAR levels above typical clinical imaging protocols caused the body temperature to increase. Furthermore, for exposure periods in excess of standard clinical MR imaging protocols, the temperature increase was insufficient to cause adverse thermal effects.[30]

IV. CHARACTERISTICS OF RF ENERGY-INDUCED HEATING: IMPLICATIONS FOR HUMAN SUBJECTS

The physical dimensions and anatomic configurations of biologic tissues in relation to the incident wavelength are important factors that determine the relative amount and pattern of RF energy that is absorbed by the human body.[1-4] For example, if the size of the tissue is large in relation to the incident wavelength, RF energy is predominantly absorbed on the surface.[1-4] If it is small relative to the wavelength, there is little absorption of RF power, and the resulting effects of heating are minimized.[1-6,19,20]

Tissue heating that results from the RF energy used for an MR procedure is primarily caused by magnetic induction, with a negligible contribution from the electric fields.[1,19,20] This ohmic heating of tissue is greatest at the surface or periphery and minimal at the center of the body of human subjects (Figure 4.1). Predictive calculations and measurements obtained in phantoms, laboratory animals, and human subjects exposed to MRI using MR systems operating at 1.5 T or less support this pattern of temperature distribution.[1,19,20]

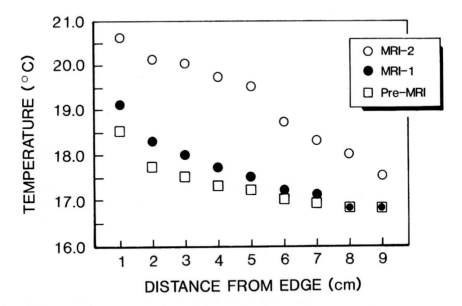

FIGURE 4.1 To study the depth of temperature changes related to RF energy-induced heating, MRI was performed on a spherical-shaped, seedless watermelon (diameter 24 cm). A specially designed thermistor needle was inserted into the watermelon immediately before (opened squares) and after MRI was performed for 30 min using a 1.5-T, 64-MHz MR system. A quadrature, transmit and receive body coil was used at whole-body averaged SARs of 1.0 W/kg (closed circles) and 2.5 W/kg (opened circles). The magnet bore temperature was 20.5°C, and the relative humidity was 45%. The findings of this experiment indicated that under these conditions there is predominantly surface or peripheral heating that occurs during RF energy-induced heating associated with MRI.

Notably, the actual increase in tissue temperature caused by exposure to RF energy is dependent on a variety of factors related to the thermoregulatory system of the individual and the surrounding environment.[1-4,7,8,10,11,14-20,21,25] Regarding the thermoregulatory system, the human body loses heat by means of convection, conduction, radiation, and evaporation when subjected to a thermal challenge. Each of these mechanisms is responsible to a varying degree for heat dissipation, as the body attempts to maintain thermal homeostasis. If these thermoregulatory effectors are not capable of totally dissipating the heat load, heat accumulates and is stored, resulting in elevation in local and/or overall tissue temperatures.

Additionally, there are various underlying health conditions that may affect an individual's ability to tolerate a thermal challenge. These conditions include cardiovascular disease, hypertension, diabetes, fever, old age, and obesity.[31-35] Various medications (diuretics, beta-blockers, calcium blockers, amphetamines, muscle relaxers, sedatives, etc.) can also greatly alter thermoregulatory responses to a heat load.[36,37] In fact, certain medications may have a synergistic effect with respect to tissue heating if the heating is specifically caused by exposure to RF radiation.[36]

The environmental conditions that exist in and around the MR system will also affect the tissue temperature changes associated with RF energy-induced heating. During the MR procedure, the amount of tissue heating that occurs is dependent upon environmental factors that include the ambient temperature, relative humidity, and air flow within the bore of the MR system.

With respect to the environmental conditions of the MR system, it has been proposed that in order to counterbalance excessive tissue heating that may occur during exposure to high levels of RF energy, patients should be "pre-cooled" before performance of MR procedures. However, the subjective perception to the environmental temperature depends on the gradient of temperature that is sensed by the peripheral thermoreceptors. Therefore, patients going from a cooler (i.e., the "pre-cooling" room) to a warmer environment (i.e., the MR system) would likely be more uncomfortable. Preliminary data obtained during recently performed experiments support this contention (unpublished observations, 1994).

V. IMPORTANT CONSIDERATIONS FOR EVALUATION OF PHYSIOLOGICAL CHANGES DURING RF ENERGY-INDUCED HEATING

Acquiring measurements of thermal and other physiologic parameters in human subjects within the harsh electromagnetic environment of the MR system is not a simple task. The static magnetic field of the MR system can easily create missiles out of conventional monitoring devices because they usually contain ferromagnetic components.[1,14,15,17,18,21] In addition, the static, gradient, and RF electromagnetic fields may adversely interfere with the proper operation of the monitoring equipment. In turn, the devices may produce subtle or substantial artifacts by generating RF noise that can distort the quality of the MR images. Therefore, temperature recording devices and physiologic monitors must be specially adapted or modified and then rigorously tested prior to use in the MR environment. Otherwise, the data pertaining to thermal and other physiologic responses may be erroneous.

Currently, there are a variety of MR compatible monitors, as well as other patient support devices, that are commercially available for use in the MR environment (see Chapter 11, Patient Monitoring in the Magnetic Resonance Environment). Every physiologic parameter that is typically recorded in the critical care area or operating room setting may be obtained during an MR procedure, including heart rate, oxygen saturation, end-tidal carbon dioxide, respiratory rate, blood pressure, cutaneous blood flow, and, most importantly, body and skin temperatures.[38-42]

For assessment of thermal responses during an MR procedure, volunteer subjects or patients have been semi-continuously or continuously monitored throughout the experimental procedures using several different types of devices.[43-54] For example, sublingual pocket or tympanic membrane temperatures have been obtained immediately before and after MR procedures using sensitive electronic thermometry or infrared devices. Notably, there is a good relationship between temperatures measured in the sublingual pocket or tympanic membrane and esophageal temperature, which is an indicator of "deep-body" or "core" temperature.

Skin temperatures have been measured immediately before and after MR procedures using highly sensitive and accurate infrared thermometry or thermographic equipment. Body and skin temperatures measured at multiple sites have been recorded before, during, and after MR procedures using a fluoroptic thermometry system that is unperturbed by electromagnetic radiation of all types, including static magnetic fields of up to 9.0 T.[42]

Heart rate, oxygen saturation, blood pressure, respiratory rate, and cutaneous blood flow, which are important physiologic variables that change in response to a thermal load, have been monitored before, during, and after MR procedures to assess the reaction of the thermoregulatory system of human subjects exposed to RF radiation-induced heating. All of these parameters may be obtained with devices that have been extensively tested and demonstrated to provide sensitive and accurate data in the MR environment.

VI. RF ENERGY-INDUCED HEATING AND MR PROCEDURES: ASSESSMENT OF VOLUNTEER SUBJECTS AND PATIENTS

As previously described, the increase in tissue temperature caused by exposure to RF energy during an MR procedure depends on multiple physiological, physical, and environmental factors. These include the rate at which RF energy is deposited, the status of the patient's thermoregulatory system, the presence of an underlying health condition or medications, and the ambient conditions within the MR system.

Although the primary cause of tissue heating during MR procedures is attributed solely to RF radiation, it should be noted that various reports have suggested that exposure to the powerful static magnetic fields used for MR procedures may also cause temperature changes.[55,56] The mechanism(s) responsible for such an effect remains unclear. Nevertheless, the results of these previously published studies warranted investigations in human subjects to determine the possible contribution of the static magnetic field to temperature changes that may be observed during an MR procedure.[57,58]

Studies were performed in human subjects exposed to a 1.5-T static magnetic field to evaluate if there was any thermal effect produced on body and/or skin temperatures.[57,58] The data revealed that there were no statistically significant alterations in any of the recorded tissue temperatures or other physiologic parameter.[57,58] Furthermore, Tenforde[59] examined this phenomenon in laboratory rodents exposed to static magnetic fields as high as 7.55 T and also reported no thermal effect. As far as the potential for production of heat by gradient magnetic fields is concerned, this is not believed to occur in association with conventional imaging parameters used for clinical MR procedures.[15,19,20,22]

With regard to the effects of RF energy-induced heating, the first study of human thermal responses associated with MR procedures was conducted by Schaefer et al.[60] Temperature changes and other physiologic parameters were assessed in volunteer subjects exposed to relatively high, whole-body averaged SARs (approximately 4.0 W/kg). The data indicated that there were no excessive temperature elevations or other deleterious physiologic consequences related to exposure to RF radiation.[60]

Several studies were subsequently conducted involving volunteer subjects and patients undergoing MR procedures with the intent of obtaining information that would be applicable to the patient population typically encountered in the MR setting.[43-50,52-54,61,62] The whole-body averaged SARs ranged from approximately 0.05 W/kg (i.e., for MR procedures involving MRI using a transmit/receive head coil) to 6.0 W/kg (i.e., for MR procedures involving the imaging of the spine or abdomen with a transmit/receive body coil).[43-54,61,62] These studies demonstrated that changes in body temperatures were relatively inconsequential (i.e., less than 0.6°C) (Figures 4.2 through 4.4). While there was a tendency for statistically significant increases in skin temperatures to occur, these were not physiologically deleterious. Furthermore, there were no substantial alterations in the hemodynamic parameters that were assessed during these investigations (i.e., heart rate, blood pressure, and cutaneous blood flow).

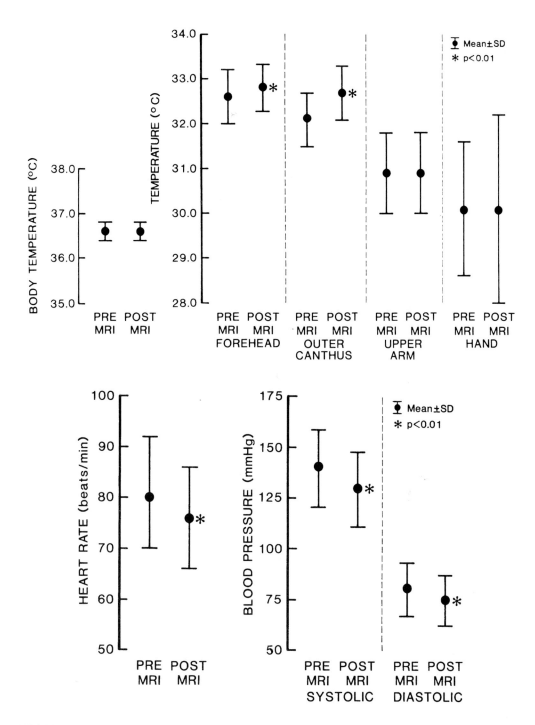

FIGURE 4.2 (Top) Average body (sublingual pocket) temperature, forehead skin temperature, outer canthus skin temperature, upper arm skin temperature, and hand skin temperature measured immediately before and after clinical MR imaging of the brain at 1.5 T/64 MHz using a head coil. There were statistically significant increases ($p < 0.01$) in body, forehead skin, and outer canthus skin temperatures (see Reference 47). (Bottom) Average heart rate and systolic and diastolic blood pressures obtained immediately before and after MRI of the brain at 1.5 T/64 MHz using a head coil. There were statistically significant decreases in each of these measured parameters associated with the MR procedure (see Reference 47).

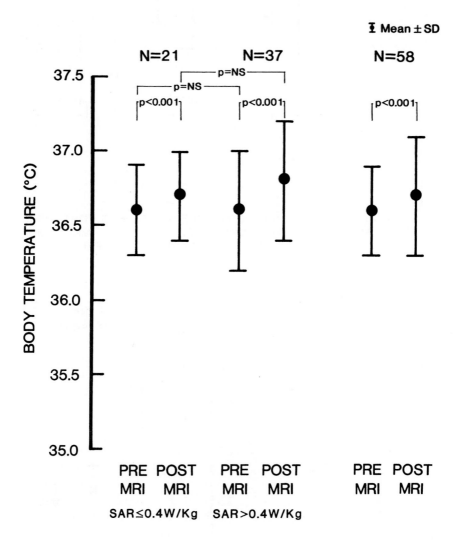

FIGURE 4.3A Average body (sublingual pocket) temperature measured immediately before and after clinical MRI performed using a 1.5-T/64-MHz MR system. Data are displayed showing the measured parameters during exposures to whole-body averaged SARs ≤0.4 and ≥0.4 W/kg, and all the data are combined (see Reference 43).

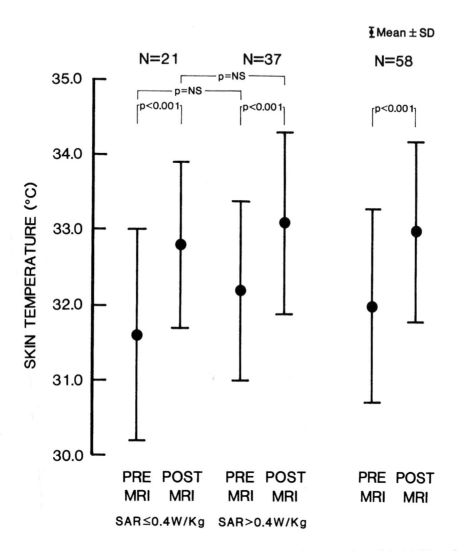

FIGURE 4.3B Average skin temperature measured immediately before and after clinical MRI performed using a 1.5-T/64-MHz MR system. Data are displayed showing the measured parameters during exposures to whole-body averaged SARs ≤0.4 and ≥0.4 W/kg, and all the data are combined (see Reference 43).

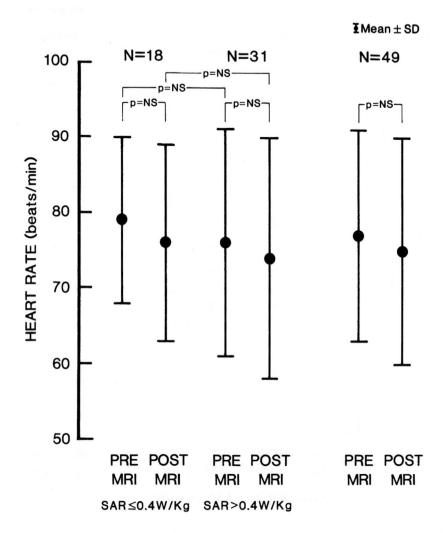

FIGURE 4.3C Average heart rate obtained immediately before and after clinical MR imaging performed using a 1.5-T, 64-MHz MR system. Data are displayed showing the measured parameters during exposures to whole-body averaged SARs ≤0.4 and ≥0.4 W/kg, and all the data are combined (see Reference 43).

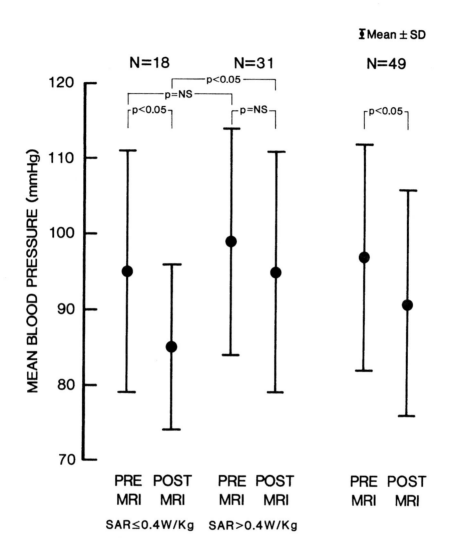

FIGURE 4.3D Average mean blood pressure obtained immediately before and after clinical MR imaging performed using a 1.5-T, 64-MHz MR system. Data are displayed showing the measured parameters during exposures to whole-body averaged SARs ≤0.4 and ≥0.4 W/kg, and all the data are combined (see Reference 43).

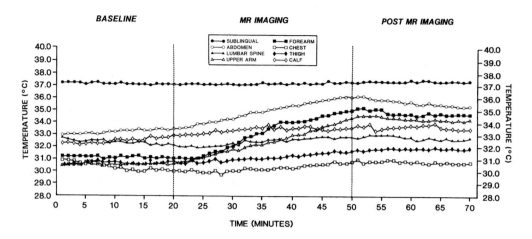

FIGURE 4.4 Body (sublingual pocket) and multiple skin temperatures measured at 1-min intervals using a fluoroptic thermometry system before (baseline), during (MRI), and after (post-MRI) MRI performed at a whole-body averaged SAR of 2.8 W/kg. Note that there was little or no change in body temperature, whereas there were slight to moderate changes in skin temperatures (depending on the site of measurement) during MRI. After MRI, some skin temperatures returned to the baseline level, whereas others remained elevated during the 20-min post-MRI evaluation period (see Reference 50).

Notably, research has indicated that there is a poor correlation between changes in body and skin temperatures vs. whole-body averaged SARs for clinical MR procedures (Figure 4.5). This finding is not surprising considering the previously mentioned myriad of variables that may alter thermal responses in a patient population. Therefore, the thermal reactions to a given SAR may be quite variable depending on the individual's thermoregulatory system and the presence of one or more underlying condition(s) that can alter or impair the ability to dissipate heat.

To date, exposure to a whole-body averaged SAR of 6.0 W/kg is the highest level of RF energy that has been reported for human subjects undergoing MR procedures.[53] In this study, Shellock et al.[53] evaluated volunteer subjects exposed to an MR procedure performed using a 1.5-T, 64-MHz MR system. Experiments were performed in cool and warm environments to characterize thermal and other physiologic responses to this high level of RF energy. The impetus for this study coincided with the advent of pulse sequences that had very high SARs associated with their use.[53]

The temperature of the tympanic membrane (i.e., an index of deep-body temperature) and seven different skin temperatures were monitored along with blood pressure, heart rate, oxygen saturation, and cutaneous blood flow.[53] Measurements were obtained immediately before, during, and after exposure to RF energy.

In the cool environment, there were statistically significant increases in tympanic membrane, abdomen, upper arm, hand, and thigh temperatures, as well as heart rate and skin blood flow (Figure 4.6). In the warm environment, there were statistically significant increases in tympanic membrane, hand, and chest temperatures, as well as systolic blood pressure and heart rate (Figure 4.6).

Importantly, the tissue temperature increases were within acceptable, safe levels. Of critical note is that these data indicated that an MR procedure performed at a whole-body averaged SAR of 6.0 W/kg can be physiologically tolerated by an individual with normal thermoregulatory function.[53]

While the data obtained to date are encouraging regarding the relative lack of substantial health effects from exposure to high SAR levels associated with MR procedures, it must be remembered that patients may have compromised thermoregulatory systems that could significantly alter their ability to handle a heat load. For example, patients with cardiovascular disease are known to poorly tolerate the effects of heating, which can lead to circulatory collapse.

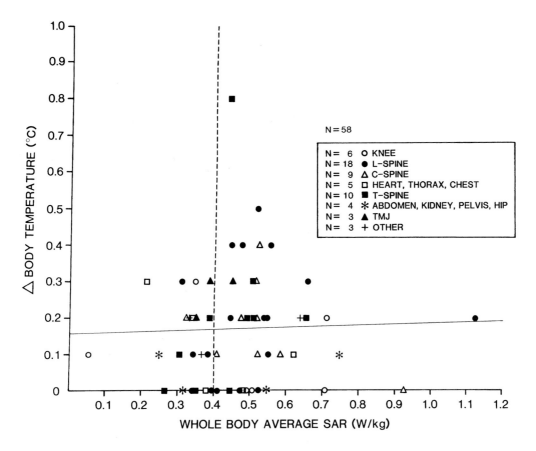

FIGURE 4.5A Changes in body temperature vs. whole-body averaged SARs during clinical MR imaging procedures. Note that there is a poor correlation between these two variables.

Can RF power deposition in a patient with cardiovascular disease place potentially unsafe stress on the cardiovascular system? For example, could an MR procedure cause an increase in skin blood flow that results in potentially excessive changes in the heart rate and/or blood pressure? At some SAR levels, this thermal stress is likely to be a problem. Therefore, studies are warranted to specifically address this potential safety issue.

VII. RF ENERGY-INDUCED HEATING AND THERMAL-SENSITIVE ORGANS

The testes and eyes of human subjects have reduced capabilities for heat dissipation and may be injured or damaged by elevated temperatures.[6,7] Therefore, the testes and eyes are primary sites of potentially harmful effects if exposure to RF radiation during an MR procedure is excessive.[6,7,11-15,17,18,46,48,49,63]

A. TESTES

Laboratory investigations have demonstrated that RF energy-induced heating may have detrimental effects on testicular function. If the exposure level to RF energy increases scrotal and/or testicular tissue temperatures between 38 to 42°C,[8] this heating may cause a reduction or cessation of spermatogenesis, impaired sperm motility, degeneration of seminiferous tubules, as well as other

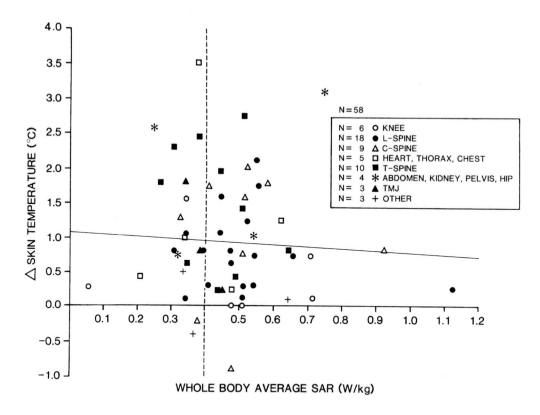

FIGURE 4.5B Changes in skin temperature vs. whole-body averaged SARs during clinical MR imaging procedures. Note that there is a poor correlation between these two variables.

abnormal conditions.[8,64] Notably, there is a direct relationship between temperature and sperm motility and viability.

The temperature of the testes correlates directly with the temperature of the scrotal skin.[64] The temperature exists because the scrotum has little or no subcutaneous fat or connective tissue, and, as such, there is no tissue mediated temperature gradient present.[64]

In 1990, Shellock et al.[48] conducted an investigation to examine the thermal effects of MR procedures performed on the scrotum to determine if excessive heating of this body part occurred. A non-contact infrared thermometer was used to measure scrotal skin temperatures (i.e., as a index to testicular temperatures) immediately before and after the MR procedures performed at relatively high SAR levels (mean, 0.72 W/kg).[48]

A statistically significant increase in scrotal skin temperature was associated with the MR procedures (pre-MRI, 30.8°C; post-MRI, 32.3°C). The highest scrotal skin temperature recorded was 34.2°C.[48] Notably, these temperature alterations were below the threshold known to alter or adversely affect the function of the testes.[8,48]

Excessive heating of the scrotum associated with an MR procedure could exacerbate a pre-existing disorder associated with increased testicular temperature (e.g., febrile illnesses, varicocele, etc.) in patients who are already oligospermic, leading to temporary or permanent sterility. Therefore, additional investigations designed to investigate these particular issues with regard to the testes are warranted, particularly if patients are subjected to MR procedures using RF energy levels (i.e., SARs) that are higher than those previously evaluated. This scenario is entirely possible considering the widespread clinical use of pulse sequences that use higher levels of RF energy (e.g., fast spin

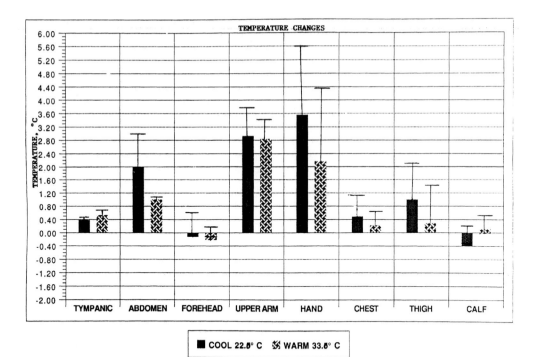

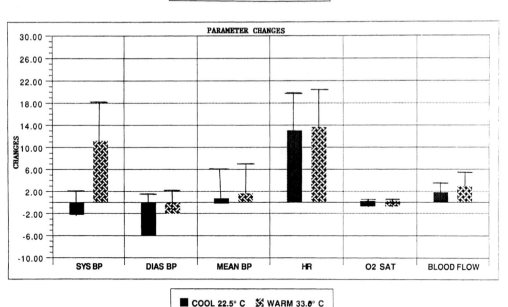

FIGURE 4.6 MR procedures performed in volunteer subjects exposed to a whole-body averaged SAR of 6.0 W/kg. The temperature of the tympanic membrane and seven different skin temperatures (abdomen, forehead, upper arm, hand, chest, thigh, and calf) were recorded (top) along with heart rate, blood pressure, oxygen saturation, and skin blood flow (bottom). Measurements were obtained with the subjects exposed to cool (22.5°C, solid bars) and warm (33°C, striped bars) MR environments. In the the cool environment, there were statistically significant increases in tympanic membrane, abdomen, upper arm, hand, and thigh temperatures, as well as heart rate and skin blood flow. In the warm environment, there were statistically significant increases in tympanic membrane, hand, and chest temperatures, as well as systolic blood pressure and heart rate (see Reference 53).

echo) and MR systems with higher static magnetic field strengths that inherently have associated higher SARs compared with conventional spin echo imaging techniques.

B. Eye

Dissipation of heat from the eye is a slow and inefficient process due to its relative lack of vascularization.[77] Acute, near-field exposures of RF radiation to the eyes or heads of laboratory animals have been shown to be cataractogenic as a result of the thermal disruption of ocular tissue.[7]

An investigation conducted by Sacks et al.[63] revealed that there were no discernible effects on the eyes of rats caused by MR procedures performed at RF energy levels that far exceeded typical levels used in the clinical setting. However, as previously indicated, it may not be acceptable to extrapolate data from laboratory animals to human subjects. For example, the coupling of RF radiation to the eye of a laboratory rat is obviously quite different compared to the situation for a human subject, especially in consideration of the size, shape, tissue volume, and relative position of the eyes on the rat compared to man.

Shellock et al.[46,49] performed two separate clinical studies to evaluate the thermal effects of RF energy-induced heating of the eye associated with MR procedures. In both of these investigations, corneal temperatures were measured using a non-contact infrared thermometer immediately before and after the MR procedures. Corneal temperature is a representative site of the average temperature of the human eye.[65]

In the first study, corneal temperatures were measured in patients undergoing MRI of the brain using a transmit/receive head coil at peak SARs ranging from 2.5 to 3.1 W/kg.[46] The greatest change in corneal temperature was 1.8°C, and the highest temperature measured was 34.4°C.

The second study examined corneal temperatures in patients with suspected ocular pathology who underwent MRI using the body coil to transmit RF energy and a special eye coil for RF reception.[49] Fast spin echo pulse sequences were used to examine the eye. The peak SARs for these sequences ranged from 3.3 to 8.4 W/kg. The greatest temperature change was 1.8°C, and the highest corneal temperature measured was 35.1°C.[49]

The findings from these two clinical investigations indicated that corneal temperatures did not exceed the upper limit of normal for the human cornea, which is 36°C.[65] Of further note is that the temperature threshold for RF radiation-induced cataractogenesis in animal models has been reported to be between 41° to 55°C for acute, near-field exposures.[6] Therefore, it does not appear that clinical MR procedures under the conditions studied by Shellock et al.[46,49] have the potential to cause thermal damage to ocular tissue. However, with higher levels of RF energy used for clinical MR procedures, the thermal effects on ocular tissue may require further assessment.

VIII. MR PROCEDURES AND "HOT SPOTS"

Theoretically, during exposure to RF energy, hot spots (i.e., excessive concentration of RF energy) may develop due to an uneven distribution of RF power in association with restrictive conductive patterns.[12,21,44,54] Obviously, an unwanted result of this would be if the RF energy-induced hot spots that occur during an MR procedure generate thermal hot spots.

Because RF radiation is mainly absorbed by peripheral tissues, surface thermography was used to study the heating pattern associated with MR procedures that were performed in volunteer subjects exposed to relatively high whole-body averaged SARs.[44,54] The findings of this research demonstrated that there was no evidence of surface thermal hot spots in the human subjects.[44,54] Apparently, the thermoregulatory system responds to any RF radiation-related hot spots by evenly distributing the thermal load utilizing the cutaneous circulation (Figure 4.7). Thus, thermal hot spots do not occur.[44,54]

There is the possibility, however, that thermal hot spots may develop internally during an MR procedure. As previously mentioned, Shuman et al.[29] reported that significant temperature

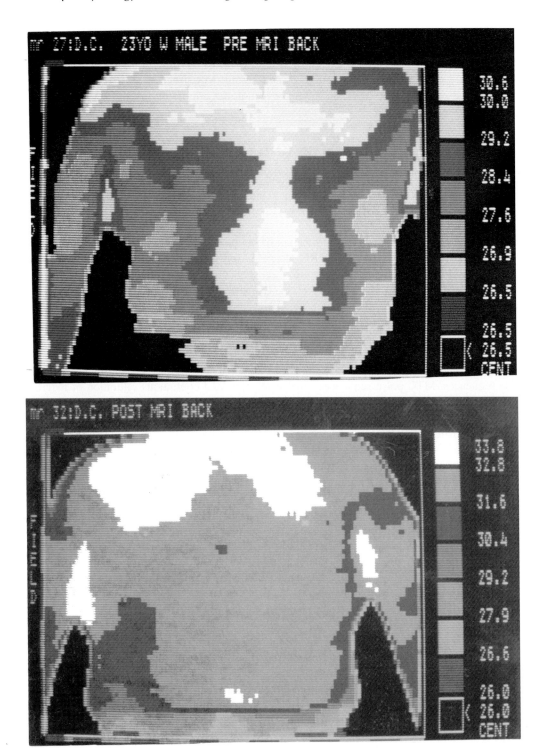

FIGURE 4.7 Surface thermography performed on the back of a volunteer immediately before (top) and after (bottom) MRI at a whole-body averaged SAR of 1.8 W/kg. Because RF radiation is mainly absorbed by peripheral tissues, surface thermography was used to study the heating pattern associated with the MR procedure. Note that after the MRI examination there was no evidence of thermal hot spots, suggesting that there is an even distribution of the thermal load by the cutaneous circulation.

increases occur in the internal organs of laboratory dogs as a result of MRI performed using relatively high SARs. These findings suggest that internal thermal hot spots may occur in association with MR procedures. Therefore, the presence of possible internal hot spots needs to be thoroughly examined in human subjects undergoing MR procedures. This could likely be accomplished by one of the MRI thermometry techniques commonly used to guide therapeutic tissue heating and cooling.[66,67]

IX. SUMMARY AND CONCLUSIONS

The characteristics of RF energy-induced heating associated with MR procedures have been presented, with an emphasis on research pertaining to human subjects. As new MR systems and clinical applications are developed, additional work is required to assess the effects of RF energy-induced heating to ensure patient safety.

Several of the pulse sequences and imaging techniques that have been developed over the last few years use relatively high levels of RF energy during their implementation.[68-70] For example, using fast spin echo (FSE) and magnetization transfer contrast (MTC) pulse sequences on high-field-strength MR systems may require levels of RF energy that easily exceed whole-body averaged SARs ranging between 5.0 and 8.0 W/kg (i.e., higher than the level currently recommended by the U.S. Food and Drug Administration).

In general, FSE pulse sequences are hybrids of rapid acquisition relaxation enhanced (RARE) pulse sequences and use higher amounts of RF energy compared to conventional spin echo sequences.[68,70] This is primarily due to the high density of 180° refocusing pulses used for these pulse sequences. MTC pulse sequences involve selective and continuous saturation of macromolecular protons by applying off-resonance RF pulses during the implementation of the technique.[69] Again, the RF power deposition is of considerable concern when MTC is performed using a high-field-strength MR system.[69] This is especially a problem during MRI of large body parts that require the transmission of RF energy using the body coil. Because both the FSE and MTC pulse sequences appear to offer important clinical advantages over conventional pulse sequences, studies are currently examining the human thermoregulatory responses to SARs that are higher than those that have been evaluated in recent years.

There are additional MR procedures that use potentially excessive levels of RF energy, including H-1 decoupling, Overhauser enhancement, and burst sequences used in MR spectroscopy.[16] Again, these techniques are particularly problematic for patients undergoing MR procedures using high-field-strength MR systems. Therefore, MR examinations that utilize these techniques will need to be carefully evaluated to determine the relative safety of performing these applications in patient populations.

Currently, there are many MR systems operating in the clinical setting with static magnetic field strengths of 3.0 and 4.0 T.[71,72] Notably, there is also an 8.0-T MR system in existence, which is the most powerful whole-body scanner in the world)[73-76] These ultra-high-field MR systems are used to perform imaging procedures, functional studies, and spectroscopy applications in human subjects.[71-76]

For a given application, the ultra-high-field MR systems are capable of generating RF power depositions that greatly exceed those associated with a 1.5-T MR system. Therefore, investigations are needed to evaluate thermal responses in human subjects to assess potential thermogenic hazards for these powerful MR devices.

Finally, additional studies are required to evaluate patients with conditions that impair heat dissipation. An ongoing effort is needed to characterize thermal and other physiologic responses for these various patient groups to ensure the safe use of MR procedures that require exposure to high levels of RF energy.

REFERENCES

1. Shellock, F.G. and Kanal, E., Bioeffects of radiofrequency electromagnetic fields, in *Magnetic Resonance: Bioeffects, Safety, and Patient Management*, 2nd edition, Lippincott-Raven Publishers, New York, 1996, chap. 3, pp. 25-48.
2. National Council on Radiation Protection and Measurements, Biological Effects and Exposure Criteria for Radiofrequency Electromagnetic Fields, Report No. 86, National Council on Radiation Protection and Measurements, Bethesda, MD, 1986.
3. Gordon, C.J., Thermal physiology, in *Biological Effects of Radiofrequency Radiation*, EPA-600/8-83-026A, U.S. EPA, Health Effects Research Laboratory, Research Triangle Park, NC, pp. 4-1 to 4-28, 1984.
4. Gordon, C.J., Effect of radiofrequency radiation exposure on thermoregulation, *ISI Atlas Sci. Plants Anim.*, 1:245-250, 1988.
5. Michaelson, S.M. and Lin, J.C., *Biological Effects and Health Implications of Radiofrequency Radiation*, Plenum Press, New York, 1987.
6. Adey, W.R., Tissue interactions with nonionizing electromagnetic fields, *Physiol. Rev.*, 61:435-514, 1981.
7. Elder, J.A., Special senses, in Biological Effects of Radiofrequency Radiation, EPA-600/8-83-026A, U.S. EPA, Health Effects Research Laboratory, Research Triangle Park, NC, pp. 5-64 to 5-78, 1984.
8. Berman, E., Reproductive effects, in Biological Effects of Radiofrequency Radiation, EPA-600/8-83-026A, U.S. EPA, Health Effects Research Laboratory, Research Triangle Park, NC, pp. 5-29 to 5-42, 1984.
9. U.S. Environmental Protection Agency, Evaluation of Potential Electromagnetic Carcinogenicity, EPA-600/6-90-005A, Office of Health and Environmental Assessment, U.S. Environmental Protection Agency, Research Triangle Park, NC, June 28, 1990.
10. O'Conner, M.E., Mammalian teratogenesis and radio-frequency fields, *Proc. IEEE*, 68:56-60, 1980.
11. Lary, J.M. and Conover, D.L., Teratogenic effects of radiofrequency radiation, *IEEE Eng. Med. Biol.*, 44:42-46, 1987.
12. Edelman, R.R., Shellock, F.G., and Ahladis, J., Practical MRI for the technologist and imaging specialist, in *Clinical Magnetic Resonance*, R.R. Edelman and J. Hesselink, Eds., W.B. Saunders, Philadelphia, 1990.
13. Persson, B.R.R. and Stahlberg, F., *Health and Safety of Clinical NMR Examinations*, CRC Press, Boca Raton, FL, 1989.
14. Shellock, F.G., Biological effects and safety aspects of magnetic resonance imaging, *Magn. Reson. Q.*, 5:243-261, 1989.
15. Kanal, E., Shellock, F.G., and Talagala, L., Safety considerations in MR imaging, *Radiology*, 176:593-606, 1990.
16. Morvan, D., Leroy-Willig, A., Jehenson, P., Cuenod, C.A., and Syrota, A., Temperature changes induced in human muscle by radiofrequency H-1 coupling:measurement with an MR imaging diffusion technique, *Radiology*, 185:871-874, 1992.
17. Shellock, F.G., MRI bioeffects and safety, in *Magnetic Resonance Imaging of the Brain and Spine*, S. Atlas, Ed., Raven Press, New York, 1990.
18. Shellock, F.G., Thermal responses in human subjects exposed to magnetic resonance imaging, *Ann. N.Y. Acad. Sci.*, 260-272, 1992.
19. Bottomley, P.A., Redington, R.W., Edelstein, W.A., et al., Estimating radiofrequency power deposition in body NMR imaging, *Magn. Reson. Med.*, 2:336-349, 1985.
20. Bottomley, P.A. and Edelstein, W.A., Power deposition in whole body NMR imaging, *Med. Phys.*, 8:510-512, 1981.
21. Shellock, F.G., Litwer, C., and Kanal, E., MRI bioeffects, safety, and patient management: a review, *Rev. Magn. Reson. Imaging*, 4:21-63, 1992.
22. Beers, J., Biological effects of weak electromagnetic fields from 0 Hz to 200 MHz: a survey of the literature with special emphasis on possible magnetic resonance effects, *Magn. Reson. Imaging*, 7:309-331, 1989.
23. Coulter, S. and Osbourne, S.L., Short wave diathermy in heating of human tissues, *Arch. Phys. Ther.*, 17:679-687, 1936.

24. Gersten, J.W., Wakim, K.G., Herrick, J.F., and Krusen, F.H., The effect of microwave diathermy on the peripheral circulation and on tissue temperature in man, *Arch. Phys. Med.*, 30:7-25, 1949.

25. Gordon, C.J., Normalizing the thermal effects of radiofrequency radiation: body mass versus total body surface area, *Bioelectromagnetics*, 8:111-118, 1987.

26. Athey, T.W., A model of the temperature rise in the head due to magnetic resonance imaging procedures, *Magn. Reson. Med.*, 9:177-184, 1989.

27. Adair, E.R. and Berglund, L.G., On the thermoregulatory consequences of NMR imaging, *Magn. Reson. Imaging*, 4:321-333, 1986.

28. Adair, E.R. and Berglund, L.G., Thermoregulatory consequences of cardiovascular impairment during NMR imaging in warm/humid environments, *Magn. Reson. Imaging*, 7:25-37, 1989.

29. Shuman, W.P., Haynor, D.R., Guy, A.W., Wesby, G.E., Schaefer, D.J., and Moss, A.A., Superficial and deep-tissue increases in anesthetized dogs during exposure to high specific absorption rates in a 1.5-T MR imager, *Radiology*, 167:551-554, 1988.

30. Barber, B.J., Schaefer, D.J., Gordon, C.J., Zawieja, D.C., and Hecker, J., Thermal effects of MR imaging: worst-case studies on sheep, *Am. J. Roentgenol.*, 155:1105-1110, 1990.

31. Drinkwater, B.L. and Horvath, S.M., Heat tolerance and aging, *Med. Sci. Sport Exercise*, 11:49-55, 1979.

32. Fennel, W.H. and Moore, R.E., Responses of aged men to passive heating, *Amer. J. Physiol.*, 67:118-119, 1969.

33. Kenny, W.L., Physiological correlates of heat intolerance, *Sports Med.*, 2:279-286, 1985.

34. Barany, F.R., Abnormal vascular reaction in diabetes mellitus, *Acta Med. Scand. Suppl.*, 304:556-624, 1955.

35. Buskirk, E.F., Lundergren, H., and Magnussen, L., Heat acclimation patterns in obese and lean individuals, *Ann. N.Y. Acad. Sci.*, 131:637-653, 1965.

36. Jauchem, J.R., Effects of drugs on thermal responses to microwaves, *Gen. Pharmacol.*, 16:307-310, 1985.

37. Shellock, F.G., Drury, J.K., Meerbaum, S., et al., Possible hypothalamic thermostat increase produced by a calcium blocker, *Clin. Res.*, 31:64A, 1983.

38. Shellock, F.G., Myers, S.M., and Kimble, K., Monitoring heart rate and oxygen saturation during MRI with a fiber-optic pulse oximeter, *Am. J. Roentgenol.*, 158:663-664, 1992.

39. Shellock, F.G., Monitoring during MRI: an evaluation of the effect of high-field MRI on various patient monitors, *Med. Electron.*, September: 93-97, 1986.

40. Holshouser, B., Hinshaw, D.B., and Shellock, F.G., Sedation, anesthesia, and physiologic monitoring during MRI, *J. Magn. Reson. Imaging*, 3:553-558, 1993.

41. Kanal, E. and Shellock, F.G., Patient monitoring during clinical MR imaging, *Radiology*, 85:623-629, 1992.

42. Wickersheim, K.A. and Sun, M.H., Fluoroptic thermometry, *Med. Electron.*, February: 84-91, 1987.

43. Shellock, F.G. and Crues, J.V., Temperature, heart rate, and blood pressure changes associated with clinical MR imaging at 1.5-T, *Radiology*, 163:259-262, 1987.

44. Shellock, F.G., Schaefer, D.J., Grundfest, W., et al., Thermal effects of high-field (1.5 Tesla) magnetic resonance imaging of the spine: clinical experience above a specific absorption rate of 0.4 W/kg, *Acta Radiol. Suppl.*, 369:514-516, 1986.

45. Shellock, F.G., Gordon, C.J., and Schaefer, D.J., Thermoregulatory response to clinical magnetic resonance imaging of the head at 1.5 Tesla: lack of evidence for direct effects on the hypothalamus, *Acta Radiol. Suppl.*, 369; 512-513, 1986.

46. Shellock, F.G. and Crues, J.V., Corneal temperature changes associated with high-field MR imaging using a head coil, *Radiology*, 167:809-811, 1988.

47. Shellock, F.G. and Crues, J.V., Temperature changes caused by clinical MR imaging of the brain at 1.5 Tesla using a head coil, *Am. J. Neuroradiol.*, 9:287-291, 1988.

48. Shellock, F.G., Rothman, B., and Sarti, D., Heating of the scrotum by high-field-strength MR imaging, *Am. J. Roentgenol.*, 154:1229-1232, 1990.

49. Shellock, F.G. and Schatz, C.J., Increases in corneal temperature caused by MR imaging of the eye with a dedicated local coil, *Radiology*, 185:697-699, 1992.

50. Shellock, F.G., Schaefer, D.J., and Crues, J.V., Alterations in body and skin temperatures caused by MR imaging: is the recommended exposure for radiofrequency radiation too conservative?, *Br. J. Radiol.*, 62:904-909, 1989.

51. Shellock, F.G., Rubin, S.A., and Everest, C.E., Surface temperature measurement by IR, *Med. Electron.*, 86:81-83, 1986.

52. Shellock, F.G., Schaefer, D.J., and Crues, J.V., Evaluation of skin blood flow, body and skin temperatures in man during MR imaging at high levels of RF energy, *Magn. Reson. Imaging*, 7(Suppl. 1):335, 1989.

53. Shellock, F.G., Schaefer, D.J., and Kanal, E., Physiologic responses to MR imaging performed at an SAR level of 6.0 W/kg, *Radiology*, 192:865-868, 1994.

54. Schaefer, D.J., Shellock, F.G., Crues, J.V., and Gordon, C.J., Infrared thermographic studies of human surface temperature in magnetic resonance imaging, in *Proceedings of the Bioelectromagnetics Society, Eighth Annual Meeting*, 1986, p. 68.

55. Sperber, D., Oldenbourg, R., and Dransfeld, K., Magnetic field induced temperature change in mice, *Naturwissenschaften*, 71:100-101, 1984.

56. Gremmel, H., Wendhausen, H., and Wunsch, F., Biologische Effeckte Statischer Magnetfelder bei NMR-Tomographic am Menschen, Wiss. Mitt. Univ. Kiel Radiol. Klinik., 1983.

57. Shellock, F.G., Schaefer, D.J., and Gordon, C.J., Effect of a 1.5 Tesla static magnetic field on body temperature of man, *Magn. Reson. Med.*, 3:644-647, 1986.

58. Shellock, F.G., Schaefer, D.J., and Crues, J.V., Effect of a 1.5 Tesla static magnetic field on body and skin temperatures of man, *Magn. Reson. Med.*, 10:371-375, 1989.

59. Tenforde, T.S., Thermoregulation in rodents exposed to high intensity stationary magnetic fields, *Bioelectromagnetics,* 7:341-346, 1986.

60. Schaefer, D.J., Barber, B.J., Gordon, C.J., et al., Thermal effects of magnetic resonance imaging, in *Book of Abstracts*, Vol. 2, Society for Magnetic Resonance in Medicine, Berkeley, CA, 1985, 925.

61. Vogl, T., Krimmel, K., Fuchs, A., et al., Influence of magnetic resonance imaging of human body core and intravascular temperature, *Med. Phys.*, 15:562-566, 1988.

62. Kido, D.K., Morris, T.W., Erickson, J.L., et al., Physiologic changes during high-field strength MR imaging, *Am. J. Neuroradiol.*, 8:263-266, 1987.

63. Sacks, E., Worgul, B.V., and Merriam, G.R., The effects of nuclear magnetic resonance imaging on ocular tissues, *Arch Ophthalmol.*, 104:890-893, 1986.

64. Kurz, K.R. and Goldstein, M., Scrotal temperature reflects intratesticular temperature and is lowered by shaving, *J. Urol.*, 135:290-292, 1986.

65. Mapstone, R., Measurement of corneal temperature, *Exp. Eye Res.*, 7:233-243, 1968.

66. Le Bihan, D., Delannoy, J., and Levin, R.L., Temperature mapping with MR imaging of molecular diffusion: application to hyperthermia, *Radiology*, 171:853-857, 1989.

67. Schwarzmaier, H.J. and Kahn, T., Magnetic resonance imaging of microwave induced tissue heating, *Magn. Reson. Med.*, 33:729-731, 1995.

68. Hennig, J., Nauerth, A., and Friedburg, H., RARE imaging: a fast imaging method for clinical MR, *Magn. Reson. Med.*, 3:823-833, 1986.

69. Balaban, R.S. and Ceckler, T.L., Magnetization transfer contrast in magnetic resonance imaging, *Magn. Reson. Q.*, 8:116-117, 1992.

70. Melki, P.S., Mulkern, R.V., Panych, L.P., and Jolesz, F.A., Comparing the FAISE method with conventional dual-echo sequences, *J. Magn. Reson. Imaging*, 1:319-326, 1991.

71. Schenck, J.F., Dumoulin, C.L., Redington, R.W., Kressel, H.Y., Elliott, R.T., and McDougall, I.L., Human exposure to 4.0-Tesla magnetic fields in a whole-body scanner, *Med. Phys.*, 19:1089-1098, 1992.

72. Ortendahl, D.A., Whole-body MR imaging and spectroscopy at 4 Tesla: where do we go from here?, *Radiology,* 169:864-865, 1988.

73. Abduljalil, A.M., Kangarlu, A., Zhang, X., Burgess, R.E., and Robitaille, P.M.L., Acquisition of human multislice MR image at 8.0 T, *J. Comput. Assist. Tomogr.*, 23:335-340, 1999.

74. Robitaille, P.M.L., Warner, R., Jagadeesh, J., Abduljalil, A.M., Kangarlu, A., Zhang, X., Burgess, R.E., Yu, Y., Yang, L., Zhu, H., Jiang, Z., Bailey, R.E., Chung, W., Somawiharja, Y., Feynan, P., and Rayner, D., Design and assembly of an 8 Tesla whole body MRI scanner, *J. Comput. Assist. Tomogr.*, 23:807-820, 1999.

75. Robitaille, P.M.L., On RF power and dielectric resonances in UHF MRI, *NMR Biomed.*, 12:318-319, 1999.

76. Kangarlu, A., Zhu, H., Burgess, R.E., Hamlin, R.L., and Robitaille, P.M.L., Cognitive, cardiac, and physiological safety studies in ultra high field magnetic resonance imaging, *Comput. Assist. Tomogr.*, 17, 1407-1416, 1999.

5 Specific Absorption Rates and Induced Current Density Distributions for Radiofrequency and Gradient Magnetic Fields Used for Magnetic Resonance Procedures

Om P. Gandhi

CONTENTS

I. INTRODUCTION

Magnetic resonance imaging (MRI) has proven to be an invaluable tool for medical diagnostic applications. As such, there is considerable interest in expanding its applications to study body functions *in vivo* by using more intense static magnetic fields (i.e., 4 to 10 T), larger and more rapidly switched magnetic field gradients (100 mT/m or more), and higher radiofrequencies (RF) up to 300 to 400 MHz. In order to optimize the design of new equipment, it is important to know the variation of internal time-varying magnetic fields because this can impact the quality of MR images. Also of interest from a patient safety consideration are the induced current densities and the rates of RF energy power deposition (specific absorption rates or SARs) in the various organs.

Currently, the worldwide safety standards for safe exposures to electromagnetic fields prescribe limits of induced current densities at low frequencies (i.e., on the order of kilohertz) associated with switched gradient magnetic fields and SARs for the RF magnetic fields (64 MHz and above).

Until recently, relatively simple homogeneous spherical, cylindrical, and disc models were used to obtain information for induced currents and SARs associated with MRI.[1-3] These models are inherently incapable of providing accurate information on the induced current densities and the SAR distributions that may occur for the critical regions of the human body.

In order to alleviate this obvious weakness of using simplistic models, the finite element method has recently been used to obtain SAR distributions in a 3256-element, anatomically based representation of the human head in the saddle-shaped head coil typically used for MRI procedures.[4] The biconjugate gradient (BCG) algorithm in combination with fast Fourier transform (FFT) previously used for the analysis of the absorption of electromagnetic power by the human body has also been used to calculate coupling to the MRI head coil for a model of the human body truncated at the neck.[5,6] However, as acknowledged by Jin et al.,[6] the high SAR in the region close to the neck may be due to the artificially truncated model used for these calculations.

Anatomy-based models have recently been developed that represent the model of the human body with voxel resolutions on the order of millimeters.[7] Also, a highly tested numerical electromagnetic method, called the finite-difference time-domain (FDTD) method,[8,9] has been modified[10] and used to calculate the SAR distributions due to RF magnetic fields of birdcage coils of dimensions typical of body and head coils used for MR systems operating at the RF of 64 MHz.[10] Since the FDTD method[8,9] is based on the complete set of Maxwell's equations, it is usable at any RF that is likely to be of interest.

This chapter describes the use of the FDTD method to obtain the SAR distributions not only at the presently used RF of 64 MHz, but also at the higher frequencies of 128 and 170 MHz that are used for investigational, very-high-field-strength MR systems. The SAR calculations are also extended for the newly proposed head coils operating at 300 to 400 MHz.[11,12] For calculations of currents induced due to switched gradient fields, the low-frequency, quasi-static impedance method, which has previously been used for a number of applications from power frequency magnetic field sources such as hair dryers and hair clippers to RF sources such as induction heaters etc., is described.[7,13–16]

II. THE FINITE-DIFFERENCE TIME-DOMAIN METHOD

The FDTD method has been described in several publications and a couple of recent textbooks.[8,9] This method has also been used successfully to obtain SARs for anatomically based models of the human body for whole-body or partial-body exposures to spatially uniform or nonuniform (far-field or near-field) electromagnetic fields from ELF to microwave frequencies.[7,13] In this method, the time-dependent Maxwell's curl equations

$$\nabla \times \mathbf{E} = -\mu \frac{\partial \mathbf{H}}{\partial t}, \qquad \nabla \times \mathbf{H} = \sigma \mathbf{E} + \varepsilon \frac{\partial \mathbf{E}}{\partial t} \tag{5.1}$$

are implemented for a lattice of subvolumes or "cells" that may be cubical or parallelepiped with different dimensions $\delta_x \delta_y \delta_z$ in x-, y-, or z-directions, respectively. The details of this method are given in several of the above-referenced publications and, therefore, will not be repeated here.

In the FDTD method, it is necessary to represent not only the scatterer/absorber, such as the human body or a part thereof, but also any near-field source(s), such as 16-rung shielded birdcage coils that are currently used in MR systems. The source–body interaction volume is subdivided into the Yee cells for which the volume-averaged electrical properties are prescribed for each of the cells of volume $\delta_x\delta_y\delta_z$. The interaction space consisting of several hundred thousand to several million cells is truncated by means of absorbing boundaries.

For the SAR calculations given in this chapter, retarded time boundary conditions have been used with the absorbing boundaries that were assumed separated by five to ten cells in each direction from the modeled volume.[17] Sixteen rungs of the birdcage coil were modeled by voxels representing the respective conductors for which the current sources were prescribed by means of magnetic fields H_x and H_y around the boundaries of the cell such that consistent with Ampere's law

$$I = \oint(\vec{H} \cdot d\vec{\ell}) \tag{5.2}$$

For the FDTD cells, this corresponds to

$$I = (H_x\delta_x + H_y\delta_y) = 2H_x\delta_x \text{ or } 2H_y\delta_x \tag{5.3}$$

since $\delta_x = \delta_y$. In order to obtain circularly polarized RF magnetic fields with the birdcage coils, progressive relative phase shifts of 22.5° are assumed between the adjacent rungs.[18] These relative phase shifts are also used in prescribing the H_x and H_y for the cells representing each of the rungs. Furthermore, it is asumed that the rungs are made of a highly conducting material such as copper, which is modeled with a conductivity $\sigma = 5.8 \times 10^7$ S/m for each of the voxels representing the rungs. Also, it is assumed for the calculations that the current passing through each of the rungs is constant and in phase from one end to the other, which is justified since the length of the rung is small compared to wavelength at the lower frequencies of 64, 128, and even 170 MHz.

For the higher frequency head coils at 300 to 400 MHz, a sinusoidally varying RF current distribution over the length of the rung is, however, taken as suggested in Vaughan et al.[11] and Zhang et al.[12] The initial fields, thus defined and assumed to be sinusoidally varying in time, are tracked in the time domain for all voxels of the interaction space. The problem is considered completed when a sinusoidal steady-state behavior for **E** and **H** is observed for the interaction space. This generally involves four to five RF cycles at the various frequencies of interest.

III. THE QUASI-STATIC IMPEDANCE METHOD

Because of the fairly low frequencies up to a few kilohertz involved in switched gradient fields, the widely used quasi-static impedance method may be used for calculations of induced current densities. For low-frequency dosimetry problems, the impedance method has been found to be highly efficient as a numerical procedure for calculations of internal current densities and induced electric fields for exposure to time-varying magnetic fields.[7,13–16] In this method, the biological body or the exposed part thereof is represented by a three-dimensional (3-D) network of impedances whose individual values are obtained from the complex conductivities $\sigma + j\omega\varepsilon$ for the various locations of the body. Since $\sigma \gg \omega\varepsilon$ for low frequencies of a few kilohertz characteristic of switched gradient fields, the network at these frequencies may be approximated by a 3-D grid of resistances whose values are given by

$$R_m^{i,j,k} = \frac{\delta_m}{\delta_n\delta_p\sigma_m^{i,j,k}} \tag{5.4}$$

where i, j, k indicate the cell indices; m is the direction which can be x, y, or z for which the resistance is calculated; $\sigma_m^{i,j,k}$ is the electrical conductivity for the cell i, j, k in the mth direction; and δ_n, δ_p are the widths of the cell in directions at right angles to the mth direction.

For exposure to time- and space-varying magnetic fields, voltages or electromotive forces (EMFs) are induced for the various loops of the 3-D resistance network whose values are given by the following expression:

$$V_m^{i,j,k} = -\frac{d}{dt}\int \mathbf{B}^{i,j,k} \cdot d\mathbf{S} = -\left(\frac{d}{dt}B_m^{i,j,k}\right)\delta_n\delta_p \qquad (5.5)$$

The initial value of the loop currents was set to zero, assuming that the external electric field was negligible.

In addition to the current densities, the x-, y-, and z-components of electric fields inside each cell can also be evaluated as

$$E_{x,y,z}^{i,j,k} = \frac{J_{x,y,z}^{i,j,k}}{\sigma^{i,j,k}} \qquad (5.6)$$

In the impedance method formulation, the conductivity for a given cell can be directionally dependent. This feature is important for calculations at ELF where highly anisotropic conductivities have been reported, particularly for the skeletal muscle.[19,20]

For the calculations reported in this chapter, the dielectric properties taken for the various RF are given in Table 5.1. Also given in the same table are the frequency-independent conductivities taken for the various tissues of the body that have been used for calculations of induced currents due to switched gradient magnetic fields. These properties have been compiled from a number of references.[19-24]

IV. MILLIMETER-RESOLUTION MODEL BASED ON MRI SCANS OF THE HUMAN BODY

A millimeter-resolution model of the human body has been developed from the MRI scans of a male volunteer of height 176.4 cm and weight 64 kg.[7] The MRI scans were taken with a resolution of 3.0 mm along the height of the body and 1.875 mm for the orthogonal axes in the cross-sectional planes. Even though the height of the volunteer was quite appropriate for an average adult male, the weight was somewhat lower than an average of 71 kg, which is generally assumed for an average male. This problem was ameliorated by assuming that the pixel dimensions for the cross sections are larger than 1.875 x 1.875 mm by the ratio of $(71/64)^{1/2} = 1.053$. By taking the larger pixel dimensions $1.053 \times 1.875 = 1.974$ mm for the cross-sectional axes, the volume of the model was increased by $(1.053)^2 = 1.109$ (i.e., by about 10.9%), which resulted in an increase of its weight to approximately 71 kg. The MRI section locations were converted into images involving 30 tissue types whose electrical properties may be prescribed at the exposure frequencies (Table 5.1).

Even for the highest frequency of 400 MHz used for the present calculations, it is not necessary to use the above-described $1.974 \times 1.974 \times 3.0$ mm resolution model. Therefore, voxels may be combined to obtain a somewhat coarser resolution model with a considerably reduced number of voxels for which the induced current and SAR calculations may be performed expeditiously.

For the calculations given in this chapter, $3 \times 3 \times 2$ voxels have been combined along x-, y-, and z-axes, respectively, to obtain a new model with somewhat larger size voxels, each of dimension $5.922 \times 5.922 \times 6.0$ mm. This new model with volume-averaged electrical properties at RF and directionally averaged conductivities at low frequencies was then used for all of the calculations given herein.

TABLE 5.1
Tissue Properties Assumed for the 5.922 × 5.922 × 6.0 mm Resolution, Anatomically Based Model[18-23]

Tissue	Mass Density 10³ kg/m³	Low Frequencies	64 MHz ε_r	64 MHz σ S/m	128 MHz ε_r	128 MHz σ S/m	170 MHz ε_r	170 MHz σ S/m	350 MHz ε_r	350 MHz σ S/m
Muscle	1.05	0.07 (horz.) 0.86 (vert.)	72.23	0.69	63.49	0.72	61.27	0.73	57.60	0.78
Fat	0.92	0.04	10.08	0.05	9.15	0.05	8.95	0.06	11.68	0.08
Bone	1.47	0.04	11.82	0.09	9.89	0.09	9.47	0.10	18.02	0.16
Cartilage	1.10	0.04	62.91	0.45	52.92	0.49	50.36	0.51	46.04	0.57
Skin	0.98	0.11	84.45	0.46	63.51	0.53	58.18	0.57	49.44	0.66
Nerve	1.04	0.12	55.06	0.31	44.06	0.35	41.11	0.37	36.06	0.43
Intestine	1.04	0.11	118.36	1.59	87.97	1.69	80.29	1.74	38.40	0.52
Spleen, pancreas	1.05	0.18	110.56	0.74	82.89	0.84	75.96	0.88	38.40	0.52
Heart	1.03	0.5	95.95	1.03	81.03	1.09	76.37	1.12	64.82	1.33
Blood	1.06	0.60	86.45	1.21	73.16	1.25	69.95	1.27	64.82	1.33
Partoid gland	1.05	0.11	82.63	0.40	63.03	0.46	58.25	0.49	50.68	0.57
Liver	1.03	0.13	80.56	0.45	64.25	0.51	59.83	0.54	38.40	0.52
Kidney	1.05	0.27	118.56	0.74	89.62	0.85	81.76	0.90	38.40	0.52
Lung	0.35	0.04	37.10	0.29	29.47	0.32	27.50	0.33	19.20	0.26
Bladder	1.03	0.20	24.59	0.29	21.86	0.30	21.13	0.30	38.40	0.52
CSF	1.01	1.66	97.31	2.07	84.04	2.14	79.13	2.17	71.71	2.24
Eye humor	1.01	1.66	69.13	1.50	69.06	1.51	69.05	1.51	69.01	1.52
Eye sclera	1.17	0.11	75.29	0.88	65.00	0.92	62.42	0.93	58.21	0.99
Eye lens	1.10	0.11	55.44	0.44	47.93	0.46	46.10	0.47	43.18	0.51
Stomach	1.05	0.11	85.82	1.59	74.90	1.69	72.26	1.74	38.40	0.52
Erectile tissue	1.04	0.11	85.49	0.98	72.65	1.04	69.50	1.07	38.40	0.52
Prostate gland, spermatic cord, testicle	1.04	0.11	84.53	0.89	72.13	0.93	69.04	0.95	38.40	0.52
Compact bone	1.20	0.04	16.68	0.06	14.72	0.07	14.20	0.07	13.28	0.09
Ligament	1.22	0.11	59.49	0.47	51.86	0.50	50.13	0.51	38.40	0.52
Brain, pineal gland, pituitary gland	1.05	0.12	82.63	0.40	63.03	0.46	58.25	0.49	50.68	0.57

V. TEST RUNS

A. FOR RF MAGNETIC FIELDS

For calculations of the SAR distributions with the $5.922 \times 5.922 \times 6.0$ mm anatomically based model of the human body described in the previous section, the dimensions of the birdcage coils which are given in Table 5.2 are used. The accuracy of the FDTD code was validated by calculating the magnetic field distributions for coils A, B, and C (defined in Table 5.2) in air, as well as for coaxially placed dielectric cylinders of diameter 40 cm for coil A and 20 cm for coils B and C, respectively, for which properties corresponding to two thirds muscle were taken. The salient features of the calculated results are summarized in Table 5.3.

Because of the limitation of space, only a few of the calculated results are shown in Figures 5.1 and 5.2. Shown in Figure 5.1 are the variations of the axial ratio H_y/H_x or H_x/H_y and the relative phase difference between H_y and H_x, which are calculated for the central transverse plane (x, y plane) for the unloaded body coil A at 64 MHz. As expected, the RF magnetic fields created for this central plane are nearly circularly polarized in the plane at a right angle to the axis of the coil.

TABLE 5.2
The Dimensions of the 16-Rung Birdcage Coils Considered for the SAR Calculations

	Body Coil A[18,25] (cm)	Head Coil B[18,25] (cm)	High Frequency Head Coil C[11,12] (cm)
Diameter of the cage with rungs	56.0	28.5	30.6
Diameter of the shield	65.5	65.5	36.4
Length of the rungs	56.0	39.3	19.0
Length of the shield	56.0	56.0	21.2
Frequencies (MHz)	64, 128, 170	64, 128, 170	300, 350, 400

TABLE 5.3
Salient Features of the FDTD-Calculated Data for 16-Rung Birdcage Coils A, B, and C of Table 5.2

	Body Coil A			Head Coil B			Head Coil C		
Frequency (MHz)	64	128	170	64	128	170	300	350	400
Empty Coils									
H| with no shield (A/m) center	6.03	6.52	6.87	12.44	12.42	12.62	8.10	8.36	8.50
H| from Biot-Savart law[26] center (A/m)	6.43	6.43	6.43	12.62	12.62	12.62	11.77	11.77	11.77
H| with outer shield (A/m) center	2.57	2.60	2.64	10.49	10.75	11.13	3.58	3.67	3.85
Coils Filled with 2/3 Muscle-Equivalent Cylinder									
Diameter of cylinder (cm)	40	40	40	20	20	20	20	20	20
Length of cylinder (cm)	82.5	82.5	82.5	65.5	65.5	65.5	33.6	33.6	33.6
Maximum layer-averaged SAR (W/kg)	5.87	8.49	14.26	62.9	164.1	179.7	61.46	72.18	74.03

Note: Assumed for the calculations is a current of 1.0 A (RMS) for each of the rungs which are fed with a progressive phase shift of 22.5° between adjacent rungs.

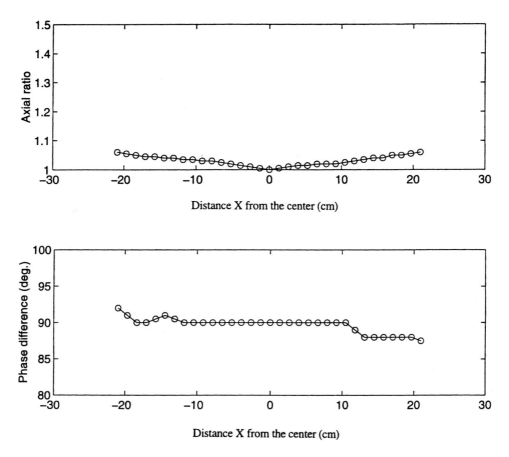

FIGURE 5.1 The axial ratio H_y/H_x or H_x/H_y and the relative phase difference between H_x and H_y for the unloaded body coil A at 64 MHz.

A perfect circularly polarized magnetic field would have had an axial ratio of 1.0 and a relative phase difference of 90° between H_y and H_x. The calculated values are certainly very close to this requirement for circularly polarized fields.

Shown in Figure 5.2 are the calculated variations of the total magnetic field $H_t = (H_x^2 + H_y^2 + H_z^2)^{1/2}$, with radius r for $z = 0$ (i.e., the central plane), and for the H_t for points along the central z-axis ($r = 0$) for the high-frequency coil C. Also shown for comparison are the measured values given by Zhang et al.[12] Similar to the design of the high-frequency coils,[11,12] 16 rungs have been taken for which the sinusoidally varying currents given by Equation 5.7 have been assumed for the calculations:

$$I(z) = I_O \cos k(z - \ell/2) \qquad (5.7)$$

where ℓ is the length of the rung for the birdcage coil C and $k = 2\pi/\lambda$ with λ being the wavelength at the RF of excitation. It should be noted that, as suggested in Vaughan et al.,[11] this current distribution is similar to that for a half wavelength dipole. Also, like the cases of lower frequency birdcage coils, a 22.5° progressive phase shift is assumed for the various rungs in order to obtain circularly polarized RF magnetic fields. As seen in Figure 5.2, agreement between the calculated and experimentally measured variations of RF magnetic fields along radial and axial directions is quite good.

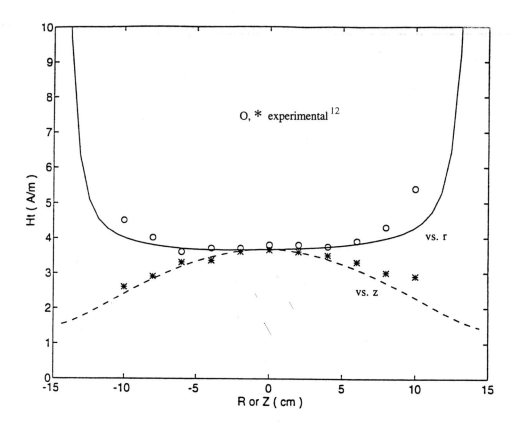

FIGURE 5.2 The FDTD-calculated variations of total magnetic field H_t vs. radius r or axial position z for an unloaded high-frequency coil C at 350 MHz. Current I = 1.0 A, and frequency = 350 MHz. Also shown for comparison are the data measured by Zhang et al.[12]

B. FOR SWITCHED GRADIENT MAGNETIC FIELDS

As aforementioned, the quasi-static impedance method has been used for calculations of induced internal current densities for the 3-D spatially varying switched magnetic fields typical of MR systems.[7,13–16] This method detailed in Section III has been tested thoroughly and has been previously used for a number of bioelectromagnetic problems.[7,13–16] For the present calculations, a Maxwell pair of single-turn loops are considered with radii 0.327 m placed at axial locations $z = \pm0.2832$ m through which equal and opposite currents $I = \pm1344.5$ A flow with trapezoidal time-domain variation shown as the insert of Figure 5.3. Note that, as desired for the Maxwell pair, the axial distance is $\sqrt{3}\ r_o$, where r_o is the radius for each of the loops.[25]

From the Biot-Savart law of electromagnetics,[26] the expressions for the vector magnetic fields $(B_x, B_y,$ and $B_z)$ which are set up for the space between the Maxwell pair as well as the other regions occupied by the patient can be written. Shown in Figure 5.3 is the variation of the total magnetic field for the various axial locations z for all of the period corresponding to the top of the $I(t)$ curve shown as the insert of Figure 5.3.

The magnetic field is purely z-directed for all of the axial locations and, as expected, shows a reversal in direction because of the oppositely directed currents in the two single-turn loops. These magnetic fields calculated for maximum equal and opposite currents of 1344.5 A should, of course, be multiplied by the time-domain variation given for $I(t)$ to obtain the switched gradient magnetic fields for the various axial locations inside and outside the Maxwell pair of loops. Three-dimensional variations of vector magnetic fields (B_x, B_y, B_z) have similarly been obtained

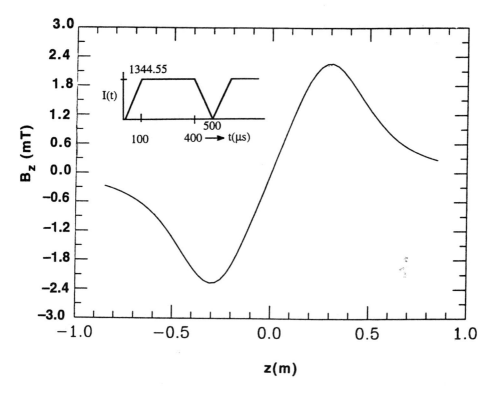

FIGURE 5.3 Axial variation of magnetic fields calculated for a Maxwell pair of oppositely directed, current-carrying, single-turn loops coaxially placed at z = ±0.2832 m. I = 1344.55 A. The trapezoidal variation of current as a function of time is shown as the insert of the figure.

for all locations occupied by the patient from the Biot-Savart law and used for calculations of induced current densities.

VI. SAR DISTRIBUTIONS FOR THE ANATOMICALLY BASED MODEL FOR MAGNETIC FIELDS

Section IV described an anatomically based model developed from the MRI scans of a male human volunteer for which was identified each of the voxels of dimensions $1.974 \times 1.974 \times 3.0$ mm with one of 30 tissues shown in Table 5.1. To reduce computer memory requirements, another model was developed with somewhat coarser cells by combining $3 \times 3 \times 2$ voxels of the higher resolution model, such that the new model has voxel dimensions of $5.922 \times 5.922 \times 6.0$ mm (nominal 6.0 mm resolution) along x-, y-, and z-directions, respectively.

This requires storing the new volume-averaged electrical properties ε_r, σ and mass densities for each of the larger voxels of this model. The SARs thus obtained for the individual larger voxels were used to calculate the layer-averaged SARs for each of the coils of interest (Figures 5.4 to 5.6). Since SARs in various tissues were also of interest, each of the larger voxels were identified with the majority of tissue in that subvolume. This naturally altered the weights of some of the tissues and organs in the nominal 6.0-mm resolution model. However, the weights of important tissues and organs in the nominal 6.0-mm resolution model were found to be within ±5% of the corresponding weights in the original $1.974 \times 1.974 \times 3.0$ mm MRI-based model.

This nominal 6.0-mm resolution, anatomically based model was used to obtain SAR distributions for the body coil A of dimensions given in Table 5.2 for RF frequencies of 64, 128, and 170 MHz. For these calculations, the body coil was assumed to be centered at a plane that is 130.6 cm

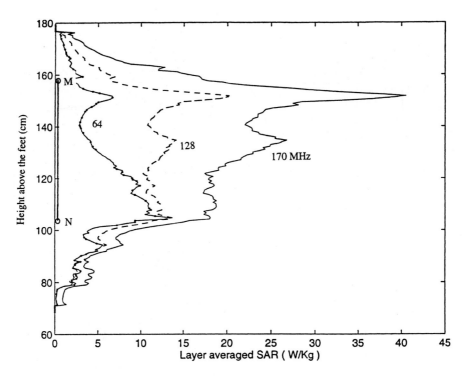

FIGURE 5.4 The layer-averaged SAR distribution for a 6.0-mm resolution, anatomically based model of the human body exposed to the birdcage body coil A. Each rung is assumed to be fed by a 1.0-A (RMS) current. The location of the coil vis-à-vis the body is indicated by points M, N along the ordinate.

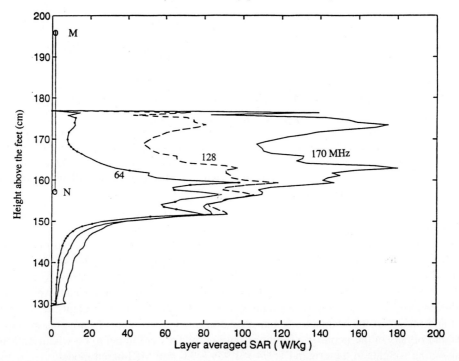

FIGURE 5.5 The layer-averaged SAR distribution for a 6.0-mm resolution, anatomically based model of the human body exposed to the head coil B. Each rung is assumed to be fed by a 1.0-A (RMS) current. The location of the coil vis-à-vis the body is indicated by points M, N along the ordinate.

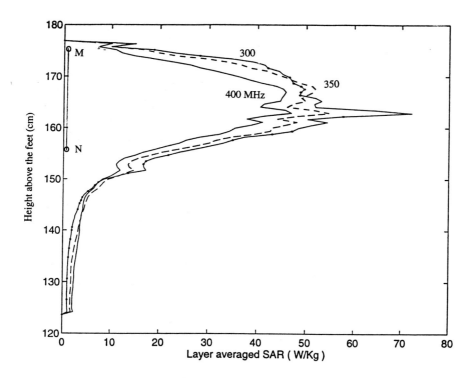

FIGURE 5.6 The layer-averaged SAR distribution for a 6.0-mm resolution, anatomically based model of the human body exposed to the head coil C. Each rung is assumed to be fed by a 1.0-A (RMS) current. The location of the coil vis-à-vis the body is indicated by points M, N along the ordinate.

above the bottom of the feet of the model, and the man model was truncated at two planes that are 70.8 and 176.3 cm above the bottom of the feet, respectively. The salient features of the calculated results are summarized in Table 5.4, and the section-averaged SAR values for the various cross sections of the body are plotted in Figure 5.4.

As expected, the higher the frequency, the higher the SARs. An $f^{1.1}$-type dependence, rather than the f^k ($k \geq 2$)-type dependence predictable from quasi-static considerations,[27,28] is observed for the calculated whole-body-averaged SARs. This result is interesting since considerably higher SARs increasingly approximately as f^2 with frequency were previously projected both by us[28] and by others.[6,27] However, most of these projections were made with quasi-static methods that are valid strictly at the lower frequencies, whereas a full-wave analysis using the FDTD method has been used for the present calculations, and this approach is certainly valid for all of the frequencies presently used or projected for MR procedures.

Table 5.5 shows the salient features of the results calculated for the head coil B of dimensions given in Table 5.2 for frequencies of 64, 128, and 170 MHz. The head coil of axial length 39.3 cm was assumed to be placed such that its central plane was coincident with the top of the head (assumed to be 176.3 cm above the bottom of the feet). Figure 5.5 shows the layer-averaged SAR distributions for this head coil at frequencies of 64, 128, and 170 MHz, respectively. As for the case of the body coil A (Table 5.4), here also the total power absorbed by the head and the head-averaged SAR varies approximately as $f^{1.2}$ rather than as f^k ($k \geq 2$), which would have been predicted from quasi-static considerations.[27,28]

Table 5.6 displays the results calculated for the high-frequency head coil C proposed by Vaughan et al.[11] of dimensions given in the last column of Table 5.2. For this coil, the SARs at the planned frequencies of 300, 350, and 400 MHz were calculated. Shown in Figure 5.6 are the layer-averaged SAR distributions for the high-frequency head coil C at frequencies of 300, 350, and 400 MHz, respectively.

TABLE 5.4
Salient Features of the Calculated Organ-Averaged SARs for the 6.0-mm Resolution, Anatomically Based Model of the Human Body Exposed to the Body Coil A

Tissue	Organ-Averaged SAR (W/kg)		
	64 MHz	128 MHz	170 MHz
Intestine	0.15	0.43	0.64
Spleen	0.13	0.38	0.96
Pancreas	0.06	0.13	0.22
Heart	0.10	0.30	0.53
Blood	0.11	0.35	0.59
Parotid gland	0.12	0.34	0.71
Liver	0.16	0.39	0.45
Kidney	0.11	0.30	0.62
Lungs	0.19	0.64	1.12
Bladder	0.03	0.07	0.15
Cerebrospinal fluid (CSF)	0.06	0.14	0.33
Aqueous humour	0.10	0.24	0.46
Stomach	0.14	0.32	0.65
Prostate gland	0.06	0.09	0.22
Pineal gland	0.05	0.12	0.30
Brain	0.04	0.10	0.23
Calculated SARs (W/kg)	**64 MHz**	**128 MHz**	**170 MHz**
Whole-body-averaged SAR	0.14	0.25	0.44
Maximum SAR for 1 kg tissue	0.37 (1.0 kg)[a]	0.83 (0.98 kg)[a]	2.17 (0.98 kg)[a]
Maximum SAR for 100 g tissue	1.52 (101 g)[a]	2.13 (90 g)[a]	4.37 (102 g)[a]

Note: Each of the rungs is assumed to be fed with a current of 1.0 A (RMS) with progressive phase shifts of 22.5° to obtain circular polarization. A duty cycle of 1/25 is assumed for the calculations.

[a] Actual weights are given in parentheses.

The salient features of the organ-averaged SARs obtained for this high frequency head coil C are summarized in Table 5.6. However, it is interesting to note that contrary to expectations, the SARs here do not increase with frequency. This is likely due to the cosinusoidal current distribution of Equation 5.7[11,12] that was assumed at these frequencies.

Since the assumed current was normalized to a maximum value of 1.0 A at the center of the rungs, a reducing spatially averaged I^2 varying as 1:0.957:0.909 was thus assumed for frequencies of 300, 350, and 400 MHz, respectively. This may be part of the reason why somewhat lower SARs have been calculated at 350 and 400 MHz as compared to the values at 300 MHz. Nevertheless, as expected, the SARs in Table 5.6 are considerably higher than those shown in Table 5.5. This was to be expected since the frequencies here are considerably higher than the highest frequency of 170 MHz used for coil B (Table 5.5).

VII. CURRENTS INDUCED IN THE HUMAN BODY MODEL FOR SWITCHED GRADIENT B-FIELDS

The 6.0-mm resolution, anatomy-based model of the human body was also used to calculate the distribution of induced current densities for switched gradient magnetic fields of the axial variation shown in Figure 5.3. Such fields are generated by a Maxwell pair of single-turn loops with oppositely

TABLE 5.5
Salient Features of the Calculated Organ-Averaged SARs for the Region of the Truncated Body for the Head Coil B at Frequencies of 64, 128, and 170 MHz

Tissue	Organ-Averaged SAR (W/kg)		
	64 MHz	128 MHz	170 MHz
Heart	0.15	0.22	0.33
Blood	0.47	1.12	1.51
Parotid gland	1.94	6.46	14.33
Liver	0.11	0.12	0.17
Lungs	0.35	0.59	0.87
Cerebrospinal fluid (CSF)	0.82	4.36	10.00
Aqueous humour	1.46	4.98	10.79
Stomach	0.16	0.16	0.29
Pineal gland	0.26	1.09	3.38
Brain	0.59	3.13	6.90
Calculated SARs (W/kg)	**64 MHz**	**128 MHz**	**170 MHz**
Whole-body-averaged SAR	0.19	0.35	0.55
Maximum SAR for 1 kg tissue	3.47 (1.0 kg)[a]	4.72 (0.96 kg)[a]	6.78 (1.03 kg)[a]
Maximum SAR for 100 g tissue	7.21 (100 g)[a]	7.92 (96 g)[a]	9.90 (100 g)[a]

Note: Each of the rungs is assumed to be fed with a current of 1.0 A (RMS) with progressive phase shifts of 22.5° to obtain circular polarization. A duty cycle of 1/25 is assumed for the calculations.

[a] Actual weights are given in parentheses.

TABLE 5.6
Salient Features of the Calculated Organ-Averaged SARs for the Region of the Truncated Body for the High-Frequency Head Coil C at Frequencies of 300, 350, and 400 MHz

Tissue	Organ-Averaged SAR (W/kg)		
	300 MHz	350 MHz	400 MHz
Blood	0.27	0.27	0.24
Parotid gland	4.28	3.65	3.04
Lungs	0.07	0.08	0.07
Cerebrospinal fluid (CSF)	3.37	3.65	3.02
Aqueous humour	3.31	2.92	2.26
Stomach	0.03	0.04	0.04
Pineal gland	1.86	2.02	1.55
Brain	2.35	2.25	1.79
Calculated SARs (W/kg)	**300 MHz**	**350 MHz**	**400 MHz**
Whole-body-averaged SAR	0.15	0.15	0.13
Maximum SAR for 1 kg tissue	2.67 (1.11 kg)[a]	2.57 (1.11 kg)[a]	2.20 (1.13 kg)[a]
Maximum SAR for 100 g tissue	4.17 (116 g)[a]	3.88 (112 g)[a]	3.29 (115 g)[a]

Note: Each of the rungs is assumed to be fed with a current of 1.0 A (RMS) with progressive phase shifts of 22.5°. A duty cycle of 1/25 is assumed for the calculations.

[a] Actual weights are given in parentheses.

directed currents varying in the time domain as shown in the insert of Figure 5.3. For this case (Figure 5.3), $dB/dt \cong 22$ T/s occurs for axial locations $z = \pm 0.2832$ m. The induced current densities were calculated using the quasi-static impedance method described in Section III.

The properties of the various tissues were assumed to be frequency independent for the low kilohertz frequencies that are involved for switched gradient magnetic fields. For the assumed time-domain variation of currents and the corresponding dB/dt of 22 T/s, the induced currents for the man model are maximum for time durations $0 \le t \le 100$ μs and $400 \le t \le 500$ μs, for the latter the induced currents being maximum but oppositely directed since $dB/dt = -22$ T/s.

For anisotropic conductivities assumed for skeletal muscle and isotropic conductivities for all other tissues (see Table 5.1), the calculated maximum induced current densities for each of the layers of the model are plotted in Figure 5.7. For these calculations, the Maxwell pair was assumed centered at a layer 108.6 cm from the bottom of the feet. The physical locations M and N corresponding to the two single-turn loops used for the Maxwell pair are shown along the ordinate in Figure 5.7. As expected, some of the highest current densities are calculated for layers close to the axial locations *M* and *N* for these loops. Maximum induced current densities as high as 386 mA/m² are calculated for some of the layers under the top loop of the Maxwell pair.

VIII. COMPARISON OF CALCULATED SARS WITH SAFETY GUIDELINES

It is informative to compare the calculated SARs for RF magnetic fields and the induced peak current densities with the safety guidelines proposed by the U.S. Food and Drug Administration

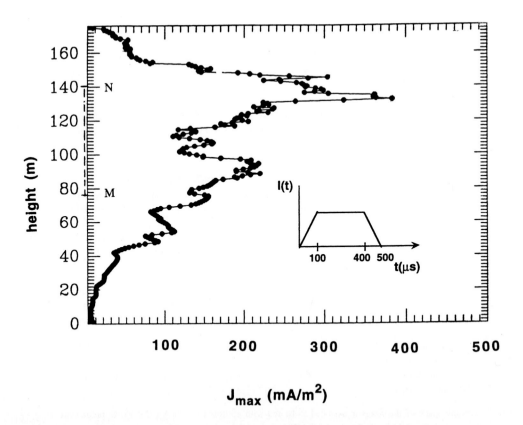

FIGURE 5.7 Peak-induced current densities for the various layers of a 6.0-mm resolution, anatomically based model of the human body. $dB/dt|_{center} = 22$ T/s.

TABLE 5.7
The NRPB Safety Guidelines for Maximum SARs for RF Magnetic Fields and Induced Current Densities for Switched Gradient Magentic Fields

Duration of Exposure (minutes)	Peak SARs in any 1 kg[a] of Tissue		
	Head	Trunk	Limbs
>30	2 W/kg	4 W/kg	6 W/kg
15–30	60 W min/kg	120 W min/kg	180 W min/kg
<15	4 W/kg	8 W/kg	12 W/kg

[a] Averaged over any 6-min period.

(FDA)[29] and the National Radiological Protection Board (NRPB, U.K.).[30] The NRPB safety guidelines for peak SARs in any 1 kg of tissue and for maximum local induced current densities are summarized in Table 5.7.

By comparing the numbers obtained for maximum 1 kg SARs in Tables 5.4 to 5.6 with the SAR guidelines in Table 5.7, one can estimate the duty cycles (assumed to be 1/25 for Tables 5.4 to 5.6) or the RF currents (assumed to be 1.0 A RMS for each of the rungs) that must not be exceeded to be within the SAR safety guidelines.

Similarly, compare the peak-induced current density J_{max} of 400 mA/m^2 obtained for an axial dB/dt = 22 T/s (Figure 5.7) with the maximum current densities that should not be exceeded according to the NRPB safety guidelines (Figure 5.7). Note that for the switched gradient fields assumed for the present calculations, $\tau = 100$ µs and $J \leq 480$ mA/m^2 from Table 5.7. The calculated J_{max} of 386 mA/m^2 is less than this prescribed upper limit for the induced current density, implying that somewhat higher dB/dt on the order of 27.4 T/s could indeed be used for $\tau = 100$ µs switched gradient fields. This compares favorably with $dB/dt \leq 2400/\tau$ (µs) for $12 \leq \tau \leq 120$ µs suggested in the FDA safety guidelines.[29]

IX. SUMMARY AND CONCLUSIONS

This chapter provides numerical procedures, such as the FDTD method and the quasi-static impedance method, that have been used to calculate the SARs and induced current densities for time-varying magnetic fields associated with MR systems currently used and those planned for the future. Based on the complete set of Maxwell's equations, the FDTD method is usable at any RF. Therefore, this method has been used for birdcage RF coils of realistic dimensions at 64 MHz (i.e., 1.5-T MR systems) and may be used for higher frequency coils operating at 300 to 400 MHz that are being planned for 8- to 10-T MR systems.

Alternatively, the impedance method is a low-frequency method and can only be used at frequencies less than about 10 MHz for physical dimensions, such as those of the human body. Therefore, this method is well suited for calculation of induced current densities for present and planned switched gradient magnetic fields of MR systems. For all of the calculations, an anatomic, tissue-segmented model of the human body has been used.

The computational methods presented in this chapter may also be used for improved designs of RF and switched gradient magnetic field coils and to ascertain the intended uniformity of the internal magnetic fields at RF. This is desirable to reduce the distortion of the MR images. As such, these methods offer a valuable tool for design of newer RF coils, both at RF being used today and the considerably higher frequencies planned for the future.

REFERENCES

1. Bottomley, P. A. et al., Estimating radiofrequency power deposition in body NMR imaging, *Magn. Reson. Med.*, 2, 336, 1985.
2. Buchli, R. et al., Increased RF power absorption in MR imaging due to RF coupling between body coil and surface coil, *Magn. Reson. Med.*, 9, 105, 1989.
3. Keltner, J. R. et al., Electromagnetic fields of surface coil in-vivo NMR at high frequencies, *Magn. Reson. Med.*, 22, 467, 1991.
4. Simunic, D. et al., Spatial distribution of high-frequency electromagnetic energy in human head during MRI: numerical results and measurements, *IEEE Trans. Biomed. Eng.*, 43, 88, 1996.
5. Borup, D. T. and Gandhi, O. P., Fast Fourier transform method for calculation of SAR distribution in finely discretized inhomogeneous models of biological bodies, *IEEE Trans. Microwave Theory Tech.*, 32, 355, 1984.
6. Jin, J. M. et al., Computation of electromagnetic fields for high-frequency magnetic resonance imaging applications, *Phys. Med. Biol.*, 41, 2719, 1996.
7. Gandhi, O. P., Some numerical methods for dosimetry: extremely low frequencies to microwave frequencies, *Radio Sci.*, 30, 161, 1995.
8. Kunz, K. S. and Luebbers, R. J., *The Finite-Difference Time-Domain Method in Electromagnetics*, CRC Press, Boca Raton, FL, 1993.
9. Taflove, A., *Computational Electrodynamics: The Finite-Difference Time-Domain Method*, Artech House, Dedham, MA, 1995.
10. Gandhi, O. P. and Chen, X. B., Specific absorption rates and induced current densities for an anatomy-based model of the human for exposure to time-varying magnetic fields of MRI, *Magn. Reson. Med.*, 41, 816, 1999.
11. Vaughan, J. T. et al., High frequency volume coils for clinical NMR imaging and spectroscopy, *Magn. Reson. Med.*, 32, 206, 1994.
12. Zhang, N. et al., An experimental study of a head coil for proton imaging and spectroscopy at 8-10 T, Society of Magnetic Resonance Imaging, Berkeley, CA, 1994.
13. Lin, J. C. and Gandhi, O. P., Computational methods for predicting field intensity, in *Handbook of Biological Effects of Electromagnetic Fields*, 2nd edition, C. Polk and E. Postow, Eds., CRC Press, Boca Raton, FL, 1996, chap. 9.
14. Gandhi, O. P. and DeFord, J. F., Calculation of EM power deposition for operator exposure to RF induction heaters, *IEEE Trans. Electromagn. Compat.*, EMC-30, 63, 1988.
15. Orcutt, N. and Gandhi, O. P., A 3-D impedance method to calculate power deposition in biological bodies subjected to time-varying magnetic fields, *IEEE Trans. Biomed. Eng.*, BME-35, 577, 1988.
16. Gandhi, O. P. et al., Currents induced in anatomic models of the human for uniform and non-uniform power-frequency magnetic fields, *Bioelectromagnetics*, 21, 2000.
17. Berntsen, S., Bajers, F., and Hornsleth, S., Retarded time absorbing boundary conditions, *IEEE Trans. Antennas Propag.*, 42, 1059, 1994.
18. Hayes, C. E. et al., An efficient, highly homogeneous radiofrequency coil for whole body NMR imaging at 1.5 Tesla, *J. Magn. Res.*, 63, 622, 1985.
19. Epstein, B. R. and Foster, K. R., Anisotropy in dielectric properties of skeletal muscle, *Med. Biol. Eng. Comput.*, 21, 51, 1983.
20. Zheng, E., Shao, S., and Webster, J. G., Impedance of skeletal muscle from 1 Hz to 1 MHz, *IEEE Trans. Biomed. Eng.*, 31, 477, 1984.
21. Geddes, L. A. and Baker, L. E., The specific resistance of biological material — a compendium of data for the biomedical engineer and physiologist, *Med. Biol. Eng.*, 5, 271, 1967.
22. Foster, K. R. and Schwan, H. P., Dielectric properties of tissues, in *Handbook of Biological Effects of Electromagnetic Fields*, 2nd edition, C. Polk and E. Postow, Eds., CRC Press, Boca Raton, FL, 1996, chap. 1.
23. Gabriel, C., Compilation of the Dielectric Properties of Body Tissues at RF and Microwave Frequencies, Report AL/OE-TR-1996-0037, Armstrong Laboratory (AFMC), Radiofrequency Radiation Division, Brooks AFB, TX, 1996.
24. Durney, C. H. et al., *Radio Frequency Radiation Dosimetry Handbook*, 4th edition, USAF SAM-TR-85-73, Brooks AFB, TX, 1986.

25. Thomas, S R., Magnets and gradient coils: types and characteristics, in *The Physics of MRI (1992 AAPM Summer School Proceedings)*, M.J. Bronskill and P. Sprawls, Eds., American Institute of Physics, Woodbury, NY, 1993.
26. Paul, C. R. and Nasar, S. A., *Introduction to Electromagnetic Field*, Second edition, McGraw-Hill, New York, 1987.
27. Roeschmann, P., Radiofrequency penetration and absorption in the human body: limitations to high-field whole-body nuclear magnetic resonance imaging, *Med. Phys.,* 14, 922, 1987.
28. Gandhi, O. P. and Chen, J. Y., Absorption and distribution patterns of RF fields, *Ann. N.Y. Acad. Sci.,* 649, 131, 1992.
29. Athey, T. W., Current FDA guidance for MR patient exposure and considerations for the future, *Ann. N.Y. Acad. Sci.,* 649, 242, 1992.
30. National Radiological Protection Board, U.K., (NRPB) Board Statement on Clinical Magnetic Resonance Diagnostic Procedures, Chilton, Didcot, Oxon, U.K., 2, 1, 1991.

6 Acoustic Noise and Magnetic Resonance Procedures

Mark McJury

CONTENTS

I. INTRODUCTION

During the operation of magnetic resonance (MR) systems, various types of acoustic noise are produced. The problems associated with acoustic noise for patients and healthcare workers range from simple annoyance and difficulties in verbal communication to heightened anxiety, temporary hearing loss, and potentially permanent hearing impairment.[1-8] Acoustic noise may pose a particular problem for specific patient groups that may be at increased risk. Patients with head injuries or psychiatric disorders, the elderly, young children, and infants may be confused or suffer from heightened anxiety during MR procedures.[2] Some patients may be taking medication that increases hearing sensitivity.[3] Neonates with immature anatomical development may be at increased risk for adverse effects associated with acoustic noise. Significant fluctuations in the vital signs of newborns have been reported during MR procedures, which may partly be attributable to acoustic noise.[4]

Aside from issues of safety, acoustic noise levels also pose a problem for the increasing numbers of researchers involved in functional magnetic resonance imaging (fMRI) studies of brain activation.

MR system-related acoustic noise will interfere with communication of activation task instructions that often must be given during scanning.

One area of particular interest is the study of auditory and language function. In these studies, the response to pure tone stimuli is analyzed.[9] Any background levels of unwanted or uncontrolled acoustic noise can interfere with the delivery of these sound stimuli and affect experimental integrity.

Acoustic noise levels during echo planar imaging (EPI) have been reported to significantly increase pure tone hearing thresholds in the optimal frequency hearing range (0.1 to 8 kHz).[10] These effects vary across the frequency range and the threshold changes dependent on the characteristics of the sequence-generated acoustic noise.[10] It may be possible to take account of, or adjust for, the MR system-induced auditory activation by using a control series of scans in task paradigms. Results have been reported on mapping auditory activation induced by MR system-induced acoustic noise.[11]

Finally, the problem of acoustic noise may also have implications for the operational costs of an MR facility. Notably, there is a potential decrease in image quality due to patient movement, resulting from being startled or being uncomfortable in association with acoustic noise. This may add to the need to repeat scans or interrupted studies that can impact adversely on the efficiency of an MR facility. For all the above reasons, it is important that the MR-generated acoustic noise is quantified and characterized as part of a safety and quality assurance program. Furthermore, any exposure to acoustic noise that is excessive must be controlled.

Exposure to acoustic noise can routinely be confined to levels within permissible limits with little effort by using passive protection. Several more sophisticated methods are also under investigation by researchers, offering perhaps more elegant solutions without the disadvantages of passive methods. This chapter will discuss acoustic noise and hearing, describe the common characteristics of MR-related acoustic noise, explain the permissible levels for acoustic noise, and present various methods used for measurement and control of this potential hazard.

II. ACOUSTIC NOISE AND HEARING

The ear is a highly sensitive, wideband receiver, with the typical frequency range for normal hearing of 2 to 20 kHz.[12] The arrival of sound waves at the ear sets up a fluctuating pressure just outside the entrance to the external auditory canal. These pressure fluctuations are then transmitted as pressure waves along the auditory canal. Normally, under slight tension, the eardrum, or tympanic membrane, is physically moved by these pressure waves.

On the other side of the membrane, three tiny bones, known as the ossicles, transmit this movement across the middle ear cavity to another membrane, the oval window, that forms the end of the spiral-shaped, fluid-filled cochlea. The vibration of the membrane and hair cells in the cochlea is transformed, via the auditory nerve, in a way not fully understood to give a sense of hearing. Figure 6.1 shows a diagram of the main components of the hearing mechanism.

At high sound intensities, the muscles that control the motion of the ossicles alter their tension, creating the acoustic reflex to protect the ear from damage. However, this reflex occurs approximately 0.5 ms after the insult, such that the ear is particularly vulnerable to impact noise of high intensity.

The human ear does not tend to discern sound powers in absolute terms, but assesses how much greater one power is than another. Combined with the very wide range of powers that exist, the logarithmic decibel scale (dB) is used when referring to sound power.

The sound level that is measured depends not only on the source, but also on the environment (e.g., the proximity of surfaces that may reflect sound). Thus, sound levels are usually quoted in terms of sound pressure level (SPL), which accounts for the environment of the measurement. Table 6.1 gives a range of SPLs for some typical sources of acoustic noise.

The sensitivity of the ear is also frequency dependent, as shown is Figure 6.2.[13] Peak hearing sensitivity occurs in the region of 4 kHz. This is also the region where potential maximum hearing loss occurs, with damage spreading into neighboring frequencies.

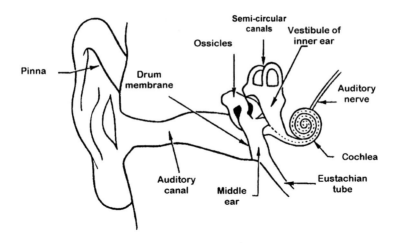

FIGURE 6.1 The main components of the human hearing mechanism. (Adapted from Bess, F.H. and Humes, L.E., *Audiology, the Fundamentals*, Williams & Wilkins, Baltimore, 1995.)

TABLE 6.1
Sound Pressure Level for Some Typical Sources of Acoustic Noise

SPL (dB)	Typical Sound Sources
140	Threshold of pain
130–20	Pneumatic drill
120	Chainsaw
110–120	Car horn at 1 m
80-90	Inside a bus
70-80	Traffic at street corner
60-70	Normal voice
50-60	Typical office
30	Whisper
0	Threshold of hearing

Since the ear is not equally sensitive to all frequencies, measured data may be weighted using the dB (A) measurement scale, which biases the meter to respond similarly to the human ear. The quality or efficiency of hearing is defined by the audible threshold, which is the SPL at which one can just begin to detect a sound. This is normally defined as 0 dB.

Acoustic noise is defined in terms of frequency spectrum (measured and indicated in hertz or Hz), intensity (indicated in decibels or dB), and duration (or time). Additionally, noise may be steady state, intermittent, impulsive, or explosive. Time-varying noise is reported in terms of L_{eq}, which is defined as the continuous SPL that contains the same sound energy as the time-varying sound over the measurement period. It can be considered as the average noise level.

Stimulation of the ear with noise has three potential effects: (1) adaptation; (2) temporary threshold shift, TTS (post-stimulation fatigue); and (3) permanent threshold shift, PTS (permanent impairment). Transient hearing loss may occur following loud noise, resulting in a TTS (a shift in audible threshold).

Brummett et al.[1] reported temporary shifts in hearing thresholds in 43% of the patients scanned without ear protection or with improperly fitted earplugs. Ulmer et al.[10] measured changes in pure tone thresholds in volunteer subjects wearing ear protection exposed to EPI sequences. Intense

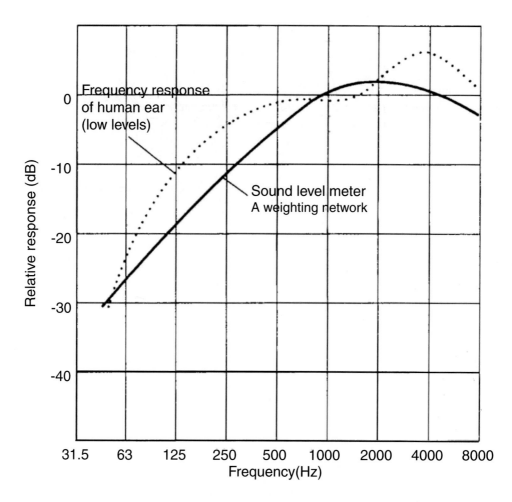

FIGURE 6.2 The frequency response of the human ear. The dashed line shows the relative frequency response of the human ear and the solid line shows the A-weighted filter approximation to this response. (From Department of Health, *Acoustics: Design Considerations*, HTM 2045, Her Majesty's Stationery Office, London, 1996. Reprinted by permission of HMSO. Copyright 1996.)

impulse noise at 0.65 kHz with cut-offs at 0.3 and 1 kHz have also been shown to generate substantial hearing threshold shifts.[14]

Recovery should be exponential and occur quickly.[1] However, full recovery can take up to several weeks if the noise insult is particularly severe. Additionally, if the noise is sufficiently damaging, this may result in a PTS at specific frequencies.[15,16]

Hearing damage from steady-state noise usually takes the form of inner ear damage; that is, destruction of the hair cells that convert acoustic energy to electrical impulses to be fed via the nervous system to the brain. These cells cannot regenerate, and therefore, the damage is irreversible.

This damage to hearing is similar to age-related hearing loss (presbycusis) in that it progresses slowly, with the hearing threshold rising. Mean hearing loss is a function of noise frequency and duration.[15] Permanent damage is primarily a risk for prolonged daily exposure to loud (>80 dB) occupational noise. Excessive noise is known to be one of the most common causes of hearing loss in the world.[15] The risk of hearing damage increases with the noise level, duration of the noise, the number of exposures to the noise, and the susceptibility of the individual.[15,16]

III. CHARACTERISTICS OF MR-RELATED ACOUSTIC NOISE

The gradient magnetic field of the MR system is the primary source of acoustic noise associated with MR procedures.[17-29] This noise occurs during the rapid alterations of currents within the gradient coils. These currents, in the presence of a strong, static magnetic field of the MR system, produce significant (Lorentz) forces that act upon the gradient coils. From basic physics, a conductor element dl carrying a current $I = I\ \underline{i}$ placed into a magnetic uniform field $B = B\ \underline{k}$ will experience a Lorentz force F per unit length given by

$$\mathbf{F} = -\mathbf{B} \times \mathbf{I} = jBI \sin\theta \tag{6.1}$$

where θ is the angle between the conductor and the field direction and $\underline{i}\ \underline{j}\ \underline{k}$ are unit vectors along the conductor, force, and magnetic field direction, respectively.

Acoustic noise, manifested as loud tapping or knocking, is produced when the forces cause motion or vibration of the gradient coils as they impact against their mountings, which then also flex and vibrate. All structures have intrinsic resonance frequencies, and these frequencies have their own modal shapes.

If the gradient coil modal shape due to deformation corresponds to the shape of the exciting Lorentz force distribution, then large coil displacements occur and result in the generation of significant acoustic noise.[29] Current designs of gradient coils are manufactured to have a high stiffness, which minimizes coil motion and thus the structural resonances of the coils.

Alteration of the gradient output (i.e., rise time or amplitude) produced by modifying the parameters of MR sequences will cause the level of gradient-induced acoustic noise to vary. This noise is enhanced by decreases in section thickness, field of view, repetition time, and echo time. The physical features of the MR system, especially whether or not it has special sound insulation, and the material and construction of coils and support structures also affect the transmission of the acoustic noise and its perception by the patient and MR system operators.

Gradient magnetic field-induced noise levels have been measured during a variety of pulse sequences for clinical MR systems with static magnetic field strengths ranging from 0.35 to 1.5 T[17-29] and up to 3.0 T on research systems.[24,28] Initial measurements of MR-related acoustic noise levels were published by Goldman et al.[17] and Hurwitz et al.[18] They reported that the sound levels varied from 82 to 93 dB on the A-weighted scale and from 84 to 103 dB on the linear scale.[18] Obviously, since the gradient magnetic field is primarily responsible for acoustic noise in the MR environment, the ability of the MR system to produce noise is dependent upon the specifications for the gradients as well as the types of imaging parameters that are available on the MR system.

Later studies performed using other MR parameters, including "worst-case" or extreme pulse sequences, showed that, perhaps unsurprisingly, fast gradient echo pulse sequences produced the greatest noise during MRI,[19-22] and three-dimensional pulse sequences, where multiple gradients are applied simultaneously, are among the loudest. Notably, acoustic noise levels in these investigations did not exceed a range of 103 to 113 dB (peak) on the A-weighted scale.[19-22]

More recent studies have been performed to include noise generated by echo planar and fast spin echo sequences.[24-27] Echo planar sequences, in collecting a complete image in one radiofrequency (RF) excitation of the spin system, require extremely fast gradient switching times and high gradient amplitudes. Thus, echo planar sequences can generate potentially high levels of acoustic noise. However, the duration of the sequence and, thus, the patient exposure are shorter than those for conventional pulse sequences.

Shellock et al.[25] reported relatively high levels of acoustic noise, ranging from 114 to 115 dB (A) on the two MR systems tested when running EPI sequences with parameters selected to represent a worst-case protocol. Nevertheless, these acoustic noise levels were within current permissible limits for MR systems. Miyati et al.[27] conducted an extensive survey of EPI sequences performed on 11 MR systems. The results of sound level measurements also found the levels to be within permissible limits.

The increased interest in diffusion and functional MRI has meant an increased interest in high field strength MR systems (i.e., mostly 3.0 and 4.0 T) with fast gradient capability (25 to 30 mT/m switching rates and high amplitudes) to acquire multi-slice EPI images of high quality. At this point, no comprehensive data are available from MR systems with static fields above 3.0 T.

Measurements of SPLs offer a limited amount of information with regard to the quality of the noise and its impact on hearing. In addition to measurements of noise level, several authors have recorded and analyzed the acoustic noise.[17,21-24,26,27] Similar noise levels and characteristics are found when comparing different clinical MR systems.[22,27] Frequency analysis of the noise shows that noise is pseudo-periodic, with variation in the degree of periodicity depending on the sequence used.[22]

For conventional pulse sequences used for MR procedures, peak noise levels are found at the low frequency region of the spectra. However, for EPI, sound levels are reported to contain a larger fraction of high frequency noise (around 4 kHz).[27] Figure 6.3 shows an example of the octave band spectra for 1.0-T (black squares) and 1.5-T (open squares) MR systems.[18,21] Spectral peaks in the sound levels are found in the range of 0.2 to 1.5 kHz.[22] Cho et al.[24] have also found that prescan noise generated high levels (100 dB, C scale) across a wide spectral range up to 4 kHz, with peaks around 2.4 kHz.

Characteristics of the frequency spectra depend on the MR system hardware and protocol parameters. The presence of acoustic dampers (e.g., encased acoustic absorbent foam surrounding the magnet) can reduce noise levels by approximately 3 dB (peak on A scale) or 9 dB (RMS A-scale).[22]

In addition to the dependence on pulse sequence parameters and MR hardware and construction, acoustic noise is dependent on the immediate environment. Noise characteristics also have a spatial dependence. Noise levels have been found to vary by 10 dB as a function of patient position along the magnet bore.[23] The presence and size of a patient may also affect the level of acoustic noise. An increase of 1 to 3 dB has been measured with a patient present in the bore of the MR system,[23]

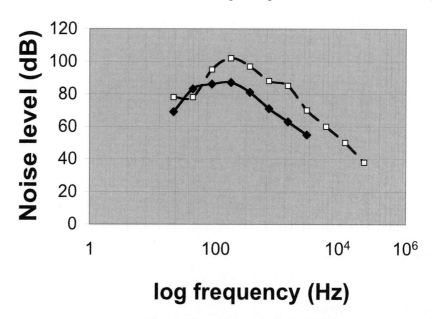

FIGURE 6.3 The octave band spectra for two MR systems: a 1.0-T Siemens Impact (black squares) and a 1.5-T Siemens Magnetom (open squares). Measurements obtained on these MR systems show that the peaks in noise intensity are at approximately 200 Hz. (From McJury, M.J., *Clin. Radiol.*, 50, 331, 1995. Reprinted by permission of Wiley-Liss, Inc., a subsidiary of John Wiley & Sons, Inc. Copyright 1997.)

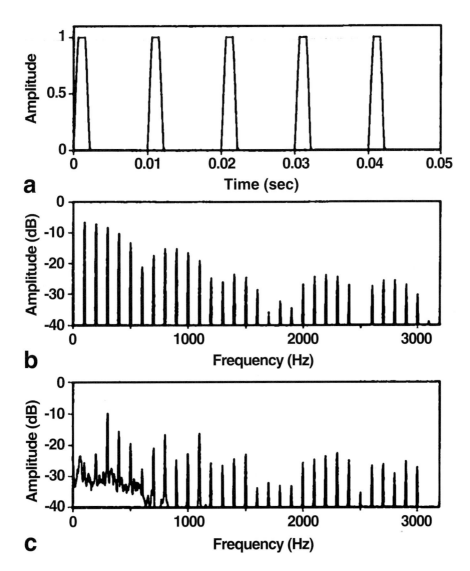

FIGURE 6.4 Gradient trapezoidal current excitation and acoustic noise response. (a) Trapezoidal current waveform time series. The signal consisted of a series of simple trapezoidal gradient pulses. (b) Fourier transform of trapezoidal time series and (c) measured acoustic response. (From Hedeen, R.A. and Edelstein, W.A., *Magn. Reson. Med.*, 37, 7, 1997. Reprinted by permission of Wiley-Liss, Inc., a subsidiary of John Wiley & Sons, Inc. Copyright 1997.)

which may be due to pressure doubling (i.e., the increase in sound pressure close to a solid object, caused when sound waves reflect and undergo in-phase enhancement).

Hedeen and Edelstein[23] demonstrated the similarity between the gradient pulse spectrum and the acquired noise spectrum, which is colored by additional system acoustic resonances (Figure 6.4). There was a good qualitative match between input signal and resulting acoustic noise spectrum. Hedeen and Edelstein[23] derived an acoustic transfer function that is independent of input and, which once determined, may be applied to any input impulse function and may then predict the generated acoustic noise.

Defining the system frequency response function (FRF) as $H(f)$, the input signal represented in the frequency domain as $G(f)$, and the resulting acoustic noise as $P(f)$, the following may be expressed:

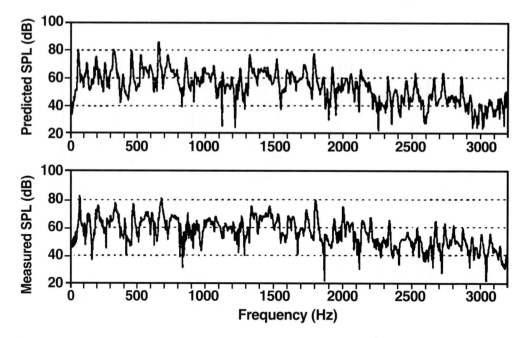

FIGURE 6.5 Predicted (top) and measured (bottom) acoustic noise spectrums, SPL, for an FSE pulse sequence. Overall predicted and measured levels are 93.1 and 92.7 dB, respectively. Thus, the good agreement over a broad spectral range is evident. (From Hedeen, R.A. and Edelstein, W.A., *Magn. Reson. Med.*, 37, 7, 1997. Reprinted by permission of Wiley-Liss, Inc., a subsidiary of John Wiley & Sons, Inc. Copyright 1997.)

$$P(f) = H(f) \cdot G(f) \tag{6.2}$$

Hedeen and Edelstein[23] applied this analysis to a fast spin echo (FSE) pulse sequence and achieved an agreement between measured and predicted noise level to within 0.4 dB (Figure 6.5).

Sellers et al.[29] also noted the similarity between gradient input and acoustic noise. To simplify the intercomparison of noise levels generated by different gradient coils and MR hardware, they concatenated measurement data into a single noise factor (NF). If the gradient slew rate (SR) is defined as

$$SR = 2A/r \tag{6.3}$$

where A is the gradient amplitude (mT/m) and r is the total rise time (ms) (maximum positive to minimum negative), then the characteristic NF for the unit can be indicated as

$$NF = SP/SR \tag{6.4}$$

where SP is the sound pressure measures in Pascals (Pa).

IV. ACOUSTIC NOISE LEVELS AND PERMISSIBLE LIMITS

Table 6.2 shows the relationship between the noise duration and recommended permissible sound levels for occupational exposures.[30,31] In the U.S., the Food and Drug Administration advises that the acoustic noise levels associated with the operation of MR systems must be less than an average of 105 dB (A) and less than a peak level of 140 dB at the patient's ear. These recommended limits

TABLE 6.2
Permissible Duration for Daily Noise Exposures, Based on OSHA Guidelines

SPL [dB(A)]	OSHA Permissable Daily Exposure Limits for Industrial Noise	OSHA Suggested Daily Exposure Limits for Non-occupational Noise
115	<15 min	<2 min
110	30 min	<4 min
105	1 h	<8 min
102	1.5 h	—
100	2 h	15 min
97	3 h	—
97	4 h	30 min
92	6 h	—
90	8 h	1 h

for acoustic noise produced during MR procedures are based on recommendations (published by Occupational Safety and Health Adminitration[31]) for occupational exposures that are inherently chronic exposures with respect to the time duration.

Comparable recommendations do not exist for non-occupational exposure to relatively short-term noise produced by medical devices. A more recent standard has been published by the International Electrotechnical Commission (IEC),[32] which specifies a lower permissible average noise level of 99 dB (A). Recently, guidelines in the U.K. were changed since the initial recommendations (by the Department of Health) on limits for MR-related acoustic noise.[33] Current guidelines issued by the British Standards Institute (BSI)[34] for the safe use of medical equipment state that exposure to acoustic noise must be restricted to levels below an average RMS noise level, $L_{Aeq,1h}$ of 99 dB (A), in line with the IEC limits. In addition, they suggest the equipment should not generate unweighted peak noise levels in excess of 140 dB in any area accessible to patients.

This would suggest that ear protection should *always* be worn by patients undergoing MR procedures in association with MR systems that produce substantial acoustic noise. Recommendations for the duration of exposure are not included.[34]

The exposure of healthcare workers in the MR environment is also a concern (e.g., those involved in interventional procedures or who remain in the room for patient management reasons or support). Shellock et al.[25] reported levels of noise at the magnet bore entrance and exit ranging from 108 to 111 dB while running EPI sequences. The acceptable duration for exposure to these noise levels is approximately 15 to 30 min[31] (see Table 6.2). This indicates that MR healthcare workers should wear ear protection if they remain in the room for longer periods. In the U.K., guidelines issued by the Department of Health recommend that ear protection be worn by the MR staff exposed to an average of 85 dB over an 8-h day.[33]

While the acoustic noise levels suggested for patients exposed during MR procedures on an infrequent and short-term temporal basis are considered to be highly conservative, they may not be appropriate for individuals with underlying health problems who may have problems with noise at certain levels or at particular frequencies. The acoustic noise produced during MR procedures represents a minimal risk to patients if ear protection is worn.

However, the possibility exists that substantial gradient magnetic field-induced noise may represent a heightened risk in certain patients who are particularly susceptible to the damaging effects of loud noises or for those with poorly fitting hearing protection. In fact, there have been unconfirmed claims of permanent hearing loss associated with MR examinations.[8] Therefore, special care is essential when controlling noise levels associated with MR procedures.

V. ACOUSTIC NOISE CONTROL TECHNIQUES

Controlling acoustic noise is generally accomplished in one of three simple ways: (1) control of noise at the source, (2) control along the path of the noise, or (3) control at the receiver. Once acoustic energy has been generated in the air, it can be difficult to control, so the control of noise at the source is arguably the typically preferred method. The noise control methods described in detail below fall into category (1), controlling noise at the source, or category (3), control at the receiver.

A. PASSIVE NOISE CONTROL

The most convenient and least expensive means of preventing problems associated with acoustic noise during MR procedures is to encourage the routine use of earplugs or headphones[1,6-8] Earplugs, when properly fitted, can abate noise by 10 to 30 dB, which is usually an adequate amount of sound attenuation for the MR environment. The use of earmuffs, headphones, or disposable earplugs has been shown to provide a sufficient decrease in acoustic noise that, in turn, would be capable of preventing the potential temporary hearing loss associated with MR procedures.[1] Notably, acoustic dampers provided by some equipment manufacturers with their MR systems may also be considered as a means of passive protection. They offer a slight reduction in noise levels (2 to 3 dB)[22] (see below).

The level and frequency range of noise attenuation will vary with the type and design of ear protection used. If data are unavailable for noise abatement, the protector should be tested. Since the designs of hearing protectors do vary, care should be taken when offering these to patients. Proper fitting instructions must be provided.

Patients who may be confused, young, or have difficulty in correctly fitting the hearing protection themselves may need additional assistance to prevent poor fitting of the device and compromised noise attenuation for these patients. If using earmuffs or headphones, they should regularly be assessed for wear to seals and be replaced as needed.

Unfortunately, earplugs, earmuffs, and headphones suffer from a number of problems. These devices hamper verbal communication with the patient during the operation of the MR system. In certain circumstances, they can also cause discomfort or hamper the immobilization of the patient's head when optimal immobilization is required for certain studies that are very sensitive to patient movement (i.e., diffusion and phase-sensitive studies).

Standard earplugs are often too large for the ear canal of young babies. Some small sizes are available (Carbot Safety Ltd., Slough, U.K.), although a snug fit is essential if noise is to be efficiently attenuated, as the study by Brummett et al.[1] clearly demonstrated.

These passive devices may attenuate noise non-uniformly over the hearing range. While high frequency sound may be well attenuated, attenuation can be poor at low frequencies. This is unfortunate, as the low frequency range is also where the peak in MR-related acoustic noise is often generated; however, this may be balanced by the lower hearing sensitivity of hearing also in this frequency range (Figure 6.2). Figure 6.6 shows the sound attenuation for a typical headphone. Note that attenuation is less efficient in the low frequency region.

In addition to this, passive protection also offers poor attenuation of noise transmitted to the patient through bone conduction.[35] The effects of conduction of vibration have been reported by Glover et al.[26] The presence of an insulating foam mattress on the patient couch has been found to reduce vibrational coupling to the patient and noise levels by around 10 dB.[26]

B. ACTIVE NOISE CONTROL (ANC)

A significant reduction in the level of acoustic noise caused by MR procedures has been accomplished by implementing the use of an active noise cancellation (ANC) or "anti-noise" technique.[17,36,37] Unlike many other noise control solutions that result in compromised performance of

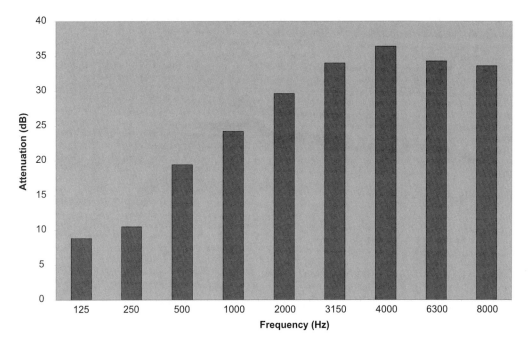

FIGURE 6.6 Noise attenuation for a typical headphone (Silenta-Sportif, Oy-Silenta, Finland). Note that attenuation is less efficient at low frequencies.

the MR procedure or hardware, this technique has a minimal impact on the performance of the MR system.

Controlling the noise from a particular source by introducing anti-phase noise to interfere destructively with the noise source (Figure 6.7) is by no means a new idea.[38,39] However, the initial results for the use of anti-noise applied to MR were disappointing. Goldman et al.[17] used a combined passive and active noise control system (i.e., an active system built into a headphone), achieving an average noise reduction of around 14 dB. This performance is similar to that of a standard passive headphone alone (Figure 6.6).

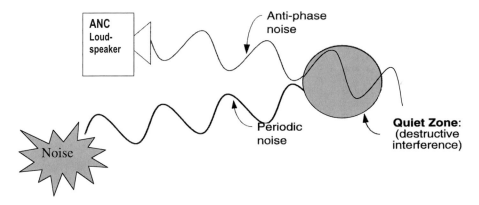

FIGURE 6.7 Principle of sound attenuation using anti-phase noise to create a zone of quiet. This diagram shows a noise (periodic) source and synthesized anti-phase noise interfering destructively in a specific region to produce a zone of quiet.

Advances in digital signal processing (DSP) technology permit efficient modern ANC systems to be realized at a moderate cost.[40] The anti-noise system involves a continuous feed-forward or feedback loop with continuous sampling of the sounds in the noise environment so that the gradient magnetic field-induced noise is attenuated (Figure 6.8). Thus, it is possible to attenuate the pseudo-periodic MR system-related noise, while allowing the transmission of vocal communication or music to be maintained. Some commercial manufacturers are currently offering ANC systems that pipe anti-noise to headphones in a manner similar to airline music systems.[29]

McJury et al.[36] reported the sound attenuation of MR-generated acoustic noise with a real-time adaptive ANC system. In the adaptive ANC controller, the system attempts to minimize the error signal power using a feedback control algorithm. If this minimization is successful, a zone of quiet will appear around the error microphone. A number of general points must be addressed by the architecture, namely, the following:

1. The use of a feedback algorithm requires that careful attention be paid to algorithm stability and numerical integrity.
2. If a reference microphone is to be used, there is a feedback path through the acoustic transfer path $H_r(f)$ that could cause stability problems.
3. A larger zone of quiet than achievable with one microphone is likely to be desirable.
4. Depending on the physical location of the reference microphone and error microphones, the noise controller may not be able to cancel random noise due to the non-causality of the architecture.

To address these points, a multi-channel, filtered-U, least mean square (LMS) algorithm was implemented, whereby more than one secondary source and error microphones are used. MR system-related noise was measured with octave band sampling and found to peak at approximately

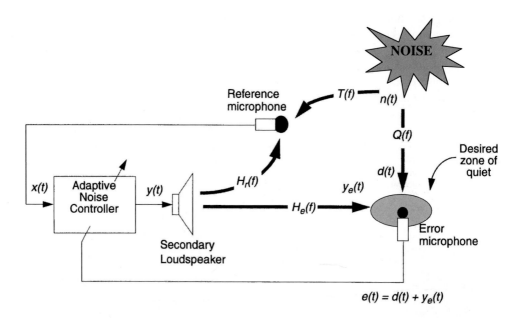

$$e(t) = d(t) + y_e(t)$$

FIGURE 6.8 A schematic of the ANC system. The acoustic transfer path from the secondary source to the error microphone is denoted as $H_e(f)$, and the feedback from the secondary source to the reference microphone is denoted $H_r(f)$. ADC represents an analog-to-digital converter, and DAC represents a digital-to-analog converter.[36] In the ANC, the system attempts to minimize the error signal power, $e(t)$, using a feedback control algorithm. If this minimization is successful, a zone of quiet will appear around the error microphone.

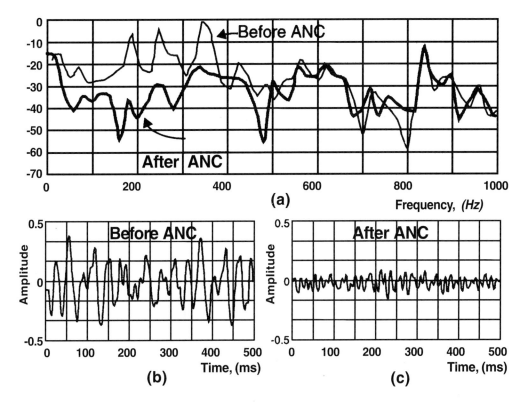

FIGURE 6.9 Results of noise cancellation for a typical clinical spin echo pulse sequence. Noise level spectra before (thin solid line) and after cancellation (heavy solid line) are shown for time and frequency domain spectra. A major disadvantage of this technique is that, if performed below optimal efficiency, at certain frequencies or in some spatial regions, noise levels may be enhanced rather than attenuated by the superposition of the additional anti-noise. (From McJury, M. et al., *Magn. Reson. Imaging*, 15, 319, 1997. Reprinted by permission of Wiley-Liss, Inc., a subsidiary of John Wiley & Sons, Inc. Copyright 1999.)

250 Hz.[21] The ANC controller was therefore optimized to control noise below 500 Hz by using a sampling rate of 2 kHz and an anti-alias filter cut-off at 700 Hz.

Acoustic noise was recorded digitally from a series of typical clinical MR protocols performed on a 1.0-T Siemens Impact. This noise was then replayed through the bench-top adaptive, real-time DSP ANC system (Motorola DSP 56001). A typical peak sound attenuation of approximately 30 dB was achieved over the frequency range from 0 to 700 Hz (Figure 6.9). A major disadvantage of this technique is that, if performed below optimal efficiency, at certain frequencies or in some spatial regions, noise levels may be enhanced rather than attenuated by the superposition of the additional anti-noise.

Chen et al.[37] used a similar bench-top adaptive technique, achieving an average noise attenuation of 18.8 dB with a cut-off of 4 kHz. They clearly showed that the use of anti-noise can efficiently cancel MR system-related noise, while leaving speech and music piped into the MR system relatively unaffected.

C. "Quiet" MRI Sequences

1. Minimizing Conventional Gradient Levels

As the dominant effect on acoustic noise levels lies with the signal details of a particular MR protocol rather than the structure of the MR system,[23] it follows that it should be possible to reduce the noise level by optimizing the choice of MR pulse sequence parameters. Simply using a spin echo (SE) sequence rather than a gradient echo (GRE) pulse sequence and running the sequence with reduced gradient parameters (rise time and amplitude) can significantly reduce the levels of acoustic noise.

Skare et al.[41] designed quiet sequences in this way and defined a simple "quietness factor" (QF) as

$$QF = RT_m/RT_s \tag{6.5}$$

where the RT_m is the gradient rise time of the modified sequence and RT_s is the original/default gradient rise time. On a 1.5-T MR system, a QF of 6 resulted in a noise attenuation of 20 dB. This procedure, however, lengthens the echo time, reduces the number of acquisition slices, and results in a longer examination time.

2. Soft Gradient Pulses

An elegant solution has been suggested by Hennel,[42] which may be applied to minimize the acoustic noise generated by a range of conventional MR pulse sequences. As mentioned above, it has been shown that the acoustic response of the gradient system to current pulses is linear.[23] Thus, the sound generated by a gradient waveform can be derived from a product of the FT of the source input and the FRF of the gradient system (see Equation 6.2). If gradient pulses are designed such that their current waveforms contain no frequencies for which the amplitude of the FRF is high, then resultant acoustic noise levels should be minimized.[42] The FRF of the gradient system in a 3.0-T MR system was measured, and a very low response was noted at low frequencies (below 200 Hz). Frequency components below this threshold should be attenuated in the acoustic spectrum of any pulse sequences.

In minimizing high frequency components in the gradient pulses, it is possible to avoid or reduce sharp transitions, such as step functions in the waveform, and replace these with more slowly varying sinusoidal transitions. This may be done by following three simple rules.

1. Use sinusoidal ramping rather than trapezoidal.
2. Maximize ramp duration (keeps cut-off frequency low for efficient band limiting).
3. Minimize the number of ramps (merge consecutive gradients on the same channel).

The use and efficiency of soft pulses are shown in Figure 6.10. With the sinusoidal ramping, high frequency acoustic components above 500 Hz are severely attenuated. Acoustic noise levels, (dB, A scale) averaged over 1 s, were measured for SE and GRE sequences as a function of echo time (Figure 6.11). Good quality images may be acquired, with sound levels dropping as echo time (TE) increases. At TEs of 30 to 50 ms, good quality images are still provided and acoustic noise levels are below ambient room noise (i.e., with the air-conditioning running, room sound levels approach 45 dB, A scale).

The are three main limitations of this technique.

1. There is an increased sensitivity of the pulse sequences to flow.
2. It is unsuitable for use with ultrafast pulse sequences (e.g., EPI).
3. Increased voltages by factor of 2 are needed to produce sinusoidal ramps instead of linear ramps.

3. Minimizing the Gradient Effects

A reduction of acoustic noise levels may also be achieved by reducing the level of gradient pulsing in a pulse sequence.[43,44] STEAM-Burst[44] is a rapid, single-shot technique based on stimulated-echoes

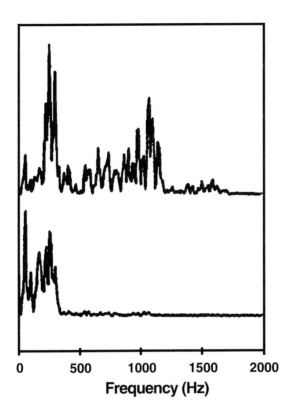

FIGURE 6.10 The efficiency of soft gradient pulses. Magnitude spectra are shown (with an arbitrary linear scale) for the sound generated by the readout gradient of a FLASH (i.e., fast GRE) pulse sequence. Data was acquired with a linear ramp, 0.5 ms duration (top plot), and a sinusoidal ramp, duration 4 ms (lower plot). With the sinusoidal ramping, high frequency acoustic components above 500 Hz are severely attenuated. (From McJury, M. et al., The use of active noise control (ANC) to reduce acoustic noise generated during MRI scanning: some initial results, *Magn. Reson. Imaging,* 15, 319, 1997. Reprinted by permission of Wiley-Liss, Inc., a subsidiary of John Wiley & Sons, Inc. Copyright 1999.)

without the rapid gradient switching necessary in other single-shot techniques such as echo planar. The STEAM-Burst sequence uses a combination of the Burst technique,[45] involving the application of multiple RF pulses under a constant gradient and subsequent refocusing of the resultant set of echoes, and the STEAM stimulated echo acquisition mode.[46] Limited data on acoustic noise measurements show peak noise attenuation of 15 dB compared with a similar EPI sequence.[44]

Although this pulse sequence offers the potential for rapid acquisition of images, it is insensitive to artifacts due to B_0 inhomogeneities, and it generates reduced levels of acoustic noise. The sequence suffers from two main problems. First, the signal-to-noise ratio (SNR) is low compared with other rapid imaging techniques. Second, the images acquired at 3.0 T have an SNR of approximately 20:1. The characteristics of this sequence's signal decay due to T_2 and diffusion effects, combined with a poor SNR, also lead to low image resolution. Thus, these pulse sequences remain more suited to specific research applications than to routine use in the clinical MR setting.

4. Techniques Utilizing Hardware Optimization

Cho et al.[24,47] developed a quiet MR technique based on a variation of the projection reconstruction method which also minimizes gradient pulsing. In conventional projection reconstruction, the frequency and phase encoding gradients remain simultaneously at a low level throughout the

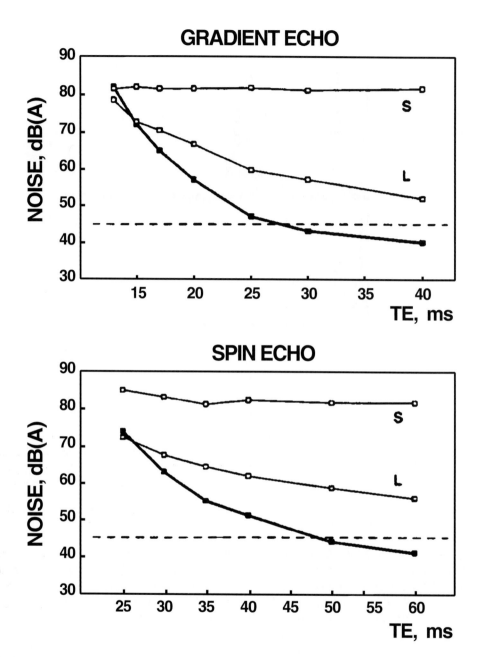

FIGURE 6.11 Acoustic noise levels for GRE and SE pulse sequences measured as a function of echo time (TE, milliseconds) at 3.0 T. The top lines in the graphs correspond to sequences using soft (S) gradient pulses. The middle lines in the graphs show sequences with linear (L) ramps of maximum duration. The bottom lines in the graphs show standard sequence default settings. The dashed line is the level of ambient room noise from the air-conditioning system. (From Hennel, F. et al., *Magm. Reson. Med.*, 42, 6, 1999. Reprinted by permission of Wiley-Liss, Inc., a subsidiary of John Wiley & Sons, Inc. Copyright 1999.)

acquisition of a line of image data.[48] Less gradient pulsing is done, and gradient amplitudes are generally lower than in conventional, two-dimensional Fourier transform imaging.

Cho et al.[24,47] reduced gradient pulsing with a projection reconstruction type of pulse sequence and replaced the two gradient pulsings with a single, mechanically rotating, direct current (DC)

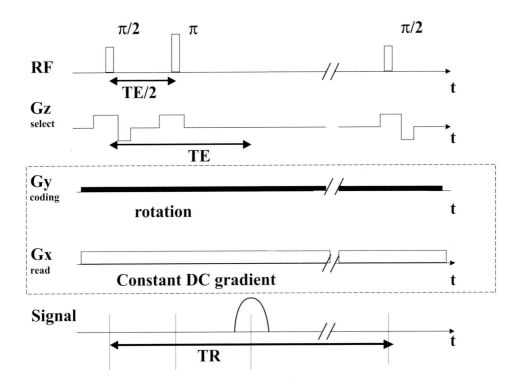

FIGURE 6.12 A schematic of the silent SE pulse sequence. Note the absence of the phase encoding gradient and the presence of the DC gradient applied in the readout direction. (From Cho, Z.H. et al., *Magn. Reson. Med.,* 39, 317, 1998. Reprinted by permission of Wiley-Liss, Inc., a subsidiary of John Wiley & Sons, Inc. Copyright 1998.)

gradient coil (Figure 6.12). In addition, the DC gradient remains on for the entirety of the image acquisition (in conventional projection reconstruction, the gradients are pulsed on for the acquisition of each line of image data).

The use of this "silent MRI" technique results in a 20.7-dB attenuation in sound level. However, the technique suffers from two important limitations. First, the slices may be selected in the z-axis, only due to the readout gradient rotating around the z-axis (i.e., no acquisition of oblique slices is possible). Second, there is a loss of slice volume at each angle of rotation, due to a tilting of the selected slice caused during gradient rotation.

D. "QUIET" MRI GRADIENT COILS

1. Active Mechanical Methods: Force-Balanced Coils

Arguably the best, if not the most technically challenging, solution to address acoustic noise is to eliminate the noise at the source by designing a quiet gradient coil. It is possible to design gradient coil windings such that all Lorentz forces generated by current pulsing are balanced (i.e., each force is effectively cancelled by one of equal magnitude at a conjugate position relative to the coil center).[28,49-51] This is, in essence, similar to using anti-phase noise to cancel a noise source.

For example, actively shielded coils are intrinsically force balanced to a degree. They are designed to have a secondary coil operate in opposition to the main primary coil in order to minimize Lorentz forces on the primary. The combination of coil design and a consideration of construction methods and materials are essential for efficient results.

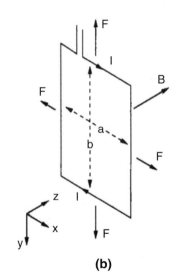

(a)

(b)

FIGURE 6.13 (a) A diagram representing two coupled line elements of conductor dl of equal mass *m* carrying equal and opposite currents. The center of mass of the system remains fixed if the spring constants κ, are equal. The system is placed in a magnetic field **B**, which gives rise to the forces, *F*, causing displacements. (b) Rectangular conductor loop carrying a current, *I*, placed in a magnetic field, **B**, such that the loop plane is normal to **B**. All forces *F* and *F′* are balanced, provided the plane of the coil is oriented perpendicular to the magnetic field direction. If these coils are coupled to similar others via non-compressive struts, then all forces in the system are balanced. If non-compressive materials are used, the conductors cannot move, and no sound is generated. (From Mansfield, P.M. et al., *Meas. Sci. Technol.,* 5, 1021, 1994. Reprinted by permission of the Institute of Physics Publishing. Copyright 1994.)

Rather than trying to mount a vibrating gradient coil to a heavy and immovable base or to somehow damp the coil, if the coil is considered an a harmonic oscillator and coupled to another back-to-back, and if masses and spring constants are equal, the center of mass of the system will be constant without the need for a heavy mount.[49] This is the principle of active force balancing which may be applied to gradient coil design (Figure 6.13).

All solids have visco-elastic properties, and this results in residual movement of the conductors, limiting the ideal noise cancellation suggested above. These movements result in compression waves propagating through the material with velocity,

$$v = (E/\rho)^{1/2} \tag{6}$$

where E is Young's modulus and ρ is the density of the material. Knowing that wave velocity and frequency are related by $v = f\lambda$, a slow wave velocity will result in a low wave frequency, above which progressive phase effects will be expected which will interfere with noise cancellation.

For optimal acoustic noise cancellation, strut material should have a large value for E and small value for ρ, resulting in a high compressional wave velocity. Thus, a light coupling structure of high strength may perform as well as a heavier structure. Composite materials have been tested and found to perform well with a frequency response up to 20 kHz (single loop coil of dimensions 30×20 cm).[49]

Using a bench-top prototype two-coil system (a square coil design measuring 40 cm along each side, powered by a 10-A sinusoidal current), the noise attenuation, when powered in balanced mode, was approximately 40 dB at 100 Hz, dropping to 0 dB at 3.5 Hz (Figure 6.14). The results of attenuation levels agree reasonably well with a theoretical prediction (curve D).[49]

Designs have also been extended and tailored to include the capability of current balancing, acoustic screening, and magnetic field screening in one coil.[28] A head gradient coil has been designed analytically using coaxial return paths to minimize localized Lorentz forces and acoustic noise. When performing EPI (3-mm slice thickness, gradient switching frequency 830 Hz, current 207 A) in a 3.0-T, whole-body MR system, noise levels of 102 dB (RMS) have been reported.[28]

The implications for gradient coil characteristics of the acoustic screening design mean a loss of gradient strength and an increase in coil inductance, thus reducing high speed performance.

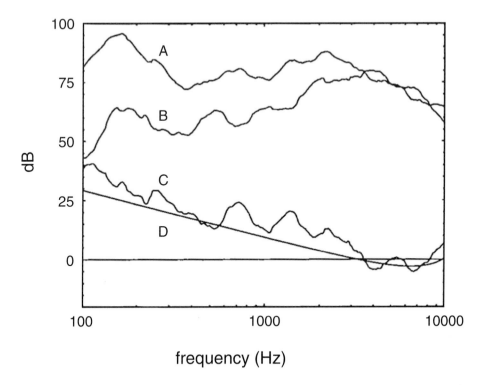

FIGURE 6.14 A plot showing SPL and attenuation dB(A) vs. f for a test coil. Curve A corresponds to the radiated sound received when one coil only is powered. Curve B is the reduced level when two coils are powered in balanced mode. Curve C is the resultant sound attenuation (the difference between curves A and B). Curve D is the theoretical prediction. The results of attenuation levels agree reasonably well with a theoretical prediction (curve D). (From Mansfield, P.M., Glover, P.M., and Bowtell, R.W., *Meas. Sci. Technol.*, 5, 1021, 1994. Reprinted by permission of the Institute of Physics Publishing. Copyright 1994.)

Estimates of the increase in inductance for a three-cylinder coil system (fully force shielded and acoustically and magnetically shielded) over a coil with only active magnetic shielding is a factor of approximately 8.

To counteract this in keeping performance constant, an increase in driver current of $\sqrt{8}$ is required, which will, in turn, increase the acoustic noise output of the coil. Throughout the data on sound generation in relatively simple gradient structures,[51] the highest sound pressure levels were noted to come from spurious resonances, thought to be due to bending and buckling of the coil structures (Chladni resonances). Designing coil systems that completely cancel acoustic noise, including contributions from these sources, is a considerable challenge.

2. Passive Coil Methods

As suggested above, greater coil stiffness should reduce mechanical vibration and associated noise. Stiffness is dependent on material properties and geometrical factors. Altering coil dimensions or materials to increase Young's modulus will help reduce acoustic noise due to vibration. Damping the coil may also attenuate the mechanical vibration. This can be achieved by using particular materials for construction or by mounting the coil in such a way that an acoustic absorber surrounds it.

Damping will be most efficient at or near resonance and, unfortunately, will reduce overall stiffness of the coil structure. Several commercial manufacturers use damping techniques for their gradient coil systems.[22,29] A reduction of around 3 dB (A), due to the use of acoustically damped commercial gradient systems, has been reported.[22]

Some other standard methods for noise attenuation used in industrial environments are enclosure and perforation.[29,52] Enclosure involves enclosing the noise source in an airtight skin, damping the source side of the enclosure, and decoupling the enclosure from the source. Perforating a noise-generating surface has been found to significantly reduce the levels of acoustic noise generated. Unfortunately, both these methods are difficult to implement efficiently in MR systems.

VI. OTHER SOURCES OF MR SYSTEM-RELATED ACOUSTIC NOISE

A. AUDITORY PERCEPTION OF RF ELECTROMAGNETIC FIELDS

When the human head is subjected to pulsed RF radiation at certain frequencies, an audible sound perceived as a click or knocking noise may be heard.[53-55] This acoustic phenomenon is referred to as "RF hearing," "RF sound," or "microwave hearing."

Thermoelastic expansion is believed to be the mechanism responsible for the production of RF hearing, whereby there is absorption of RF energy that produces a minute temperature elevation (i.e., approximately $1 \times 10^{-6}°C$) over a brief time period (i.e., approximately 10 μs) in the tissue of the head.[53-55] Subsequently, a pressure wave is induced that is sensed by the hair cells of the cochlea via bone conduction. In this manner, the pulse of RF energy is transferred into an acoustic wave within the human head and sensed by the hearing organs.

The sounds that occur with RF hearing appear to originate from within or near the back of the human head, regardless of the orientation of the head in the RF field. The actual type of noise that is heard varies with the RF pulse width and repetition rate. The relative loudness is dependent on the total energy per pulse. RF energy-related acoustic noise has been observed at frequencies ranging from 216 to 7500 MHz.[53-55]

RF hearing is mathematically predictable from classical physics and has been studied and characterized in laboratory animals and human subjects. Individuals involved with the use of microwaves in industrial and military settings commonly experience RF hearing. With specific reference to the operation of MR systems, RF hearing has been found to be associated with frequencies ranging from 2.4 to 170 MHz.[53]

The gradient magnetic field-induced acoustic noise that occurs during MR procedures is significantly louder than the sounds associated with RF hearing. Therefore, noises produced by the RF auditory phenomenon are effectively masked and not perceived by patients or MR operators.[53] There is also no evidence of any detrimental health effects related to the presence of RF hearing. However, Roschmann[53] recommends an upper level limit of 30 kW applied peak pulse power of RF energy for head coils and 6 kW for surface coils used during MR imaging or spectroscopy to avoid RF-evoked SPLs in the head increasing above the discomfort threshold of 110 dB.

B. Noise from Subsidiary Systems

Room air conditioners, fans for patient comfort, and cryogen reclamation systems associated with superconducting magnets for MR systems are the main sources of ambient acoustic noise found in the MR environment. Cryogen reclamation systems are devices that are effectively used to minimize the loss of cryogens and function on a continuous basis, producing sounds that are considerably less than those associated with the activation of the gradient magnetic fields during MR procedures. Therefore, this acoustic noise may, at the very most, be a mild annoyance to patients or MR system operators in the MR environment.

VII. SUMMARY AND CONCLUSIONS

MR procedures can generate significant levels of acoustic noise.[17-29] This noise can be an annoyance, hinder communication with staff, and at high levels presents a safety hazard to patients and MR healthcare workers that must be measured and controlled.

Many groups have measured and analyzed the acoustic noise associated with MR procedures.[17-29] Acoustic noise levels increase with changes in imaging parameters, including a decrease in section thickness, field of view, and gradient ramp time and an increase in the gradient amplitude. Environment, hardware design, presence of patient in the magnet, and patient position also affect noise levels recorded.

Although many options are available for noise control, the use of simple passive protection in the form of earplugs or defenders should be sufficient to bring noise levels well within permissible limits[30-34] for the great majority of patients. However, care must be taken to ensure that passive protection is properly fitted and in good condition.[1]

Current documents regarding permissible limits vary, but a general consensus or rule of thumb appears to set a permissible average noise level at the patients ear of 99 dB (A).[32,34] Noise levels outside the magnet bore are lower and present reduced risks for an MR healthcare worker present during the MR procedure.

Passive methods of course have limitations, and several more elegant solutions are possible and under investigation by researchers.[17,36-44,47,49-51] These methods range from simply optimizing the MR procedure to be used in terms of gradient parameters,[41-44] to the utilization of anti-noise systems or redesigning of gradient coils themselves.[28,36,37,49-51]

As with many aspects of MRI, the specifications for achieving high noise attenuation often run counter to fast acquisition of high quality diagnostic images, and compromises must be made. Optimizing procedures to lengthen gradient ramp times, lower amplitudes, or minimize pulsing can result in sequences with reduced performance.[41-44] Designing gradient coils that are force balanced to minimize acoustic resonances will compromise performance in terms of increasing inductance and loss of gradient strength.[28,49-51]

The solution that presents a minimal impact on the performance of the MR system is ANC using anti-noise.[36,37] This is a promising technique, but an optimal system is yet to be fully investigated on routine clinical systems.

Current trends in MR are for increasing static magnetic field strengths and improved gradient performance for rapid clinical imaging applications. Both of these developments will result in increases in MR-generated acoustic noise levels. This will mean an increasing interest in acoustic noise control methods and warrants continued investigation of these techniques.

REFERENCES

1. Brummett, R. E., Talbot, J. M., and Charuhas, P., Potential hearing loss resulting from MR imaging, *Radiology*, 169, 539, 1988.
2. Quirk, M. E., Letendre, A. J., Ciottone, R. A., and Lingley, J. F., Anxiety in patients undergoing MR imaging, *Radiology*, 170, 464, 1989.
3. Laurell, G., The combined effect of noise and cisplatin, *Ann. Otol. Rhinol. Laryngol.,* 1001, 969, 1992.
4. Philbin, M. K., Taber, K. H., and Hayman, L. A., Preliminary report: changes in vital signs of term newborns during MR, *Am. J. Neuroradiol.,* 17, 1033-1036, 1996.
5. Kanal, E., Shellock, F. G., and Talagala, L., Safety considerations in MR imaging, *Radiology*, 176, 593, 1990.
6. Shellock, F. G. and Kanal, E., Policies, guidelines, and recommendations for MR imaging safety and patient management, *J. Magn. Reson. Imag.,* 1, 97, 1991.
7. Shellock, F. G., Litwer, C. A., and Kanal, E., Magnetic resonance imaging: bioeffects, safety, and patient management, *Rev. Magn. Reson. Med.,* 4, 21, 1992.
8. Kanal, E., Shellock, F. G., and Sonnenblick, D., MRI clinical site safety survey: phase I results and preliminary data (abstr.), *Magn. Reson. Imag.,* 7, 106, 1988.
9. Strainer, J. C., Ulmer, J. L., Yetkin, F. Z., Haughton, V. M., Daniels, D. L., and Millen, S. J., Functional MR of the primary auditory cortex: an analysis of pure tone activation and tone discrimination, *Am. J. Roentgenol.*, 18, 601, 1997.
10. Ulmer, J. L., Biswal, B. B., Mark, L. P., Mathews, V. P., Prost, R., Millen, S., Garman, J. N., and Horzewski, D., Acoustic echoplanar scanner noise and pure tone hearing thresholds: the effects of sequence repetition times and acoustic noise rates, *J. Comput. Assist. Tomogr.,* 22, 480, 1998.
11. Bandettini, P. A., Jesmanowicz, A., Van Kylen, J., Birn, R. A., and Hyde, J., Functional MRI of brain activation induced by scanner acoustic noise, *Magn. Reson. Med.,* 39, 410, 1998.
12. Bess, F. H. and Humes, L. E., *Audiology, the Fundamentals*, Williams & Wilkins, Baltimore, 1995.
13. Department of Health, *Acoustics: Design Considerations*, HTM 2045, Her Majesty's Stationery Office, London, 1996.
14. Hetu, R., Laroche, C., Quoc, H. T., LePage, B., and St. Vincent, J., The spectrum of impulse noise and the human ear response, in *Noise-Induced Hearing Loss*, Dancer, A.L., Henderson, D., Salvi, R.J., and Hamernik, R.P., Eds., Mosby, St. Louis, 1992, p. 361.
15. Alberti, P., Noise and the ear, in *Adult Audiology*, Stephens, D., Ed., Butterworths, London, 1987.
16. Mills, J. H., Effects of noise on auditory sensitivity, psychophysical tuning curves and suppression, in *New Perspectives on Noise Induced Hearing Loss*, Hamernik, R.P., Henderson, D., and Salvi, R., Eds., Raven Press, New York, 1982.
17. Goldman, A. M., Gossman, W. E., and Friedlander, P. C., Reduction of sound levels with antinoise in MR imaging, *Radiology*, 173, 549, 1989.
18. Hurwitz, R., Lane, S. R., Bell, R. A., and Brant-Zawadzki, M.N., Acoustic analysis of gradient-coil noise in MR imaging, *Radiology*, 173, 545, 1989.
19. Shellock, F. G., Morisoli, S. M., and Ziarati, M., Measurement of acoustic noise during MR imaging: evaluation of six "worst-case" pulse sequences, *Radiology*, 191, 91, 1994.
20. McJury, M., Blug, A., Joerger, C., Condon, B., and Wyper, D., Acoustic noise levels during magnetic resonance imaging scanning at 1.5 T, *Br. J. Radiol.,* 64, 413, 1994.
21. McJury, M. J., Acoustic noise levels generated during high field MR imaging, *Clin. Radiol.*, 50, 331, 1995.
22. Counter, S. A., Olofsson, A., Grahn, H. F., and Borg, E., MRI acoustic noise: sound pressure and frequency analysis, *J. Magn. Reson. Imag.,* 7, 606, 1997.
23. Hedeen, R. A. and Edelstein, W. A., Characteristics and prediction of gradient acoustic noise in MR imagers, *Magn. Reson. Med.,* 37, 7, 1997.
24. Cho, Z. H., Park, S. H., Kim, J. H., Chung, S. C., Chung, S. T., Chung, J. Y., Moon, C. W., Yi, J. H., and Wong, E. K., Analysis of acoustic noise in MRI, *Magn. Reson. Imag.,* 15, 815, 1997.

25. Shellock, F. G., Ziarati, M., Atkinson, D., and Chen, D. Y., Determination of gradient magnetic field-induced acoustic noise associated with the use of echo planar and three-dimensional fast spin echo techniques, *J. Magn. Reson. Imag.*, 8, 1154, 1998.

26. Glover, P., Hykin, J., Gowland, P., Wright, J., Johnson, J., and Mansfield, P. M., An assessment of the intrauterine sound intensity level during obstetric echo-planar magnetic resonance imaging, *Br. J. Radiol.*, 68, 1090, 1995.

27. Miyati, T., Banno, T., Fujita, H., Mase, M., Narita, H., Imazawa, I., and Ohuba, S., Acoustic noise analysis in echo planar imaging: multi-center trial and comparison with other pulse sequences, *IEEE Trans. Med. Imaging*, 18, 773, 1999.

28. Bowtell, R. W. and Peters, A., Analytic approach to the design of transverse gradient coils with co-axial return paths, *Magn. Reson. Med.*, 41, 600, 1999.

29. Sellers, M. B., Pavlids, J. D., and Carlberger, T., MRI acoustic noise, *Int. J. Neuroradiol.*, 2, 549, 1996.

30. U.S. Food and Drug Administration, Magnetic resonance diagnostic device: panel recommendation and report on petitions for MR reclassification, *Fed. Regist.*, 53, 7575, 1988.

31. Occupational Safety and Health Administration (OSHA), Occupational Noise Exposure, 29 C.F.R., pt. 1910.95, 1988.

32. International Electrotechnical Commission, Particular Requirements for the Safety of Magnetic Resonance Equipment for Medical Diagnosis, IEC Standard, 601-2-33, 1, 1995.

33. Department of Health, *Guidelines for Magnetic Resonance Diagnostic Equipment in Clinical Use*, Her Majesty's Stationery Office, London, 1993.

34. British Standards Institute, Specification for Magnetic Resonance Equipment for Medical Diagnosis, British Standard, 5724, section 2.33, 1996.

35. Naughton, R.F., The measurement of hearing by bone conduction, in *Modern Developments in Audiology*, Jerger, J., Ed., Academic Press, New York, 1963.

36. McJury, M., Stewart, R.W., Crawford, D., and Toma, E., The use of active noise control (ANC) to reduce acoustic noise generated during MRI scanning: some initial results, *Magn. Reson. Imag.*, 15, 319, 1997.

37. Chen, C. K., Chiueh, T. D., and Chen, J. H., Active cancellation system of acoustic noise in MR imaging, *IEEE Trans. Biomed. Eng.*, 46, 186, 1999.

38. Lueg, P., Process of silencing sound oscillations, U.S. Patent 2,043,416, 1936.

39. Chaplain, G. B. B., Anti-noise: the Essex breakthrough, *Chart. Mech. Eng.*, 30, 41, 1983.

40. Elliot, S. J. and Nelson, P. A., The acoustic control of sound, *Electr. Comm. Eng. J.*, 2, 127, 1990.

41. Skare, S., Nordell, B., Jakobeeus, C., Mosskin, M., Blennow, M., and Flodmark, O., An incubator and 'quiet' pulse sequences for MRI examination of premature neonates, *Proc. Soc. Magn. Reson.*, 1727, 1996.

42. Hennel, F., Giard, F., and Loenneker, T., 'Silent' MRI with soft gradient pulses, *Magn. Reson. Med.*, 42, 6, 1999.

43. Jakob, P. M., Schlaug, G., Griswold, M., Lovblad, K. O., Thomas, R., Ives, J. R., Matheson, J. K., and Edelman, R. R., Functional burst imaging, *Magn. Reson. Med.*, 40, 614, 1998.

44. Cremillieux, Y., Wheeler-Kingshott, C. A., Briguet, A., and Doran, S. J., STEAM-Burst: a single-shot multi-slice imaging sequence without rapid gradient switching, *Magn. Reson. Med.*, 38, 645, 1997.

45. Hennig, J. and Hodapp, M., Burst imaging, *MAGMA*, 1, 39, 1993.

46. Frahm, J., Merboldt, K., Hanicke, W., and Haase, A., Stimulated echo imaging, *J. Magn. Reson. Imag.*, 64, 81, 1985.

47. Cho, Z. H., Chung, S. T., Chung, J.Y., Park, S. H., Kim, J. S., Moon, C. H., and Hong, I. K., A new silent magnetic resonance imaging using a rotating DC gradient, *Magn. Reson. Med.*, 39, 317, 1998.

48. Lauterbur, P.C., Image formation by induced local interactions: example employing nuclear magnetic resonance, *Nature*, 242, 190, 1973.

49. Mansfield, P.M., Glover, P. M., and Bowtell, R.W., Active acoustic screening: design principles for quiet gradient coils in MRI, *Meas. Sci. Technol.*, 5, 1021, 1994.

50. Bowtell, R. W. and Mansfield, P. M., Quiet transverse gradient coils: Lorentz force balancing designs using geometric similitude, *Magn. Reson. Med.*, 34, 494, 1995.

51. Mansfield, P. M., Glover, P. M., and Beaumont, J., Sound generation in gradient coil structures for MRI, *Magn. Reson. Med.*, 39, 539, 1998.

52. Mulholland, K. A., Noise control, in *The Noise Handbook*, Tempest W., Ed., Academic Press, New York, 1985, p. 282.
53. Roschmann, P., Human auditory system responses to radio frequency energy in RF coils for magnetic resonance at 2.4 to 170 MHz, *Magn. Reson. Med.,* 21, 197, 1991.
54. Elder, J.A., Special senses, in Biological Effects of Radio Frequency Radiation, EPA-600/8-83-026F, U.S. Environmental Protection Agency, Health Effects Research Laboratory, Research Triangle Park, NC, 1984, p. 570.
55. Postow, E. and Swicord, M. L., Modulated fields and "window" effects, in *CRC Handbook of Biological Effects of Electromagnetic Fields*, Polk, C. and Postow, E., Eds., CRC Press, Boca Raton, FL, 1989, p. 425.

7 Safety Considerations of Siting and Shielding for Magnetic Resonance Systems

Robert A. Bell

CONTENTS

I. INTRODUCTION

Safety is often interpreted as minimizing patient and employee physical risk. Although monitoring physical hazards is clearly an important facet, another important risk may be the lack of patient access to potentially life-saving diagnostic imaging technology. If magnetic resonance (MR) diagnostic services are unavailable because they are not financially viable in the general medical marketplace, patients will be deprived of this powerful non-invasive technology. Therefore, a thorough treatment of safety concerns must include the consideration of operational and financial risks as well as conventional MR environment-related hazards in the comprehensive plan for siting and shielding the MR system.

A broad scope of siting and shielding information is required due to the wide range of magnet types and system configurations. Thus, this chapter will concentrate on the following important siting- and shielding-related safety topics: (1) the choice of location for the MR system; (2) the types of magnets used for various MR systems; (3) magnetic fringe field considerations; (4) dynamic magnetic fields (gradients) shielding and siting considerations; (5) radiofrequency (RF) field containment issues; (6) cryogenic-related issues; (7) structural support for the MR system, (8) pre-owned (used) MR systems; (9) mobile MR systems; and (10) employee training, education, and quality control. Other siting and shielding considerations for MR systems will also be presented.[1-5]

II. IMPORTANT FUNDAMENTAL STEPS

Six key steps to save time and money and to prevent headaches are outlined below. Each step should be considered carefully before committing to a specific type of MR system or location for this equipment.

A. DETERMINE YOUR NEEDS

The initial review of potential locations for the MR system should begin with a thorough assessment of the patient population and the medical need the MR system is designed to serve. If a significant number of inpatients or special cases (e.g., pediatric, cardiac, stroke, critical care, or research patients) are anticipated, location within the radiology department or similar support service will minimize transport and maximize the availability of radiologists and ancillary medical services. If such cases are expected to represent less than 10 to 20% of all MR examinations, placement in an imaging center can often provide increased efficiency and throughput for standard outpatient studies.

Picture Archiving and Communications Systems (PACS) can overcome radiology coverage and image transfer problems that may arise in remote locations. Parking, a perennial problem at hospitals, is also more easily addressed in the outpatient setting. However, stand-alone facilities generally require duplication of reception and other personnel services. Medical supervision for administration of contrast agents, sedation, coverage of code blue situations, and other similar cases must also be considered. The overall economic impact must be evaluated in deciding between in-house or free-standing outpatient installation.

B. EDUCATE YOURSELF REGARDING NEW TECHNOLOGY

In the past, the technical aspects of the MR system, especially the magnet, usually determined the site location. Notably, large magnetic fringe fields, bulky magnetic shields, heavy loads, and frequent cryogen deliveries previously eliminated many MR system sites that may have offered better access or more efficient operation. However, advances in active shielding techniques now allow placement of most MR systems in almost any setting.

Indeed, modern, "compact," high-field-strength MR systems usually are lighter and have smaller magnetic fringe fields than low-field-strength "open" MR systems. Thus, any assertion that an MR system (high-field-strength or low-field-strength system) cannot fit into a selected site should be challenged until this is confirmed by siting experts from at least two different vendors.

C. Explore All Reasonable Alternatives

The adage "Commit in haste, repent at leisure" emphasizes an important point. It should be remembered that MR facilities usually have useful lifetimes of 10 or more years. Therefore, extra time should be taken to consider as many opportunities as possible before committing to a particular site location for the MR system.

D. Anticipate Future Needs

Throughout most of the 1980s, head and spine studies represented more than 95% of all magnetic resonance imaging (MRI) examinations in the U.S. As of this year (i.e., 2001), the volumes of MRI studies of the upper and lower extremities now equal that for head studies at most MR facilities.

Thus, it may be prudent to anticipate an increase in MRI examination volume from non-traditional sources such as body studies, early stroke evaluation, cardiac, functional, therapy planning and evaluation, surgical pre-planning, spectroscopy, and others. The site location for the MR system should be selected accordingly.

E. Utilize Vendor Expertise

The MR system vendors employ some of the most capable and experienced siting talent in the industry. Part of the MR system selection process should incorporate a review of potential locations by siting experts from each of the vendors under consideration. Allow them to be creative, and assess their abilities based on the thoroughness of their findings. However, it should be remembered that the vendor siting experts will seek sites that offer advantages to the special features of their specific MR system which may not pertain to others of a similar static magnetic field strength.

F. Distribute Your Risk

Once the MR system vendor has been selected, it is best to contractually obligate the company to pay for any later changes to the site plans they may require and that they should have reasonably noted during the review and approval of the final drawings.

III. CHOICE OF LOCATION

Selecting the location for the MR system is as important as the choice of the particular type of MR system. Obviously, this depends on the proper evaluation of many variables. Ensuring that all of these are considered for each possible site requires thorough planning. Establishing a matrix of concerns can simplify the process. Each entry should be weighted to reflect its order of importance. Typical categories and issues are listed in Table 7.1 and include the following:

- **Patient access** — Can patients conveniently reach the location? Does adequate wheel-chair and gurney access exist?
- **Convenience to radiology department** — Can radiologists be readily available for consultation or for code blue situations? If suggested Medicare supervision rules are enacted, are radiologists available to monitor MRI contrast injections?
- **Interference from environment** — What potential electrical or mechanical interference might exist? Are there sources of vibration? Are large moving metal masses (e.g., elevators, loading dock, ambulance route, etc.) near the site? Are there large metal structures nearby (I-beams, cast iron drainage, etc.)?

TABLE 7.1
Recommended Evaluation Categories
for MR System Site Planning

Patient access
Convenience to radiology department
Interference from environment
Magnetic fringe field impact
Structural support
Availability of utilities
Parking
Architectural esthetics
Delivery route (magnet/cryogens)
Space available
Comparative cost considerations

- **Magnetic fringe field impact** — What devices (instruments, computers, monitors, etc.) are planned for the space nearby? Does a life-flight helicopter fly close to the site? Are any non-controlled areas impacted by fields of 5 gauss or greater?
- **Structural support** — Is the present floor loading sufficient to support the system? What seismic anchoring may be needed?
- **Availability of utilities** — What will it cost to bring adequate power, cooling water, telephone service, and other necessary utilities and services to the site?
- **Parking** — Because MRI examinations tend to be predominantly used by outpatients, is sufficient parking available for the anticipated patient volume? Does the local traffic pattern allow reasonable access to this parking?
- **Architectural aesthetics** — If new construction or significant renovation is anticipated, will the changes conflict with the general architectural plan? Can the MRI facility serve as an architectural statement emphasizing a commitment to state-of-the-art imaging?
- **Delivery route** — Can magnet components be delivered to the site? Is there a route for cryogen dewars? If the magnet of the MR system had to be replaced, what walls or other structures would need to be disturbed?
- **Space available** — Is the available space adequate for all of the planned functions (e.g., waiting and reception rooms, patient dressing room, radiologist's interpretation area, etc.)? Is there space for a computer room near the MR system room? Has storage space been considered? What opportunities for expansion exist if additional MR systems are desired?
- **Comparative cost considerations** — What are the relative cost components of each location? Can the overall financial plan bear the cost of the preferred site? Does this choice have financial implications for other projects in the vicinity? What savings may be effected with minor modifications? To what extent do site cost factors vary among the vendors?

IV. TYPES OF MAGNETS

A. SUPERCONDUCTING MAGNETS

The majority of MR systems in the U.S. utilize a superconducting design.[1] The passage of electricity through an aligned group of superconducting coils, bathed in liquid helium, creates an area of magnetic homogeneity down the common centers of the coils. Superconducting magnets allow the highest field strengths and have the most stable fields of all current magnet designs. Generally, the higher the field strength for the static magnetic field, the better the image quality (i.e., as a result of a higher signal-to-noise ratio) and the shorter the examination time. Field strength, stability, and homogeneity are basic requirements of many advanced imaging techniques.

Superconducting magnets typically enjoy the lowest risk of obsolescence and longest useful lifetimes. In modern MR systems, cryogens (the liquefied gases used to chill the coils) are typically replenished only once every 2 to 3 years. "Active shielding," which is additional coils placed outside the normal field windings, is used to counteract the spread of external magnetism, markedly reducing fringe fields for high-field-strength MR systems. Notably, the resulting compact, high-field-strength designs have shortened the length of the magnet bore for MR systems by as much as 3 ft compared to older versions of the superconducting MR systems. However, the tubular superconducting magnet design remains more constrained on the sides, which may exacerbate psychological distress reactions for certain patients. Another consideration for modern superconducting magnet-based MR systems is that the inherent higher level of technology often translates into somewhat higher service costs.

B. Permanent Magnets

MR systems with permanent magnets rely on magnetism arising from the permanent alignment of domains within iron or other ferromagnetic materials. The most common alloys used for these magnets are combinations of boron, neodymium, and iron. These MR systems do not require electricity to produce the static magnetic field and do not need cryogens.

The designs of these MR systems often incorporate flat magnet disks suspended above and below the patient, allowing access and open viewing on the sides. Unfortunately, these MR systems usually are limited in field strength to approximately 0.3 T and can be highly temperature sensitive. Most of these particular MR systems are heated above room temperature to enhance field stability.

The lower static magnetic field strengths of MR systems with permanent magnets have a reduced signal-to-noise and longer imaging times compared to MR systems with high static magnetic field strengths. Gradient strength and slew rate are usually constrained due to eddy currents induced in the magnet pole pieces of these MR systems. Additionally, the implementation of advanced MRI techniques is problematic or not possible on permanent MR systems due to the lower signal-to-noise and/or gradient limitations. Specialty or dedicated extremity MR systems designed and optimized for imaging extremities typically utilize permanent magnets.

C. Resistive Magnets

Early resistive magnet designs for MR systems used loops of copper wire aligned in the same arrangement similar to the present-day superconducting MR systems. However, since the wire exhibited some degree of resistance, electricity had to be continuously supplied, and heat was produced. The result was a practical upper bound in field strength of about 0.25 T due to limitations in electrical supply and cooling water.

Most current resistive magnet designs use the same technology, but orient the coils horizontally above and below the patient in a fashion similar to permanent magnet designs. Although these units must be supplied with electricity and cooling water, they share most of the other advantages of permanent units (open on the sides and relatively low service costs) and are lighter in weight. However, they also share the limitations of permanent magnet-based MR systems.

D. Hybrid Magnets

A number of MR system vendors have produced iron-core magnets in which the static magnetic field strength is boosted by external resistive or superconducting coils. Such innovative magnet designs have achieved fields of up to 0.7 T, while keeping weight and electrical consumption within acceptable levels. These so-called high-field-strength, open MR systems allow enhanced signal-to-noise performance, but may be subject to the temperature and gradient problems found in permanent and resistive units. They may also be more sensitive to vibration than other MR systems.

V. MAGNETIC FRINGE FIELD CONSIDERATIONS

The magnet of the MR system creates fields not only within the instrument, but also outside it. The extent of these fringe magnetic fields can vary enormously depending on field strength, system design, and the inherent system shielding method. Theses fringe fields do not vary with time (static fields). At low levels, such fringe fields are not known to be harmful. Indeed, we are all exposed to the Earth's magnetic field, which ranges from approximately 0.1 to 1 gauss depending on the proximity to the magnetic poles.

However, at higher levels, static magnetic fields can be hazardous. General categories of potential problems include the following:

1. Interactions might occur with components of cardiac pacemakers or implantable cardio-verter defibrillator devices, causing them to malfunction and potentially endanger the patient or individual.
2. Blood flowing within a magnetic field can generate electrical potentials (magneto-hydro-dynamic effect) that complicate cardiac monitoring and can, at very high fields, produce arrythmias or other variations of normal cardiac function.
3. Ferromagnetic materials (e.g., certain aneurysm clips, foreign bodies, etc.) within the patient or individual may move, causing injury.
4. Ferromagnetic objects brought into the MR system room (tools, scalpels, pens, gas tanks, etc.) can be accelerated into the magnet, causing injury to patients or MR system operators.
5. Magnetic fringe fields may cause alterations in the function of monitoring or diagnostic equipment located in rooms near the MR system. Prime examples are nuclear medicine cameras, computer tomography (CT) scanners, linear accelerators, high resolution color cathode ray tubes (CRTs), and magnetoencephalography units.
6. Magnetic fringe fields may be altered by moving metal objects near the MR system, yielding variations in image quality. Elevators, large trucks or ambulances, subway trains, and similar objects can significantly perturb images if they are too close to the magnet.

Responding to these concerns, the U.S. Food and Drug Administration (FDA) recommended the policy that all persons must be informed and given proper warning when entering a static magnetic field of 5 gauss or greater. Some have argued this fringe field level is too low,[2] noting that other sources of static magnetic fields exceeding 5 gauss exist in everyday life (e.g., telephone handsets, "Walkman" earphones, electric subway trains, "refrigerator" magnets, etc.).

Table 7.2 highlights some of the interactions for various devices that may be encountered with magnetic fringe fields of the MR system. Other possible fringe field problems will vary according to the type of MR system. A complete discussion of these are beyond the scope of this chapter.

VI. RF FIELD CONTAINMENT CONSIDERATIONS

MR systems utilize powerful RF pulses to alter the macroscopic magnetic behavior of the patient's tissues. MR images are then created from magnetic oscillations at radiofrequency fields detected using antenna coils. For these reasons, MR system rooms are usually lined with an electrically conductive layer of material that grounds RF signals impinging upon it. This RF shield or Faraday cage protects MR images from outside electrical signals and limits the potential for the MRI-related RF pulses to interfere with normal radio and television transmissions outside the MR system suite.

TABLE 7.2
Static Magnetic Fringe Field Limits for Various Devices

Device	Maximum Static Fringe Field (mT)
Mechanical/analog watches	3
Magnetic data media (diskettes, credit cards, magnetic tape)	2
Computers	2
Monochrome CRTs, video monitors	0.5
Pacemakers, implantable cardioverter defibrillators (ICDs)	0.5
Metal detector	0.3
Videotape storage (long term)	0.2
Color CRTs, video monitors	0.1
Linear accelerators	0.1
CT scanner	0.1
Image intensifier, nuclear camera, positron emission tommography (PET), cyclotron	0.05

The specifications for RF shielding vary according to vendor requirements. In general, most specify at least 100-dB attenuation for electrical wave and 90 dB for magnetic component, with a ground isolation of at least 100 Ω. RF shielding material is commonly a thin copper sheet, but other conductive materials such as iron and aluminum have been used.

It is important to recognize that the integrity of the RF shield rests upon the electrical contact of its components. Corrosion at the junction of panels or at an RF door that has lost some of its sealing components (e.g., small leaves of metal that make contact with the door jam) may allow RF leakage, resulting in significant image artifacts. These usually appear as dotted lines perpendicular to the frequency-encoded axis and can vary with time. If the MR system room has been subjected to water damage (e.g., from a broken pipe, flooding, etc.), it is advisable to have the RF screen checked for possible damage.

VII. CRYOGENIC-RELATED ISSUES

The liquefied gases used to keep a superconducting system below critical temperatures can pose a significant risk to the unwary. These materials are extremely cold (i.e., –352°F for liquid nitrogen and –452°F for liquid helium) and can cause severe frostbite or even loss of extremities if mishandled.

Under the unusual occurrence of a magnet quench (i.e., the loss of cryogens due to the loss of superconductivity), these liquids rapidly become gaseous and expand to approximately 650 to 700 times their liquid volume. The gases typically egress from the magnet vent with a loud roaring sound. The venting system must be designed to handle this sudden pressure increase, and the outlet must be located so as not to endanger anyone outside the MRI facility. Should the venting system fail, gaseous nitrogen and/or helium could enter the MR system room, forming a dense white cloud from the ceiling downwards. Anyone in the MR system room must be evacuated immediately, since the cloud will displace air and be unbreathable.

In many MR system rooms the door opens inward. Therefore, venting escaping gases into this space can pressurize it and render the door inoperable. In this event, some vendors recommend breaking the window into the MR system room to relieve the pressure and opening the door once the pressure is reduced. Obviously, MR system operators must be properly trained regarding handling of this situation, particularly with regard to patient management, in the event of a magnet quench.

VIII. STRUCTURAL SUPPORT

MR systems can weigh a little as a few tons for new compact designs or specialty magnets to over 40 tons for older systems with large passive magnetic shields. Indeed, some MR systems exceed 200 tons in weight. Therefore, floor support must be properly designed to carry such large loads.

In earthquake-prone regions, appropriate seismic anchoring should also be applied. These considerations should be the responsibility of the architect, with assistance from the MR system vendor.

The significant weight and dimension of some MR system components necessitates a plan for delivery. It is important to ensure a delivery path that can handle both the size and weight of the MR system and ancillary equipment.

Vibration of the MR system can cause diffuse phase-encoded artifacts that degrade image quality. Structural planning should incorporate a review of vibration sources and possibly a field check to verify local conditions. Most MR system vendors do not warrant system performance if vibration is larger than specified limits. Both steady state and transient vibration should be assessed for the proposed MR system site.

IX. PRE-OWNED MR SYSTEMS

MR technology has undergone an astounding transition in the past 3 years. The expansion of the low-field-strength, open market segment prompted many high-field-strength vendors to develop compact or "second-generation open" units to address anxious or claustrophobic patients. Their efforts have markedly shrunk magnetic fringe fields; decreased cryogen boil-off rates (and, hence, costs); reduced system weight; and, in the case of one vendor, entirely eliminated the need for a separate computer room. Compact units preserve the signal-to-noise and high homogeneity advantages of high-field-strength MR systems, while allowing many previously impossible locations to now be utilized.

The shift to short-bore magnet technology has generated a very active market for used MR systems that are available at reasonable prices. No longer can computer or gradient upgrades transform an older system into the latest version; the magnet itself must be replaced to achieve all "new" capabilities. Thus, older units with excellent clinical capabilities are now available at a fraction of the cost of new units.

However, there are some drawbacks to these "inexpensive" MR systems. They generally have higher service and cryogen costs, they require more extensive magnetic shielding, they become obsolete faster, and they are somewhat more claustrophobic. Those considering used MR systems usually accept a larger financial risk in siting, maintenance, and obsolescence in return for a lower equipment price.

Care must be taken in the evaluation of opportunities for used MR systems. For example, consider the following:

1. Can the site for the pre-owned MR system be used in the preferred location without excessive expense or disruption to surrounding activities?
2. Will the referring physicians accept the clinical limitations of the older, pre-owned MR system?
3. Does the financial incentive of a used purchase more than offset the reduced service and cryogen costs over 5 years and the warranty of a new MR system?
4. Are there throughput or other operational advantages of a new system that are not available for the older, pre-owned MR system?

These and other important questions should be addressed in the process of exploring new vs. used MR systems.

X. MOBILE MR SYSTEMS

The market for mobile MR systems has also been transformed. Initially, mobile MR systems served customers who could not afford their own equipment or felt the long-term financial commitment of purchasing an MR system was unduly risky. MRI is now a thoroughly established diagnostic modality. Additionally, accurate tools exist for predicting the patient volume for MRI procedures. Thus, the risk of purchase has greatly diminished. Also, as the used MR system market expands, better equipment is financially available to the limited volume sites that previously relied upon mobile MR systems.

Most new, mobile MR systems contain fringe magnetic fields that are contained within the van, allowing continuous operation "at field" (i.e., without the need to ramp the system down and then up again for relocation to a different site). As such, siting concerns have decreased. Smaller fringe fields and lighter vans are easier to place on the hospital campus or at the free-standing, outpatient center. However, the older, mobile MR systems continue to have substantial fringe fields that require attention. Obviously, consideration of the specifications for a given MR system proposed for use in a mobile configuration is vital to avoid siting problems and other related issues.

XI. EDUCATION AND QUALITY CONTROL

Many MR environment-related injuries tend to occur from the lack of knowledge and proper training of the MR healthcare workers or support individuals rather than the result of inherent or unknown hazards. It is virtually impossible for the MR system vendor to control local staff carrying ferromagnetic objects into the MR system room where they are attracted by the magnet. Thus, ongoing staff education in the safe and efficient use of the MR system is an important facet of any safety program and is the responsibility of the managers, operators, and owners of the MR facility.

Quality control should also incorporate safety concerns. Staff turnover can often leave gaps in knowledge that may result in dangerous actions. Ensuring staff training is as important as verifying optimal technical performance for the MR system. The opportunity to learn from previous mistakes and to pass the knowledge to others can benefit everyone. Accreditation by agencies such as the American College of Radiology can also be beneficial to verify that technologists and radiologists have the proper credentials to perform their respective tasks.

XII. OTHER SITING CONSIDERATIONS

A. SITE PLANNING

The ease with which patients move through the MRI process directly influences their safety at the site and the cost-effectiveness of the operation. The design of the site must reflect a lucid plan that addresses all components of the MRI experience, including scheduling, reception, patient screening, patient preparation, scanning, and report generation. Since patient throughput can be severely impacted by poor site planning, workflow design should reflect anticipated MRI patient volume increases[5] and new applications. Often a consultant with significant MRI experience can help to locate problems in plans before they become concrete.

B. EFFICIENT PATIENT THROUGHPUT

The average MR facility now spends more than one hour per MRI examination, performance that is well below that of more efficient sites (i.e., less than 30 min per examination). For MR facilities that appear to spend excessive time on MRI procedures, consideration should be given to conducting an operations audit to disclose potential bottlenecks in patient flow or other impediments to effective throughput.

C. SPECIAL NEEDS

MR facilities that utilize unusual or unique equipment such as interventional MR systems,[3] anesthesiology systems, or dedicated extremity magnets[4] have unique siting and safety concerns. Federal legislation, including the Americans with Disabilities Act, has also specified that access be provided for those in wheelchairs (patients and staff members) and other disabled individuals. These important factors must be incorporated into site planning for the MR facility.

D. PURCHASE TERMS AND CONDITIONS

Successful site development requires a coordinated effort between the customer and MR system vendor. The best guarantee of a workable partnership is to have clearly defined obligations for both parties. Unfortunately, most equipment contracts are authored by vendors and, consequently, usually reflect their needs disproportionately. Consider amending vendor "boilerplate" with provisions, defining topics such as

1. The assistance and responsibility of the vendor in regard to the preparation and review of site plans
2. The responsible party for applications and other on-site educational assistance
3. The responsible party for technologist training
4. The quality assurance and performance testing program
5. The MR system's "uptime" guarantee
6. The service capabilities (response time, backup, local stocking of parts, etc.) of the MR system vendor

XIII. CONCLUSION

Various important safety issues in the comprehensive planning for siting and shielding of MR systems have been reviewed. These topics, when carefully considered and properly addressed prior to site construction or system selection, will help to clarify the process and contribute to a safe environment for patients and MR healthcare workers.

REFERENCES

1. Bell, R. A., Economics of MRI technology, *J. Magn. Reson. Imaging*, 6, 10, 1996.
2. Budinger, T. F., Biological and environmental hazards, in *Magnetic Resonance Imaging of the Body*, Higgins, C. B. and Hricak, H., Eds., Raven Press, New York, 1987, p. 539.
3. Jolesz, F. A., Interventional and intraoperative MRI: a general overview of the field, *J. Magn. Reson. Imaging*, 8, 3, 1998.
4. Peterfy, C. G., Roberts, T., and Genant, H. K., Dedicated extremity MR imaging, *Magn. Reson. Imaging Clin. North Am.*, 6, 849, 1998.
5. Bell, R. A., Tools of the trade for cost-effective MRI, *Diagn. Imaging,* April, 49, 1997.

8 Magnetic Resonance Procedures and Pregnancy

Patrick M. Colletti

CONTENTS

I. INTRODUCTION

Magnetic resonance imaging (MRI) has been used to evaluate obstetrical, placental, and fetal abnormalities in pregnant patients for more than 15 years. While a survey conducted in 1988 by Kanal et al.[1] showed that 36% of magnetic resonance (MR) facilities did not perform MRI examinations in pregnant patients because of the increased need to assess and manage this patient group, the use of MRI has become more commonplace. Notably, MRI is now recognized as a beneficial diagnostic tool and is utilized to assess a wide range of diseases and conditions that affect the pregnant patient as well as the fetus.

Initially, there were substantial technical problems with the use of MRI, primarily due to the presence of image degradation from fetal motion. However, several technological improvements, including the development of high-performance gradient systems and rapid pulse sequences, have provided major advances that are especially useful for imaging pregnant patients. Thus, high-quality MRI studies for obstetrical and fetal applications may now be accomplished routinely in the clinical setting.

Because of the importance and prevalence of MR procedures in pregnant patients, it is crucial to understand the safety aspects of this technology and the possible bioeffects associated with the presence of the electromagnetic fields used for MR. Therefore, this chapter will discuss pregnancy and MR safety, will present an overview of various clinical MR applications for pregnant patients, and will provide guidelines for the use of MR during pregnancy. Additionally, recommendations for pregnant healthcare workers will be discussed.

II. PREGNANCY AND MR SAFETY

The use of diagnostic imaging is often required in pregnant patients. Thus, it is not surprising that the question of whether or not a patient should undergo an MR procedure during pregnancy arises frequently. Unfortunately, there have been too few studies directed toward determining the relative safety of using MR procedures in pregnant patients. The main safety issues are related to the possible bioeffects of the static magnetic field of the MR system, the risks associated with exposure to the gradient magnetic fields, the potential adverse effects of the radiofrequency (RF) electro-magnetic fields, and the possible adverse effects related to the combination of these three different electromagnetic fields.

Notably, the MR environment-related risks are difficult to assess for pregnant patients due to the number of possible permutations of the various factors that are present in this setting (e.g., differences in field strengths, pulse sequences, etc.). This becomes even more complicated because new hardware and software are continually being developed for clinical MR systems.

Recommendations for the use of MR procedures in pregnant patients provided by regulatory agencies and professional organizations have been somewhat limited.

- 1983, the British Nuclear Regulatory Policy Bureau — "It might be prudent to exclude women (from MRI) during the first three months of pregnancy."[2]
- 1989, U.S. Food and Drug Administration — "The safety of MRI when used to image fetuses and infants has not been established."[3]
- 1991, Safety Committee for the Society of Magnetic Resonance Imaging — "MR imaging may be used in pregnant women if other non-ionizing forms of diagnostic imaging are inadequate or if the examination provides important information that would otherwise require exposure to ionizing radiation (e.g., fluoroscopy, CT, etc.). Pregnant patients should be informed that, to date, there has been no indication that the use of clinical MR imaging during pregnancy has produced deleterious effects."[4] This policy has also been adopted by the American College of Radiology and is now considered a "Standard of Care"[5] with reference to pregnant patients.

A. BASIC RESEARCH AND ANIMAL STUDIES

MRI exposes the patient and fetus to a static magnetic field, rapidly changing gradient magnetic fields and gradient noise, and RF irradiation. The overall effects of this electromagnetic energy on the human fetus are not easily determined. Consider the following:

- The strength of the static magnetic field of the MR system is known (e.g., 1.5 T).
- The gradient amplitude (e.g., 20 mT/m) and slew rate, dB/dt (e.g., 3 T/s), may be determined at the location of the fetus for a given pulse sequence; however, several different pulse sequences are typically used during an MRI examination.
- RF energy deposition and absorption will vary considerably with the MR system, RF coil, and the pulse sequence that is used. Common pulse sequences used for fast fetal imaging, such as single-shot fast spin echo, employ multiple rapid RF pulses and would be expected to deposit much more RF energy compared to the use of gradient echo pulse sequences.

- RF absorption varies considerably within the human body. For example, approximately 87% of the RF energy would be deposited in the outer one third of the body.[6] Thus, ignoring "hot spot" RF energy deposition, the embryo or fetus should receive a relatively small RF exposure during MRI.
- Heating is the only well-established mechanism for RF bioeffects.[7] The fetus has a large surface area-to-volume ratio. Convective heat transfer to the amniotic fluid, with its relatively high heat capacity, should enhance fetal cooling, if needed.
- The relatively "deep" anatomic position of the fetus and the surrounding amniotic fluid could help to reduce the effects of gradient noise.
- In addition, the stage of pregnancy is very important with regard to the potential risk to the embryo or fetus, and spontaneous adverse outcomes are very common[8] (see Table 8.1).

TABLE 8.1
Spontaneous Adverse Outcomes of Pregnancy[8]

Period	Risk	Spontaneous Occurrence Rate
Day 1-10	Reabsorption	30%
Day 10-50	Abnormal organogenesis	4-6%
>Day 50	Intra-uterine growth retardation	4%

There have been a number of laboratory and clinical research investigations conducted to determine the effects of the use of MRI during pregnancy. Most of the laboratory studies showed no evidence of injury or harm to the fetus (Table 8.2), while a few studies reported adverse outcomes for laboratory animals (Table 8.3). By comparison, there have been relatively few studies performed in humans exposed to MRI or the MR environment *in utero* (Table 8.4). Each of these investigations reported no adverse outcomes for human subjects. For example, Baker et al.[26] reported no demonstrable increase in disease, disability, or hearing loss in 20 children examined *in utero* with echoplanar MRI for suspected fetal compromise. Myers et al.[27] reported no significant reduction in fetal growth vs. matched controls in 74 volunteer subjects exposed *in utero* to echo-planar MRI at 0.5 T.

TABLE 8.2
Safety of MRI in Pregnancy — Non-Adverse Outcomes

Study	Findings
McRobbie and Foster, 1985[9]	No change in litter number or growth rate in mice exposed to gradients ranging from 3.5-12 kT/s
Teskey et al., 1987[10]	No change in stress reactivity or survivability in rats repeatedly exposed *in utero*
Heinrichs et al., 1988[11]	No embryo toxicity or teratogenesis with prolonged exposure (BLB/c mice, midgestational, 0.35 T)
Kay et al., 1988[12]	No adverse effects (*Xenopus laevis* embryo, long-term exposure, 1.5 T)
Tyndall, 1990[13]	MRI exposure does not add to low-level X-ray irradiation-induced teratogenesis in C57B1/6J mice at 1.5 T
Murkami et al., 1992[14]	No change in pregnancy outcomes for mice exposed to 6.3 T for 1 h per day from days 7 to 14
Malko et al., 1994[15]	No change in cell density (yeast cells grown at 1.5 T)
Yip et al., 1994[16] Yip et al., 1995[17]	No change in survival, migration, and proliferation; no effect on axonal growth in chick embryos exposed to simulated imaging conditions at 1.5 T
Tablado et al., 2000[18]	No testicular abnormalities in mice continually exposed *in utero* from day 7 to birth at 0.7 T

TABLE 8.3
Safety of MRI in Pregnancy — Adverse Outcomes

Study	Findings
Tyndall and Sulik, 1991[19]	At least twofold increased incidence of eye malformations (C57B16J mice, 10% spontaneous eye malformations, gestational day 7, 1.5 T for 36 min)
Tyndall, 1993[20]	Increased teratogenicity with reduced crown-rump length and craniofacial size in C57B1/6J mice exposed to clinically realistic MRI at 1.5 T
Yip et al., 1994[21]	"Trend toward higher abnormality and mortality rates" in chick embryos exposed to simulated imaging conditions at 1.5 T
Carnes et al., 1996[22]	Fetal weight reduction (11%) in mice exposed for 8 h in midgestation at 4.7 T
Nara et al., 1996[23]	Reduced spermatogenesis and embryogenesis in Webster mice exposed *in utero* to 1.5 T for 30 min

TABLE 8.4
Safety of MRI in Pregnancy — Non-Adverse Outcomes in Humans

Study	Findings
Johnson et al., 1990[24]	No change in fetal heart rate or Doppler-determined umbilical artery blood flow (humans, 10–20 weeks, 0.5 T)
Kanal et al., 1993[25]	No increase in adverse reproductive outcomes (280 pregnant female MRI workers)
Baker et al., 1994[26]	No increase in disease or disability, no hearing loss in 20 children at 3 years after *in utero* exposure to echo-planar MRI at 0.5 T
Myers et al., 1998[27]	No significant decrease vs. matched controls in fetal growth in 74 volunteers exposed *in utero* to echo-planar MRI up to five times at 0.5 T
Vadeyar et al., 2000[28]	No change in fetal heart rate in human volunteers at term (37–41 weeks), echo-planar MRI at 0.5 T

A longer term study is ongoing. A survey of reproductive health among 280 pregnant MR healthcare workers performed by Kanal et al.[25] showed no substantial increase in common adverse reproductive outcomes.

In consideration of the literature published to date, there apparently are discrepancies with respect to the experimental findings of the effects of electromagnetic fields used for MR procedures and the pertinent safety aspects of pregnancy. These discrepancies may be explained by a variety of factors, including the differences in the scientific methodology used for the experiment, the type of organism examined, and the variance in exposure duration as well as the conditions of the exposure to the electromagnetic fields. Obviously, additional investigations are warranted before the risks associated with exposure to MR procedures can be absolutely known and properly characterized.

B. MR Contrast Agents and Pregnancy

The placenta is very vascular with a large blood pool. Thus, MR contrast agents show prominent placental localization when used during MRI examinations (Figure 8.1). The currently approved MR contrast agents are of low molecular weight (Table 8.5) and readily cross the placental barrier.

Massive doses of these agents have been shown to cause post-implantation fetal loss, retarded development, increased locomotive activity, and skeletal and visceral abnormalities in experimental animals (Table 8.6). Thus, the U.S. Food and Drug Administration lists parenteral MR contrast agents as "PREGNANCY CATEGORY C." Statements such as "adequate and controlled studies in pregnant woman have not been conducted" and *this agent* "should only be used during pregnancy

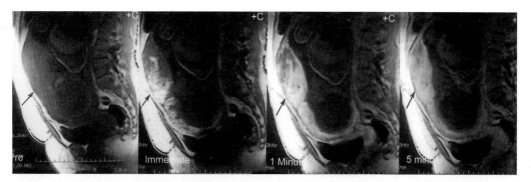

FIGURE 8.1 Dynamic contrast enhancement of the placenta (arrow) in a 28-year-old pregnant woman at 30 weeks. Note the rapid, heterogeneous enhancement.

TABLE 8.5
Currently Approved MRI Contrast Agents

Agent	Molecular Weight
Gadopentetate dimeglumine (Magnevist™, Berlex, Wayne, NJ)	938
Gadoteridol (ProHance™, Bracco, Princeton, NJ)	559
Gadodiamide (Omniscan™, Nycomed Amersham, Princeton, NJ)	574
Gadovesetamide (OptiMARK™, Mallinkrodt, St. Louis, MO)	661
Mangafodipar (Teslascan™, Nycomed Amersham, Princeton, NJ)	757
Ferumoxide (Feridex IV™, Berlex, Wayne, NJ)	83, in particles of 80–160 nm (would not cross placental barrier)

TABLE 8.6
Safety of MRI Contrast Agents in Pregnancy[a]

Post-implantation fetal loss in rats (ProHance, 33× human dose for 12 days)

Retarded development in rats (Magnevist, 2.5× human dose) and in rabbits (Magnevist, 7.5–12.5× human dose for 12 days)

Increased locomotor activity in rats (ProHance, 20–33× human dose for 12 days)

Skeletal and visceral abnormalities in rabbits (Omniscan, 5× human dose)

Teratogenicity in rabbits at doses 6× the usual cleared dose (Feridex I.V.)

Fetotoxic and embryotoxic in rats and rabbits ("Teslascan, …must not be given to pregnant women.") (Package insert)

Reduced birth weight in mice at 0.5 mmol/day for 5 weeks; reduced fetal weight, abnormal liver lobules, delayed ossification, and delayed development in rats at 10× human dose for days 7-17; not seen at 1× human dose/day; Forelimb flexion-contractions, cardiovascular abnormalities in rabbits at 1-4× human dose/day 6-18 (OptiMARK)

[a] Data from package inserts of ProHance, Magnevist, Omniscan, OptiMARK, Feridex, and Teslascan.

if the potential benefit justifies the potential risk to the fetus" are typically noted in package inserts for MR contrast agents.

After intravenous administration of gadolinium chelates, a portion of the agent localizes to the placenta, and, from there, a small portion reaches the fetus. If the fetal kidneys are developed (beyond 7 weeks), the gadolinium chelate is excreted into the fetal bladder (Figure 8.2), where it is voided into the amniotic fluid. From there, some of the contrast material is swallowed by the fetus, where it passes through the fetal gut and reenters the amniotic fluid.[25] Based on adult studies, fetal intestinal absorption is not expected. The potential for breakdown of the gadolinium chelate bond, while theoretically possible, seems unlikely.

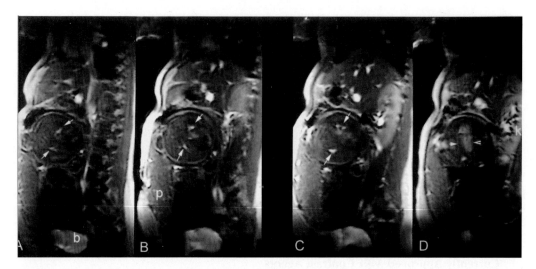

FIGURE 8.2 Contrast enhanced spoiled gradient echo MR of the fetus at 32 weeks shows fetal renal enhancement (arrows) (A, B, C) and fetal bladder (arrowheads) (D). Also shown are the maternal kidney (k), the bladder (b), and the placenta (p).

III. CLINICAL APPLICATIONS OF MR PROCEDURES IN PREGNANT PATIENTS

A. NON-PELVIC IMAGING

The pregnant patient is subject to most of the same brain, spine, body, and musculoskeletal conditions as the non-pregnant patient.[29] In addition, abnormalities associated with pregnancy, such as toxemia (Figure 8.3) and sagittal sinus thrombosis (Figure 8.4), can occur. Pituitary adenomas may show growth during pregnancy (Figure 8.5). Obviously, medical imaging is frequently required to assess and manage patients with these conditions. Because MRI does not use ionizing radiation, it is particularly suited as an alternative to computed tomography (CT), especially in cases where the use of ultrasound is unsatisfactory and inappropriate.

1. Brain Imaging

Besides the brain conditions associated with pregnancy, common cerebral conditions such as tumor, infarction, hemorrhage (Figure 8.6), arteriovenous malformation, and aneurysm may occur during pregnancy. These are also best evaluated with MRI testing. MR contrast agents should be reserved for patients in whom diagnosis (i.e., metastasis) or therapy (i.e., brain tumor therapy prior to surgery) is needed immediately (Figures 8.7 to 8.9). Diffusion-weighted imaging is useful if acute cerebral infarction is suspected. MR angiography is helpful to screen for cerebral aneurysm in pregnant patients with a family history of aneurysm in preparation for the stress of vaginal delivery.

2. Spine Imaging

MRI should be reserved for specific cases of suspected disc extrusion, in which surgery would be performed during the pregnancy. The use of MRI is also appropriate for the evaluation of spinal tumor, unstable fracture (Figure 8.10), infection, syrinx, or arteriovenous (AV) malformation (Figure 8.11), all of which would affect immediate therapy or mode of delivery (caesarean section vs. vaginal delivery).

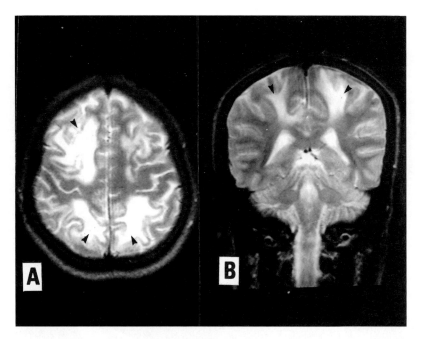

FIGURE 8.3 A 32-year-old woman presents with hypertension and headaches at 34 weeks of pregnancy. Axial (A) and coronal (B) T2-weighted (TR 2500, TE 100) views of the brain show white matter edema (arrowheads). Diagnosis: toxemia of pregnancy. (From Colletti, P.M. and Sylvestre, P.B., *Magn. Reson. Imaging Clin. North Am.*, 2, 291, 1994. With permission.)

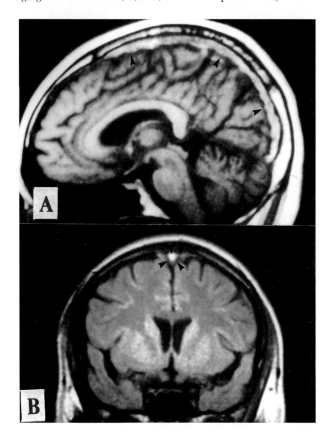

FIGURE 8.4 A 22-year-old woman presents with severe headache at 12 weeks of pregnancy. She has a history of hyperemesis gravidarium. Sagittal (A) and axial (B) T1-weighted (TR 400, TE 20) views show high signal in the sagittal sinus (arrowheads). The pregnancy was terminated, and she improved on anticoagulant therapy. Diagnosis: sagittal sinus thrombosis. (From Colletti, P.M. and Sylvestre, P.B., *Magn. Reson. Imaging Clin. North Am.*, 2, 291, 1994. With permission.)

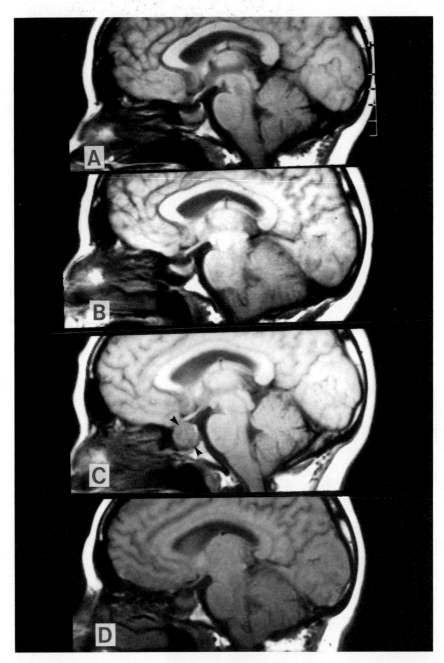

FIGURE 8.5 A 36-year-old woman presents with headache at 14 weeks of pregnancy. She has a history of pituitary microadenoma treated with bromocriptine. Sagittal T1-weighted (TR 400, TE 20) views of the brain at 2 years (A) and 1 year (B) prior to the pregnancy show no pituitary mass. The examination during pregnancy (C) shows pituitary enlargement (arrowheads). A follow-up study at 1-year post-pregnancy (D) shows a reduction in pituitary size. Diagnosis: pituitary enlargement in pregnancy. (From Colletti, P.M. and Sylvestre, P.B., *Magn. Reson. Imaging Clin. North Am.*, 2, 291, 1994. With permission.)

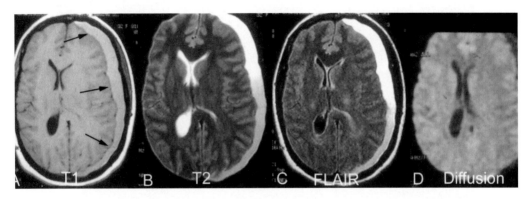

FIGURE 8.6 A 23-year-old woman presents with severe headache and lethargy at 18 weeks of pregnancy. Axial T1-weighted (A), T2-weighted (B), FLAIR (C), and diffusion weighted images (D) show a prominent left-sided subdural hematoma (arrows) with midline shift. The subdural hematoma was evacuated, and the patient improved. Diagnosis: non-traumatic subdural hematoma.

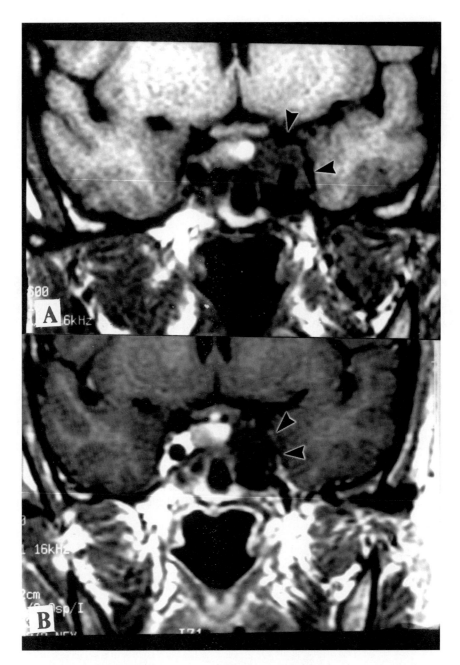

FIGURE 8.7 A 28-year-old woman presents with blurred vision in the left eye at 25 weeks of pregnancy. Non-enhanced (A) and contrast enhanced (B) coronal T1-weighted (TR 600, TE 20) views show a non-enhancing, left cavernous sinus mass (arrows). An epidermoid was resected after delivery at 34 weeks. Diagnosis: cavernous sinus epidermoid. (From Colletti, P.M. and Sylvestre, P.B., *Magn. Reson. Imaging Clin. North Am.*, 2, 291, 1994. With permission.)

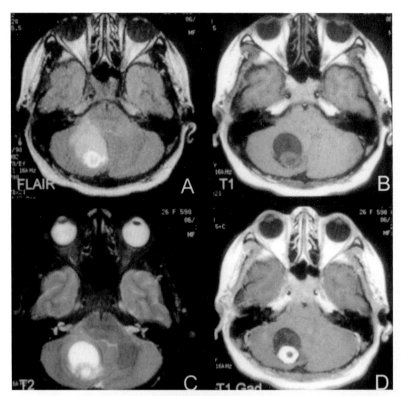

FIGURE 8.8 A 26-year-old woman presents with headache and dizziness at 8 weeks of pregnancy. FLAIR (A), T1-weighted (B), and T2-weighted (C) images show a right cerebellar cystic mass with a solid enhancing (D) nodule. The pregnancy was terminated, and a right posterior fossa craniectomy was performed to resect a cystic astrocytoma. Diagnosis: cerebellar cystic astrocytoma.

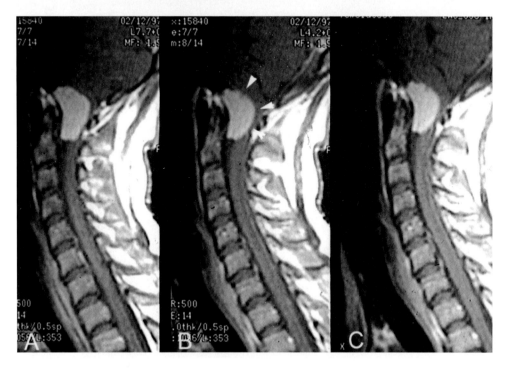

FIGURE 8.9 A 32-year-old woman presents with increasing weakness and lethargy at 22 weeks of pregnancy. Contrast enhanced sagittal T1-weighted (TR 400, TE 20) views (A, B, C) of the craniovertebral junction show a large, enhancing foramen magnum mass. A meningioma was resected. Diagnosis: foramen magnum meningioma.

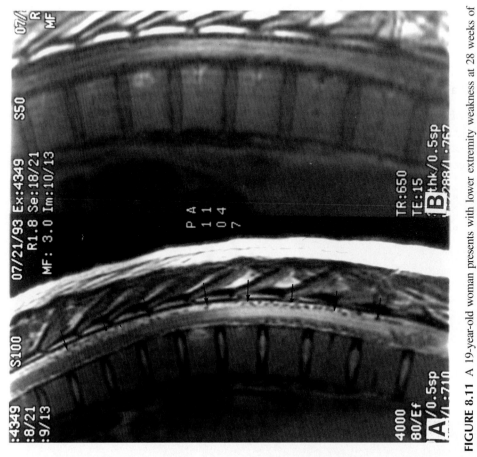

FIGURE 8.11 A 19-year-old woman presents with lower extremity weakness at 28 weeks of pregnancy. Sagittal T2-weighted (TR 4000, TE$_{eff}$ 80) FSE images (A) show an extensive spinal arteriovenous malformation (arrows). A post-contrast T1-weighted (TR 650, TE 15) view (B) did not add to the diagnosis. Diagnosis: spinal arteriovenous malformation. (From Colletti, P.M. and Sylvestre, P.B., *Magn. Reson. Imaging Clin. North Am.*, 2, 291, 1994. With permission.)

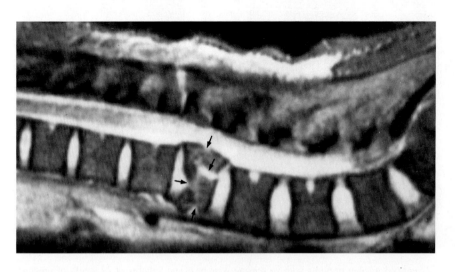

FIGURE 8.10 A 20-year-old woman was thrown out of a second story window at 28 weeks of pregnancy. Sagittal gradient echo image shows fractures of the anterior, middle, and posterior columns of the L-2 vertebra (arrows). Diagnosis: burst fracture. (From Colletti, P.M. and Sylvestre, P.B., *Magn. Reson. Imaging Clin. North Am.*, 2, 291, 1994. With permission.)

3. Head and Neck Imaging

MRI of the head and neck may be advantageous as compared to CT because of its lack of ionizing radiation and lesser need for the use of contrast agents.

4. Chest and Cardiovascular Imaging

Hilar and mediastinal nodes can be shown easily with MRI (Figure 8.12) without the use of ionizing radiation or contrast agents. Cardiovascular MRI is ideal to demonstrate and confirm abnormalities such as coarctation of the aorta, aortitis, aortic dissection, and arterial myxoma in the pregnant patient. Echocardiography remains the standard, non-invasive cardiac imaging modality, particularly in the pregnant patient.

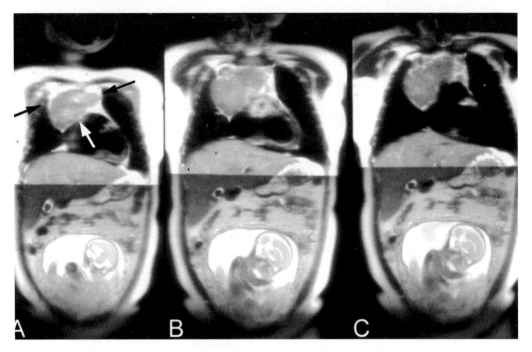

FIGURE 8.12 A 24-year-old woman presents with a right neck mass at 27 weeks of pregancy. Biopsy revealed low-grade lymphoma. Whole-body, single-shot fast spin echo (ssFSE) MRI (A, B, C) shows extensive mediastinal adenopathy (arrows). No abdominal or pelvic disease is seen. Gallstones and the fetus are seen. Diagnosis: lymphoma.

5. Abdominal Imaging

Sonography is the examination of choice for abdominal imaging in the pregnant patient, particularly to evaluate for hepatobiliary and renal lesions. The absence of ionizing radiation gives MRI an advantage over CT, particularly to evaluate the liver, pancreas, and retroperitonium. Large lesions such as tumors, pseudocysts (Figure 8.13), and abscesses (Figure 8.14) are shown well with MRI. A fatty liver in pregnancy may also be evaluated with MRI.

6. Musculoskeletal Imaging

MRI is useful in the evaluation of musculoskeletal abnormalities in selected patients in whom intervention is required during pregnancy. Routine knee and shoulder examinations can often be delayed until after delivery, but the evaluation of suspected infection[30] (Figure 8.15) or neoplasm (Figure 8.16) must often be performed immediately.

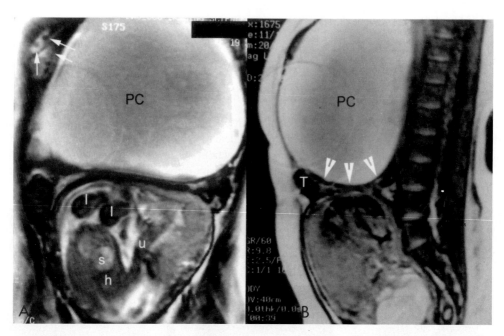

FIGURE 8.13 A 19-year-old woman presents with severe abdominal pain and as "large for dates" at 26 weeks of pregnancy. Ultrasonography showed a large cystic mass. Its relation to pelvic organs could not be determined. A coronal fast gradient echo subsecond image (A) shows a large pseudocyst (PC). Several gallstones are seen (arrows). Details of the fetus (f) are seen, including the upper (u) and lower (l) extremities, stomach (s), and heart (h). A sagittal fast gradient echo image (B) again shows the pseudocyst (PC). The transverse colon (T) and mesocolon (arrowheads) separate this cyst from the uterus and pelvic structures. Gallstones, pancreatitis, and a pseudocyst were found at surgery. (From Colletti, P.M. and Sylvestre, P.B., *Magn. Reson. Imaging Clin. North Am.*, 2, 291, 1994. With permission.)

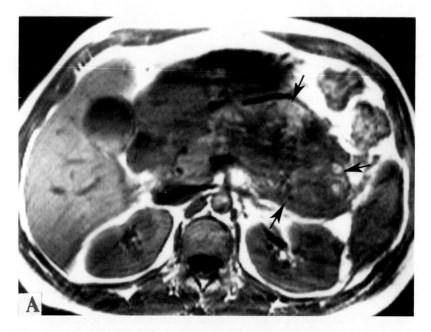

FIGURE 8.14 A 28-year-old woman presents with abdominal pain and fever at 12 weeks of pregnancy. An axial T1-weighted (TR 500, TE 20) abdominal study (A) shows an edematous pancreas (arrows). (From Colletti, P.M. and Sylvestre, P.B., *Magn. Reson. Imaging Clin. North Am.*, 2, 291, 1994. With permission.) (*continued*)

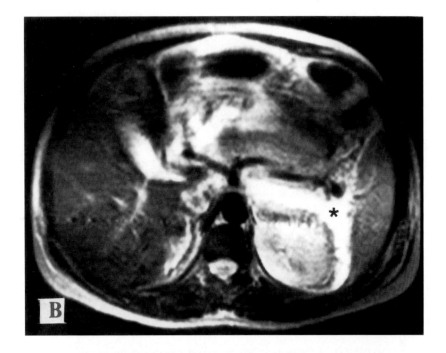

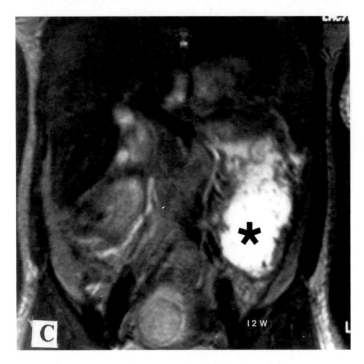

FIGURE 8.14 (CONTINUED) A 28-year-old woman presents with abdominal pain and fever at 12 weeks of pregnancy. An axial T2-weighted (TR 2200, TE 100) view (B) shows fluid in the anterior pararenal space (*). This is confirmed on a coronal T2-weighted (TR 2200, TE 80) view (C). One liter of inflammatory fluid was aspirated with ultrasound guidance. The patient's pain and fever subsided. (From Colletti, P.M. and Sylvestre, P.B., *Magn. Reson. Imaging Clin. North Am.*, 2, 291, 1994. With permission.)   (*continued*)

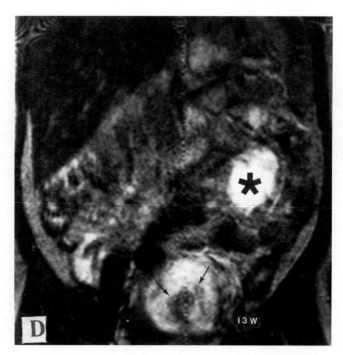

FIGURE 8.14 (CONTINUED) A 28-year-old woman presents with abdominal pain and fever at 12 weeks of pregnancy. One liter of inflammatory fluid was aspirated with ultrasound guidance. The patient's pain and fever subsided. Follow-up coronal examination at 13 weeks (D) shows reduction in the anterior pararenal space fluid (*). The fetus (arrows) is seen. Diagnosis: pancreatic phlegmon. (From Colletti, P.M. and Sylvestre, P.B., *Magn. Reson. Imaging Clin. North Am.*, 2, 291, 1994. With permission.)

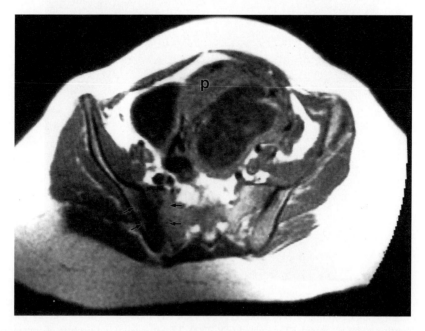

FIGURE 8.15 A 22-year-old woman with a history of intravenous drug abuse presents with severe right sacroiliac pain and fever at 14 weeks of pregnancy. An axial T1-weighted (TR 500, TE 20) view of the pelvis shows a pregnant uterus (p = placenta) along with an abnormal low signal right sacroiliac joint (arrows). Diagnosis: *S. aureus* sacroiliitis. (From Colletti, P.M. and Sylvestre, P.B., *Magn. Reson. Imaging Clin. North Am.*, 2, 291, 1994. With permission.)

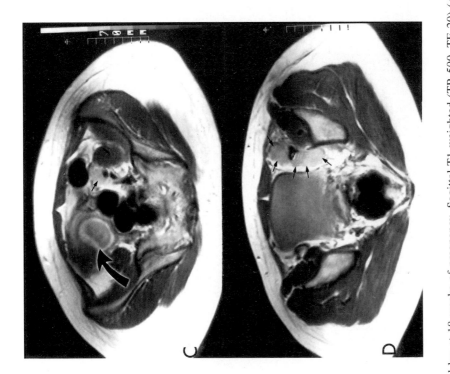

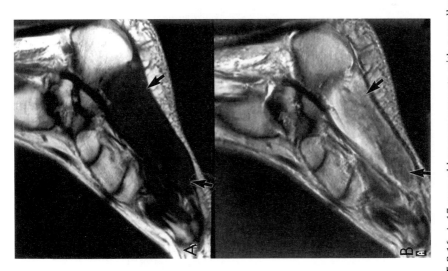

FIGURE 8.16 A 17-year-old woman presents with a swollen left foot and leg at 18 weeks of pregnancy. Sagittal T1-weighted (TR 500, TE 20) (A) and T2-weighted (TR 2000, TE 80) (B) views of the left foot show a mass (arrows). Axial T1-weighted (TR 400, TE 20) (C, D) images show the fetus on the right (curved arrow) and left iliac adenopathy (arrows). (From Colletti, P.M. and Sylvestre, P.B., *Magn. Reson. Imaging Clin. North Am.*, 2, 291, 1994. With permission.)   *(continued)*

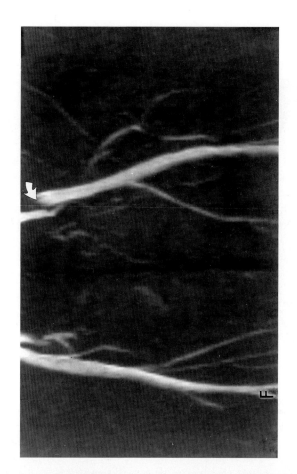

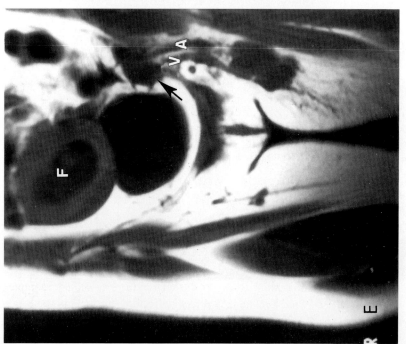

FIGURE 8.16 (CONTINUED) A 17-year-old woman presents with a swollen left foot and leg at 18 weeks of pregnancy. A coronal T1-weighted (TR 400, TE 20) view (E) shows the relationship of the mass (arrow) to the femoral artery (A) and vein (V); fetus (F). A two-dimensional time-of-flight venogram shows near total occlusion of the left iliac vein (white curved arrow) by the mass. Pregnancy was terminated at 20 weeks. Diagnosis: rhabdomyosarcoma. (From Colletti, P.M. and Sylvestre, P.B., *Magn. Reson. Imaging Clin. North Am.*, 2, 291, 1994. With permission.)

B. Pelvic Imaging

Pregnancy can accelerate the growth of benign and malignant pelvic masses. A common diagnostic differential decision involves the separation of uterine abnormalities such as leiomyoma from adnexal lesions, including ovarian cysts and neoplasms. Occasionally, sonography has difficulty with this distinction, particularly in larger lesions. MRI may better delineate and characterize these abnormalities[31,32] (Figures 8.17 to 8.19). Breath-held MR images obtained using pulse sequences to acquire relative T1 and T2 weighting are useful to localize and characterize lesions.

MR angiography may be used to demonstrate pelvic, arterial (Figure 8.20), and venous abnormalities in the pregnant patient. An enlarged uterus may cause markedly reduced flow in the inferior vena cava and iliac veins with extensive collateral vessel formation (Figure 8.21A) during the third trimester. Blood vessels may be exquisitely shown using two-dimensional time-of-flight MR angiography with superior saturation. Normal fetal vessels may also be visualized with this technique (Figure 8.21B).

Furthermore, MRI may be useful to demonstrate pelvic abnormalities related specifically to pregnancy, such as placenta acretea, abruptio placentae, chorioangioma, ectopic pregnancy, and abdominal pregnancy (Figure 8.22). MR pelvimetry[33] is often used as an alternative to radiographic or CT pelvimetry.

C. Imaging of the Fetus

There have been a number of institutional review board-approved MRI studies of fetal abnormalities.[24,34-68] Fetal sedation is no longer considered necessary to perform good fetal MRI. While gross fetal motion may cause image degradation, much of the difficulty in fetal imaging is due to maternal respiration. Current techniques generally utilize breath-held imaging with single-shot fast spin echo (ssFSE) techniques[69-78] (Figures 8.23 to 8.25) along with fast gradient refocused echo or fast spoiled gradient echo imaging techniques. Echo-planar techniques have also shown considerable success in fetal imaging.

Because the very abnormal fetus often has reduced fat due to growth retardation, MR images obtained in these cases may show relatively poor anatomic detail. Brain myelination *in utero* may be demonstrated using T1- and T2-weighted images. Normal fetal structures such as the brain, face, spine, heart, liver, stomach, intestines, and bladder are seen routinely. Often, the fetal genitalia are identified. Obviously, these structures are much more easy to evaluate in later pregnancy, although with higher quality faster techniques, reasonable detail can be obtained by the mid-second trimester.

The use of MRI can confirm most sonographically detected gross fetal abnormalities such as hydrocephalus, anencephaly, meningocele, omphalocele, gastroschisis, and teratoma. Subtle anomalies such as limb abnormality are more difficult to detect, but even these are demonstrated occasionally with current imaging techniques. MRI gives information not apparent on sonography in approximately 10% of the cases. This is most often seen in the fetal brain, but, again with current techniques, occasionally fetal lungs, fetal diaphragm, fetal liver, and fetal kidneys may be better shown with MR procedures.

A recent study was conducted by Coakley et al.[78] to determine the effect of using MRI findings for the management of complex fetal disorders. These disorders included congenital high-airway obstruction syndrome, congenital hemochromatosis, unilateral cerebellar deficiency in association with congenital diaphragmatic hernia, and severe facial disfigurement secondary to a giant anterior neck mass. The results of this investigation indicated that using MRI in the evaluation of complex fetal disorders provides incremental information that may directly affect management in a substantial proportion of cases.[78] In other cases, MRI findings may help supplement or confirm indeterminate or equivocal ultrasound findings.

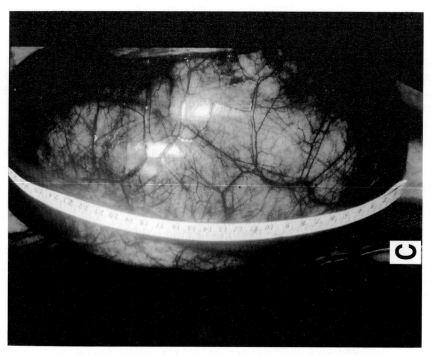

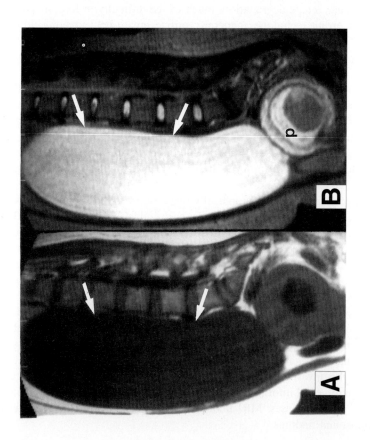

FIGURE 8.17 A 32-year-old woman presents as large for dates at 12 weeks of pregnancy. Ultrasound showed a very large cystic mass superior to the uterus. Sagittal T1-weighted (TR 400, TE 20) (A) and T2-weighted (TR 2000, TE 80) (B) views show a large cystic mass separate from the uterus (p = placenta). At surgery, a 30-cm cyst was resected (C). Diagnosis: giant corpus luteum cyst in pregnancy. (From Colletti, P.M. and Sylvestre, P.B., *Magn. Reson. Imaging Clin. North Am.*, 2, 291, 1994. With permission.)

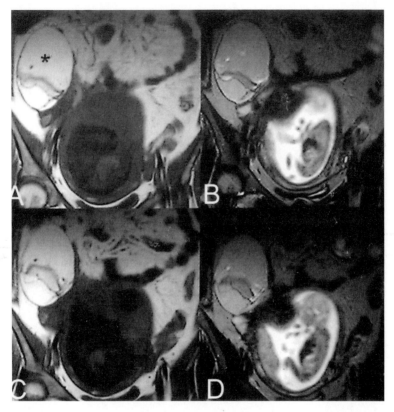

FIGURE 8.18 A 23-year-old woman presents as large for dates at 20 weeks of pregnancy. Ultrasound showed a right midabdominal complex mass. Coronal T1-weighted (A, C) and T2-weighted (B, D) images show a right abdominal complex mass containing high signal fat and low signal septa. Diagnosis: dermoid.

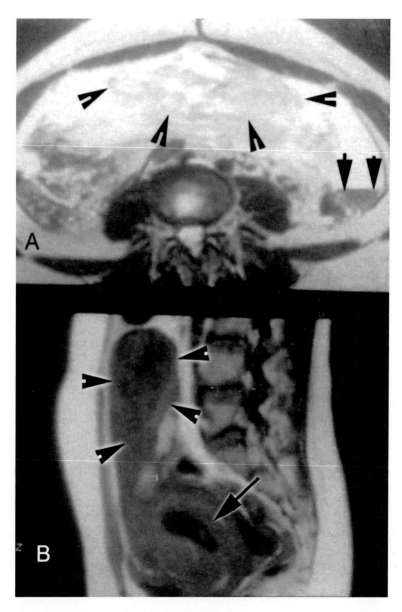

FIGURE 8.19 A 19-year-old woman presents with abdominal pain and large for dates at 13 weeks of pregnancy. Ultrasound showed a pelvic mass and ascites. An axial T2-weighted (TR 3500, TE_{eff} 90) view (A) shows ascites with layering of low signal blood products in the left paracolic gutter (arrows). A large omental mass is seen anteriorly (arrowheads). A sagittal T1-weighted (TR 400, TE 20) view shows the omental mass (arrowheads) superior to the pregnant uterus (arrow). (From Colletti, P.M. and Sylvestre, P.B., *Magn. Reson. Imaging Clin. North Am.*, 2, 291, 1994. With permission.) (*continued*)

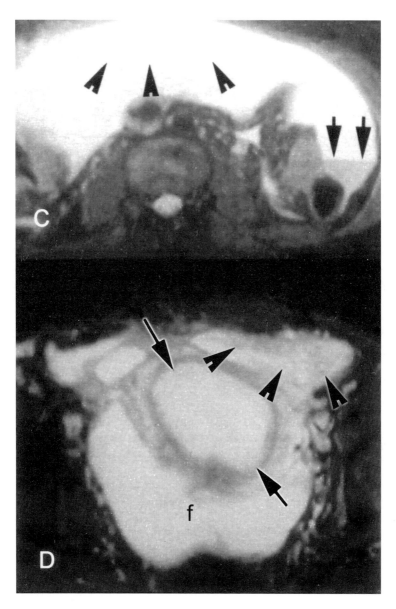

FIGURE 8.19 (CONTINUED) A 19-year-old woman presents with abdominal pain and large for dates at 13 weeks of pregnancy. Ultrasound showed a pelvic mass and ascites. Axial fast inversion recovery (STIR) images (C, D) confirm the findings. f = fluid. Diagnosis: embryonal cell cancer, probably ovarian with hemorrhagic ascites and omental metastasis. (From Colletti, P.M. and Sylvestre, P.B., *Magn. Reson. Imaging Clin. North Am.*, 2, 291, 1994. With permission.)

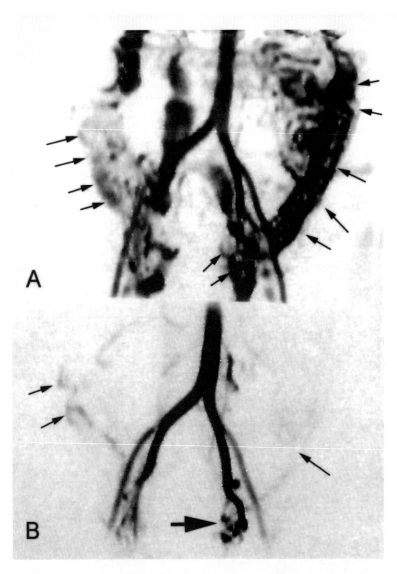

FIGURE 8.20 A 35-year-old woman with a history of a pelvic arteriovenous malformation presents at 28 weeks of pregnancy. Two-dimensional time-of-flight (A) and three-dimensional phase contrast (B), venc = 80 cm/s, MR angiograms show the extensive pelvic AVM (arrows). Large supplying vessels are seen on the phase contrast study (curved arrow). The images were used to help plan for cesarean delivery due to failure of progression of labor. Diagnosis: pelvic AVM. (From Colletti, P.M. and Sylvestre, P.B., *Magn. Reson. Imaging Clin. North Am.*, 2, 291, 1994. With permission.)

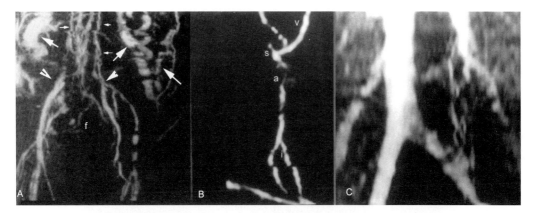

FIGURE 8.21 A 32-year-old woman presents with markedly swollen legs at 30 weeks of pregnancy. Two-dimensional time-of-flight MR angiography with superior saturation (A) shows apparent occlusions of the iliac veins (curved arrows) and extensive collateral vessels (large arrows), including epidural vessels (small arrows). Fetal (f) vessels also are seen. Targeted MIP display of the fetal vessels (B) shows flow in the superior to inferior direction due to superior presaturation and cephalic presentation: v = brachiocephalic veins, s = superior vena cava, a = aorta, i = iliac arteries. A two-dimensional time-of-flight examination with superior presaturation performed immediately after delivery (C) shows normal veins with normal left iliac vein narrowing. Diagnosis: extrinsic compression of the iliac veins and inferior vena cava by the pregnant uterus. (From Colletti, P.M. and Sylvestre, P.B., *Magn. Reson. Imaging Clin. North Am.*, 2, 291, 1994. With permission.)

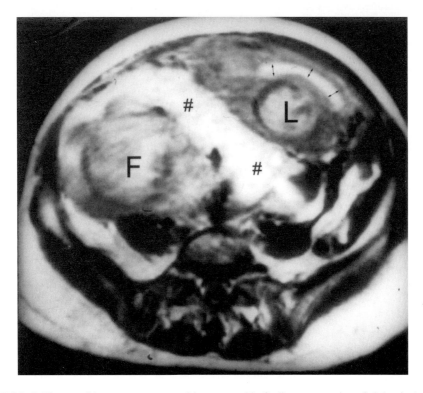

FIGURE 8.22 A 22-year-old woman presents with sonographic findings suggestive of abdominal pregnancy at 32 weeks pregnancy. An axial proton density-weighted (TR 2000, TE 20) view shows the uterus on the left side (endometrial cavity = double arrows) with a prominent leiomyoma (L). The fetus (F) is separated from the uterus by fluid (#). An abdominal pregnancy was successfully surgically delivered. (From Colletti, P.M. and Sylvestre, P.B., *Magn. Reson. Imaging Clin. North Am.*, 2, 291, 1994. With permission.)

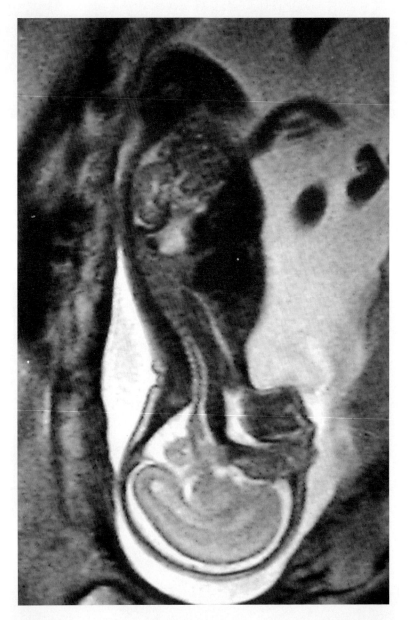

FIGURE 8.23 Breath-held, 11-s ssFSE sagittal view shows normal fetal anatomy at 24 weeks.

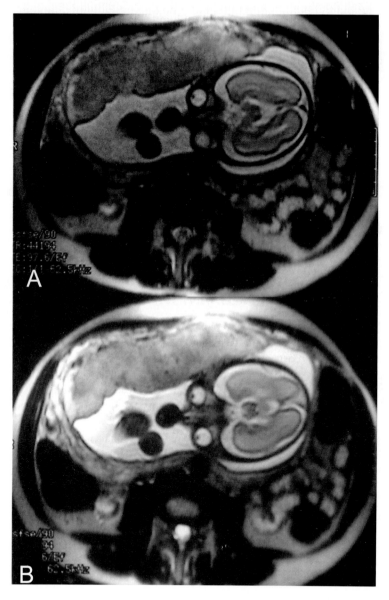

FIGURE 8.24 Axial, breath-held, 12-s ssFSE views show normal fetal anatomy at 28 weeks. Images at the level of the fetal midbrain (A) and pons (B) are seen.

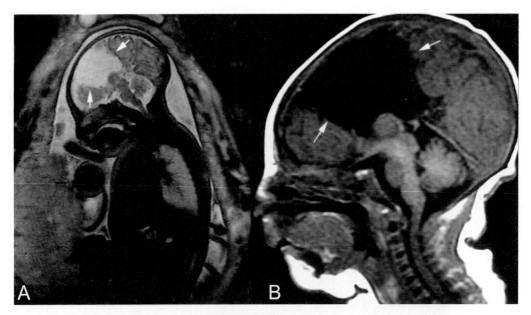

FIGURE 8.25 A coronal, breath-held, 11-s ssFSE view (A, inverted for display) at 32 weeks of pregnancy shows agenesis of the corpus callosum and a large midline cleft (arrows). A sagittal T1-weighted (TR 400, TE 18) view of the newborn on day 3 confirms these findings.

IV. RECOMMENDED GUIDELINES FOR THE USE OF MR PROCEDURES IN PREGNANT PATIENTS

Basically, MR procedures may be used in pregnant patients to address important clinical problems or to manage potential complications for the patient or fetus. The MR procedure should be conducted using a verbal and written informed consent procedure. The pregnant patient should be informed that, based on the currently available data, there is no indication that the use of clinical MRI during pregnancy produces deleterious effects.[5] As previously indicated, this standard policy has been adopted by the American College of Radiology and is considered to be the "standard of care" with respect to the use of MR procedures in pregnant patients.

The overall decision to utilize an MR procedure in a pregnant patient involves answering a series of important questions, including the following (Figure 8.26 supplies a flowchart summarizing these decisions):[29]

- Is the patient pregnant?
- Is sonography satisfactory for diagnosis?
- Is the MR procedure appropriate to address the clinical question?
- Can the MR procedure be delayed until later in pregnancy (second or third trimester) or until after delivery?
- Is obstetrical intervention prior to the MR procedure a possibility? That is, is termination of pregnancy a consideration? Is early delivery a consideration?
- Is an MR contrast agent essential to diagnosis and treatment?

V. PREGNANT HEALTHCARE WORKERS IN THE MR ENVIRONMENT

Pregnant healthcare workers rarely find themselves in the MR system during acquisition of imaging data. Thus, there is little or no exposure to the gradient and RF electromagnetic fields. The main exposure to the pregnant healthcare worker is to a static magnetic field, with time and distance

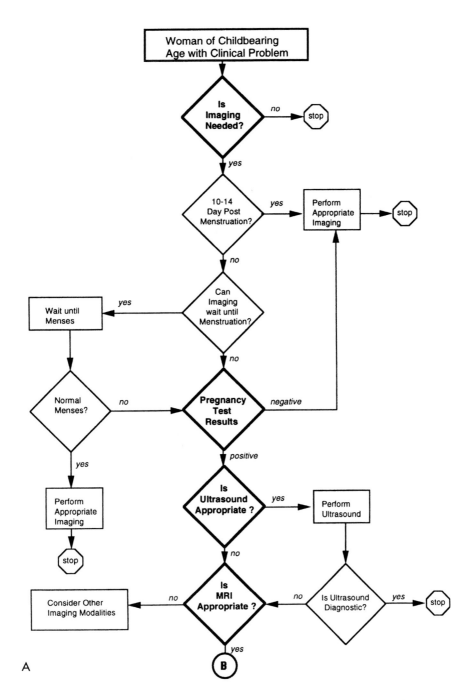

FIGURE 8.26 (A and B) Decision-making flowchart for the use of MRI in the pregnant patient. (From Colletti, P.M. and Sylvestre, P.B., *Magn. Reson. Imaging Clin. North Am.*, 2, 291, 1994. With permission.) (*continued*)

from the magnet being the major variations. Notably, the pregnant technologist might be within a static magnetic field of several hundred gauss or more each working day for prolonged periods of time. However, this level of exposure to the magnetic field is not considered to be deleterious or injurious to the embryo or fetus.

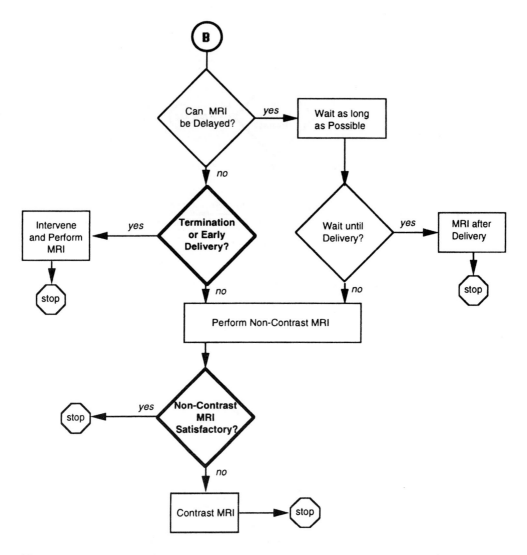

B

FIGURE 8.26 (CONTINUED) (A and B) Decision-making flowchart for the use of MRI in the pregnant patient. (From Colletti, P.M. and Sylvestre, P.B., *Magn. Reson. Imaging Clin. North Am.*, 2, 291, 1994. With permission.)

Because of the concern for pregnant MRI technologists and other healthcare workers to be present in the MR environment, a survey of reproductive health among female MR system operators was conducted in 1990 by Kanal et al.[25] Questionnaires were sent to all female MR technologists and nurses at the majority of clinical MR facilities in the U.S.

The findings from this extensive epidemiological investigation were reassuring insofar as that there did not appear to be any deleterious effects from exposure to the static magnetic field component of the MR system.[25] Although Kanal et al.[25] showed that there is no increase in adverse outcomes of pregnancies in MRI workers, it would be reasonable to limit the amount of time spent by the pregnant worker within the magnet room. For example, the pregnant physician, anesthesiologist, or nurse anesthetist probably would be advised against monitoring the patient from within the MR system during image acquisition.

A guideline is recommended that permits the pregnant MRI technologist or healthcare worker, regardless of the pregnancy trimester, to perform MR procedures, as well as to enter the MR system room, and to attend to the patient. Importantly, the technologists or healthcare worker should not remain within the MR system room or magnet bore during the actual operation of the MR system.

It is especially important for MR healthcare workers that are involved in interventional or MR-guided examinations to adhere to this recommendation because it may be necessary for them to be directly exposed to the MR system's electromagnetic fields at levels similar to those used for patients. Notably, these particular recommendations are not based on indications of adverse effects, but rather from a conservative point of view and in consideration of the fact that there currently is insufficient data pertaining to the combined effects of the electromagnetic fields of the MR system.

VI. SUMMARY AND CONCLUSIONS

The information pertaining to the safety aspects of MR procedures for pregnant patients has been presented along with a discussion of the important clinical applications for this diagnostic imaging technique. In cases where the referring physician and radiologist can defend that the findings of the MR examination has the potential to change or alter the care or management of the mother or fetus, the MR procedure (i.e., MRI, angiography, functional MRI, or spectroscopy) may be performed with verbal and written informed consent.

With regard to the use of MR procedures in pregnant patients, this diagnostic technique should not be withheld for the following cases:

- Patients with active brain or spine signs and symptoms requiring imaging
- Patients with cancer requiring imaging
- Patients with chest, abdomen, and pelvic signs and symptoms of active disease when sonography is non-diagnostic
- In specific cases of suspected fetal anomaly or complex fetal disorder

With regard to pregnant healthcare workers and the MR environment, the following should be considered:

- Pregnant MRI technologists have not been shown to be at increased risk of adverse outcomes from occupational exposure to static magnetic fields.
- Pregnant MR healthcare workers, especially those involved in interventional or MR-guided procedures, should minimize the time spent within the MR system and the room itself.

REFERENCES

1. Kanal, E., Shellock, F.G., and Sonnenblick, D., MRI clinical site safety: phase I results and preliminary data, *Magn. Reson. Imaging,* 7(Suppl. 1), 106, 1988.
2. National Radiological Protection Board, Revised guidance on acceptable limits of exposure during nuclear magnetic clinical imaging, *Br. J. Radiol.,* 56, 974, 1983.
3. U.S. Food and Drug Administration, Guidelines for Evaluating Electromagnetic Exposure Risk Trials of Clinical NMR Systems, Center for Devices and Radiological Health, Rockville, MD, 1982.
4. Shellock, F.G. and Kanal, E., Policies, guidelines, and recommendations for MR imaging safety and patient management, *J. Magn. Reson. Imaging,* 1, 97, 1991.
5. Shellock, F.G. and Kanal, E., Magnetic resonance procedures and pregnancy, *Magnetic Resonance Bioeffects, Safety, and Patient Management,* Second Edition, Lippincott-Raven, Philadelphia, 1996, chapter 4, p. 49.

6. Schaefer, D.J., Safety aspects of radiofrequency power deposition in magnetic resonance, *Magn. Reson. Imaging Clin. N. Am.*, 6, 775, 1998.

7. Elder, J. E., Special senses, in Biological Effects of Radio-Frequency Radiation, II, Elder, J.E. and Cahill, D.P., Eds., EPA-600/8-83-026A: 5-64-5-78, U.S. Environmental Protection Agency, Washington, D.C., 1984, pp. 64-78.

8. Wilcox, A., Weinberg, C., O'Connor, J., et al., Incidence of early loss of pregnancy, *N. Engl. J. Med.*, 319, 189-194, 1988.

9. McRobbie, D. and Foster, M.A., Pulsed magnetic field exposure during pregnancy and implications for NMR foetal imaging: a study with mice, *Magn. Reson. Imaging*, 3, 231, 1985.

10. Tesky, G.C., Ossenkopp, K.P., Prato, F.S., and Sestini, E., Survivability and long-term stress reactivity levels following repeated exposure to nuclear magnetic resonance imaging procedures in rats, *Physiol. Chem. Phys. Med. NMR*, 19, 43, 1987.

11. Heinrichs, W.L., Fong, P., Flannery, M., Meinrichs, S.C., et al., Midgestational exposure of pregnant BALB/c mice to magnetic resonance imaging conditions, *Magn. Reson. Imaging*, 6, 305, 1988.

12. Kay, H.H., Herfkens, R.J., and Kay, B.K., Effect of magnetic resonance imaging on *Xenopus laevis* embryogenesis, *Magn. Reson. Imaging*, 6, 501-506, 1988.

13. Tyndall, D.A., MRI effects on the teratogenicity of x-irradiation in the C57BL/6J mouse, *Magn. Reson. Imaging*, 8, 423, 1990.

14. Murakami, J., Toril, Y., and Masuda, K., Fetal developmet of mice following intrauterine exposure to a static magnetic field of 6.3 T, *Magn. Reson. Imaging*, 10, 433, 1992.

15. Malko, J.A., Constatinidis, I., Dillehay, D., et al., Search for influence of 1.5 T magnetic field on growth of yeast cells, *Bioelectromagnetics*, 15, 495, 1987.

16. Yip, Y.P., Capriotti, C., Talagala, S.L., and Yip, J.W., Effects of MR exposure at 1.5 T on early embryonic development of the chick, *J. Magn. Reson. Imaging*, 4, 742, 1994.

17. Yip, Y.P., Capriotti, C., and Yip, J.W., Effects of MR exposure on axonal outgrowth in the sympathetic nervous system of the chick, *J. Magn. Reson. Imaging*, 4, 457, 1995.

18. Tablado, L., Soler, C., Nunez, M., et al., Development of mouse testis and epididymis following intrauterine exposure to a static magnetic field, *Bioelectromagnetics*, 21, 19, 2000.

19. Tyndall, R.J. and Sulik, K.K., Effects of magnetic resonance imaging on eye development in the C57BL/6J mouse, *Teratology*, 43, 263, 1991.

20. Tyndall, D.A., MRI effects on craniofacial size and crown-rump length in C57BL/6J mice in 1.5T fields, *Oral Surg. Oral Med. Oral Pathol.*, 76, 655, 1993.

21. Yip, Y.P., Capriotti, C., Norbash, S.G., Talagala, S.L., and Yip, J.W., Effects of MR exposure on cell proliferation and migration of chick motor neurons, *J. Magn. Reson. Imaging*, 4, 799, 1994.

22. Carnes, K.I. and Magin, R.L., Effects of in utero exposure to 4.7T MR imaging conditions on fetal growth and testicular development in the mouse, *Magn. Reson. Imaging*, 14, 263, 1996.

23. Nara, V.R., Howell, R.W., Goddu, S.M., et al., Effects of a 1.5T static magnetic field on spermatogenesis and embryogenesis in mice, *Invest. Radiol.*, 31, 586, 1996.

24. Johnson, I.R., Stehling, M.K., Blamire, A., et al., Study of the internal structure of the human fetus in utero by echo-planar magnetic resonance imaging, *Am. J. Obstet. Gynecol.*, 163, 601, 1990.

25. Kanal, E., Gillen, J., Evans, J.A., et al., Survey of reproductive health among female MR workers, *Radiology*, 187, 395, 1993.

26. Baker, P.N., Johnson, I.R., Harvey, P.R., et al., A three-year follow-up of children imaged in utero with echo-planar magnetic resonance, *Am. J. Obstet. Gynecol.*, 170(1), 32-33, 1994.

27. Myers, C., Duncan, K.R., Gowland, P.A., et al., Failure to detect intrauterine growth restriction following in utero exposure to MRI, *Br. J. Radiol.*, 71, 549, 1998.

28. Vadeyar, S.H., Moore, R.J., Strachan, B.K., et al., Effect of fetal magnetic resonance imaging on fetal heart rate patterns, *Am. J. Obstet. Gynecol.*, 182, 666, 2000.

29. Colletti, P.M. and Sylvestre, P.B., Magnetic resonance imaging in pregnancy, *Magn. Reson. Imaging Clin. North Am.*, 2, 291, 1994.

30. Wilbur, A.C., Langer, B.G., and Spigos, D.G., Diagnosis of sacroiliac joint infection in pregnancy by magnetic resonance imaging, *Magn. Reson. Imaging*, 6, 341, 1988.

31. Weinreb, J.C., Brown, C.E., Lowe, T.W., et al., Pelvic masses in pregnant patients, MR and US imaging, *Radiology*, 159, 717, 1986.

32. McCarthy, S.M., Stark, D.D., Filly, R.A., et al., Uterine neoplasms, MR imaging, *Radiology,* 170, 125, 1989.

33. Stark, D.D., McCarthy, S.M., Filly, R.A., et al., Pelvimetry by magnetic resonance imaging, *Am. J. Roentgenol.,* 144, 947, 1985.

34. Angtuaco, T.L., Shah, H.R., Mattison, D.R., et al., MR imaging in high-risk obstetric patients. A valuable complement to US, *Radiographics,* 12, 91, 1992.

35. Benson, R.C., Colletti, P.M., Platt, L.D., et al., MR imaging of fetal anomalies, *Am. J. Roentgenol.,* 156, 1205, 1991.

36. Brown, C.E.L. and Weinreb, J.C., Magnetic resonance imaging appearance of growth retardation in a twin pregnancy, *Obstet. Gynecol.,* 71, 987, 1988.

37. Carswell, H., Fast MRI of fetus yields considerable anatomic detail, *Diagn. Imaging,* November 11-12, 1988.

38. Catizone, F.A., Gesmundo, G., Montemagno, R., et al., The non-invasive methods of prenatal diagnosis: the role of ultrasound and MRI, *J. Perinat. Med.,* 19, 42, 1991.

39. Colletti, P.M. and Platt, L.D., When to use MRI in obstetrics, *Diagn. Imaging,* 11, 84, 1989.

40. De Clyn, K., Degryse, H., Slangen, T., et al., MRI in the prenatal diagnosis of bilateral renal agenesis, *Fortschr. Geb. Rontgenstr.,* 150, 104, 1989.

41. Deans, H.E., Smith, F.W., Lloyd, D.J., et al., Fetal fat measurement by magnetic resonance imaging, *Br. J. Radiol.,* 62, 603, 1989.

42. Dinh, D.H., Wright, R.M., and Hanigan, W.C., The use of magnetic resonance imaging for the diagnosis of fetal intracranial anomalies, *Child Nerv. Syst.,* 6, 212, 1990.

43. Dunn, R.S. and Weiner, S.N., Antenatal diagnosis of sacrococcygeal teratoma facilitated by combined use of Doppler sonography and MR imaging, *Am. J. Roentgenol.,* 156, 1115, 1991.

44. Fitamorris-Glass, R., Mattrey, R.F., and Cantrell, C.J., Magnetic resonance imaging as an adjunct to ultrasound in oligohydramnios, *J. Ultrasound Med.,* 8, 159, 1989.

45. Fraser, R., Magnetic resonance imaging of the fetus. Initial experience [letter], *Gynecol. Obstet. Invest.,* 29, 255, 1990.

46. Gardens, A.S., Weindling, A.M., Griffiths, R.D., et al., Fast-scan magnetic resonance imagin of fetal anomalies, *Br. J. Obstet. Gynecol.,* 98, 1217-1222, 1991.

47. Hill, M.C., Lande, I.M., and Larsen, J.W., Jr., Prenatal diagnosis of fetal anomalies using ultrasound and MRI, *Radiol. Clin. North Am.,* 26, 287-307, 1988.

48. Horvath, L. and Seeds, J.W., Temporary arrest of fetal movement with pancuronium bromide to enable antenatal magnetic resonance imaging of holosencephaly, *Am. J. Roentgenol.,* 6, 418-420, 1989.

49. Lenke, R.R., Persutte, W.H., and Nemes, J.M., Use of pancuronium bromide to inhibit fetal movement during magnetic resonance imaging, *J. Reprod. Med.,* 34, 315-317, 1989.

50. Mansfield, P., Stehling, M.K., Ordidge, R.J., et al., Study of internal structure of the human fetus in utero at 0.5T, *Br. J. Radiol.,* 13, 314-318, 1990.

51. Mattison, D.R., Angtuaco, T., Miller, F.C., et al., Magnetic resonance imaging in maternal and fetal medicine, *J. Perinatol.,* 9, 411-419, 1989.

52. Mattison, D.R. and Angtuaco, T., Magnetic resonance imaging in pernatatl diagnosis, *Clin. Obstet. Gynecol.,* 31, 353-389, 1988.

53. Mattison, D.R., Kay, H.H., Miller, R.K., et al., Magnetic resonance imaging: a noninvasive tool for fetal and placental physiology, *Biol. Reprod.,* 38, 39-49, 1988.

54. McCarthy, S.M., Filly, R.A., Stark, D.D., et al., Magnetic resonance imaging of fetal anomalies in utero, early experience, *Am. J. Roentgenol.,* 145, 677-682, 1985.

55. McCarthy, S.M., Filly, R.A., Stark, D.D., et al., Obstetrical magnetic resonance imaging, fetal anatomy, *Radiology,* 154, 427-432, 1985.

56. Powell, M.C., Worthington, B.S., Buckley, J.M., et al., Magnetic resonance imaging (MRI) in obstetrics. II. Fetal anatomy, *Br. J. Obstet. Gynaecol.,* 95, 38-46, 1988.

57. Smith, F.W., Magnetic resonance tomography of the pelvis, *Cadiovasc. Intervent. Radiol.,* 8, 367-376, 1986.

58. Smith, F.W., Kent, C., Abramovich, D.R., et al., Nuclear magnetic resonance imaging — a new look at the fetus, *Br. J. Gynaecol.,* 92, 1024-1033, 1985.

59. Smith, F.W. and Sutherland, H.W., Magnetic resonance imaging: the use of the inversion recovery sequence to display fetal morphology, *Br. J. Radiol.,* 61, 338-341, 1988.

60. Stehling, M.K., Mansfield, P., Ordidge, R.J., et al., Echoplanar magnetic resonance imaging in abnormal pregnancies, *Lancet*, July, 157, 1989.

61. Toma, P., Lucigrai, G., Dodero, P., et al., Prenatal detection of an abdominal mass by MR imaging performed while the fetus is immobilized with pancuronium bromide, *Am. J. Roentgenol.*, 154, 1049, 1990.

62. Toma, P., Lucigrai, G., Ravegnai, M., et al., Hydrocephalus and porencephaly: prenatal diagnosis by ultrasonography and MR imaging, *J. Comp. Assist. Tomogr.*, 14, 843, 1990.

63. Turner, R.J., Hankins, G.V.D., Weinreb, J.C., et al., Magnetic resonance imaging and ultrasonography in antenatal evaluation of cojoined twins, *Am. J. Obstet. Gynecol.*, 77, 529, 1986.

64. Vila-Coro, A.A. and Dominguez, R., Intrauterine diagnosis of hydroencephaly by magnetic resonance imaging, *Magn. Reson. Imaging*, 7, 105-107, 1989.

65. Weinreb, J.C., Lowe, T., Cohen, J.M., et al., Human fetal anatomy: MR imaging, *Radiology*, 157, 715-720, 1985.

66. Weinreb, J.C., Lowe, T., Santos-Ramos, R., et al., Magnetic resonance imaging in obstetric diagnosis, *Radiology*, 154, 157-161, 1985.

67. Wenstrom, K.D., Williamson, R.A., Weiner, C.P., et al., Magnetic resonance imaging of fetuses with intracranial defects, *Obstet. Gynecol.*, 77, 529-532, 1991.

68. Williamson, R.A., Weiner, C.P., Yuh, W.T.C., et al., Magnetic resonance imaging of anomalous fetuses, *Obstet. Gynecol.*, 71, 952, 1988.

69. Levine, D., Hatabu, H., Gan, J., et al., Fetal anatomy revealed with fast MR sequences, *Am. J. Roentgenol.*, 167, 905, 1996.

70. Garden, A.S., Griffiths, R.D., Weindling, A.M., et al., Fast-scan magnetic resonance imaging in fetal visualization, *Am. J. Obstet. Gynecol.*, 164, 1190, 1991.

71. Amin, R.S., Nikolaids, P., Kawashima, A., et al., Normal anatomy of the fetus at MR imaging, *Radiographics*, 19, S201, 1999.

72. Huppert, B.J., Brandt, K.R., Ramin, K.D., et al., Single-shot fast spin-echo MR imaging of the fetus: a pictorial essay, *Radiographics*, 19, S215, 1999.

73. Levine, D., Barnes, P.D., Sher, S., et al., Fetal fast MR imaging: reproducibility, technical quality, and conspicuity of anatomy, *Radiology*, 206, 549, 1998.

74. Levine, D., Barnes, P.D., and Edelman, R.R., Obstetric MR imaging, *Radiology*, 211, 609, 1999.

75. Yanashita, Y., Namimoto, T., Abe, Y., et al., MR imaging of the fetus by HASTE sequence, *Am. J. Roentgenol.*, 168, 513, 1997.

76. Colletti, P.M., Computer-assisted imaging of the fetus with magnetic resonance imaging, *Comput. Med. Imaging Graphics*, 20, 491, 1996.

77. Tsuchiya, K., Katase, S., Seki, T., et al., Short communication: MR imaging of fetal brain abnormalities using HASTE sequence, *Br. J. Radiol.*, 69, 668, 1996.

78. Coakley, F. V., Hricak, H., Filly, R.A., Barkovich, A.J., and Harrison, M.R., Complex fetal disorders: effect of MR imaging on management-preliminary clinical experience, *Radiology*, 213, 691, 1999.

9 FDA Guidance for Magnetic Resonance System Safety and Patient Exposures: Current Status and Future Considerations

Loren A. Zaremba

CONTENTS

I. INTRODUCTION

The development of magnetic resonance (MR) as a diagnostic radiological modality occurred during the period that the U.S. Food and Drug Administration (FDA) was first given authority to regulate medical devices. Lauterbur published his paper describing a technique for generating images using MR in 1973, and by 1979 experimental systems were capable of producing whole-body images.[1] The FDA was given the authority to regulate medical devices through the Medical Device Amendments of 1976. As a result, the development of FDA guidance and policies relating to MR provides an interesting study in the application and progression of the medical device law, as well as the advancement of MR technology.

This chapter provides a brief overview of the FDA's authority over medical devices in the U.S., the regulatory mechanisms incorporated within that authority, and the limitations of the FDA's authority. It also describes the mechanisms that have recently been developed to facilitate the device review process and to increase industry and user participation in policy development.

Additionally, this chapter provides a history of FDA regulatory activity relating to MR devices. That is followed by a discussion of the present international standard for MR equipment safety and current FDA policies and activities. Finally, there is a discussion of the challenges confronting the FDA in establishing MR safety standards and guidelines for the future.

II. FDA AUTHORITY AND REGULATORY MECHANISMS

The Medical Device Amendments of 1976 to the Food, Drug and Cosmetic Act provide the basis for FDA regulation of medical devices, including those involving MR. This law is primarily administered by the Center for Devices and Radiological Health (CDRH), one of the five centers within the FDA. The Medical Device Amendments grandfathered all existing devices on the market and established three classes relating to their degree of risk and the means needed to ensure their safety and effectiveness.

Class I devices involve minimum risk and require only general controls (e.g., good manufacturing practices and prohibitions against mislabeling and adulteration). Class II devices are those for which general controls are insufficient, but for which there is sufficient information to permit the development of standards. Prior to introducing most Class II devices into commerce, a manufacturer must submit a premarket notification [510(k)] demonstrating that the device is substantially equivalent to a pre-1976 device or a legally marketed post-1976 device. Premarket notifications are also required for some Class I and Class III devices. It should be noted that in a 510(k), the FDA is not approving a device that is found to be substantially equivalent. If a device is found to be substantially equivalent, it is "cleared for market."

Class III devices are those for which sufficient information is not yet available to develop standards. Manufacturers of such devices generally must submit a premarket approval (PMA) application demonstrating that the device is safe and effective. However, a humanitarian device exemption (HDE) may be submitted for devices that are intended for use in diseases that affect fewer than 4000 individuals in the U.S. per year. A clinical study is generally required as part of a PMA. Since the FDA reviews the data supporting the safety and efficacy of a Class III device, these devices are approved by the FDA. If a study involves a significant risk to patients, the manufacturer must submit an investigational device exemption (IDE) to the FDA prior to beginning clinical studies. A local institutional review board (IRB) makes the initial determination regarding whether a study involves significant risk. However, the IRB decision is subject to review by the FDA.

A point that is commonly misunderstood is that the FDA's authority applies only to manufacturers. For example, the FDA may ask manufacturers to provide information to users regarding the spatial distribution of the static magnetic field surrounding a scanner and to advise the user to establish a controlled access zone at the 5 gauss line in the instruction manuals provided with the system. However, the FDA does not inspect sites and cannot require users to establish a controlled access zone. Authority for such activities resides with state government agencies.

Another common misconception is that FDA approval or marketing clearance of a device ensures that insurance reimbursement will be provided. The FDA has no control over private or public insurance providers. In the case of government reimbursement, Medicare and Medicaid payments are controlled by the Health Care Financing Administration (HCFA). In some cases, the HCFA has utilized FDA approval or clearance as a necessary condition for reimbursement, but this is not always the case.

For example, the HCFA reimbursed women for MR imaging (MRI) examinations to diagnose silicone breast implant leakage for several years before a manufacturer received marketing clearance for this specific intended use. Most MR system manufacturers had obtained marketing clearance for general breast imaging and did not submit applications for the specific intended use of detecting silicone leakage from implants. Even today, most MR manufacturers have not requested clearance for this indication, but MR is regarded as the gold standard for the assessment of silicone breast implant leakage.

Since the passage of the Medical Device Amendments, the FDA's authority over medical devices has twice been revised. The first revision was the Safe Medical Devices Act (SMDA) of 1990, and the second was the Food and Drug Administration Modernization Act (FDAMA) of 1997. Under the SMDA, administrative requirements such as the summaries of safety and effectiveness and statements of indications for use were introduced for premarket notifications.

The FDAMA introduced the more general concept of special controls (e.g., voluntary standards) as a means for ensuring the safety and efficacy of Class II devices. The increased use of voluntary standards in the review of medical devices has effectively increased industry and user participation in the regulatory process, since both groups, as well as the FDA, generally participate in the development of these standards

Several years ago a re-engineering effort was started at the CDRH that resulted in the development of new mechanisms to facilitate the introduction of medical devices into the marketplace. These mechanisms include alternatives to traditional premarket notifications: the special and abbreviated 510(k)s,[2] and third party review.[3] Special 510(k)s are limited to modifications of previously cleared devices and are reviewed in 30 days by the agency rather than the 90 days allowed for traditional submissions. Special 510(k)s are particularly appropriate for many MR devices, since they are often improvements of previously cleared devices.

The abbreviated 510(k) allows a manufacturer to certify that the device will comply with the provisions of applicable endorsed standards prior to marketing.[4] Test data demonstrating compliance need not be provided. This is intended to reduce the amount of information that must be supplied in the 510(k) and the time required for review. Abbreviated 510(k)s are also appropriate for MR devices because there are several applicable standards, such as International Electrotechnical Commission (IEC) 60601-2-33 and the standards developed by the National Electrical Manufacturers Association (NEMA).

The Third Party Review program allows manufacturers of designated devices to have their 510(k) reviewed by a third party that has been certified for this purpose by the CDRH. The agency then has 30 days to review the third party recommendation. MR devices have been designated as eligible for third party review.

As a part of the re-engineering effort at the CDRH, good guidance practices (GGPs) have also been developed and implemented. The CDRH used guidance documents for a number of years to communicate its recommendations regarding the information that should be supplied in 510(k)s and other subjects. However, there were no formal internal procedures for guidance development. Under the GGPs, a formal internal procedure for guidance development has been established which includes posting on the agency's website and an opportunity for public comment on new draft guidance documents.

III. HISTORY OF FDA REGULATORY ACTIVITY RELATING TO MR

A. CLASS III DEVICES

When manufacturers first brought MR devices to market in the early 1980s they were placed in Class III, requiring clinical studies to demonstrate safety and effectiveness and the submission of a PMA. In 1982, the FDA issued its first guidance relating to MR devices in the form of recommendations for IRBs overseeing clinical trials.[5] To avoid the risk of excessive radiofrequency (RF) heating associated with MR procedures, the FDA recommended that the specific absorption rate (SAR) be limited to 0.4 W/kg averaged over the body and 2.0 W/kg averaged over any 1 g of tissue. The recommended upper limit for the rate of change of the gradient magnetic field, dB/dt, was 3 T/s to avoid peripheral nerve stimulation (PNS), and the limit for the main static field was set at 2.0 T. An IDE was required for studies in which any of these levels was exceeded. Notably, these levels are considered very conservative by current standards.

B. RECLASSIFICATION AND THE 1988 MR DIAGNOSTIC DEVICE 510(K) GUIDANCE

In 1987, 13 manufacturers of MR devices petitioned the FDA to reclassify their devices. The petitions were reviewed by the Radiological Devices Panel later that year, and the panel recommended reclassification to Class II. The FDA implemented this recommendation in July 1988. The description of the reclassified device is contained in Title 21 of the Code of Federal Regulations, where all medical device classifications are listed. The reclassified device is described in section 892.1000 and is formally called a magnetic resonance diagnostic device (MRDD). The description is as follows:

892.1000 Magnetic Resonance Diagnostic Device

A magnetic resonance diagnostic device is intended for general diagnostic use to present images which reflect the spatial distribution and/or magnetic resonance spectra which reflect frequency and distribution of nuclei exhibiting nuclear magnetic resonance. Other physical parameters derived from the images and/or spectra may be produced. The device includes hydrogen-1 (proton) imaging, sodium-23 imaging, hydrogen-1 spectroscopy, phosphorus-31 spectroscopy and chemical shift imaging (preserving simultaneous frequency and spatial information).

The term "magnetic resonance diagnostic device" was used to include both imaging and spectroscopy.

Prior to the submission of these petitions, MR device manufacturers, under the auspices of NEMA, had begun to develop standard test methods for the measurement of MR performance parameters, including signal-to-noise ratio, geometric distortion, slice thickness and spacing, and image uniformity. The NEMA standards demonstrated the availability of sufficient information for standards development as required for a Class II device. The MR Technical Committee of NEMA has continued to develop standard test methods relating to the safety and performance of MR devices. Eight such standards have been developed to date,[6] and the FDA has participated in the NEMA standards development process since its inception.

In August 1988, the FDA issued its first "Guidance for the Content and Review of a Magnetic Resonance Diagnostic Device 510(k) Application" (the 1988 MRDD guidance). The principal elements of this document from a safety standpoint are Attachment I, "Safety Parameter Action Levels," and Attachment II, "Required Elements in the Labeling for a Magnetic Resonance Diagnostic Device." The "Safety Parameter Action Levels" represented a departure from the 1982 IRB guidance in that manufacturers were allowed two options to satisfy agency safety concerns.

A manufacturer could either limit operation to levels where the safety parameters were below specified levels or provide valid scientific evidence to establish the safety of operating at the intended levels. The safety parameters were static field strength, SAR, dB/dt, and acoustic noise. Temperature and PNS could be used in place of SAR and dB/dt, respectively. The limit for static field strength remained at 2.0 T, as in the 1982 IRB guidance.

Two alternative limits were provided for the safety parameter for time-varying fields, dB/dt. A manufacturer could show that (1) the maximum dB/dt was less than 6 T/s (twice the limit in the 1982 IRB guidance) or (2) the maximum dB/dt was less than a specified level that depended on pulse duration. The latter limit was 20 and 60 T/s for axial and transverse gradients, respectively, for pulse durations greater than 120 μs (which applied to virtually all systems at the time as well as today).

The limits in the second alternative were based on calculations by Reilly,[7,8] which have more recently been shown to be in reasonably good agreement with experimental values for the PNS threshold. However, a safety factor was also applied to Reilly's results. The rationale for using a threefold higher limit for transverse gradients was that the net flux (which is through the transverse plane of the patient for the imaging component of the gradient field) is zero for these gradients in a solenoid-type magnet. This rationale turned out to be erroneous, as discussed below.

As a third alternative, a manufacturer could use PNS as the safety parameter and demonstrate by an adequate margin of safety (at least a factor of three) that PNS would not occur.

It is now known that the PNS threshold for a *dB/dt* pulse duration of 0.25 μs is about 60 T/s and is less for longer pulse durations. Consequently, the third alternative was actually a more restrictive limit for most MR systems at that time. Of course, the alternative remained to provide valid scientific evidence to establish the safety of operating an MR system at the intended levels, and a manufacturer could argue that operating at the threshold of PNS would not be unsafe.

With regard to RF energy-induced heating during an MRI examination, the safety parameter action levels for a whole-body-averaged SAR remained at 0.4 W/kg. A new peak SAR limit of 3.2 W/kg was introduced for the head, and the local limit for 1 g of tissue was quadrupled to 8.0 W/kg.

As an alternative, an MR system manufacturer could utilize temperature rise as a safety parameter. In this case, the manufacturer would have to demonstrate that the temperature rise would be less than 1°C in the body core, and localized heating would be less than 38°C in the head, 39°C in the trunk, and 40°C in the extremities. Notably, the temperature rise criterion was utilized immediately by all high-field-strength (i.e., 1.0 to 1.5 T) MR system manufacturers. High-field-strength MR systems were already operating well above 0.4 W/kg in 1988.

A recommendation for gradient field-induced acoustic noise was not included in the 1982 IRB guidance. In the 1988 guidance, the manufacturer was requested to demonstrate that the noise level was "below the level of concern established by pertinent Federal Regulatory or other recognized standard setting organizations." If the acoustic noise was not below this level, it was recommended that the manufacturer suggest steps (e.g., earplugs) to alleviate the noise perceived by the patient.

Attachment II, "Required Elements in the Labeling for a Magnetic Resonance Diagnostic Device," included lists of indications, cautions, contraindications, warnings, and precautions. In addition, it was recommended that the operator's manual contain a description of the recommended training, a procedure for removing patients from the magnet, quality assurance procedures, recommended maintenance schedules, and specifications for the system. A site planning guide was also suggested, containing recommendations that the user establish a warning zone where the magnetic field exceeds 5 G and that venting be provided for superconducting systems in the event of a magnet quench or other similar problem.

In addition to safety-related items, the 1988 guidance recommended that information relating to imaging performance be submitted in a 510(k). This information was based on the NEMA standards and includes signal-to-noise ratio, image uniformity, geometric distortion, slice profile, thickness, and interslice spacing. Sample clinical images were also to be provided for each coil.

C. THE MR GUIDANCE UPDATE FOR *dB/dt*

Significant improvements in equipment capabilities occurred in the years following the introduction of the first clinical MR systems. In particular, the speed and strength of gradients increased dramatically. By the early 1990s, manufacturers were beginning to introduce echo-planar imaging capabilities on their clinical systems. However, in 1993, a report was published that PNS was being experienced by subjects and patients during echo-planar imaging procedures when gradients in the antero-posterior (A-P) direction were applied.[9]

A closer examination of the situation revealed that the imaging component of the gradient field (i.e., the component in the direction of the main static field) was not producing the stimulation.[10–12] Cylindrical magnet configurations generally use saddle coils for generating the transverse gradients.

Directly below the saddle coils, at both ends of the imaging volume, these coils tend to look like a Helmholtz pair, and the gradient field is almost completely in the transverse direction (e.g., in the A-P direction for the A-P gradient).

Thus, the A-P gradient produces a field in the A-P direction that interacts with the relatively large area available in the coronal plane of the patient. The result is a large flux change resulting in high currents in the body and a high propensity for stimulation.

The 1988 MRDD guidance did not specify a method for measuring dB/dt, but the FDA had been using a method developed by NEMA. This method involved positioning a search coil in the transverse plane. Consequently, only the imaging component of the gradient field was measured. Thus, the FDA was receiving test data in 510(k)s that was not directly related to the mechanism that was producing stimulation in clinical systems (i.e., the transverse component of the gradient). Furthermore, the FDA had cleared the InstaScan echo-planar MR system for market with a dB/dt for the transverse gradient of 60 T/s, since this was permitted under the 1988 MRDD guidance that allowed the dB/dt for the transverse gradient to be three times stronger than for the axial gradient.

In order to attempt to correct this situation, the FDA issued a draft MRI guidance update for dB/dt in early 1995 for public comment. The principal features of this guidance were that manufacturers were to submit estimates of the maximum $d|B|/dt$ rather than dB_z/dt, where $|B|$ is the magnitude of the gradient field and B_z is the imaging component.

Also, if $d|B|/dt$ exceeded 20 T/s, a study using volunteer subjects would be conducted to determine if PNS could be induced. If so, the MR system would be equipped with a warning to the MR system operator when PNS was imminent. The latter feature was similar to a warning which was required by the new international standard (IEC 60601-2-33) at 20 T/s (the upper limit of the normal operating mode).[13] However, by 1995, human PNS data had been acquired, indicating that the stimulation threshold was well above 20 T/s for the sub-500-μs gradient pulse rise times that were being used at the time. The FDA believed that requiring a warning at 20 T/s would be unnecessary and that MR system operators would tend to ignore it.

A public meeting of the FDA Radiological Devices Panel was held in the fall of 1995, and the guidance was finalized with minor revisions. Representatives of the NEMA MR Technical Committee testified at that meeting and made the important point that PNS was not harmful. However, they maintained that painful stimulation must be avoided in MR exams. This point was incorporated into the guidance, and it has carried over into the latest revision of the IEC standard as discussed below. This was a significant departure from the 1988 MRDD guidance that stated that PNS was to be avoided by a safety factor of three.

IV. THE CURRENT IEC STANDARD 60601-2-33

Work began on IEC 60601-2-33, "Particular Requirements for the Safety of Magnetic Resonance Equipment for Medical Diagnosis," in the early 1990s and was finalized in July 1995. This document is discussed here because the FDA participated in its development, and it has had a significant influence on current FDA policies and guidance relating to MR. Additionally, it is hoped that the FDA will eventually be able to rely entirely on this standard for its MR safety requirements. However, it should be kept in mind that the FDA has been given the responsibility for ensuring both the safety and efficacy of medical devices. Since the IEC standard does not address efficacy (i.e., imaging performance), the FDA will continue to be required to establish its own criteria in this area.

In terms of labeling requirements, the IEC standard contains essentially the same indications, contraindications, precautions, and warnings as the 1988 FDA guidance discussed above. However, it does not contain the 1988 FDA recommendations relating to quality assurance procedures and maintenance.

The most unique feature of the IEC standard is the establishment of three modes of operation relating to RF energy-induced heating and dB/dt; the normal operating mode, first level controlled (FLC) operating mode, and second level controlled (SLC) operating mode.

The normal operating mode is suitable for all patients and requires only routine monitoring. The FLC mode is defined in the standard as operation at levels that "may cause undue physiological stress." Operation of the MR system in this mode requires medical supervision. This can be in the form of the direct consent of a medical practitioner or conformity with a set of criteria established by a medical practitioner. Confirmation by the operator is required to enter the FLC mode.

The SLC mode is defined as operation at levels that "may produce significant risk." Operation in this mode requires IRB approval. Manufacturers are required to restrict access to this mode (e.g., by means of the use of a password).

The upper limit of the normal operating mode for dB/dt is, for practical purposes, identical to the 1988 FDA guidance. It should be noted that the IEC incorporated the 1993 version of NEMA MS-7 for measuring dB/dt. Consequently, limits are actually stated in terms of dB_z/dt.

For RF energy-induced heating, the whole-body-averaged SARs have upper limits for the normal and FLC modes of operation at levels of 1.5 and 4.0 W/kg, respectively. For the SAR in the head, the upper limit of the normal mode is 3.0 W/kg. There is no FLC mode, so anything higher is considered the SLC mode. The local tissue SAR is limited to 8.0 W/kg in the head and torso and 12.0 W/kg in the extremities in the normal operating mode. There is also no FLC mode for local SAR.

The multi-level operating mode scheme is not applied to static magnetic field strength and acoustic noise. Static magnetic field strength is only addressed in subclause 6.8.2, "Instructions for Use." This subclause states that for equipment capable of whole body examinations above 2.0 T or a locally set limit, "the instructions shall state that it is essential that operation above that level be performed only under an approved IRB protocol and vital body functions should be monitored." A single upper limit of 140 dB is applied to peak acoustic noise. However, the instructions for use must advise the MR system operator to provide hearing protection to patients for operation above an acoustic noise level of 99 dBA.

V. CURRENT FDA GUIDANCE

A. BIOCOMPATIBILITY OF MATERIALS

In February 1996, the FDA responded to a request by the NEMA MR Technical Committee that biocompatibility studies not be required in 510(k) submissions for external RF coil assemblies (e.g., surface coils) used with MR systems. In its response, the agency stated that biocompatibility data need not be provided for external RF coil assemblies and other MR components that are not intended to come in contact with the body. Such data also need not be provided for devices that come in contact with the skin, if the materials used for patient contact in their final finished form have a history of safe use.

In such cases, the manufacturer should document the use of the material in a legally marketed predicate device. However, biocompatibility data is required for MR devices that incorporate a non-routinely used material and for devices that are intended for invasive use (e.g., endocavitary coils). The type of data required in such cases depends on the nature of the contact, as described in ISO-10933 "Biological Evaluation of Medical Devices Part 1: Evaluation and Testing." In cases where biocompatibility data are required for materials, they may be incorporated by reference.

B. MR SOFTWARE

In August 1997, the FDA responded to a request from the NEMA Magnetic Resonance Section that MR software be reclassified from moderate to minor level of concern. In this response, the agency distinguished between software that is used for control of the MR procedure, image reconstruction, and image processing. Software used for image reconstruction and processing will generally be considered a minor level of concern. However, software that performs scan control functions (e.g., regulation of the output of the RF and gradient subsystems and estimation of SAR and *dB/dt*) will be considered as a moderate level of concern for those systems capable of reaching the FLC mode of IEC 60601-2-33. Premarket notifications for moderate level of concern software should contain a detailed description of the algorithms and a summary of the verification and validation testing.

C. Significant Risk Criteria

Criteria for determining if an MR examination involved significant risk (SR), thus requiring an IDE, was issued by the FDA in 1982, during the period when MR devices were Class III and subject to premarket approval. In the years following, the hardware capabilities of MR devices increased dramatically. At the same time, additional information was obtained regarding the physiological effects of human exposure in the MR environment.

In order to update the information available to sponsors and IRBs regarding the FDA's policies relating to significant risk in MR studies, a new guidance document entitled "Guidance for Magnetic Resonance Diagnostic Devices — Criteria for Significant Risk Investigations" was issued on September 29, 1997.[14] The new SR criteria are based on the IEC standard and studies conducted on advanced MR systems.

In the 1997 criteria, the SR level for static magnetic field strength was increased from 2.0 to 4.0 T. The IEC standard currently requires that studies conducted above 2.0 T be reviewed by an IRB. However, it should be noted that review by an IRB does not mean that the study requires an IDE. An IDE is only required if the IRB or the FDA determines that the study involves significant risk. As of this publication, human volunteers have been subjected to static magnetic fields as high as 8.0 T in research systems, and, thus far, no significant adverse effects have been observed.[15] Consequently, consideration may be given to raising the SR level for static magnetic field strength above 4.0 T.

For gradient fields, the approach was taken to use physiologic response rather than the device operating parameter, such as *dB/dt*, as the SR criterion. Since mild PNS is not considered harmful, painful stimulation was used as the criterion. Nerve stimulation is a function of pulse duration, waveform, gradient direction, region of the anatomy exposed, and numerous other factors. Consequently, it was not considered practical to attempt to specify SR in terms of operating parameters. In addition, although information was rapidly accumulating regarding the relationship between MR operating parameters and mild PNS, very little information was available regarding painful stimulation at the time.

For RF energy-induced heating, the upper limits of the FLC mode were adopted as the SR criteria. This is somewhat conservative, since the IEC standard only requires IRB review at these levels. However, the IEC had defined the SLC mode as one that may involve SR, and insufficient information was available to establish the safety of operation at higher levels. For acoustic noise, the IEC upper limit of 140 dB was adopted.

D. The 1998 MRDD 510(k) Guidance

In November 1998, the FDA issued a revision of the 1988 MRDD guidance for 510(k) submissions, and this is currently in use.[16] The purpose of this document was to summarize the changes in FDA policies relating to MR safety parameters that had occurred since reclassification and to harmonize the FDA with the international standard, IEC 60601-2-33, to the greatest extent possible.

In the 1998 MRDD guidance, the FDA recommends that manufacturers utilize the IEC operating mode scheme. If the value of SAR or *dB/dt* is such as to enter the FLC mode, a clear indication of this should be displayed on the console and a deliberate action of the operator should be required to start the MR procedure. A means should be provided to ensure that the values of *dB/dt* and SAR do not exceed the upper limits of the FLC mode. Equipment that is capable of operating in the SLC mode should have security measures that control entry into this mode, such as a lock, password, or other protective device.

However, in the case of time-varying magnetic fields (dB/dt), the FDA's recommended limits for the operating modes and measurement methodology differ from that of the IEC. In the July 1995 version of the IEC standard, the ranges of dB/dt values that define the operating modes did not reflect recent data. Based on these data, the lower limit of the FLC mode is too low and may cause operators to ignore the warning. On the other hand, the upper limit is well above the pain threshold. Also, only the component of the gradient in the direction of the main static field (the component used to spatially encode the image) is measured in the determination of dB/dt. Consequently, the FDA decided to use the MRI guidance update for dB/dt to define the operating mode limits. That is, the upper limit of the normal operating mode corresponds to the PNS threshold, and the upper limit of the FLC mode corresponds to the threshold of severe discomfort or pain.

In July 1997, the NEMA MR Technical Committee revised NEMA MS-7, "Measurement Procedure for Time-Varying Gradient Fields (dB/dt) for Magnetic Resonance Imaging Systems," to include a method of measuring the peak modulus sum of all magnetic field vectors, $d|B|/dt$. This method is recommended in the 1998 MRDD guidance. The revised version of NEMA MS-7 permits the measurement of dB_z/dt in cases where it is less than 20 T/s, which is also acceptable to the FDA.

In the 1998 MRDD guidance, the FDA recognizes that the technology of these devices is still advancing, and information relating to safe operation continues to accrue. In order to ensure that technologically advanced devices that may benefit patients are not kept from the market, the FDA offers a manufacturer the option of demonstrating that the physiological response of the patient is within safe limits. This alternative was also available in the 1988 MRDD guidance.

The NEMA standards MS-1 through 8[6] are recognized by the FDA, and they are endorsed for use in 510(k)s. They are as follows:

MS-1 Determination of Signal-to-Noise Ratio (SNR)
MS-2 Determination of Two-Dimensional Geometric Distortion
MS-3 Determination of Image Uniformity
MS-4 Acoustic Noise Measurement Procedure
MS-5 Determination of Slice Thickness
MS-6 Characterization of Special Purpose Coils
MS-7 Measurement Procedure for Time-Varying Gradient Fields (dB/dt)
MS-8 Characterization of the Specific Absorption Rate

MS-4, 7, and 8 are safety related. However, the remaining standards are used in the evaluation of imaging performance. This is within the FDA's responsibility for ensuring efficacy as well as safety. Generally, the performance of the new device is compared with the predicate to determine substantial equivalence.

For the most part, the FDA relies upon laboratory data (i.e., phantom measurements in accordance with the NEMA standards). However, in order to evaluate the efficacy of an MR device, the FDA also generally requests sample clinical images, if applicable. Most MR devices are submitted to the FDA with general claims (e.g., whole-body imaging or imaging of a specific anatomic region). However, if a more specific claim is made, a clinical study may be required. An example of this was the clearance of diffusion weighted imaging for stroke detection. Another special case where human studies are required is for gradient systems that produce a dB/dt in excess of 20 T/s. In such cases, the FDA recommends that a manufacturer conduct limited volunteer studies to determine if PNS is possible. If so, these studies should ascertain the level at which the operator should be notified of this possibility. The study should also confirm that painful stimulation does not occur.

If an MR device application involves the use of a drug (e.g., an MRI contrast agent), the manufacturer should provide evidence that the indications for use of the device are within the scope of the approved use of the drug. A number of years ago, the CDRH signed a memorandum of understanding (MOU) with the Center for Drug Evaluation and Research (CDER). In this MOU, the CDRH agreed to ensure that a device would only be cleared for market if the intended use was consistent with the approved use of any associated drug.

MRI contrast agents have been approved by the CDER for the visualization of lesions, but have not yet been approved for the evaluation of vasculature. Consequently, the CDRH is presently unable to clear MR devices for the evaluation of cerebral and myocardial perfusion. Another example is the use of contrast-enhanced MR angiography in the evaluation of peripheral vasculature.

The labeling information requested in the 1998 MRDD guidance is essentially identical to that requested in the previous 1988 MRDD guidance. A section relating to software information has been added. As noted above, software utilized for image reconstruction or processing (including sequences) is considered to be a minor level of concern. However, software that performs scan control functions, such as regulating the output of the RF or gradients or estimating the SAR or dB/dt, are considered as a moderate level of concern. A description of the information to be submitted in either case is contained in the "Guidance for the Content of Premarket Submissions for Software Contained in Medical Devices" issued on May 20, 1998.[17]

E. MR SAFETY AND COMPATIBILITY

MR safety and compatibility has been an issue from earliest days of clinical MR, when it was realized that patients with ferromagnetic or electromagnetically active implants were at risk in the MR environment. However, it has become an issue of increasing importance as the interventional or intraoperative use of MR has increased. Initially, MR guidance was used for minimally invasive procedures such as needle biopsies. However, recently it has been used in surgical procedures of increasing complexity, such as identifying tumor margins to ensure complete resection. Such procedures require MR compatible surgical tools, patient monitoring devices, and anesthesiology equipment.

The FDA has been evaluating devices intended for use with MR for a number of years as part of the IDE, 510(k), and PMA processes. Much of this activity has been performed by members of the CDRH MR working group, which has developed FDA policies in this area and attempted to ensure uniformity of reviews. The FDA's approach to the evaluation of MR compatibility is discussed in "A Primer on Medical Device Interactions with Magnetic Resonance Imaging Systems," which was released for comment in February 1997.[18]

Many of the manufacturers of implants and devices intended for use in interventional and intraoperative MR procedures are unfamiliar with MR technology. Consequently, the primer contains an overview of basic MR theory as well as a discussion of the components of an MR system and their potential interactions with medical devices. The document makes the distinction between MR safety and MR compatibility. A device that is "MR safe" is one that will not present a hazard in the MR environment. A device that is "MR compatible" is MR safe and, in addition, will not interfere with the operation of the MR system, nor itself be adversely affected.

The primer states the FDA's policy that any claims of MR safety or compatibility should be accompanied by test data or other scientific evidence. The document contains some general notes on testing, but does not specify detailed test methods. These are currently being developed by The American Society for Testing and Materials (ASTM) under subcommittee F04.15.11.

The primer also states the FDA's policy that labeling for a device that claims to be MR safe or compatible should contain a summary of the conditions under which the device was tested and the test results. The purpose of this information is to enable users to determine if they will be using the device beyond the conditions under which it was tested. This is especially important in view of the fact that MR hardware capabilities are steadily improving, resulting in an increasing severity of the exposure conditions for any medical devices brought into the MR environment.

For most medical devices, a manufacturer is only required to submit information relating to MR safety or compatibility if one of these is claimed for the device. However, in February 1997, the Office of Device Evaluation initiated a policy requiring that any submission for an implanted device must include a statement by the manufacturer regarding the MR safety and compatibility of that implant. This policy was instituted because MR use has increased dramatically and most people will require a MR examination at some time in their lives. Any person who is considering an implant should be aware of whether the implant will preclude his or her ability to undergo an MR examination in the future.

VI. FUTURE CONSIDERATIONS

A. THE FORTHCOMING REVISION OF THE IEC STANDARD

In February 1997, the secretary of SC 62 B submitted a proposal to the IEC to revise IEC 60601-2-33 to include new information that had not been included in the original version of that standard. The areas to be addressed were the ranges of values for the *dB/dt* and SAR operating modes and interventional MRI. Working Group 28 was formed to develop this revision. The working group completed a committee draft (CD) late in 1999 and submitted this draft for national comment.

The most extensive proposed revisions developed by the working group are to the provisions of the standard relating to *dB/dt*. The objectives of these provisions as stated in the draft are to prevent cardiac stimulation and intolerable PNS in any operating mode and to minimize painful stimulation in the normal operating mode.

Intolerable stimulation is defined as the level at which the patient will request that the scan be terminated. Painful stimulation is defined as a level tolerable to the patient when properly informed and motivated.

These objectives represent a change in attitude toward PNS in MR examinations. The change is justified by the fact that hundreds of volunteers have experienced painful stimulation in human studies with no harmful effects. As noted in the objectives, cardiac stimulation is obviously hazardous and to be avoided in all operating modes. Intolerable PNS is obviously undesirable because it leads to termination of the examination.

The new proposed *dB/dt* requirements are similar to the 1995 MRI guidance update for *dB/dt* in that they permit a manufacturer to perform a "direct determination" to demonstrate compliance. In a direct determination, the manufacturer would conduct a study using human volunteers. The upper limits for the normal and FLC mode would then be based on the median PNS threshold determined in that study. In the CD, the upper limit of the normal mode would be 80% of the median PNS threshold and the upper limit of the FLC operating mode would be 100% of the median PNS threshold.

However, in the case of whole-body gradients, a manufacturer may also use default *dB/dt* values as the limits of the normal and FLC operating modes. The default values are based on extensive human studies data for whole-body gradients that are now available. Many of these studies were conducted to obtain marketing clearance from the FDA. The working group examined the data for whole-body gradients and determined that a best fit to the median PNS threshold as a function of pulse duration was given by the function $dB/dt = 22.8\ \text{T/s}\ (1 + 0.4/t)$, where t is the pulse duration in milliseconds. As in the direct determination method, the upper limit of the normal mode would be 80% of this value, and the upper limit of the FLC mode would be 100%. For special purpose (e.g., head or extremity) gradients, the manufacturer could use direct determination or default values of the electric field.

The principal problem faced by the working group in defining the upper limit of the normal and FLC modes for *dB/dt* is the variability in human response. This is the reason for the relatively narrow gap between the upper limits for the normal and FLC modes (i.e., 20% of the median PNS threshold).

Intuitively, one would think that it would be possible to define the upper limit of the FCL mode well above the PNS threshold. However, as noted in the rationale for this section, available data indicates that at the mean PNS threshold (the proposed upper limit of the FLC mode), 5% of the patients may experience intolerable PNS (A-P gradient). This is probably the upper limit of acceptability in normal clinical operation.

One would also think that it would be possible to use a higher limit for the normal operating mode. However, at 80% of the mean PNS threshold, the committee estimated that painful stimulation could still occur in almost 2% of patients (A-P gradients). It may be possible to circumvent the problem presented by the variability in human response by applying a test sequence prior to examination. Such sequences are currently used to adjust the equipment parameters for optimal operation. This alternative will be considered by the working group before the standard is finalized.

It should be noted that in the CD, dB/dt refers to the rate of change of the magnitude of the gradient field. This is consistent with the approach in the 1995 MRI guidance update for dB/dt. In cases where gradients are applied simultaneously, the magnitude of the B field includes contributions from the combined gradients. When gradients are applied simultaneously, the CD requires that compliance be assessed using a quadratic addition rule or a properly validated alternative summation rule. The quadratic addition rule includes weighting factors to correct for the fact that the left-right gradient and head-foot gradients have higher PNS thresholds than the A-P gradient and, thus, are somewhat less effective. In the 1995 version of the IEC standard, the issue of simultaneous combined gradients in different directions was incorporated in the test method, which required simultaneous pulsing of all three gradients.

With respect to RF energy-induced heating, the CD permits the alternative of either limiting temperature rises or SAR, which is the same as the current FDA guidance. A core temperature rise of greater than 1°C would place a system in the SLC mode, requiring IRB approval. The whole-body-averaged SAR limit for the normal operating mode would also be increased from 1.5 to 2.0 W/kg.

The operating mode scheme would be applied to static magnetic field strength. Fields up to 2.0 T would be considered in the normal mode, fields from 2.0 to 4.0 T would be in the FLC mode, and fields above 4.0 T would be in the SLC mode. This is more consistent with the current FDA SR criteria than the current version of the IEC standard, which requires IRB approval above 2.0 T.

B. CHALLENGES IN ESTABLISHING SAFETY STANDARDS FOR THE FUTURE

Since the beginning of MR as a diagnostic modality, there has been a concern that the development of the technology would be limited by human tolerance to such effects as RF energy-induced heating and stimulation by time-varying magnetic fields. In the early years, safety limits were very conservative, but this did not limit MR system performance because the equipment was not capable of reaching these limits.

One of the greatest problems with early MR was the length of time needed to acquire an image. This was not only an economic disadvantage and a source of patient discomfort, but it had serious adverse effects on image quality due to physiological motion. To increase the speed of image acquisition, it has been generally necessary to increase the RF power input to the patient and the speed and strength of the gradients. Increased RF power deposition and gradient output are also essential in clinical techniques such as MR angiography, echo-planar, and diffusion weighted imaging.

As the speed of MR has increased, safety limits have risen. It is interesting to note that in the FDA's 1982 recommendations to IRBs, whole-body-averaged SAR above 0.4 W/kg was considered a significant risk. In the current version of IEC 60601-2-33, a whole-body-averaged SAR of 1.5 W/kg is considered safe for all patients, and a whole-body-averaged SAR of 4.0 W/kg is considered safe for patients with normal thermoregulatory capacity.

The significant risk level for dB/dt was 3 T/s in 1982, compared to a normal mode limit of 20 T/s in the current IEC standard. The limit of 20 T/s will undoubtedly be increased in the revision of this standard currently under consideration. In the CD, a time-dependent limit is proposed to take advantage of the fact that the PNS threshold increases with decreasing pulse duration. In the current draft revision, the normal mode limit would be increased to 36 T/s for a pulse duration of 0.4 ms, an increase of almost a factor of 2 over the current limit and a factor of 12 over the 1982 recommendation.

Until now, MR safety limits have increased largely as a result of increased knowledge of human tolerance levels. Early guidelines generally incorporated a large safety factor to account for uncertainties, and it has been possible to reduce these safety factors as data on human response has increased. However, at some point, this knowledge will be substantially complete, and such increases will no longer be possible. At that time, it will be necessary for manufacturers to turn their attention to engineering solutions. For example, speed is especially important in cardiac applications, and smaller gradient coils have been utilized for cardiac imaging. Because of its smaller size, the output of such a gradient coil can be very high without inducing nerve stimulation. One manufacturer has marketed a system with a dual gradient configuration. The second set of gradient coils covers a smaller region and is intended for applications where very high resolution is needed. The draft revision of the IEC standard provides for special purpose gradient coils by allowing a manufacturer to satisfy a limit on the induced electric field rather than *dB/dt*.

Another key challenge in the development of safety standards and guidelines for MR is anticipating the direction the technology will take and ensuring that the standards and guidelines can account for the new developments. An example of this is the development of higher field strength, open, vertical field magnets. A great deal of time and effort has been spent studying PNS in cylindrical magnets. It is likely that stronger gradients will be developed for the vertical field configurations in the near future because they are important in many clinical applications. When this occurs, PNS may become possible in these MR systems. However, the gradient coil designs for a vertical field magnet are different from those for cylindrical magnets, and the PNS data for cylindrical magnets may not be applicable.

It is important that safety standards and guidelines be written with sufficient flexibility so as to be applicable to new MR system designs and not hinder their introduction into the marketplace. This has been done in the draft revision of the IEC standard by allowing direct determination of the upper limits of the normal and first level controlled operating modes for gradient output and the establishment of limits on the induced electric field.

VII. CONCLUSIONS

In the past 20 years, MR has developed into a major radiological modality to the point where it has become the gold standard for the diagnosis of a number of disorders and conditions. During this period, there have been major changes in safety standards and guidelines. In general, recommended exposure limits have risen significantly as a result of our increased knowledge regarding the biological effects of the static, RF, and time-varying magnetic fields employed in MR. One of the most important lessons that has been learned during this time period is that it is important to include flexibility and alternatives in safety standards and guidelines so that the benefits of technical advances in MR are available to patients as soon as possible without compromising their safety.

REFERENCES

1. Zickler, P., Device focus: magnetic resonance imaging, *Med. Device Res. Rep.,* 1(3), 8, May/June 1994, Association for the Advancement of Medical Instrumentation.
2. Center for Devices and Radiological Health, The new 510(k) paradigm — alternative approaches to demonstrating substantial equivalence in premarket notifications, available on the Food and Drug Administration website at http://www.fda.gov/cdrh/ode/parad510.html.

3. Center for Devices and Radiological Health, Third party review program information, available on the Food and Drug Administration website at http://www.fda.gov/cdrh/dsma/3rdpty.html.

4. Center for Devices and Radiological Health, Standards program, available on the Food and Drug Administration website at http://www.fda.gov/cdrh/stdsprog.html.

5. Athey, T. W., FDA regulation of the safety of MR devices: past, present and future, *Magn. Reson. Imaging Clin. North Am.*, 6, 791, 1998.

6. National Electrical Manufacturers Association, NEMA Standards Publications No. MS 1 through 8, available from the National Electrical Manufacturers Association, 1300 North 17th Street, Suite 1847, Rosslyn, VA 22209 or through the NEMA website at http://www.nema.org.

7. Reilly, J. P., Peripheral nerve stimulation by induced electric currents: exposure to time varying magnetic fields, *Med. Biol. Eng. Comput.*, 27, 101, 1989.

8. Reilly, J. P., Peripheral nerve and cardiac excitation by time-varying magnetic fields: a comparison of thresholds, Final Report, Metatec, MT90–100, Silver Spring, MD.

9. Ehrhardt, J. C., Lin, C. S., Magnotta, V. A., et al., Neural stimulation in a whole body echo-planar imaging system, in Abstracts of the 12th Annual Meeting of the Society for Magnetic Resonance in Medicine, Berkeley, p. 1372, 1993.

10. Schaefer, D. J., Dosimetry and effects of MR exposure to RF and switched magnetic fields, *Ann. N.Y. Acad. Sci.*, 649, 225, 1992.

11. Schaefer, D. J., Safety aspects of switched gradient fields, *Magn. Reson. Imaging Clin. North Am.*, 6, 731, 1998.

12. Bourland, J. D., Nyenhuis, J. A., and Schaefer, D. J., Physiologic effects of intense MR imaging gradient gields, *Neuroimaging Clin. North Am.*, 9, 363, 1999.

13. International Electrotechnical Commission, Particular requirements for the safety of magnetic resonance equipment for medical diagnosis, IEC 60601-2-33, July 1995, available through the IEC website at http://www.iec.ch.

14. Center for Devices and Radiological Health, Guidance for magnetic resonance diagnostic devices — criteria for significant risk investigations, available on the Food and Drug Administration website at http://www.fda.gov/cdrh/ode/magdev.html.

15. Kangarlu, A., Burgess, R. E., Zhu, H., et al., Cognitive, cardiac and physiological safety studies in ultra high field magnetic resonance imaging, *Magn. Res. Imaging*, 17, 10, 1407, 1999.

16. Center for Devices and Radiological Health, Guidance for the submission of premarket notifications for magnetic resonance diagnostic devices, available on the Food and Drug Administration website at http://www.fda.gov/cdrh/ode/95.html.

17. Center for Devices and Radiological Health, Guidance for the content of premarket submissions for software contained in medical devices, available on the Food and Drug Administration website at http://www.fda.gov/cdrh/ode/57.html.

18. Center for Devices and Radiological Health, A primer on medical device interactions with magnetic resonance imaging systems, available on the Food and Drug Administration website at http://www.fda.gov/cdrh/ode/primerf6.html.

10 Claustrophobia, Anxiety, and Emotional Distress in the Magnetic Resonance Environment

Randy L. Gollub and Frank G. Shellock

CONTENTS

I. INTRODUCTION

The increasing availability and capabilities of magnetic resonance (MR) studies to improve medical diagnosis and prognosis have dramatically increased the number of MR procedures performed worldwide. Thus, many more first-time and repeat patients are undergoing MR examinations for an ever-widening spectrum of medical indications. Notably, increasing proportions of these procedures are performed on patients suffering from unstable medical and psychological illnesses. For many of the millions of patients who undergo MR procedures every year, the experience may cause great emotional distress. The referring physicians, radiologists, and technologists are best prepared to manage affected patients if they understand the etiology of the problem and know the appropriate maneuver or intervention to implement for treatment of the condition.[1]

This chapter will review the incidence of psychological distress in the MR environment, discuss the impact of emotional distress for patients undergoing MR procedures, characterize the sources and types of distress, and present specific measures documented to minimize dysphoric sensations.

II. INCIDENCE OF DISTRESS IN THE MR ENVIRONMENT

In this chapter, we define psychological distress in the MR environment to include all subjectively unpleasant experiences that are directly attributable to the MR procedure. Distress for the patient undergoing an MR procedure can range from mild anxiety, which can be managed simply with minimal reassurance, to a full-blown panic attack, which requires psychiatric intervention. Severe psychological distress reactions to MR examinations, namely, anxiety and panic attacks, are typically characterized by the rapid onset of at least four of the following clinical signs: fear of losing control or dying, nausea, paresthesias, palpitations, chest pain, faintness, dyspnea, feeling of choking, sweating, trembling, vertigo, or depersonalization.[2]

Many symptoms of a panic attack mimic overactivity of the sympathetic nervous system,[3] prompting concern that catecholamine responses may precipitate cardiac arrhythmias and/or ischemia in susceptible patients during the MR procedure.[4] However, this has not been reported in a clinical MR setting or any other similar situation. Nevertheless, it is advisable that, in a medically unstable patient, physiologic monitoring be a routine component of the MR procedure. Preemptive efforts to minimize patient distress are the most important factors in preventing or containing a panic attack in susceptible patients.

In its mildest form, distress is the normal amount of anxiety any reasonable person will experience when undergoing a diagnostic procedure. Moderate distress, severe enough to be described as a dysphoric psychological reaction, has been reported by as many as 65% of the patients examined by MR imaging.[5-8] The most severe forms of psychological distress described by patients are claustrophobia and anxiety or panic attacks.[3,5-12]

Claustrophobia is a disorder characterized by the marked, persistent, and excessive fear of enclosed spaces.[2] In such affected individuals, exposure to enclosed spaces such as the MR environment, but no other situations or stimuli, almost invariably provokes an immediate anxiety response that in its most extreme form is indistinguishable from a panic attack described above.

The actual incidence of distress in the MR environment is highly variable across studies, in part reflecting differences in outcome measures used to measure distress. Some studies indicate that as many as 20% of individuals attempting to undergo an MR imaging procedure cannot complete it due to serious distress such as claustrophobia or other similar sensations.[13,14] In contrast, others report that as few as 0.7% of individuals have incomplete or failed MR procedures due to distress.[8,15] A reasonable estimate of the number of patients that experience distress that compromises either their own well-being or the diagnostic utility of the MR procedure is 3 to 5% of all studies.

Notably, there are no perfect predictors of distress in the MR environment. In fact, different studies cite opposing results, such as which gender has greater difficulty tolerating the MR studies.[15,16] Obviously, these differences may reflect cultural, socioeconomic, or other influences.

III. THE IMPACT OF EMOTIONAL DISTRESS IN THE MR ENVIRONMENT

Patient distress can contribute to adverse outcomes for the MR procedure. These adverse outcomes include unintentional exacerbation of patient distress; a compromise in the quality, and, thus, the diagnostic power of the imaging study; and decreased efficiency of the imaging facility due to delayed, cancelled, or prematurely terminated studies. Patient compliance during an MR procedure, such as the ability to remain in the MR system and hold still long enough to complete the study, is of paramount importance to achieving a high quality, diagnostic examination.

If a good quality study cannot be obtained, the patient may require an invasive diagnostic examination in place of the safer, less painful, and less risky MR procedure. Thus, for the distressed patient unable to undergo an MR procedure, there are typically clinical, medico-legal, and economic-related considerations and implications.

Increasing pressure to use MR system time efficiently to cover the costs of expensive diagnostic imaging equipment puts greater stress on both staff and patients. The ability of referring physicians, radiologists, and technologists to detect patient distress at the earliest possible time, to discover the source of the distress, and then provide appropriate intervention can greatly improve patient comfort, quality of imaging studies, and efficiency of the MR facility.[1]

A motion artifact disrupting the MR image quality is frequently the result of patient distress; that is, the distressed patient becomes agitated and finds it difficult to remain motionless during the MR procedure. Motion artifacts can compromise the diagnostic power of an MR procedure. A recent study in 297 first-time outpatients undergoing MR imaging demonstrated that approximately 13% of all MR studies showed motion artifacts (i.e., unrelated to normal body pulsations), and about half of these impaired the diagnostic quality of the examination.[8]

Excessive anxiety with accompanying tremors, trembling, jaw clenching, and other related body movements has been presumed to contribute to motion artifacts in MR images. Dantendorfer et al.[8] attempted to investigate this directly and found that, while specific measures of anxiety do not predict motion artifacts, reported concerns about the MR equipment did predict motion artifacts. These results support the interpretation that adequate patient education about the MR procedure is one of the most important aspects to minimizing distress and the associated adverse outcomes.

IV. FACTORS THAT CONTRIBUTE TO DISTRESS IN THE MR ENVIRONMENT

Many factors contribute to distress experienced by certain patients undergoing MR procedures. Most commonly cited are concerns about the physical environment of the MR system. Also well documented are the anxieties associated with the underlying medical problem necessitating the MR procedure. Notably, certain individuals, such as those with psychiatric illnesses, may be predisposed to suffer greater distress due to MR procedures.

The physical environment of the MR system is clearly one important source of distress to patients. Sensations of apprehension, tension, worry, claustrophobia, anxiety, fear, and even panic attacks have been directly attributed to the confining dimensions of the interior of the MR system. For example, for certain types of MR systems, the patient's face may be 3 to 10 in. from the inner portion of the MR system, prompting feelings of uncontrolled confinement and detachment.[3,5-14,17-21]

Similar distressing sensations have been attributed to other aspects of the MR environment, including the prolonged duration of the MR examination, the gradient magnetic field-induced acoustic noise, the temperature and humidity within the MR system, and the distress related to the restriction of movement.[3-14,17-23] Gradient field-induced noise may be sufficiently intense to cause transient hearing threshold shifts in as many as 43% of patients undergoing MR procedures.[24] Obviously, noise itself can be a source of stress and, thus, particularly troublesome to certain patients undergoing MR procedures. Other studies have reported stress related to the administration of an intravenous MRI contrast agent.[3,5-7,9-14,17-23,25] Additionally, the MR system may produce a feeling of sensory deprivation, which is also known to be a precursor of severe anxiety states.[10]

MR systems that have an architecture that utilizes a vertical magnetic field offer a more open design that is presumed to reduce the frequency of distress associated with MR procedures. The latest versions of these so-called "open" MR systems, despite having static magnetic field strengths of 0.3 T or lower, have improved technology (i.e., faster gradient fields, optimized surface coils, etc.) that permit acceptable image quality for virtually all types of standard diagnostic imaging procedures (Figure 10.1). Notably, 0.7- and 1.0-T open MR systems have recently become commercially available, and these newly designed systems may be more acceptable to patients with feelings of distress (Figure 10.1). Also, the latest generation, high-field-strength (1.5-T) MR systems have shorter and wider bore configurations (Figure 10.1).

Interestingly, in direct contraindication to the presumed advantage of the open MR systems, Datendorfer et al.[8] reported absolutely no difference between a standard 1.5-T MR system (Siemens Magnetom SP-65™, Siemens Corporation, Iselin, NJ) and a more open 0.5-T MR system (Philips Gyroscan P-5™, Philips Medical Systems, Shelton, CT) in the incidence of adverse reactions (i.e., pre- or post-scan anxiety, claustrophobia, aborted studies, or motion artifacts). Clearly, more studies that directly address this issue are warranted.

In 1993, a specially designed, low-field-strength (0.2-T) MR system (Artoscan™, General Electric Medical Systems and Lunar Corporation, Madison, WI and Esaote, Genoa, Italy) became

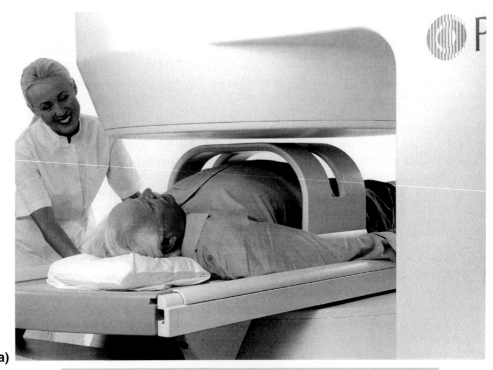

(a)

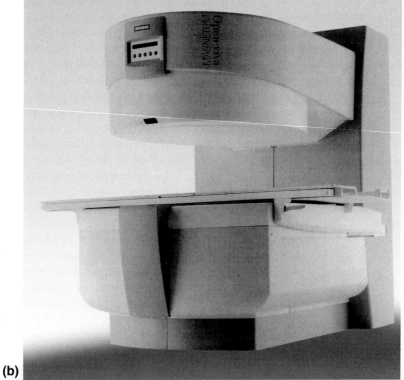

(b)

FIGURE 10.1 Examples of various types of MR system configurations that represent more open designs that may be more acceptable to patients with psychological distress. Examples of open MR systems: (a) 0.23-T, Proview MR System [Marconi Medical Systems (formerly Picker Medical Systems) Cleveland, OH]; (b) 0.2-T, MAGNETOM Open Viva (Siemens Medical Systems, Inc., Iselin, NJ).   (*continued*)

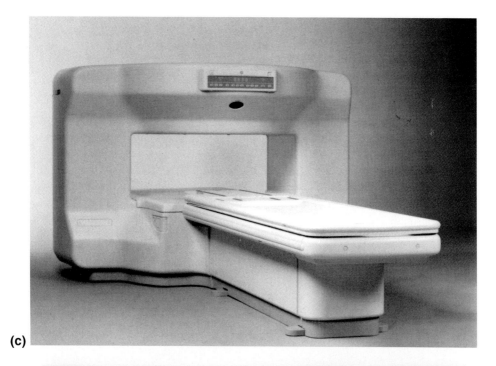

(c)

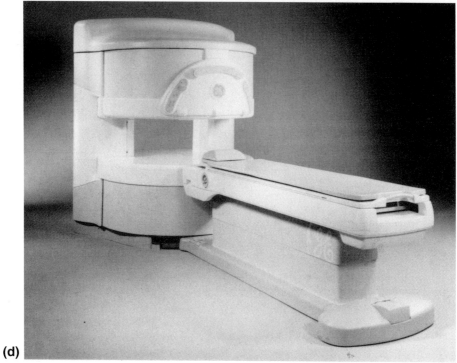

(d)

FIGURE 10.1 (CONTINUED) Examples of various types of MR system configurations that represent more open designs that may be more acceptable to patients with psychological distress. Examples of open MR systems: (c) 0.2-T, Signa Profile/i Open MRI (General Electric Medical Systems, Milwaukee, WI). Examples of newly developed, open, high-field-strength MR systems: (d) 0.7-T, Signa OpenSpeed MR System (General Electric Medical Systems).   (*continued*)

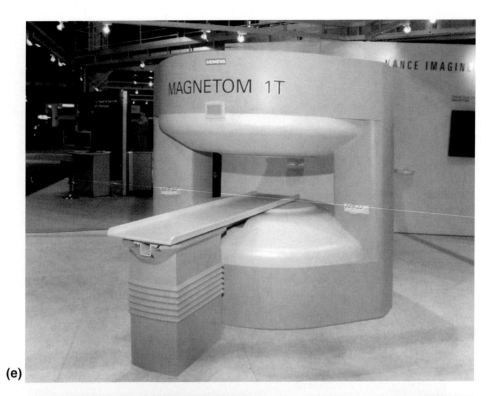

(e)

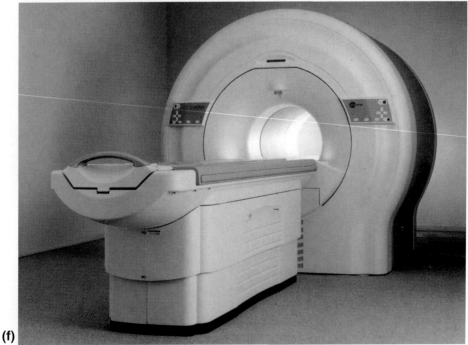

(f)

FIGURE 10.1 (CONTINUED) Examples of various types of MR system configurations that represent more open designs that may be more acceptable to patients with psychological distress. Example of newly developed, open, high-field-strength MR system: (e) 1.0-T, MAGNETOM Open Magnetic Resonance (MR) Scanner (Siemens Medical Systems, Inc.). Examples of the latest generation, high-field-strength MR systems that have shorter, wider bore configurations: (f) 1.5-T, Eclipse MR System (Marconi Medical Systems).   (*continued*)

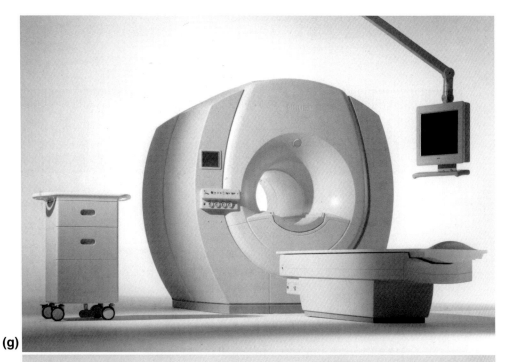

(g)

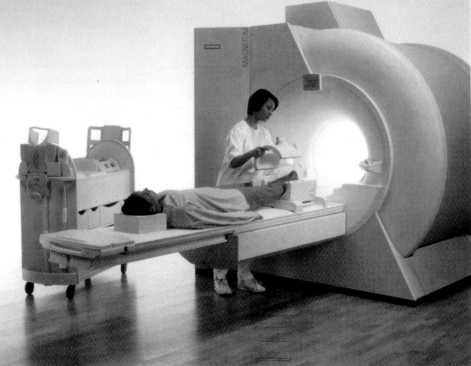

(h)

FIGURE 10.1 (CONTINUED) Examples of various types of MR system configurations that represent more open designs that may be more acceptable to patients with psychological distress. Examples of the latest generation, high-field-strength MR systems that have shorter, wider bore configurations: (g) 1.5-T, Gyroscan Intera (Philips Medical Systems, Shelton, CT); (h) 1.5-T, MAGNETOM, Symphony MR System (Siemens Medical Systems, Inc.). *(continued)*

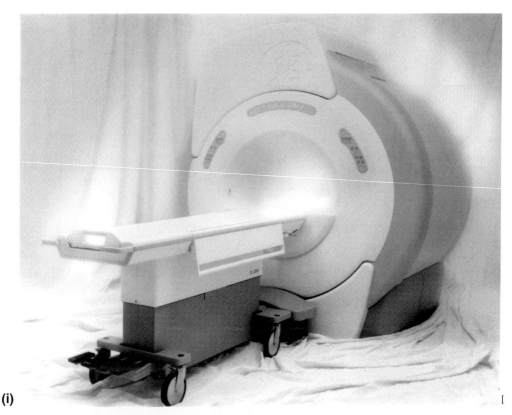

(i)

FIGURE 10.1 (CONTINUED) Examples of various types of MR system configurations that represent more open designs that may be more acceptable to patients with psychological distress. Examples of the latest generation, high-field-strength MR systems that have shorter, wider bore configurations: (i) 1.5-T, Signa MR/i MR System (General Electric Medical Systems).

commercially available for MR imaging of extremities. The use of this dedicated extremity MR system provides an accurate, reliable, and relatively inexpensive means (i.e., in comparison to the use of a whole-body MR system) of evaluating various types of musculoskeletal abnormalities. Therefore, utilization of the extremity MR system to assess musculoskeletal pathology is a viable and acceptable alternative to the use of whole-body MR systems.[26] This is particularly the case, since the image quality and diagnostic capabilities for the evaluation of the knee and other extremities has been reported to be comparable to mid- or high-field-strength MR systems for certain musculoskeletal applications.[26]

The architecture of the extremity MR system has no confining features or other aspects that would typically create patient-related problems (Figure 10.2). This is because only the body part that requires imaging is placed inside the magnet bore during the MR examination.

A preliminary study reported that 100% of the MR examinations that were initiated were completed without being interrupted or cancelled for patient-related problems.[26] The unique design of the extremity MR system likely contributed to the totally successful completion of MR procedures in the patients of this study. Furthermore, these findings represent a dramatic improvement compared with the published incidence of patient distress that tends to interrupt or prevent the completion of MR procedures using whole-body MR systems.[26] A more recently developed, dedicated extremity MR system also permits MR imaging of the shoulder (Figure 10.2).

Adverse psychological reactions are sometimes associated with the MR procedures simply because the examination may be perceived by the patient as a "dramatic" medical test that has an

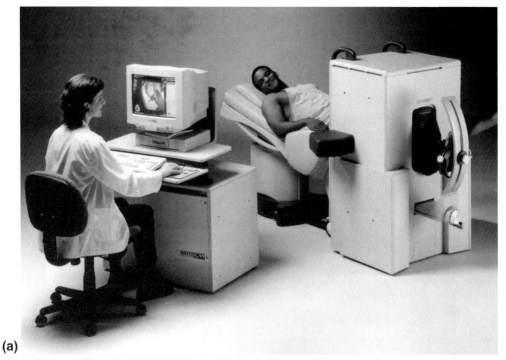

(a)

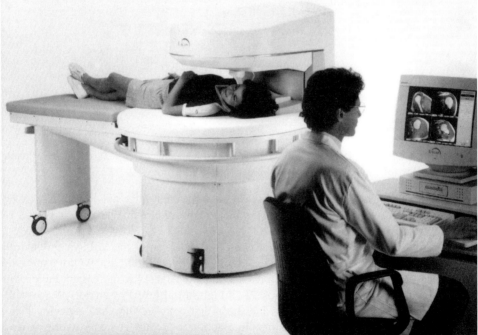

(b)

FIGURE 10.2   Dedicated extremity MR system that has no substantial confining features. (a) This MR system (Artoscan-M Dedicated Extremity MRI System, General Electric Medical Systems and Lunar Corporation, Madison, WI and Esaote, Genoa, Italy), which was designed and optimized for musculoskeletal imaging (i.e., foot, ankle, calf, knee, thigh, hand, wrist, forearm, and elbow), is unlikely to produce psychological distress in patients. (b) Recently developed, dedicated extremity MR system that also permits MR imaging of the shoulder (E-Scan Open Extremity MRI System, General Electric Medical Systems and Lunar Corporation; a version of this MR system called the MAGNETOM Jazz is also commercially available from Siemens Medical Systems, Inc.).   (*continued*)

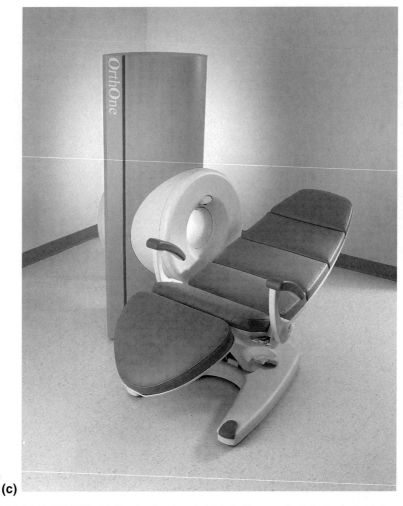

(c)

FIGURE 10.2 (CONTINUED) (c) Newly developed, high-field-strength (1.0-T), dedicated extremity MR system (OrthoOne, ONI, Inc. North Andover, MA).

associated uncertainty of outcome, such that there may be a fear of the presence of disease or other abnormality.[5,10] In fact, any type of diagnostic imaging procedure may produce a certain amount of anxiety for the patient.[18]

For example, Thorp et al.[14] found that, with the exception of the MR system environment issue (i.e., the confined space), patients undergoing computed tomography compared to those undergoing MR imaging had similar feelings that the procedure was unpleasant. Patients finding the experience difficult tended to be those with high initial levels of anxiety, those with little experience with diagnostic procedures, and those that believed they had cancer.[14] This study underscores the need for direct professional interaction to prepare and educate the patient prior to any form of diagnostic imaging examination. Improved patient compliance was reported in a recent study that directly investigated the impact of more detailed patient education on adverse outcomes from MR mammography, a procedure known to have an atypically high rate of non-compliance.[27]

Patients with pre-existing psychiatric disorders may be at greater risk for experiencing distress in the MR environment. One problem that arises more often in this population is the refusal of the prescribed MR procedure by the patient. Frequently, the cause for refusal is an inadequate understanding of why the procedure was ordered and what the procedure actually involves.

No specific reports of the differential frequency of distress or adverse outcomes for MR procedures in these patients compared to non-psychiatrically impaired patients has been published to date. However, specific inquiry should be made to identify patients with pre-existing anxiety disorders including claustrophobia, generalized anxiety disorder, post-traumatic stress disorder, and obsessive-compulsive disorder in order to increase anxiety-minimizing efforts in these patients (see below).

Patients with other psychiatric illnesses such as depression or any illness complicated by thought disorder such as schizophrenia and manic-depressive disorder may also be at increased risk for distress in the MR environment. Patients with psychiatric illnesses may, under normal circumstances, be able to tolerate the MR environment without a problem, as is clear from the thousands who participate in clinical neuroimaging research studies each year.[28] However, the increased stress due to their medical illness or fear of medical illness may exacerbate their psychiatric symptoms to such an extent that they may have difficulty complying with MR procedures. At the very least, patients with psychiatric illnesses may require more time and patience to provide the appropriate level of preparatory information.

V. TECHNIQUES TO MINIMIZE PATIENT DISTRESS IN THE MR ENVIRONMENT

We outline here a stepwise set of procedures for minimizing subjective distress for all patients undergoing MR procedures. Certain measures to alleviate patient distress should be employed for all studies. A number of other measures may be required if the patient is experiencing significant distress due to factors as described above. Finally, other distress-alleviation techniques will only be necessary for patients with co-existing psychiatric illness or other special problems. Coordination of these efforts among the referring physician, the radiologist, the MR technologist, and the MR facility support staff is crucial. Many of these methods have been described in the literature and are summarized in Table 10.1.[3-5,7,9,11,12,16,21-23,27,29-33]

TABLE 10.1
Recommended Techniques for Managing Patients with Distress Related to MR Procedures

1.	Prepare and educate the patient concerning specific aspects of the MR examination (e.g., MR system dimensions, gradient noise, intercom system, etc.).
2.	Allow an appropriately screened relative or friend to remain with the patient during the MR procedure.
3.	Maintain physical or verbal contact with the patient during the MR procedure.
4.	Use MR-compatible headphones to provide music to the patient and to minimize gradient magnetic field-induced noise.
5.	Use an MR-compatible monitor to provide a visual distraction to the patient.
6.	Use a virtual reality environment system to provide audio and visual distractions.
7.	Place the patient in a prone position inside the MR system.
8.	Position the patient feet first instead of head first into the MR system.
9.	Use special mirrors or prism glasses for the patient.
10.	Use a blindfold so that the patient is not aware of the close surroundings.
11.	Use bright lights inside and at either end of the MR system.
12.	Use a fan inside the MR system to provide adequate air movement.
13.	Use lemon or vanilla scented oil or other similar aromatherapy so that the patient can comfortably experience olfactory stimulation.
14.	Use relaxation techniques such as controlled breathing or mental imagery.
15.	Use systematic desensitization.
16.	Use medical hypnosis.
17.	Use a sedative or other similar medication.

A. For All Patients Undergoing MR Procedures

Referring clinicians should take the time to explain the rationale for the MR procedure and what he/she expects to learn from the results with respect to the implications for treatment and prognosis. Importantly, the clinician should schedule time with the patient to communicate the results of the MR procedure.

The single most important step is to educate the patient about the specific aspects of the MR examination that are known to be particularly difficult. This includes conveying, in terms that are understandable to the patient, the internal dimensions of the MR system, the level of gradient magnetic field-induced acoustic noise to expect, and the estimated time duration of the examination.

Studies have documented a decrease in the incidence of premature termination of MR procedures when patients are provided with more detailed information regarding the examination.[27] This may be effectively accomplished by means of providing the patient time to view an educational videotape or written brochure supplemented by a question and answer session with an MR-trained healthcare worker prior to the MR procedure.

Some authors have proposed adding a pre-scan "fear assessment" to help predict patients who will experience psychological problems related to the MR procedure.[13,17,18] Such a brief questionnaire could be used to help elicit questions and concerns from patients and to provide guidance to staff about which distress minimization strategies are most likely to be effective for the patient.

Upon entering the MR facility, patients who are treated with respect and are welcomed into a calm environment will report less distress. Many details of patient positioning in the MR system can increase comfort and minimize distress. Taking time to ensure comfortable positioning with adequate padding and blankets to alleviate undue discomfort or pain from positioning is also important. Adequate ear protection should be provided routinely to decrease acoustic noise from the MR system. Demonstration of the two-way intercom system to reassure the patient that the MR staff can hear them when they speak and can speak to them can also be very reassuring.

B. For Mildly to Moderately Distressed Patients

If a patient continues to experience distress after the aforementioned measures are implemented, additional interventions are required. Frequently, all that is necessary to successfully complete an MR examination is to allow an appropriately screened relative or friend to remain with the patient during the procedure. A familiar person in the MR system room often helps patients who are anxious because they develop an increased sense of security.[12,22] If a supportive companion is not present, then simply having the MR staff maintain verbal contact via the intercom system or physical contact by having a staff person remain in the MR system room with the patient during the examination will frequently decrease psychological distress.[7,12,22]

Placing the patient in a prone position inside the MR system so that the patient can visualize the opening of the bore provides a sensation of being inside a device that is more spacious and alleviates the "closed-in" feeling associated with the supine position.[22] Prone positioning of the patient may not be a practical alternative if MR imaging requires the use of flat local coils or if the patient has underlying medical conditions (e.g., shortness of breath, the presence of chest tubes, etc.) that preclude lying flat. Another method of positioning the patient that may help is to place the individual feet first instead of head first into the MR system.

MR system-mounted mirrors or prism glasses can be used to permit the patient to maintain a vertical view of the outside of the MR system in order to minimize phobic responses. Using a blindfold so that the patient is not aware of the close surroundings has also been suggested to be an effective technique for enabling anxious patients to successfully undergo MR procedures.[12,22]

The environment of the MR system may be changed to optimize the management of apprehensive patients.[12] For example, the presence of higher lighting levels tends to make most individuals feel less anxious. Therefore, the use of bright lights at either end of and inside the MR system can produce a less imposing environment for the patient. In addition, using a fan inside the MR system to provide more air movement will help reduce the sensation of confinement and lessen any tissue heating that may result when high levels of radiofrequency (RF) power absorption are used for MR imaging.[12] Some MR staff members have reported that placing a cotton pad moistened with a few drops of essential lemon or vanilla oil or other similar form of aromatherapy in the MR system for the patient to receive olfactory stimulation can also reduce distress.

Electronic devices that utilize compressed air to transmit music or audio communication through headphones have been developed specifically for use with MR systems.[30,31,34,35] MR-compatible music/audio systems may be acquired from a commercial vendor or can be made by adapting an airplane pneumatic earphone headset.[30,35] MR-compatible music systems can be used to provide calming music to the patient and, with the proper design, can help to minimize exposure to gradient magnetic field-induced acoustic noise (Figure 10.3). Reports have indicated that the use of these devices has been successful in reducing symptoms of anxiety in patients during MR procedures.[31,34] In addition, it is now possible to provide visual stimulation to the patient via special goggles.[35] Use of visual stimuli to distract patients may also reduce distress. Finally, a new system has been developed to provide a virtual reality environment for the patient that may likewise serve as an acceptable means of audio and visual distraction from the MR procedure (Figure 10.4).

C. FOR SEVERELY DISTRESSED OR CLAUSTROPHOBIC PATIENTS

Patients who are at high risk for severe distress in the MR environment and can be identified as such by their referring clinician or by the scheduling MR staff could be offered the opportunity to have pre-MR procedure behavioral therapy. MR procedures that were conducted in patients that previously refused or were unable to tolerate the MR environment have been reported to be successful as a result of treatment with relaxation techniques,[9,33] systematic desensitization,[11] and

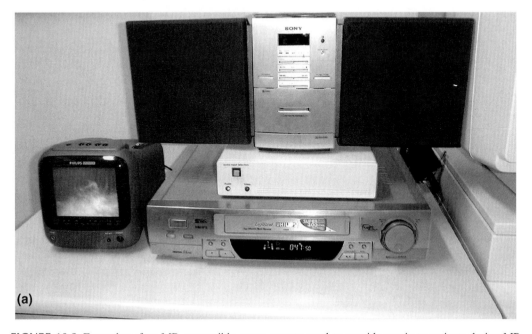

(a)

FIGURE 10.3 Examples of an MR-compatible stereo system used to provide music to patients during MR procedures. (a) The Commander XG MRI Audio System is shown interfaced with a video system (optional).

(continued)

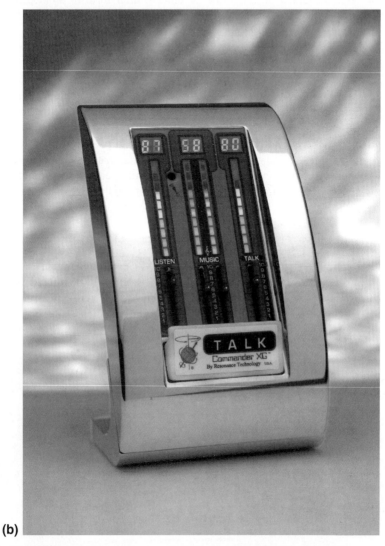

(b)

FIGURE 10.3 (CONTINUED) Examples of an MR-compatible stereo system used to provide music to patients during MR procedures. (b) The Commander XG MRI Audio System has features that include a remote control two-way intercom, a talk button that fades out music and enables the patient microphone, a digital display that shows the patient audio level, a multi-CD changer, a dual cassette deck, and an AM/FM tuner.

(*continued*)

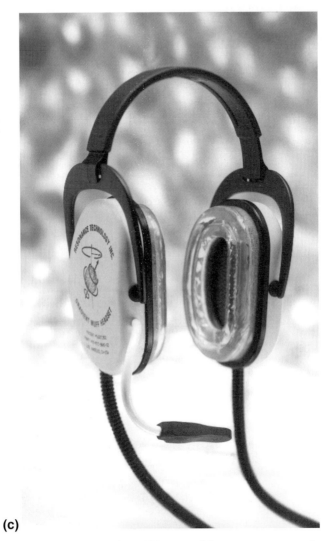

(c)

FIGURE 10.3 (CONTINUED) Examples of an MR-compatible stereo system used to provide music to patients during MR procedures. (c) The Commander XG MRI Audio System audio system features a special headset that blocks 30 dB of the acoustic noise.   (*continued*)

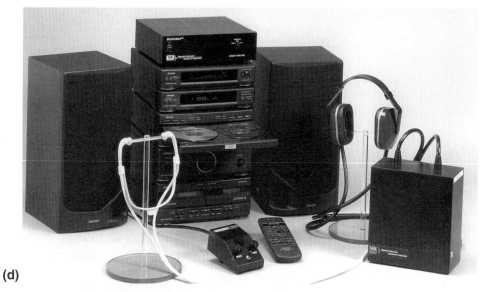

(d)

FIGURE 10.3 (CONTINUED) Examples of an MR-compatible stereo system used to provide music to patients during MR procedures. (d) The MUSICBOX™ System has features that include an over-the-ear headset for noise reduction, an integrated intercom, a multi-CD changer, a graphic equilizer, a dual cassette deck, an AM/FM tuner, and an auxilliary output for functional MRI applications.

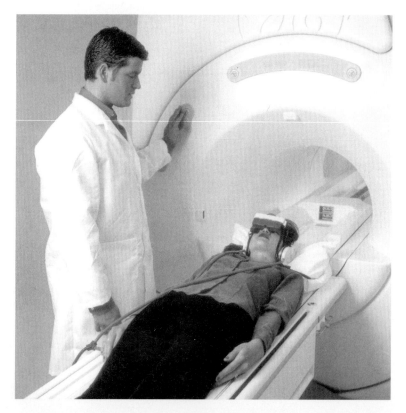

FIGURE 10.4 The MR-compatible audiovisual system, MRVision 2000 (Resonance Technology, Van Nuys, CA). This special system may be used during the MR procedure to provide the patient with audio and visual distractions. The visor/goggles fit easily into all standard head coils.

medical hypnosis.[21, 23, 32] Quirk et al.[9] reported that psychological preparation which included information about the examination and the use of relaxation strategies (i.e., breathing relaxation techniques, visualization of pleasant images, performance of mental exercises, etc.) was more effective for reducing anxiety in patients compared to providing information alone.

Klonoff et al.[11] provided a detailed example of one successful systematic desensitization protocol. This was conducted prior to the MR procedure and involved having the patient lie on the floor at home with her head in a box. The size of the box was incrementally decreased until it approximated the internal dimensions of the MR system. Additionally, the patient was required to gradually increase the amount of time she could tolerate spending with the box over her head, until it equaled 50 to 60 min, to approximate the maximum time needed for MR imaging. The patient also wore prism glasses that permitted her to have a direct view in the vertical plane during MR imaging. After four treatment sessions, the patient was able to successfully undergo MR imaging.[11] Notably, because of the time involved with systematic desensitization, this technique of preparing the distressed patient for an MR procedure may not be practical for most MR facilities.

Medical hypnosis has been demonstrated to be a successful means of treating phobias[29] and, not surprisingly, has been used as an effective intervention to enable a claustrophobic or anxious patient to complete MR examinations.[21,23,32] Successful hypnotherapy requires a trained medical hypnotist and a willing, trance-susceptible patient. Therefore, identifying the appropriate patient that would benefit from being hypnotized before and during the MR procedure and having a hypnosis therapist available for treatment are prerequisites for instituting this technique of patient management. There is a secondary effect of using hypnosis for patients with psychological disorders undergoing MR procedures insofar as patients have reported feeling a general reduction in anxiety in their everyday lives after undergoing hypnosis for MR imaging.[21]

In the majority of MR facilities, patients that are severely affected by claustrophobia, anxiety, or panic attacks in response to MR procedures are usually pharmacologically sedated when other attempts to counteract their distress fail. Using short-acting sedatives such as lorazepam, diazepam, alprazolam, intranasal midazolam, or one of the newer anxiolytic medications may be the only means of managing patients with a high degree of anxiety related to the MR procedure. Published reports of the rate of pharmacological sedation for patients undergoing MR procedures range from 2 to 14%.[8,16]

A study conducted by Avrahami[3] in patients with panic attacks who were unable to undergo MR imaging reported that treatment with intravenous diazepam caused the symptoms to disappear rapidly and permitted completion of the examination in every case. However, the use of sedatives in patients prior to and during MR procedures may not be required in all instances, nor is it always practical.[1]

Of special note, anxious patients with a history of substance abuse who are in recovery programs may not be willing to take mind altering medications because this is typically contraindicated in their treatment. These patients should be referred for behavioral therapy before MR procedures. In all cases, one or more of the recommended, non-medication-related techniques indicated in Table 10.1 should be attempted before immediately electing to use a sedative in distressed patients in the MR environment.

Sedation in the MR environment is not a totally benign procedure. Confusion and respiratory compromise, as well as other untoward reactions, have been reported in response to relatively modest doses of commonly employed sedatives.[6,9] If a sedative or other similar drug is used in a patient in preparation for an MR procedure, it should be understood that the use of this medication involves several important patient management considerations.[19] For example, the time when the patient should be administered the medication for optimal effect prior to the examination should be considered along with the possibility that there may be an adverse reaction to the drug.[19] Provisions should be available for an area to permit adequate recovery of the patient after the MR procedure. The patient should also have someone available to provide transportation from the MR facility after receiving medication.

VI. SUMMARY AND CONCLUSIONS

The advances in MR technology coupled with the advances in clinical applications of MR procedures to aid in the diagnosis and management of an ever-increasing number of medical conditions will ensure that the number of patients undergoing MR procedures continues to increase each year. Thus, the number of patients at risk for experiencing distress during these procedures will continue to increase.

We described the types of distress and the negative consequences that patient distress can have on the outcome of the MR procedure. Most importantly, we outlined simple and effective strategies for minimizing and perhaps eliminating this distress for many patients. Patient education about the MR procedure is perhaps the single most important measure to minimize distress and the associated adverse outcomes. It is not unreasonable to expect that adherence to the outlined measures will greatly improve patient comfort and, thereby, greatly reduce the number of aborted or poor quality studies.

REFERENCES

1. Shellock, F.G., Claustrophobia, anxiety, and panic disorders associated with MR procedures, in *Magnetic Resonance: Bioeffects, Safety, and Patient Management.*, Shellock, F.G., and Kanal, E., Eds., Lippincott-Raven Press, New York, 1996, 65.
2. *Diagnostic and Statistical Manual of Mental Disorders*, 4th ed., American Psychiatric Association, Washington, D.C., 1994.
3. Avrahami, E., Panic attacks during MR imaging: treatment with IV diazepam, *Am. J. Neuroradiol.*, 11, 833, 1990.
4. Brennan, S.C., Redd, W.H., Jacobsen, P.B., et al., Anxiety and panic during magnetic resonance scans, *Lancet*, 2, 521, 1988.
5. Granet, R.B. and Gelber, L.J., Claustrophobia during MR imaging, *N.J. Med.*, 87, 479, 1990.
6. Quirk, M.E., Letendre, A.J., Ciottone, R.A., et al., Anxiety in patients undergoing MR imaging, *Radiology*, 170, 463, 1989.
7. Shellock, F.G. and Kanal, E., Policies, guidelines, and recommendations for MR imaging and patient management, *J. Magn. Reson. Imag.*, 1, 97, 1991.
8. Dantendorfer, K., Amering, M., Bankier, A., et al., A study of the effect of patient anxiety, perception and equipment on motion artifacts in magnetic resonance imaging, *Magn. Reson. Imag.*, 15, 301, 1997.
9. Quirk, M.E., Letendre, A.J., Ciottone, R.A., et al., Evaluation of three psychological interventions to reduce anxiety during MR imaging, *Radiology*, 173, 759, 1989.
10. Flaherty, J.A. and Hoskinson, K., Emotional distress during magnetic resonance imaging, *N. Engl. J. Med.*, 320, 467, 1989.
11. Klonoff, E.A., Janata, J.W., and Kaufman, B., The use of systematic desensitization to overcome resistance to magnetic resonance imaging (MRI) scanning, *J. Behav. Ther. Exp. Psychiatry*, 17, 189, 1986.
12. Weinreb, J., Maravilla, K.R., Peshock, R., et al., Magnetic resonance imaging: improving patient tolerance and safety, *Am. J. Roentgenol.*, 143, 1285, 1984.
13. Melendez, C. and McCrank, E., Anxiety-related reactions associated with magnetic resonance imaging examinations, *J. Am. Med. Assoc.*, 270, 745, 1993.
14. Thorp, D., Owens, R.G., Whitehouse, G., et al., Subjective experiences of magnetic resonance imaging, *Clin. Radiol.*, 41, 276, 1990.
15. Sarji, S.A., Abdullah, B.J., Kumar, G., et al., Failed magnetic resonance imaging examinations due to claustrophobia, *Australas. Radiol.*, 42, 293, 1998.
16. Murphy, K.J. and Brunberg, J.A., Adult claustrophobia, anxiety and sedation in MRI, *Magn. Reson. Imag.*, 15, 51, 1997.
17. Kilborn, L.C. and Labbe, E.E., Magnetic resonance imaging scanning procedures: development of phobic response during scan and at one-month follow-up, *J. Behav. Med.*, 13, 391, 1990.

18. MacKenzie, R., Sims, C., Owens, R.G., et al., Patient's perceptions of magnetic resonance imaging, *Clin. Radiol.*, 50, 137, 1995.
19. Moss, M.L., Boungiorno, P.A., and Clancy, V.A., Intranasal midazolam for claustrophobia in MRI, *J. Comput. Assist. Tomogr.,* 17, 991, 1993.
20. Duluca, S.A. and Castronovo, F.P., Hazards of magnetic resonance imaging, *Am. Fam. Physician*, 41, 145, 1990.
21. Friday, P.J. and Kubal, W.S., Magnetic resonance imaging: improved patient tolerance utilizing medical hypnosis, *Am. J. Clin. Hypn.*, 33, 80, 1990.
22. Hricak, H. and Amparo, E.G., Body MRI: alleviation of claustrophobia by prone positioning, *Radiology*, 152, 819, 1984.
23. Phelps, L.A., MRI and claustrophobia, *Am. Fam. Physician*, 42, 930, 1991.
24. Brummett, R.E., Talbot, J.M., and Charuhas, P., Potential hearing loss resulting from MR imaging, *Radiology*, 169, 539 1988.
25. Thomsen, H.S., Frequency of acute adverse events to a non-ionic low-osmolar contrast medium: the effect of verbal interview, *Pharmacol. Toxicol.*, 80, 108, 1997.
26. Shellock, F.G., Stone, K.R., Resnick, D., et al., Subjective perceptions of MRI examinations performed using an extremity MR system, *Signals*, 32, 16, 2000.
27. Youssefzadeh, S., Eibenberger, K., Helbich, T., et al., Reduction of adverse events in MRI of the breast by personal patient care, *Clin. Radiol.*, 52, 862, 1997.
28. Rauch, S.L. and Renshaw, P.F., Clinical neuroimaging in psychiatry, *Harv. Rev. Psychiatry*, 2, 297, 1995.
29. McGuinness, T.P., Hypnosis in the treatment of phobias: a review of the literature, *Am. J. Clin. Hypn.*, 26, 261, 1984.
30. Axel, L., Simpler music/audio system for patients having MR imaging, *Am. J. Roentgenol.*, 151, 1080, 1988.
31. Miyamoto, A.T. and Kasson, R.T., Simple music/audio system for patients having MR imaging, *Am. J. Roentgenol.*, 151, 1060, 1988.
32. Simon, E.P., Hypnosis using a communication device to increase magnetic resonance imaging tolerance with a claustrophobic patient, *Mil. Med.*, 164, 71, 1999.
33. Lukins, R., Davan, I.G., and Drummond, P.D., A cognitive behavioural approach to preventing anxiety during magnetic resonance imaging, *J. Behav. Ther. Exp. Psychiatry*, 28, 97 1997.
34. Slifer, K.J., Penn-Jones, K., Cataldo, M.F., et al., Music enhances patient's comfort during MR imaging, *Am. J. Roentgenol.*, 156, 403, 1991.
35. Savoy, R.L., Ravicz, M.E., and Gollub, R., The psychophysiological laboratory in the magnet: stimulus delivery, response recording, and safety, in *Functional MRI*, Springer-Verlag, Berlin, 1999, 347.

11 Patient Monitoring in the Magnetic Resonance Environment

Frank G. Shellock

CONTENTS

I. INTRODUCTION

Conventional monitoring equipment and accessories were not designed to operate in the harsh magnetic resonance (MR) environment where static, gradient, and radiofrequency (RF) electromagnetic fields could adversely affect or alter the operation of those devices.[1] Fortunately, various monitors and other patient support devices have been developed or specially modified to perform properly during MR procedures.[1-29] Thus, commercially available, MR-compatible monitors and other devices can be used routinely for patients in the MR environment.[1-29]

MR healthcare workers must carefully consider the ethical and medico-legal ramifications of providing proper patient care, which includes identifying patients who require monitoring in the MR environment and following a proper protocol to ensure their safety by using appropriate equipment, devices, and accessories.[30-36] The early detection and treatment of complications that may occur in high-risk, critically ill, or sedated patients undergoing MR procedures can prevent relatively minor problems from becoming life-threatening situations.[36]

This chapter provides recommendations and guidelines for patient monitoring. In addition, techniques, equipment, and devices that may be used to monitor and support patients in the MR environment are described.

II. RECOMMENDATIONS AND GUIDELINES FOR PATIENT MONITORING

A. GENERAL POLICIES AND PROCEDURES

In general, monitoring during an MR examination is indicated whenever a patient requires observations of vital physiologic parameters due to an underlying health problem or whenever a patient is unable to respond or alert the MR imaging (MRI) technologist or other healthcare worker regarding pain, respiratory problems, cardiac distress, or other difficulty that might arise during the examination.[1-3] In addition, a patient should be monitored if there is a greater potential for a change in physiologic status during the MR procedure.[1-3] Besides patient monitoring, various support devices and accessories may be needed for use with a high-risk patient to ensure safety.[1-36]

With the advent of newer types of MR applications, such as MR-guided biopsies and surgical procedures, there is an increased need to monitor patients.[37,38] Additionally, patients undergoing MR procedures using MR systems that utilize echo planar imaging (EPI) techniques or with static magnetic fields greater than 2.0 T should be monitored continuously to ensure their safety due to potential risks that may be encountered.

Because of the widespread use of MR contrast agents and the potential for adverse effects or idiosyncratic reactions to occur, it is prudent to have MR-compatible monitoring equipment and accessories readily available for the proper management and support of patients who may experience side effects.[1-3] This is emphasized because adverse events, while extremely rare, may be serious or even fatal.

In 1992, the Safety Committee of the Society for Magnetic Resonance Imaging published guidelines and recommendations concerning the monitoring of patients during MR procedures.[2] This information indicates that all patients undergoing MR procedures should, at the very least, be visually (e.g., using a camera system) and/or verbally (e.g., using an intercom system) monitored and that patients who are sedated, anesthetized, or unable to communicate should be physiologically monitored and supported by the appropriate means.[2] Severe injuries and fatalities have occurred in association with MR procedures and may have been prevented with the proper use of monitoring equipment and devices.[1] Of note is that guidelines issued by the Joint Commission on Accreditation of Healthcare Organizations (JCAHO) indicate that patients who receive sedatives or anesthetics require monitoring during the administration and recovery from these medications.[30] Other organizations similarly recommend the need to monitor certain patients using proper equipment and techniques.[31-33] Table 11.1 summarizes the patients who may require monitoring and support during MR procedures.

B. SELECTION OF PARAMETERS TO MONITOR

The proper selection of the specific physiologic parameter(s) that should be monitored during the MR procedure is crucial for patient safety. Various factors must be considered, including the patient's

TABLE 11.1
Patients that May Require Monitoring and Support During MR Procedures

1.	Patients who are physically or mentally unstable
2.	Patients who have compromised physiologic functions
3.	Patients who are unable to communicate
4.	Neonatal and pediatric patients
5.	Sedated or anesthetized patients
6.	Patients undergoing MR-guided interventional procedures
7.	Patients undergoing MR procedures using experimental MR systems (e.g., MR systems with static magnetic field strengths that exceed 2.0 T, etc.)
8.	Patients who may have a reaction to an MR contrast agent
9.	Critically ill or high-risk patients

medical history and present condition, the use of medication and possible side effects, as well as the aspects of the MR procedure to be performed.[1-3,11,14,20,23,30-33,35,36] For example, if the patient is to receive a sedative, it is mandatory to monitor respiratory rate, apnea, and/or oxygen saturation.[30-33,35,36] If the patient requires general anesthesia during the MR procedure, monitoring multiple physiologic parameters is required.[1,3,30-36]

Policies and procedures for the management of the patient in the MR environment should be comparable to those used in the operating room or critical care setting, especially with respect to monitoring and support requirements. Specific recommendations for physiologic monitoring of patients during MR procedures should be developed in consideration of "standard of care" issues, as well as in consultation with anesthesiologists and other similar specialists.[1-3,30-33,35,36]

C. Personnel Involved in Patient Monitoring

Only healthcare workers with appropriate training and experience should be responsible for monitoring patients during MR procedures. This includes several facets of training and experience. The healthcare worker must be well acquainted with the operation of the monitoring equipment and accessories used in the MR environment and should be able to recognize equipment malfunctions, device problems, and recording artifacts. Furthermore, the person responsible for monitoring the patient should be well versed in screening patients for conditions that may complicate the procedure. For example, patients with asthma, congestive heart failure, obesity, obstructive sleep apnea, and other underlying conditions are at increased risk for experiencing problems during sedation.[36] Also, this healthcare worker must be able to identify and manage adverse events using appropriate equipment and procedures in the MR environment.[36]

If a sedated patient suddenly exhibits a rapid decline in oxygen saturation, the healthcare worker should be able to assess the patient for potential causes and rapidly determine if intervention is necessary. At the very minimum, the individual should be capable of recognizing and responding quickly to contact an emergency team in the event that an adverse event is experienced by the patient.

Additionally, there must be policies and procedures implemented to continue appropriate physiologic monitoring of the patient by trained personnel after the MR procedure is performed. This is especially needed for a patient recovering from the effects of a sedative or general anesthesia.

The monitoring of physiologic parameters and management of the patient during an MR procedure may be the responsibility of one or more individuals depending on the level of training for the healthcare worker and in consideration of the condition, medical history, and procedure that is to be performed for the patient. These individuals include anesthesiologists, nurse anesthetists, nurses, MR technologists, or radiologists.[1-3,30-33,35,36]

D. Emergency Plan

The development, implementation, and regular practice of an emergency plan that addresses and defines the activities, use of equipment, and other pertinent issues pertaining to a medical emergency are important for patient safety in the MR environment.[35] For example, a plan needs to be developed for handling patients if there is the need to remove them from the MR system room to perform cardiopulmonary resuscitation in the event of a cardiac or respiratory arrest.[35] Obviously, taking necessary equipment such as a cardiac defibrillator, intubation instruments, or other similar devices near the MR system could pose a substantial hazard to the patients and healthcare workers if these are not safe for use in the MR environment. Appropriate healthcare workers that are in charge of the code blue team, "running" the code, maintaining the patient's airway, administering drugs, recording events, and conducting other emergency-related duties must be identified, trained, and continuously practiced in the performance of these critical activities.

For outpatient or mobile MR facilities, it may be necessary to have an advanced agreement with outside emergency personnel and an acute care hospital willing to take care of their patients. Typically, MR facilities not affiliated with or in close proximity to a hospital must contact paramedics to handle medical emergencies and to transport patients to the hospital for additional care. Therefore, personnel responsible for summoning the paramedics, notifying the hospital, and performing other integral activities must be designated beforehand to avoid problems and confusion during an actual emergent event.[35]

III. TECHNIQUES AND EQUIPMENT FOR PATIENT MONITORING AND SUPPORT

Physiologic monitoring and support of patients is not a trivial task in the MR environment. A variety of potential problems and hazards exist. Furthermore, the types of equipment for patient monitoring and support must be considered carefully and implemented properly to ensure the safety of both patients and MR healthcare workers.

A. Potential Problems and Hazards

Several potential problems and hazards are associated with the performance of patient monitoring and support in the MR environment. Physiologic monitors and accessories that contain ferromagnetic components (e.g., transformers, outer casings, etc.) may be strongly attracted by the static magnetic field used in the MR system, posing a serious "missile" hazard to patients and MR healthcare workers.[1-3,21,25] Additionally, the MR system may be damaged as a result of being struck by a "flying" monitor or similar device.[1,3,11,13,14,21,26]

If possible, devices that have ferromagnetic components should be permanently fixed to the floor and properly labeled with warning information to prevent them from being moved too close to the MR system. All personnel involved with MR procedures should be aware of the importance of the placement and use of the equipment, especially with regard to the hazards of moving portable equipment too close to the MR system.

RF fields from the MR system can significantly affect the operation of monitoring equipment, especially equipment with displays that involve electron beams (i.e., CRTs) or video display screens (with the exception of those with liquid crystal displays — LCDs). In addition, the monitoring equipment itself may emit spurious noise that, in turn, produces distortion or artifacts on the MR images (Figure 11.1).

Physiologic monitors that contain microprocessors or other similar components may leak RF, producing electromagnetic interference which can substantially alter MR images.[1,3] To prevent adverse RF-related interactions between the MR system and physiologic monitors, RF-shielded cables, RF filters, special outer RF-shielded enclosures, or fiber-optic techniques can be utilized to prevent image-related problems in the MR environment.[1,3,9,11,14,17,19-21,26,27,29,36,39]

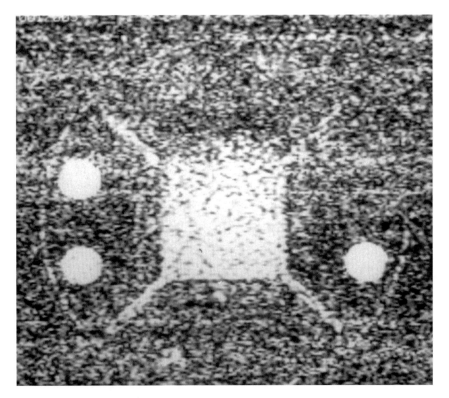

FIGURE 11.1 MR image of a fluid-filled phantom showing severe image artifacts and distortion caused by spurious RF noise associated with the operation of a monitor in the MR environment. This phantom was scanned using a T1-weighted pulse sequence.

During the operation of MR systems, electrical currents may be generated in the conductive materials of monitoring equipment that are used as part of the interface to the patient.[1,3] These currents may be of sufficient magnitude to cause excessive heating and thermal injury to the patient.[1-3,41-47] Numerous first, second, and third degree burns have occurred in association with MR procedures that were directly attributed to the use of monitoring devices.[1,3,41-47] These thermal injuries have been associated with the use of electrocardiographic lead wires, plethysmographic gating systems, pulse oximeters, and other types of monitoring equipment and accessories comprised of wires, cables, or similar components made from conductive materials.[1,3,41-47] Several safety procedures that should be followed to prevent burns associated with the use of monitors and other devices during MR procedures are described in Chapter 14, "The Magnetic Resonance Imaging Environment and Implants, Devices, and Materials."

It should be noted that for a manufacturer to have an approved claim from the U.S. Food and Drug Administration with regard to their device being designated as "MR safe" or "MR compatible," comprehensive pre-clinical *ex vivo* testing is required. (The terms MR safe and MR compatible are defined as follows: a device is considered MR safe if, when placed in the MR environment, it presents no additional risk to a patient, individual, or MR system operator from magnetic interactions, heating, or induced voltages, but may affect the quality of the diagnostic information on MR scans. A device is considered MR compatible if it is MR safe, its use in the MR environment does not adversely impact the image quality, and it performs its intended function when used in the MR environment according to its specifications in a safe and effective manner.) Therefore, in consideration of potential problems and hazards associated with the use of monitoring equipment and accessories, it is important to closely follow the instructions and recommendations from the manufacturers with regard to the use of the devices in the MR environment.

B. Monitoring Equipment and Support Devices

This section describes the physiologic parameters that may be assessed in patients during MR procedures using MR-compatible monitoring equipment. In addition, various devices and accessories that are useful for the support and management of patients are presented.

1. Electrocardiogram and Heart Rate

Monitoring the patient's electrocardiogram (ECG) in the MR environment is particularly challenging because of the inherent distortion of the ECG waveform that occurs.[1,3,11,18,22,27,48-50] This effect is observed as blood, a conductive fluid, flows through the large vascular structures in the presence of the static magnetic field of the MR system.[38] The resulting induced-biopotential is seen primarily as an augmented T-wave amplitude, although other nonspecific waveform changes are also apparent on the ECG.[1,3,38,49] Since altered T-waves or ST segments may be associated with cardiac disorders, static magnetic field-induced ECG distortions may be problematic. For that reason, it may be necessary to obtain a baseline recording of the ECG prior to placing the patient inside the MR system along with a recording obtained immediately after the MR procedure to determine the cardiac status of the patient.[1,3]

Additional artifacts caused by the static, gradient, and RF electromagnetic fields can severely distort the ECG, making observation of morphologic changes and detection of arrhythmias quite difficult (Figure 11.2). To minimize some of these artifacts, a variety of filtering techniques — active and passive — may be used.

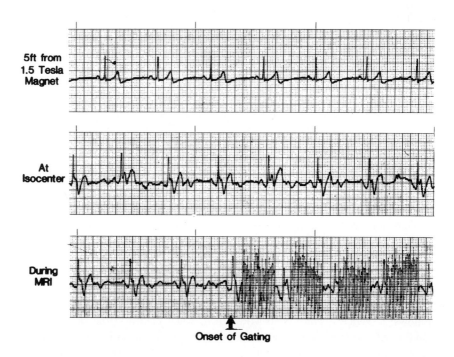

FIGURE 11.2 ECG recorded in the MR environment 5 ft from the 1.5-T magnet (top panel), at isocenter (middle panel), and inside the MR system during MRI (bottom panel). Note the augmented T-wave resulting from the induced flow potential as well as the other nonspecific changes caused by the static magnetic field of the MR system. During MRI, Onset of Gating, there is severe distortion of the electrocardiographic waveform.

Active techniques involve the use of low pass filters or the electronic suppression of noise which decreases the artifacts from the gradient and RF electromagnetic fields, while maintaining the intrinsic qualities of the ECG. Passive techniques include the use of special cable and lead preparation methods along with the proper placement of leads that will minimize the artifacts seen on the ECG in the MR environment.[49]

Rokey et al.[18] described the use of a specially designed time-varying filter developed to reduce artifacts associated with the gradient magnetic field of the MR system. This device utilizes a telemetry system to preserve the low-frequency isolation between the inside and outside of the RF shield of the MR system room.[18]

ECG artifacts that occur in the MR environment may also be decreased substantially by implementing several simple techniques which include the following:[1,3,16,18,19,27,49,50]

1. Using ECG electrodes that have minimal metal
2. Selecting electrodes and cables that contain no ferromagnetic metals
3. Placing the limb electrodes in close proximity to one another
4. Placing the line between the limb electrodes and leg electrodes parallel to the magnetic field flux lines
5. Maintaining a small area between the limb and leg electrodes
6. Placing the area of the electrodes near or in the center of the MR system
7. Twisting or braiding the ECG cables

The use of MR-safe ECG electrodes is strongly recommended to ensure patient safety and proper recording of the ECG in the MR environment.[22] Accordingly, ECG electrodes have been specially developed for use during MR procedures to protect the patient from potentially hazardous conditions. These ECG electrodes were also designed to reduce MRI-related artifacts[22] (see Chapter 14, "The Magnetic Resonance Imaging Environment and Implants, Devices, and Materials").

It is well known that the use of standard ECG electrodes, leads, and cables may cause heating which results in patient burns at the electrode sites.[1,3,11,41-45,47] Electrical current is generated by the ECG patient cable acting as an antenna in the RF field during the operation of the MR system. Thus, patient burns may occur because it is difficult to entirely insulate the ECG electrodes from the patient.

To prevent burns from occurring in patients during MR procedures, a special fiber-optic ECG recording technique was developed (Magnetic Resonance Equipment Corporation, Bay Shore, NY). This fiber-optic ECG system acquires the ECG waveform using an MR-safe transceiver that resides in the MR system bore along with the patient and is located very near the ECG electrodes (Figure 11.3). A module digitizes and optically encodes the patient's ECG waveform and transmits it out from the MR system to the monitor using a fiber-optic cable. The use of this fiber-optic ECG technique eliminates the potential for burns incurred with hard-wired ECG systems by removing the conductive patient cable and its antenna effect which are typically responsible for excessive heating.

Besides using an ECG monitor, the heart rate of patients undergoing MR procedures may be determined continuously using various types of MR-compatible devices, including a photoplethysmograph and a pulse oximeter.[1,3,11,13,17-20,49] A noninvasive heart rate and blood pressure monitor (see section below) can also be utilized to obtain intermittent or semi-continuous recordings of the heart rate during MR procedures.[1,3,11]

2. Blood Pressure

Conventional, manual sphygmomanometers may be adapted for use during MR procedures. This is typically accomplished by lengthening the tubing from the cuff to the device so that the mercury

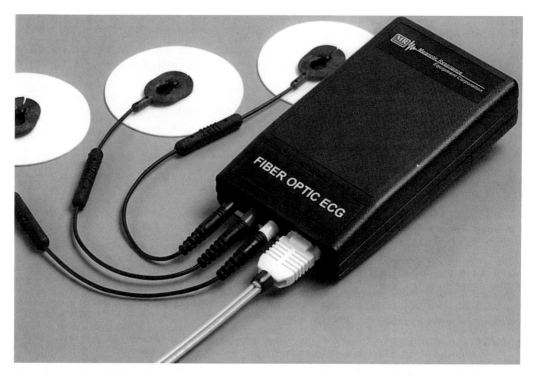

FIGURE 11.3 Fiber-optic ECG system used to record the ECG in patients undergoing MR procedures (Magnetic Resonance Equipment Corporation, Bay Shore, NY). The use of this fiber-optic ECG technique eliminates the potential for burns incurred with hard-wired ECG systems by removing the conductive patient cable and its antenna effect which are responsible for heating.

column and other primary components can be positioned an acceptable distance (e.g., 8 to 10 ft from the bore of a 1.5-T MR system) from the fringe field of the MR system.[1,3,11,13,14,19]

Blood pressure measuring devices that incorporate a spring gauge instead of a mercury column may be adversely affected by magnetic fields, causing them to work erroneously in the MR setting.[1,3,19] Therefore, spring-gauge blood pressure devices should undergo pre-clinical testing before being used to monitor patients undergoing MR procedures.

Blood pressure monitors that use noninvasive techniques, such as the oscillometric method, may be used to obtain semi-continuous recordings of systolic, diastolic, and mean blood pressures as well as pulse rate.[1,3,11] These devices can be utilized to record systemic blood pressure in adult, pediatric, and neonate patients by selecting the appropriate size for the blood pressure cuff (Figure 11.4).

Noninvasive blood pressure monitors have been modified for use during MR procedures by lengthening the hose or tubing that connects the blood pressure cuff to the monitor in order to position the monitor a suitable distance from the static magnetic field of the MR system.[1,3,11] Any metallic connectors between the cuff and hose are removed and replaced with plastic fittings. These modifications are typically performed by the manufacturers of these devices.

It should be noted that the intermittent inflation of the blood pressure cuff from an automated, noninvasive blood pressure monitor may disturb lightly sedated patients, especially pediatric or neonate patients, causing them to move and disrupt the MR procedure. For this reason, the use of a noninvasive blood pressure monitor may not be the best instrument to conduct physiologic monitoring in every type of patient.

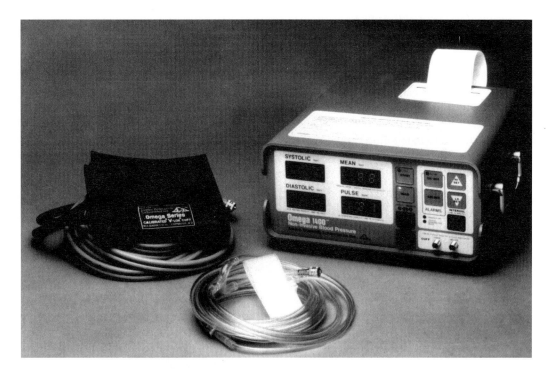

FIGURE 11.4 MR-compatible heart rate and blood pressure monitor. This device uses the oscillometric technique to obtain semi-continuous recordings of heart rate, systolic, diastolic, and mean blood pressures (In-Vivo Research, Inc., Orlando, FL).

3. Intravascular, Intracardiac, and Intracranial Pressures

Direct monitoring of intravascular, intracardiac, or intracranial pressures may be performed in patients during MR procedures using specially designed, fiber-optic pressure transducers or non-ferromagnetic, micromanometer-tipped catheters.[6,9,11,39] These monitoring devices are unaffected by the electromagnetic fields used for MR procedures and are capable of invasively recording pressures that are comparable to those obtained using conventional recording equipment.[6,9,11,39]

Invasive pressure monitoring may also be accomplished using the standard technique, whereby an additional length of pressure tubing is applied to place the transducer and recording device in an acceptable position relative to the MR system. Additional modifications of the equipment may be required to prevent distortion of the MR images when this monitoring technique is utilized to record pressures invasively.[1,3,11]

Monitoring intracranial pressure (ICP) is essential in the management of severe head injuries. Unfortunately, most conventional ICP monitors are not compatible with the electromagnetic fields associated with MRI. Recently, Macmillan et al.[39] examined the accuracy and repeatability of an ICP monitor (Codman MicroSensor, Johnson & Johnson Professional, Inc., Raynham, MA) during MRI. While the operation of this ICP monitor created a reduction in the signal-to-noise ratio during certain MR procedures (e.g., T2-weighted imaging and proton spectroscopic imaging), the resulting images were considered to be radiologically interpretable. Thus, the Codman MicroSensor ICP was considered to be sufficiently accurate and free of artifact generation to be used during most clinical MRI applications.[39] The use of this device greatly enhances the monitoring and safety for patients with severe head injuries requiring MR procedures.

4. Respiratory Rate and Apnea

Because respiratory depression and upper airway obstruction are frequent complications associated with the use of sedatives and anesthetics, monitoring techniques that detect a decrease in respiratory rate, hypoxemia, or airway obstruction should be used during the administration of these drugs.[1,3,11,31-36] This is particularly important in the MR environment because visual observation of the patient's respiratory efforts is often difficult to accomplish, especially for the patients in conventional, closed-configured MR systems.

Respiratory rate monitoring can be performed during MR procedures by various techniques. The impedance method that utilizes chest leads and electrodes (similar to those used to record the ECG) can be used to record respiratory rate. This technique of recording respiratory rate measures a difference in electrical impedance induced between the leads that correspond to changes in respiratory movements. Unfortunately, the electrical impedance method of assessing respiratory rate may be inaccurate in pediatric patients because of the small volumes and associated motions of the relatively small thorax area.

Respiratory rate may also be monitored during MR procedures using a rubber bellows placed around the patient's thorax or abdomen (i.e., for "chest" or "belly" breathers).[1,3,11] The bellows is attached to a remote pressure transducer that records body movement changes associated with inspiration and expiration.[47] However, the bellows monitoring technique, like the electrical impedance method, is only capable of recording body movements associated with respiratory efforts. Therefore, these techniques of monitoring respiratory rate do not detect apneic episodes related to upper airway obstruction (i.e., absent airflow despite respiratory effort) and may not provide sufficient sensitivity for assessing patients during MR procedures. For this reason, assessment of respiratory rate and identification of apnea should be accomplished using other, more appropriate monitoring devices.

Respiratory rate and apnea may be monitored during MR procedures using an end-tidal carbon dioxide monitor or a capnometer (Figures 11.5 and 11.6). These devices measure the level of carbon

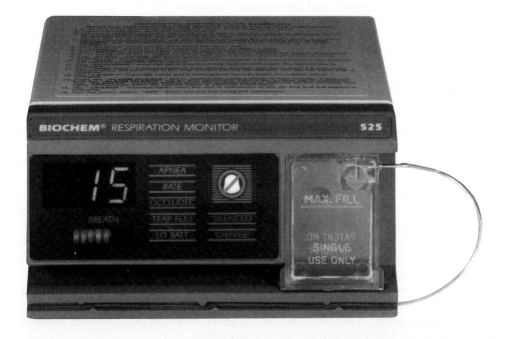

FIGURE 11.5 MR-compatible end-tidal carbon dioxide monitor used to record respiratory rate and to detect apnea (Biochem International, Waukesha, WI).

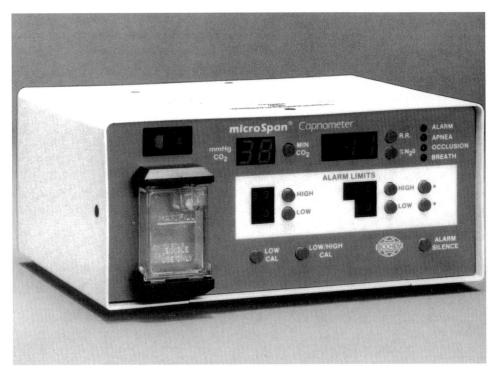

FIGURE 11.6 MR-compatible capnometer used to record respiratory rate, detect apnea, and record various gas exchange parameters (Biochem International, Waukesha, WI).

dioxide during the end of the respiratory cycle (i.e., end-tidal carbon dioxide), when carbon dioxide is at its maximum level. Additionally, capnometers provide quantitative data with respect to end-tidal carbon dioxide that is important for determining certain aspects of gas exchange in patients. The waveform provided on the end-tidal carbon dioxide monitors is also useful for assessing whether the patient is having any difficulty breathing. The interface between the patient for the end-tidal carbon dioxide monitor and capnometer is a nasal or oro-nasal cannula that is made out of plastic. Obviously, this interface prevents any potential adverse interaction between the monitor and the patient during an MR procedure.

5. Oxygen Saturation

Oxygen saturation is a crucial variable to measure in sedated and anesthetized patients.[1,3,11,31-36] This physiologic parameter is measured using pulse oximetry, a monitoring technique that assesses the oxygenation of tissue. A pulse oximeter is utilized to record oxygen saturation. Because oxygen-saturated blood absorbs differing quantities of light compared with unsaturated blood, the amount of light that is absorbed by the blood can be readily used to calculate the ratio of oxygenated hemoglobin to total hemoglobin, which is displayed as the oxygen saturation. Additionally, the patient's heart rate may be calculated by measuring the frequency at which pulsations occur as the blood moves through the vascular bed. Thus, the pulse oximeter determines oxygen saturation and pulse rate on a continuous basis by measuring the transmission of light through a vascular measuring site such as the earlobe, fingertip, or toe.

The use of pulse oximetry is considered by anesthesiologists as the standard practice for monitoring sedated or anesthetized patients.[31,32,33-36] Therefore, using a pulse oximeter to monitor sedated patients during MR procedures should be a required procedure implemented by MRI facilities.

Commercially available, specially modified pulse oximeters that have hard-wire cables have been used to monitor sedated patients during MR procedures with moderate success. Unfortunately, these pulse oximeters tend to work intermittently during the operation of the MR system, primarily due to interference from the gradient and/or RF electromagnetic fields. Of greater concern is the fact that many patients have been burned using pulse oximeters with hard-wire cables, presumably as a result of excessive current being induced in inappropriately looped conductive cables attached to the patient probes of the pulse oximeters.[1,3,24,42,46]

Fortunately, pulse oximeters have been developed that use fiber-optic technology to obtain and transmit the physiologic signals from the patient[24] (Figure 11.7). These devices operate without interference from the electromagnetic fields used for MR procedures. It is physically impossible for a patient to be burned by the use of a fiber-optic pulse oximeter during an MR procedure because there are no conductive pathways formed by any metallic materials that connect to the patient.[1,3,24] There are several different MR-compatible, fiber-optic pulse oximeters that are commercially available for use in the MR environment (Table 11.2).

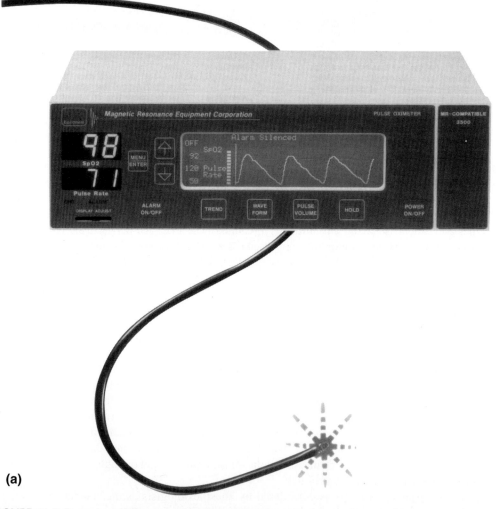

(a)

FIGURE 11.7 Examples of MR-compatible, fiber-optic pulse oximeters used to record heart rate and oxygen saturation: (a) Magnetic Resonance Equipment Corporation, Bay Shore, NY.   (*continued*)

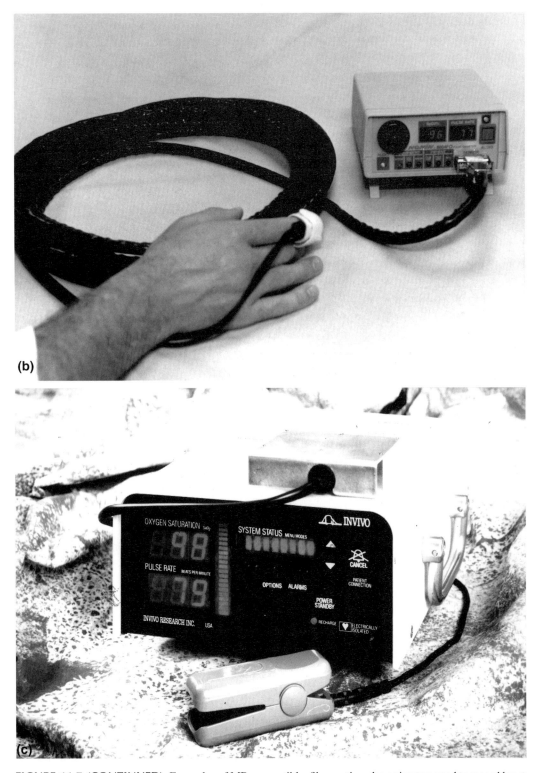

FIGURE 11.7 (CONTINUED) Examples of MR-compatible, fiber-optic pulse oximeters used to record heart rate and oxygen saturation. (b) Nonin Medical, Inc., Plymouth, MN; (c) In-Vivo Research, Inc., Orlando, FL.

TABLE 11.2
List of Manufacturers and Suppliers of Monitors and Support Devices for Use in the MR Environment*

Company and Location	Product(s)
Biochem International Waukesha, WI	Monitoring equipment
Datex-Engstrom Instrumentarium Corp. Helsinki, Finland	Monitoring equipment
Datex-Ohmeda Inc. Madison, WI	Anesthesia equipment
Groupe Bruker Odam Wissembourg, France	Monitoring equipment
In-Vivo Research, Inc. Orlando, FL	Monitoring equipment
Luxtron Santa Clara, CA	Temperature monitor
Magnetic Resonance Equipment Corporation Bay Shore, NY	Monitoring equipment
MedPacific Seattle, WA	Monitoring equipment
Medrad Indianola, PA	Monitoring equipment
MIPM — GMBH Munchen, Germany	Monitoring equipment
MR Resources, Inc. Gardner, MA	Monitoring equipment, accessories
Nonin Medical, Inc. Plymouth, MN	Monitoring equipment
North American Draeger Telford, PA	Monitoring equipment, anesthesia equipment
Ohmeda, Inc. Madison, WI	Anesthesia equipment
Omnivent Topeka, KS	Ventilator
Penlon Oxon, England	Ventilator, monitoring equipment
Vasomed, Inc. St. Paul, MN	Blood flow monitor

* *Note:* These monitors and devices may require modifications to make them MR-compatible. Consult manufacturers to determine additional information related to compatibility with specific MR systems.

6. Cutaneous Blood Flow

Monitoring blood flow through the cutaneous capillaries provides a means of assessing tissue perfusion, which is an indirect method of determining the circulatory status of the patient. The laser Doppler velocimetry method may be used to noninvasively monitor cutaneous blood flow in patients during MR procedures.[1,3,11,43]

When using laser Doppler velocimetry, a low power beam of laser light is delivered to the tissue via a fiber-optic probe. As the light moves through the tissue, the moving red blood cells impart a Doppler frequency shift of photons. A pair of optical fibers collects the light signals carrying the information on the velocity and density of red blood cells in the cutaneous capillary

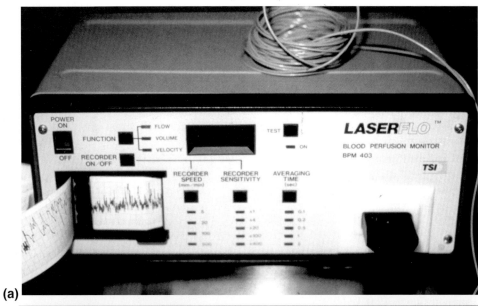

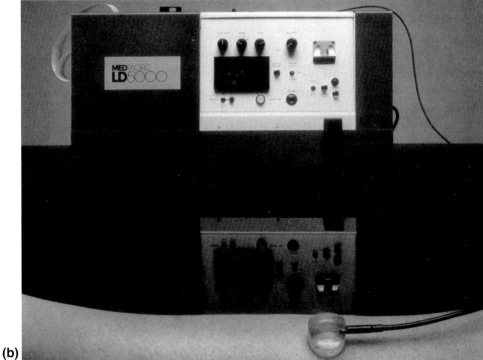

FIGURE 11.8 MR-compatible cutaneous blood flow monitors. These devices use a fiber-optic technique to record cutaneous blood flow, velocity, and volume. (a) LaserFlo Blood Perfusion Monitor, BPM 403 (Vasomed, Inc., St. Paul, MN); (b) MEDPACIFIC LD 5000 (MedPacific, Seattle, WA).

bed. Thus, cutaneous blood flow, blood volume, and velocity can be monitored for patients in the MR environment using this technique.[1,3,11]

Monitors that record cutaneous blood flow use fiber-optic cables along with a special probe that is attached to the patient using double-sided adhesive tape (Figure 11.8). Skin surface areas that have a relatively high cutaneous blood flow, such as the toe, foot, finger, hand, or ear, provide the best results for monitoring this physiologic parameter during MR procedures.

7. Temperature

There are several reasons to monitor skin and/or body temperatures during MR procedures. These include recording temperatures in neonates with inherent problems retaining body heat (a tendency that is augmented during sedation), in patients during MR procedures that require high levels of RF power, and in patients with underlying conditions that impair their ability to dissipate heat.[1,3]

Skin and body temperatures may be monitored during MR procedures using a variety of techniques.[1,3,11,26,28] However, it should be noted that the use of hard-wire, thermistor, or thermocouple-based techniques to record temperatures in the MR environment may cause artifacts or erroneous measurements due to direct heating of the temperature probes. Nevertheless, if properly modified, temperature recordings may be accomplished in the MR setting using specially modified, hard-wire leads and thermistors.[26]

A more effective and easier technique of recording temperatures during MR procedures is the use of a fluoroptic thermometry system.[1,3,11,28] Experiments and clinical studies have shown that this method is both safe and reliable and can be used with MR systems that have static magnetic field strengths up to 12.0 T.[1,3,11,28]

The fluoroptic monitoring system has several important features that make it particularly useful for temperature monitoring during MR procedures (Figure 11.9). The device incorporates fiber-optic probes that are small but efficient in carrying optical signals over long paths, provides noise-free applications in electromagnetically hostile environments, and has fiber-optic components that will not pose a risk to patients.[28]

Recently, a new fiber-optic thermometry system designed specifically for use in the MR environment has been developed (Magnetic Resonance Equipment Corporation, Bay Shore, NY). This device is currently undergoing review by the U.S. Food and Drug Administration as an MR-compatible device and, thus, may soon be available for use during clinical MR procedures.

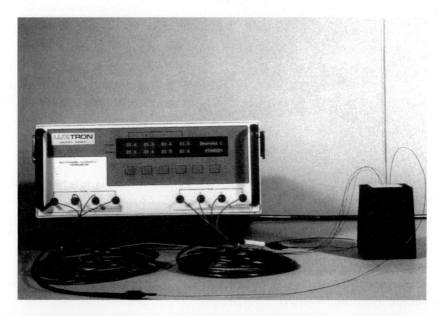

FIGURE 11.9 MR-compatible fluoroptic thermometry system (Luxtron, Santa Clara, CA) used to record temperatures in the MR environment.

8. Multi-Parameter, Physiologic Monitoring Systems

In certain cases, it may be necessary to monitor several different physiologic parameters simultaneously in patients undergoing MR procedures.[1,3,36] While several different stand-alone units may be used to accomplish this task, the most efficient means of recording multiple parameters is by utilizing a monitoring system that permits the measurement of different physiologic functions such as heart rate, respiratory rate, blood pressure, and oxygen saturation (Figure 11.10).

Currently, there are a number of multi-parameter patient monitoring systems that are MR compatible (Table 11.2). Typically, these devices are designed with components positioned within the MR system room and incorporate special circuitry to substantially reduce the artifacts that affect the recording of ECG and other physiologic variables, making them also useful for the performance of "gated" MR procedures.

9. Ventilators

Devices used for mechanical ventilation of patients typically contain mechanical switches, microprocessors, and ferromagnetic components that may be adversely effected by the electromagnetic fields used by MR systems.[1,3-5,8,10-13,15-17,25] Ventilators that are activated by high-pressure oxygen and controlled by the use of fluidics (i.e., no requirements for electricity) may still have ferromagnetic parts that can malfunction as a result of interference from MR systems.

MR-compatible ventilators have been modified or specially designed for use during MR procedures performed in adult as well as neonatal patients.[1,3-5,8,10-13,15-17,25] (Figure 11.11). These devices tend to be constructed from nonferromagnetic materials and have undergone pre-clinical evaluations to ensure that they operate properly in the MR environment without producing artifacts on MR images.

10. Additional Devices and Accessories

A variety of devices and accessories are often necessary for support and management of high-risk or sedated patients in the MR environment. MR-compatible gurneys, oxygen tanks, stethoscopes, suction devices, infusion pumps, power injectors, and other similar devices and accessories may be obtained from various manufacturers and distributors listed in Table 11.2. Additionally, there are MR-compatible gas anesthesia systems available that have been designed for use in patients undergoing MR procedures (Table 11.2).

IV. SEDATION

Whenever sedatives are used, it is imperative to perform physiologic monitoring to ensure the safety of the patient.[31-36] In addition, it is important to have the necessary equipment readily available in the event of an emergency. Obviously, these requirements should also be followed for patients undergoing sedation in the MR environment.

A. General Considerations

There is controversy regarding who should be responsible for performing sedation of patients in the MR environment.[36] (For the sake of discussion, the terms "sedation" and "anesthesia" are used interchangeably since they are actually part of the same continuum.[36] Thus, when a patient is *sedated*, he/she may actually be *anesthetized*, and all of the associated risks are present.[36]) Obviously, there are medical, regulatory, administrative, and financial issues to be considered.[30-36]

In general, for patients that do not have conditions that may complicate sedation procedures, a nurse under the direction of a radiologist may be responsible for preparing, sedating, monitoring, and recovering these cases in the MR environment.[36] However, for patients that have serious medical

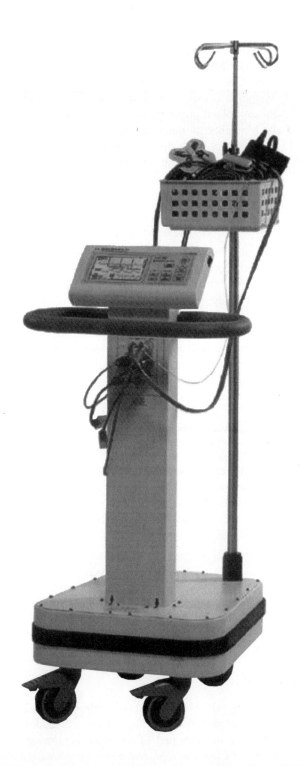

(a)

FIGURE 11.10 Examples of multi-parameter monitoring systems. (a) Omni-Track 3150 MRI, Patient Monitoring System (In-Vivo Research, Inc., Orlando, FL). *(continued)*

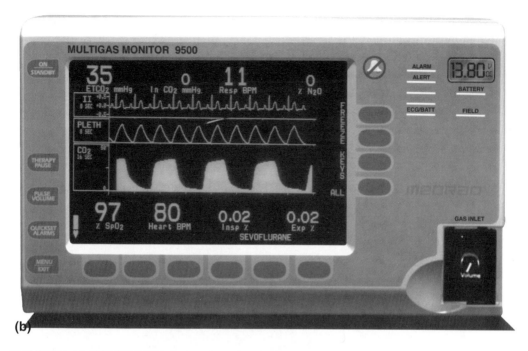

FIGURE 11.10 (CONTINUED) Examples of multi-parameter monitoring systems. (b) Monitor 9500 Multigas Monitor, Remote Control and Display (Medrad, Indianola, PA).

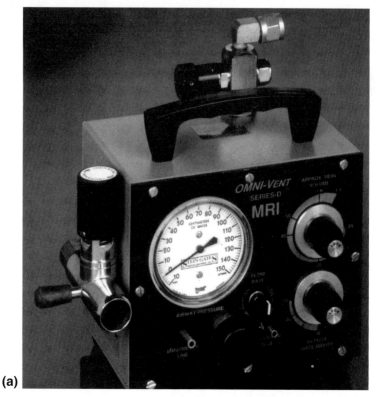

FIGURE 11.11 Examples of MR-compatible support devices and accessories. (a) Ventilator, Omni-Vent, Series D, MRI (Omnivent, Topeka, KS). *(continued)*

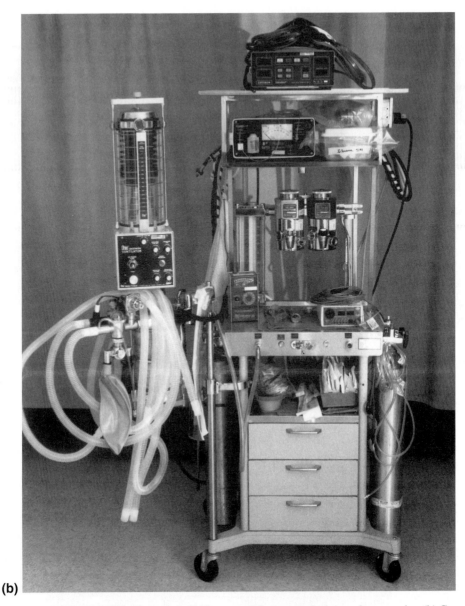

(b)

FIGURE 11.11 (CONTINUED) Examples of MR-compatible support devices and accessories. (b) Gas anesthesia machine shown as close up.   (*continued*)

or other unusual problems, it is advisable to utilize anesthesia consultation to properly manage these individuals before, during, and after MR procedures.

In addition, with regard to the use of sedation in the MR environment, the MRI facility should establish policies and guidelines for patient preparation, monitoring, sedation, and management during the post-sedation recovery period.[36] These policies and guidelines should be based on the standards set forth by the American Society of Anesthesiologists (ASA), the American College of Radiology (ACR), the American Academy of Pediatrics Committee on Drugs (AAP-COD), and the Joint Commission on Accreditation of Healthcare Organizations (JCAHO).[30,31-36]

For example, the Practice Guidelines for Sedation and Anesthesia from the ASA[32,35,36] indicate that a person must be present who is responsible for monitoring the patient if sedative or anesthetic medications are used. Furthermore, the following aspects of patient monitoring must be performed:

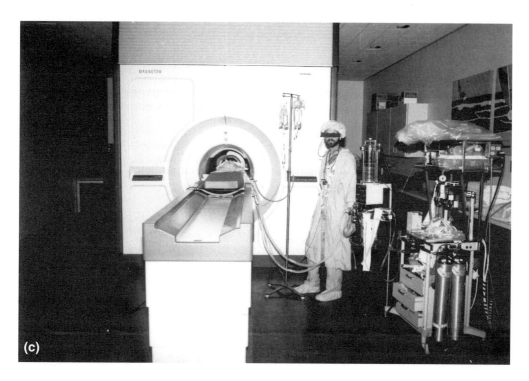

FIGURE 11.11 (CONTINUED) Examples of MR-compatible support devices and accessories. (c) Gas anesthesia machine shown in MR environment.

(1) visual monitoring, (2) assessment of the level of consciousness, (3) evaluation of ventilatory status, (4) oxygen status assessed via the use of pulse oximetry, and (5) determination of hemodynamic status via the use of blood pressure monitoring and electrocardiography if significant cardiovascular disease is present in the patient. Notably, the healthcare worker must be able to recognize complications of sedation such as hypoventilation and airway obstruction as well as be able to establish a patent airway for positive-pressure ventilation.

B. PATIENT PREPARATION

Special patient screening must be conducted to identify conditions that may complicate sedation in order to properly prepare the patient for the administration of a sedative.[36] This screening procedure should request important information from the patient which includes the following:[36] major organ system disease (e.g., diabetes, pulmonary, cardiac, or hepatic disease); prior experience or adverse reactions to sedatives or anesthetics; current medications; allergies to drugs; and a history of alcohol, substance, or tobacco abuse.

In addition, the NPO (nothing by mouth) interval for the patient must be determined to reduce the risk of aspiration during the procedure.[36] The ASA "Practice Guidelines Regarding Preoperative Fasting"[32] recommend a minimum NPO periods of 2 h for clear liquids, 4 h for breast milk, 6 h for infant formula, and six hours for a "light meal." The NPO period is extremely important because sedatives depress the patient's gag reflex. Unfortunately, the NPO status is often overlooked by outpatient MRI facilities.[36]

C. ADMINISTRATION OF SEDATION

A thorough discussion of sedation techniques, especially with regard to the use of various pharmacologic agents, is outside the scope of this chapter. Therefore, interested readers are referred to the excellent, comprehensive review of this topic written by Reinking Rothschild,[36] a board certified anesthesiologist with extensive experience sedating patients in the MR environment.

D. Documentation

During the use of sedation, written records should be maintained that indicate the patient's vital signs as well as the name, dosage, and time of administration for all drugs that are given to the patient. The use of a time-based, anesthesia-type record, such as that recommended by Reinking Rothschild,[36] is the best means of maintaining written documentation for sedation of patients in the MR environment.

E. Post-Sedation Recovery

After sedation, medical care of the patient that underwent sedation must continue.[36] This is especially important for pediatric patients because certain medications have relatively long half-lives (e.g., chloral hydrate, pentobarbitol, etc.).[36] Therefore, an appropriate room with monitoring and emergency equipment must be available to properly manage these patients.

Prior to allowing the patient to leave the MRI facility, the patient should be alert, oriented, and have stable vital signs.[36] In addition, a responsible adult should accompany the patient home. Written instructions that include an emergency telephone number should be provided to the patient.[31,32,36]

V. SUMMARY AND CONCLUSIONS

The care and management of high-risk, critically ill, or sedated patients in the MR environment presents special challenges. These challenges are related to requirements for MR-compatible equipment and devices as well as the need for MRI facilities to implement proper policies and procedures to handle these patients.

MR-compatible monitoring equipment and support accessories are commercially available from several manufacturers and distributors. Importantly, MRI facilities need to carefully consider the implementation of policies, procedures, and guidelines that have been developed and recommended by well-established professional organizations.[30–33,35]

REFERENCES

1. Shellock, F. G. and Kanal, E., *Magnetic Resonance: Bioeffects, Safety, and Patient Management*, 2nd ed., Lippincott-Raven Press, New York, 1996.
2. Kanal, E. and Shellock, F. G., Policies, guidelines, and recommendations for MR imaging safety and patient management. Patient monitoring during MR examinations, *J. Magn. Reson. Imaging,* 2, 247, 1992.
3. Shellock, F. G., Magnetic resonance: safety, bioeffects, and patient monitoring, in *Open Field Magnetic Resonance Imaging*, Gronemeyer, D. H. W. and Lufkin, R. B., Eds., Springer-Verlag, Heidelberg, 1998, p. 127.
4. Barnett, G. H., Roper, A. H. D., and Johnson, A. K., Physiological support and monitoring of critically ill patients during magnetic resonance imaging, *J. Neurosurg.,* 68, 246, 1988.
5. Boutros, A. and Palicek, W., Anesthesia for magnetic resonance imaging, *Anesth. Analg.,* 66, 367, 1987.
6. Dell'Italia, L. J., Carter, B., Millar, H., and Pohost, G. M., Development of a micromanometer-tip catheter to record high-fidelity pressures during cine-gated NMR without significant image distortion, *Magn. Reson. Med.,* 17, 119, 1991.
7. Fisher, D.M., Litt, W., and Cote, C.J., Use of oximetry during MR imaging of pediatric patients, *Radiology,* 178, 891-892, 1991.
8. Dunn, V., Coffman, C. E., McGowan, J. E., and Ehrardt, J. C., Mechanical ventilation during magnetic resonance imaging, *Magn. Reson. Imaging,* 3, 169, 1985.

9. Roos, C. F. and Carrol, F. E., Fiber-optic pressure transducer for use near MR magnetic fields, *Radiology,* 156, 548, 1985.

10. Geiger, R. S. and Cascorbi, H. F., Anesthesia in an NMR scanner, *Anesth. Analg.,* 63, 619, 1984.

11. Holshouser, B., Hinshaw, D. B., and Shellock, F. G., Sedation, anesthesia, and physiologic monitoring during MRI, *J. Magn. Reson. Imaging,* 3, 553-558, 1993.

12. Hubbard, A., Markowitz, R., Kimmel, B., Kroger, M., and Bartko, M., Sedation for pediatric patients undergoing CT and MRI, *J. Comput. Assist. Tomogr.,* 16, 33, 1992.

13. Karlik, S., Heatherley, T., Pavan, F., et al., Patient anesthesia and monitoring at a 1.5 T MRI installation, *Magn. Reson. Med.,* 7, 210, 1988.

14. McArdle, C., Nicholas, D., Richardson, C., and Amparo, E., Monitoring of the neonate undergoing MR imaging: technical considerations, *Radiology,* 159, 223, 1986.

15. McGowan, J. E. and Erenberg, A., Mechanical ventilation of the neonate during magnetic resonance imaging, *Magn. Reson. Imaging,* 7, 145, 1989.

16. Mirvis, S. E., Borg, U., and Belzberg, H., MR imaging of ventilator-dependent patients: preliminary experience, *Am. J. Roentgenol.,* 149, 845, 1987.

17. Rejger, V. S., Cohn, B. F., Vielvoye, G. J., and De-Raadt, F. B., A simple anesthetic and monitoring system for magnetic resonance imaging, *Eur. J. Anesthesiol.,* 6, 373, 1989.

18. Rokey, R. R., Wendt, R. E., and Johnston, D. L., Monitoring of acutely ill patients during nuclear magnetic resonance imaging: use of a time-varying filter electrocardiographic gating device to reduce gradient artifacts, *Magn. Reson. Med.,* 6, 240, 1988.

19. Roth, J. L., Nugent, M., Gray, J. E., et al., Patient monitoring during magnetic resonance imaging, *Anesthesiology,* 62, 80, 1985.

20. Selden, H., De Chateau, P., Ekman, G., et al., Circulatory monitoring of children during anesthesia in low-field magnetic resonance imaging, *Acta Anesthesiol.,* 34, 41, 1990.

21. Shellock, F. G., Monitoring vital signs in conscious and sedated patients during magnetic resonance imaging: experience with commercially available equipment, *Book of Abstracts,* Society of Magnetic Resonance in Medicine, Berkeley, CA, 1986, p. 1030.

22. Shellock, F. G., MRI and ECG electrodes, *Signals,* 29, 10, 1999.

23. Shellock, F. G., Monitoring sedated patients during MRI (letter), *Radiology,* 177, 586, 1990.

24. Shellock, F. G., Myers, S. M., and Kimble, K., Monitoring heart rate and oxygen saturation during MRI with a fiber-optic pulse oximeter, *Am. J. Roentgenol.,* 158, 663, 1991.

25. Smith, D. S., Askey, P., Young, M. L., and Kressel, H. Y., Anesthetic management of acutely ill patients during magnetic resonance imaging, *Anesthesiology,* 65, 710, 1986.

26. Taber, K. and Layman, H., Temperature monitoring during MR imaging: comparison of fluoroptic and standard thermistors, *J. Magn. Reson. Imaging,* 2, 99, 1992.

27. Wendt, R. E., Rokey, R., Vick, G. W., and Johnston, D. L., Electrocardiographic gating and monitoring in NMR imaging, *Magn. Reson. Imaging,* 6, 89, 1988.

28. Wickersheim, K. A. and Sun, M. H., Fiberoptic thermometry and its applications, *J. Microwave Power,* 2, 94, 1987.

29. Taber, K. H., Thompson, J., Coveler, L. A., and Hayman, L. A., Invasive pressure monitoring of patients during magnetic resonance imaging, *Can. J. Anesth.,* 40, 1092, 1993.

30. Joint Commission on Accreditation of Healthcare Organizations, Accreditation Manual for Hospitals, 1993.

31. American Academy of Pediatrics Committee on Drugs, Guidelines for monitoring and management of pediatric patients during and after sedation for diagnostic and therapeutics procedures, *Pediatrics,* 89, 1100, 1992.

32. A Report by the ASA Task Force on Sedation and Analgesia by Non-Anesthesiologists, Practice guidelines for sedation and analgesia by non-anesthesiologists, *Anesthesiology,* 84, 459, 1996.

33. American College of Radiology, ACR standard for the use of intravenous conscious sedation, and ACR standard for pediatric sedation/analgesia, in *1998 ACR Standards,* American College of Radiology, Reston, VA, 1998, p. 123.

34. Menon, D. K., Peden, C. J., Hall, A. S., Sargentoni, J., et al., Magnetic resonance for the anesthetist, Part II: anesthesia and monitoring in MR units, *Anesthesia,* 47, 508, 1992.

35. Jorgensen, N. H., Messick, J. M., Gray, J., Nugent, M., and Berquist, T. H., ASA monitoring standards and magnetic resonance imaging, *Anesth. Analg.,* 79, 1141, 1994.

36. Reinking Rothschild, D., Sedation for open magnetic resonance imaging, in *Open MRI,* Rothschild, P. A. and Reinking Rothschild, D., Eds., Lippincott, Williams & Wilkins, Philadelphia, 2000, p. 39.

37. Jolesz, F. A., Morrison, P. R., Koran, S. J., Kelly, R. J., et al., Compatible instrumentation for intraoperative MRI: expanding resources, *J. Magn. Reson. Imaging,* 8, 8, 1998.

38. Lewin, J. S., Interventional MR imaging: concepts, systems, and applications in neuroradiology, *Am. J. Neuroradiol.,* 20, 735, 1999.

39. Macmillan, C. S., Wild, J. M., Andrews, P. J., Marshall, I., et al., Accuracy of a miniature intracranial pressure monitor, its function during magnetic resonance scanning, and assessment of image artifact generation, *Neurosurgery,* 45, 188, 1999.

40. ECRI, Health Devices Alert, A new MRI complication?, *Health Devices Alert,* May 27, 1, 1988.

41. ECRI, Thermal injuries and patient monitoring during MRI studies, *Health Devices Alert,* 20, 362, 1991.

42. Kanal, E., and Shellock, F. G., Burns associated with clinical MR examinations, *Radiology,* 175, 585, 1990.

43. Kanal, E., and Shellock, F. G., Patient monitoring during clinical MR imaging, *Radiology,* 185, 623, 1992.

44. Keens, S. J. and Laurence, A. S., Burns caused by ECG monitoring during MRI imaging, *Anesthesiology,* 51, 1188, 1996.

45. Brown, T. R., Goldstein, B., and Little, J., Severe burns resulting from magnetic resonance imaging with cardiopulmonary monitoring. Risks and relevant safety precautions, *Am. J. Phys. Med. Rehabil.,* 72, 166, 1993.

46. Bashein, G. and Syrory, G., Burns associated with pulse oximetry during magnetic resonance imaging, *Anesthesiology,* 75, 382, 1991.

47. Heinz, W., Frohlich, E., and Stork, L., Burns following magnetic resonance tomography, *Z. Gastroenterol.,* 37, 31, 1999.

48. Teneforde, T. S., Gaffey, C. T., Moyer, B. R., and Budinger, T. F., Cardiovascular alterations in Maccaca monkeys exposed to stationary magnetic fields. Experimental observations and theoretical analysis, *Bioelectromagnetics,* 4, 1, 1983.

49. Dimick, R.N., Hedlund, L.W., Herfkens, R,F,, et al., Optimizing electrocardiographic electrode placement for cardiac-gated magnetic resonance imaging, *Invest. Radiol.,* 22, 17-22, 1987.

50. Damji, A.A., Snyder, R.E., Ellinger, D.C., et al., RF interference suppression in a cardiac synchronization system operating in a high magnetic field NMR imaging system, *Magn. Reson. Imaging,* 6, 637-640, 1988.

12 Safety of Magnetic Resonance Contrast Agents*

Val M. Runge

CONTENTS

I. INTRODUCTION

In the last 10 years, the use of intravenous contrast media in magnetic resonance (MR) has become well-established in clinical practice. Intravenous contrast media provide critical additional diagnostic information in many instances. Gadolinium chelates constitute the largest group of MR

---

* Portions of this chapter are reprinted with permission from Runge, V.M., *J. Magn. Reson. Imaging*, 12:205–213, 2000, *J. Magn. Reson. Imaging*, 10:489–495, 1999; and *Contrast Enhanced Magnetic Resonance Imaging*, Rung, V.M., Ed., The University Press of Kentucky, Lexington, 1997.

contrast media and are considered to be very safe. These agents are thought to be safer than nonionic iodinated contrast agents.

Unlike X-ray agents, gadolinium chelates are not nephrotoxic. Minor adverse reactions, including nausea (1 to 2% for all agents) and hives (<1% for all agents), occur in a very low percentage of cases. Healthcare personnel must be aware of the potential, although extremely uncommon, for severe anaphylactoid reactions following intravenous administration of MR contrast media and should be prepared if complications arise.

There are currently six MR contrast agents for intravenous administration with widespread approval and use. These include four gadolinium chelates (gadopentetate dimeglumine, gadoteridol, gadodiamide, and gadoterate meglumine), one manganese chelate (mangafodipir trisodium), and one iron particle (superparamagnetic iron oxide). Because of market size and commercial reasons, not all of these are available in every country. However, these six are the most common contrast agents used today in clinical practice. Of these, the first four (the gadolinium chelates) dominate the market. Of the gadolinium agents, the first three (gadopentetate dimeglumine, gadoteridol, and gadodiamide) have the greatest market share (in part because gadoterate meglumine is not available in the U.S.).

This chapter focuses on safety issues regarding the six intravenous contrast agents with widespread use worldwide. The safety of oral contrast media will also be discussed, although these agents are used much less frequently.

Two additional intravenous agents deserve mention, as they have recently been approved in a number of countries: gadobenate dimeglumine and gadobutrol. The first, gadobenate dimeglumine (Gd BOPTA or MultiHance™, Bracco Diagnostics, Princeton, NJ), will soon be available for general use.[1,2] MultiHance™ will likely be marketed for whole-body and MR angiographic applications, with clinical trials having been conducted for imaging of the central nervous system, liver, and MR angiography. It has a major advantage over the currently available gadolinium chelates in liver imaging due to its dual renal and hepatobiliary clearance. Weak protein binding also makes this agent superior in MR angiography and in conventional MR imaging of the central nervous system.

Gadobenate dimeglumine has been approved in most of Europe at this time and is pending approval in the U.S. and the Far East. Its safety profile appears similar to that of the gadolinium chelates that preceded it in approval.

The other agent that has been approved in a limited number of countries to date is gadobutrol (Gd DO3A-butriol or Gadovist™, Schering AG).[3,4] Gadobutrol is a macrocyclic ring chelate and, thus, is similar to gadoteridol. Although this chelate could be used for broad applications, only limited approval has been sought for commercial reasons.

Gadobutrol is approved at a 1.0-M concentration in Switzerland and Australia, with approval pending in the European Community. Of the gadolinium chelates on the market, only gadoteridol and gadobutrol can be formulated at 1.0 M. This is twice the standard concentration and has advantages in perfusion and angiographic imaging.

Two other gadolinium chelates (gadoversetamide and gadoxetic acid disodium) have either already been or will soon be submitted for approval in various countries across the world. Both are distributed to the extracellular space, the first being excreted only by the kidney and the second by both the kidney and the liver. The first is nonionic and the second carries a charge of −2 and is formulated as a disodium salt. Gadoversetamide (Optimark™, Mallinckrodt Inc.) is a linear chelate, with intended use in whole-body MR at a concentration of 0.5 M and a dose range of 0.1 to 0.3 mmol/kg.[5] It is most similar in this regard to gadodiamide.

Gadoversetamide recently received approval for clinical use in the U.S. in the central nervous system and liver at a dose of 0.1 mmol/kg. The second agent, gadoxetic acid disodium (Gd EOB-DTPA or Eovist™, Schering AG), has a very high hepatobiliary excretion. Initial clinical trials and early publications have focused on the use of this agent for liver imaging.[6-9]

Several other iron particles are also in various stages of clinical development.[10-12] Since the near-term impact of these agents in terms of market share is likely to be much less, they will not be further discussed.

II. GADOLINIUM CHELATES

A. GADOPENTETATE DIMEGLUMINE (GD DTPA OR MAGNEVIST®, BERLEX LABORATORIES AND SCHERING AG)

Gadopentetate dimeglumine was approved for clinical use in the late 1980s (1988 for head only, U.S.). In the U.S., the current approval is only for a dose of 0.1 mmol/kg. The injection rate must not exceed 10 ml/15 s. In Europe, a dose of up to 0.3 mmol/kg can be given. As this was the first agent approved, many early clinical trials demonstrated its utility. In particular, it was quickly evident that enhancement provided important differential diagnostic information and enabled lesion recognition with otherwise isointense masses.

Early publications recognized that intravenous contrast administration should significantly extend the diagnostic potential and specificity of MR, as has been subsequently shown.[13] The structure of the agent is that of a long linear ligand (DTPA, with a charge of –5, Figure 12.1) that wraps around and tightly binds the gadolinium ion (with a charge of +3). This gives a net charge of –2 for the metal chelate, which is counterbalanced by the presence of two methyl glucamines, each carrying a charge of +1.

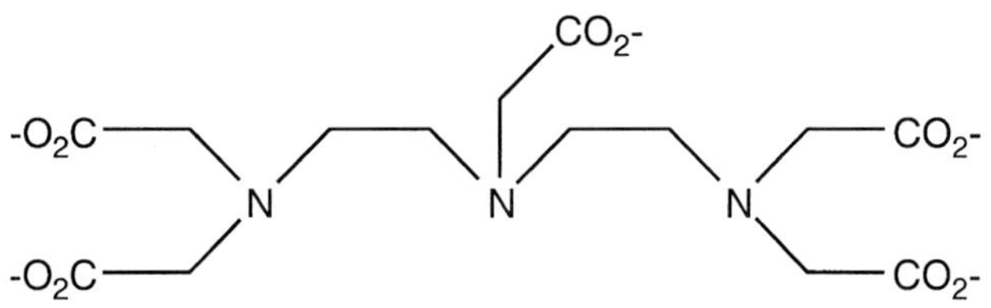

FIGURE 12.1 Ligand structure for DTPA, the chelate in gadopentetate dimeglumine (Magnevist).

U.S. clinical trials involving 1068 patients were reported in 1990.[14] A dose of 0.1 mmol/kg was administered in these trials. The three most common adverse reactions, characterized by the investigators as probably, possibly, or remotely related to contrast administration, were headache (3.6%), injection site coldness (3.6%), and nausea (1.5%). In the overall trial, adverse reactions were reported in 19.9% of the patients.

The only laboratory abnormality noted was a mild, transient (and asymptomatic) increase in serum iron (26% of men, 18% of women) and bilirubin levels (3% of men and women), which peaked at 2 to 4 h following intravenous injection. These changes most likely reflect mild transient hemolysis, due to free gadolinium ion.

In subsequent clinical trials, with gadopentetate dimeglumine reformulated using a greater excess of ligand, there was no change in serum iron and bilirubin levels. Nelson et al. reported adverse reactions in a patient population of 15,496 in 1995.[15] In this study, the rate of adverse reaction was 3.7% in patients with a history of asthma or allergy. The rate increased to 6.3% in patients with previous reactions to iodinated contrast media. The rate of adverse reaction also showed an injection rate dependency, with a reaction rate of 2.2% when administered slowly and 2.9% when administered rapidly.

The extended clinical experience with more than five million applications was reported in 1994.[16] Gadopentetate dimeglumine has an excellent and well-documented safety profile after intravenous injection. This is regardless of age and renal status. This agent is at least as safe as nonionic X-ray contrast media.

B. GADOTERIDOL (GD HP-DO3A OR PROHANCE®, BRACCO DIAGNOSTICS)

Gadoteridol was the second gadolinium chelate approved for intravenous injection. U.S. Food and Drug Administration (FDA) approval came in late 1992. The agent is approved for doses of 0.1 to

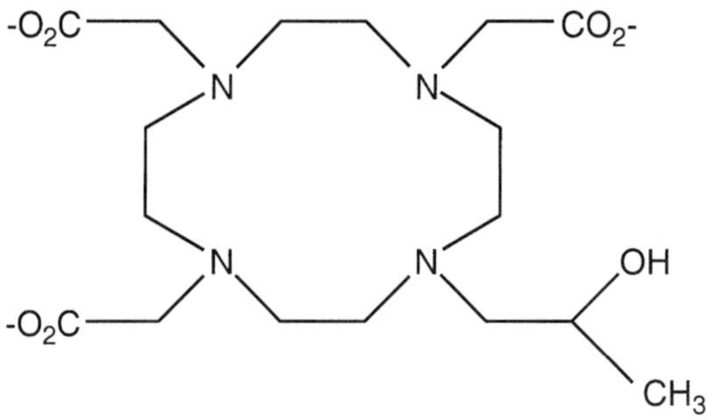

FIGURE 12.2 Ligand structure for HP-DO3A, the chelate in gadoteridol (ProHance).

0.3 mmol/kg worldwide, given either by slow infusion or as a bolus injection. Efficacy was demonstrated to be high, typical of gadolinium chelates with extracellular distribution.

For example, in phase III clinical trials, more diagnostic information was judged to be present post-contrast (as compared to pre-contrast) in 73% of brain and 68% of spine exams (in patients with confirmed disease). A change in diagnosis was considered likely from pre- to post-contrast in 29% and 34% of these brain and spine exams, respectively.

The structure of the agent is that of a rigid macrocyclic ligand (HP-DO3A, with a charge of −3, Figure 12.2) that lies like a crown over and tightly binds the gadolinium ion (with a charge of +3). This gives a net charge of zero for the chelate, which is thus neutral or nonionic.

U.S. clinical trials involving 411 patients were reported in 1991.[17] A dose of 0.1 mmol/kg was administered. Adverse reactions were reported in 7.1% of patients. Reactions possibly or probably related to contrast administration occurred in 18 patients (4.4%). The two most common reactions were taste sensation (1.4%) and nausea (1.2%). Unlike the trials with gadopentetate dimeglumine, serum iron and bilirubin changes were not seen, due to the very high kinetic and thermodynamic stability of this metal chelate. Results in European trials were similar.[18]

The U.S. clinical trial experience involving 1709 patients was reported in 1995.[19] In this trial, which included contrast doses of up to 0.3 mmol/kg, adverse events were reported in 6.9% of patients. Events possibly, probably, or definitely related to contrast administration occurred in 4.6%. The most common adverse events were taste sensation (1.2%) and nausea (1.1%). This study also examined children and bolus injection.

High-dose clinical trials conducted in the U.S., which included 67 patients, were reported in 1994.[20] In these trials, a cumulative dose of 0.3 mmol/kg was given as two bolus injections of 0.1 and 0.2 mmol/kg, separated by 30 min. Adverse reactions were reported in 6.0% of patients. Reactions possibly or probably related to contrast administration occurred in 3.0% (two patients, three total events, which included nausea, hypotension, and taste sensation).

An update from all clinical trials performed in the U.S. and Europe (2481 patients) was published in 1997.[21] Adverse reactions were seen with an incidence of 6.6%, irrespective of relationship to contrast administration. Nausea (1.5%), taste sensation (0.9%), and headache (0.6%) were the most frequently reported adverse events.

By 1997, gadoteridol had been used safely in over one million patients.[22] Like gadopentetate dimeglumine, this agent has an excellent safety profile. Likewise, it can be used regardless of age and renal status. Due to the macrocyclic nature of the ligand, the metal chelate is more stable *in vivo* and releases less gadolinium.

C. GADODIAMIDE (GD DTPA-BMA OR OMNISCAN®, NYCOMED INC.)

Gadodiamide was approved for clinical use in the U.S. in early 1993. The approved dose is 0.1 mmol/kg. An additional dose of 0.2 mmol/kg may be given within 20 min of the first dose, if indicated. This agent is approved for bolus injection.

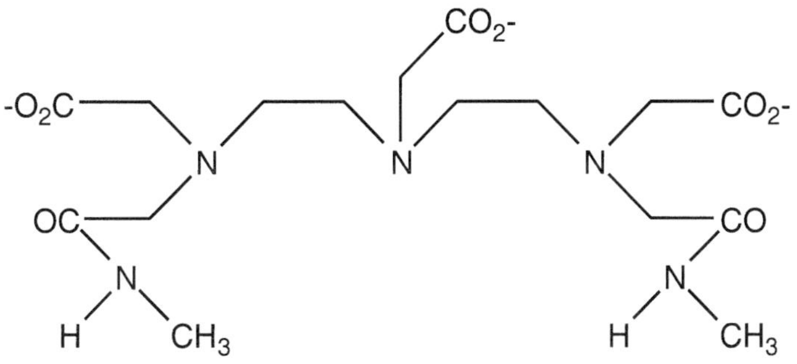

FIGURE 12.3 Ligand structure for DTPA-BMA, the chelate in gadodiamide (Omniscan).

The structure of the agent is that of a long linear ligand (DTPA-BMA, Figure 12.3) that wraps around and binds the gadolinium ion. The presence of two methyl amides differentiates the ligand from DTPA and lowers the charge from –5 to –3. Thus, this metal chelate (like gadoteridol) is also neutral or nonionic.

U.S. clinical trials involving 439 patients were reported in 1991.[23] A dose of 0.1 mmol/kg was administered. Adverse reactions were reported in 10.5% of patients. Of all reactions, nausea was the third most common (1.6%).

D. GADOTERATE MEGLUMINE (GD DOTA OR DOTAREM™, GUERBET)

Gadoterate meglumine is approved for clinical use in many parts of the world, but not in the U.S.. The structure of this agent, like gadoteridol, is that of a rigid macrocyclic ligand that binds gadolinium very tightly. However, the ligand (DOTA) carries a charge of –4, as opposed to the –3 charge of HP-DO3A (Figure 12.4). This gives a net charge of –1 for the metal chelate, which is counterbalanced by the presence of methyl glucamine (a sugar ammonium cation) carrying a charge of +1.

In a randomized, double-blind comparison in Europe (300 patients), clinical tolerance was found to be similar with gadoterate meglumine when compared to gadopentetate dimeglumine.[24] Adverse events were noted in 17.3 and 19.3% of patients, respectively, for the two contrast agents.

In a larger comparative study (also double-blind and randomized), 1038 patients were examined and questioned 1 hour after contrast injection.[25] Adverse reactions were reported in 0.97% of the gadoterate meglumine and 0.77% of the gadopentetate dimeglumine patient groups. Gadoterate meglumine is considered as safe as gadopentetate dimeglumine and has similar diagnostic efficacy.

III. DIFFERENTIATION OF THE GADOLINIUM CHELATES

The four gadolinium chelates available worldwide cannot be differentiated in terms of their enhancement effect (Table 12.1). The T1 and T2 relaxivities, which determine enhancement on MR, are

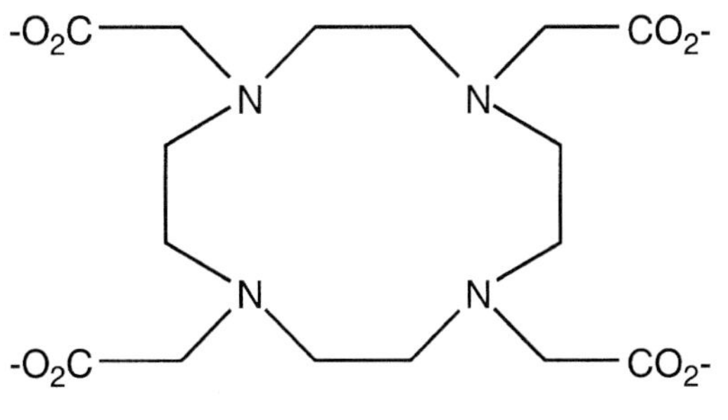

FIGURE 12.4 Ligand structure for DOTA, the chelate in gadoterate meglumine (Dotarem).

TABLE 12.1
Physicochemical Properties of the Gadolinium Chelates

Trade Name	Chemical Formula	Ligand Class	T1 Relaxivity	Log Keq	$k(\text{obs}')\text{s}^{-1}$	Osmolality (mOsmol/kg)	Viscosity (cP) at 37°C
Magnevist	Gd DTPA	Linear	3.8	22.2	1.2×10^{-3}	1960	2.9
ProHance	Gd HP-DO3A	Macrocycle	3.7	23.8	6.3×10^{-5}	630	1.3
Omniscan	Gd DTPA-BMA	Linear	3.8	16.9	$> 2 \times 10^{-2}$	783	1.4
Dotarem	Gd DOTA	Macrocycle	—	24.0	2.1×10^{-5}	1400	—

Note: Log *Keq* is the thermodynamic equilibrium constant (higher values are better), and $k(\text{obs}')\ \text{s}^{-1}$ is the acid dissociation rate (a measure of kinetic stability; lower values are better).

not statistically different. Enhancement of normal and abnormal tissue will be the same with any of the four agents, providing that the dose is held constant.

On the basis of osmolality and viscosity, the agents can be differentiated (Table 12.1). Gadoteridol and gadodiamide have the lowest osmolality and viscosity, in part since they are nonionic.[26] With iodinated agents, low osmolality and viscosity are important positive features. The significance of these parameters is less in MR, where lower volumes of contrast are generally used. Gadopentetate dimeglumine has the highest osmolality and viscosity. The chelate has a charge of –2, requiring formulation with two salts, each carrying a charge of +1. The values for osmolality and viscosity for gadoterate meglumine are intermediate between the two groups. This chelate carries a charge of –1 and is thus formulated with only a single positive sugar salt.

The difference in viscosity of the agents is quite evident clinically when injecting by hand. Both gadoteridol and gadodiamide can be administered very rapidly with little pressure exerted upon the plunger. Gadopentetate dimeglumine requires substantially more pressure to inject and is difficult to inject quickly (by hand) when using small-diameter catheters. If a power injector is used, the difference in viscosity between agents is important only if the pressure cutoff is reached (due to resistance in the line).

Osmolality also differentiates these agents in terms of a very important adverse effect — pain and tissue necrosis following inadvertent extravasation. Gadopentetate dimeglumine, due to its high osmolality, can cause pain and tissue sloughing when extravasated upon injection. This has been demonstrated in animals[27,28] and observed (pain) incidentally in man.[29] Caution should be used when injecting gadopentetate dimeglumine, particularly with a power injector. The difference between agents in this regard is not widely appreciated.

The safety of the gadolinium chelates is largely based upon their stability *in vivo*. The chelates were designed to bind the gadolinium ion extremely tightly, thus assuring near complete renal excretion of the intact chelate (with less than 1% of the injected dose remaining 1 week following injection). A major safety concern in development of this class of agents is the possible release of free gadolinium *in vivo*. This heavy metal is extremely toxic. Gadolinium is not a trace element found normally in the body.

As with osmolality and viscosity, the four agents can be differentiated in terms of stability *in vitro* and *in vivo*. On the basis of kinetic and thermodynamic stability (both basic chemical properties), gadoteridol is by far the best agent and gadodiamide is the worst (Table 12.1). The higher *in vitro* stability of the macrocyclic ring chelates (gadoteridol and gadoterate meglumine), as compared to the linear chelates (gadopentetate dimeglumine and gadodiamide), leads more importantly to higher *in vivo* stability.

Copper and zinc ions in the body can substitute for the gadolinium ion (transmetallation), leading to the release of gadolinium, which is of course undesirable. Transmetallation has been observed both *in vitro*[30,31] and *in vivo*.[32,33]

The release of gadolinium *in vivo* has been assessed in a number of ways. Using radiolabeled chelates, it has been demonstrated in experimental animals that retention in the body of gadolinium is substantially greater and prolonged with gadopentetate dimeglumine and gadodiamide (particularly the latter). In a relatively recent study, urine samples were taken before and after intravenous injection of gadoteridol, gadopentetate dimeglumine, or gadodiamide at 0.1 mmol/kg in healthy volunteers.[34] The urine was then assayed for zinc using inductively coupled, plasma atomic emission spectrometry. A statistically significant difference was noted between the three agents, with zinc excretion (percent injected dose in parentheses) highest for gadodiamide (0.4%), intermediate for gadopentetate dimeglumine (0.07%), and lowest for gadoteridol (0.009%).

The safety concern again voiced by this chapter is the possibility that transmetallation, following intravenous contrast injection, will result in the deposition of gadolinium within the body. *In vivo*, both gadopentetate dimeglumine and gadodiamide inhibit the zinc (Zn)-dependent angiotensin-converting enzyme (ACE).[35] This effect is also attributed to transmetallation. Gadoteridol and gadoterate meglumine, both macrocyclic ring-shaped chelates, are exceptionally inert, a very favorable feature given the safety concern with release of gadolinium ion from a chelate.

For the gadolinium chelates there appears to be no correlation between release of gadolinium ion and minor adverse events. All currently approved agents have comparable profiles in terms of the number of patients suffering from nausea or hives, both reactions accepted as secondary to contrast injection (although occurring in a very small number of patients). Despite the theoretical concern regarding *in vivo* release of gadolinium from these chelates, no harmful effects in humans have been reported to date due to free gadolinium deposition resulting from clinical use of the agents.

Transmetallation is also a potential problem with mangafodipir trisodium, an agent discussed in detail subsequently. Although the metal in this agent is manganese (not gadolinium) and much less toxic, the compound rapidly dechelates *in vivo*.[36-38]

A. Urticaria

The four gadolinium chelates currently in clinical use all cause hives (urticaria) in slightly less than 1% of patients. These four diagnostic agents cannot be differentiated on this basis. For reference, the incidence rate is quoted from similar clinical trial publications. With gadopentetate dimeglumine, a "rash" (which was considered to be a treatment-related reaction) was noted in 0.3% of 1068 patients.[14] With gadoteridol, "urticaria" (possibly or probably related to contrast injection) was noted in 0.2% of 411 patients.[17] With gadodiamide, urticaria (which was considered to be probably related to contrast injection) was noted in 0.7% of 439 patients.[23] With gadoterate meglumine, "pruritus" was noted in 0.4% of 518 patients.[25]

B. Anaphylactoid Reactions

The first publication of a severe anaphylactoid reaction to an intravenous gadolinium chelate injection, specifically gadopentetate dimeglumine, was in 1990.[39] The case occurred in the U.S. It is now known that such reactions do occur, but with a very low incidence. Thus, it is not surprising that the first documented reaction was observed some time after approval (1988 in the U.S.) and not in clinical trials. Notably, the patient involved had a history of asthma and previous allergic reaction (respiratory distress) to iodinated contrast media.[40]

In late 1990, a second anaphylactoid reaction was reported in the literature.[41] The review of systems in this case was negative for asthma, allergies, or known drug sensitivities. Another case study in late 1990 reported five adverse reactions in 344 patients (for a rate of 1.5%), with one that was anaphylactoid in nature.[42] Communications at that time with the manufacturer documented five known anaphylactoid reactions, with an estimated 1.1 million doses given and, thus, a frequency of 1 per 200,000 doses.

A report from France in 1992 documented another severe anaphylactoid reaction following intravenous administration of gadopentetate dimeglumine.[43] This patient also had a history of allergies (pollen) and prior anaphylactoid reactions to iodinated contrast media.

A report in 1993 documented the development of laryngeal edema following gadopentetate dimeglumine injection in Japan in a patient with bronchial asthma.[44] The authors suggested tightening the indications for contrast use in patients with an allergic disposition. Also stated was that gadopentetate dimeglumine should be used with the same care as iodinated contrast media in regard to development of possible anaphylactoid reactions.

A second severe reaction was reported in Japan in 1993 in a patient with a history of a mild adverse reaction during a prior study with gadopentetate dimeglumine.[45] A fatal reaction to gadopentetate dimeglumine was reported in 1995.[46]

Gadoteridol was approved for clinical use in 1992. Case reports appeared in 1993[47] and 1994,[48] documenting life-threatening anaphylactoid reactions with this agent as well. The authors emphasized that resuscitation equipment and properly trained personnel should be available when gadolinium chelates are administered. A life-threatening anaphylactoid reaction after intravenous injection of gadoterate meglumine was reported in 1996.[49] Given the later approval and lower market share of this agent (which has never been sold in the U.S.), the later date of this publication is not surprising.

A review article in 1994 estimated the rate of severe reactions with gadopentetate dimeglumine to be 1 in 350,000 to 450,000.[50] This number comes from the 1991 manufacturer's report, which detailed six anaphylactoid reactions in 13,439 patients (0.0003%).[51] In this study, Niendorf et al.[51] also reported that the risk of adverse reactions was substantially higher (3.7 times) in patients with a history of iodinated contrast media reaction.

In a subsequent series of 21,000 patients reviewed in 1996, two severe reactions to gadopentetate dimeglumine were reported. The incidence of severe anaphylactoid reactions in this large academic study was thus 0.01% or 1 in 10,000.[52] Of the 36 patients in this group with adverse reactions, four had a history of adverse reaction to iodinated contrast media. For reference, Caro et al. in 1992 reported the risk of life-threatening events to be 0.031% with low-osmolarity iodinated radiographic contrast media.[53]

Although the rate may be lower for severe reactions with gadolinium chelates as opposed to iodinated contrast media, it bears repeating that personnel must be trained and equipment must be readily available for management and/or resuscitation of patients receiving intravenous gadolinium chelate injection for MR imaging. Furthermore, patients with a history of reaction to iodinated contrast media are at greater risk for an adverse reaction to a gadolinium chelate. This is unfortunately not common knowledge among practitioners in the U.S.

IV. ANOTHER METAL CHELATE

A. Mangafodipir Trisodium (Mn DPDP or Teslascan®, Nycomed Inc.)

The structure of this agent is that of a large linear ligand (DPDP, with a charge of –5, Figure 12.5) that wraps around and binds the manganese ion (with a charge of +2). This gives a net charge of –3 for the metal chelate, which is counterbalanced by the presence of three sodiums, each carrying a charge of +1. The osmolality is 298 mOsmol/kg water and the viscosity is 0.8 cP at 37°C. Following intravenous injection, the manganese ion is distributed largely to the liver, pancreas, and kidneys.[54]

In phase I clinical trials with mangafodipir trisodium, facial flushing and warmth were observed in 35 of 40 subjects, and dose-dependent increases in heart rate and blood pressure were also seen.[55]

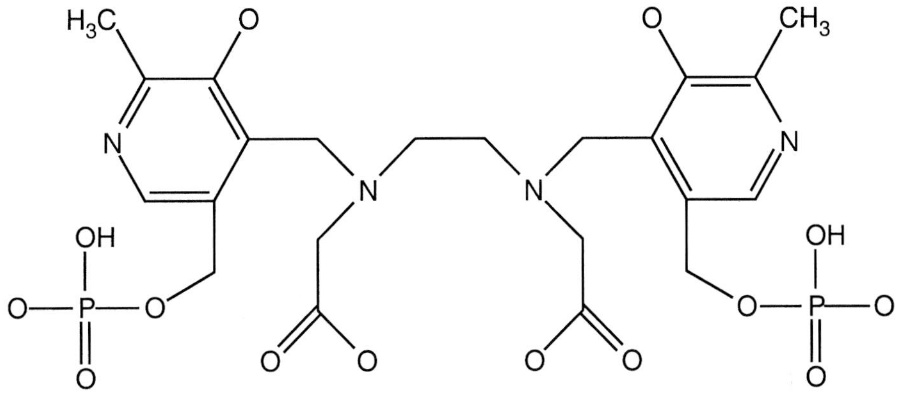

FIGURE 12.5 Ligand structure for DPDP, the chelate in mangafodipir trisodium (Teslascan).

Subsequent clinical trials were conducted with lower doses and slower intravenous injections. These resulted in fewer side effects.[56]

In the first large patient series reported with this agent, minor side effects were found in 38 of 141 patients (27%).[57] Among the different adverse events, flushing and warmth were reported most frequently (21 of 141). Three patients suffered from nausea (2.1%). In a 20-patient series reported in 1992, 6 patients reported side effects that included flushing, feelings of warmth, and/or metallic taste.[58] Mangafodipir trisodium is also known to cause a transient decrease in alkaline phosphatase levels. The agent has five major metabolites *in vivo*, which are created by dephosphorylation and transmetallation with zinc.[59] In a phase III study of 82 patients, published in 1997, mild to moderate adverse events were noted in 17% of the patients.[60] European phase III clinical trials, reported in 1997, included 624 patients. Adverse events were reported in 7% of the patients.[61]

Mangafodipir trisodium should be considered as a separate class of MR contrast media, distinctly different from the gadolinium chelates. The active component is manganese, not gadolinium. The agent also dechelates *in vivo*, with the manganese ion rapidly incorporated into hepatocytes. For the gadolinium chelates, stability of the complex *in vivo* is of the utmost importance. The dechelation of mangafodipir trisodium accounts for the high incidence of flushing as well as the enhancement of the intestinal mucosa and the pancreas.[62,63]

DPDP, the ligand, does not facilitate transport of manganese into any organ except the kidney. Following release from the chelate, the manganese (II) ion binds to human serum proteins. The presence of DPDP reduces the distribution to the heart immediately following injection, improving cardiovascular tolerance.[64] In regard to excretion, approximately 15% of the manganese ion contained in the initial injection is eliminated in the urine by 24 h and an additional 59% in the feces by 5 days (package insert).

The approved dose in the U.S. for this MR contrast agent is 5 µmol/kg (0.1 ml/kg), with the injection to be given over a 1 min period. In clinical trials, imaging was performed at 15 min, 4 h, and 24 h post-injection. Post-contrast, there is moderate enhancement of normal liver parenchyma. In one small clinical trial (examining mangafodipir trisodium), the liver signal-to-noise ratio increased from 28 ± 3 pre-contrast to 40 ± 2 post-contrast on T1-weighted gradient echo images. In the same study, the lesion-liver contrast-to-noise ratio increased (in magnitude) from 7 ± 1 pre-contrast to 23 ± 3 post-contrast.[65]

Although the instability of the complex *in vivo* has raised concerns regarding potential toxicity from the manganese ion, there is no clinical evidence to support any such effect. However, free manganese is known to accumulate in the brain and can cause a Parkinsonism-like syndrome. In preclinical trials, mangafodipir trisodium also caused, at the highest doses tested, skeletal abnormalities in fetal rats and an increased rate of fetal demise in rabbits. The manganese ion is felt to be the causative agent in this instance. The fetal demise was seen at more than ten times the clinical dose.

V. PARTICULATE AGENTS

A. FERUMOXIDES

Ferumoxides, large superparamagnetic iron oxide particles, are used in two formulations across the world. In the U.S., the agent is sold as Feridex® (Ferumoxides, Berlex Laboratories) and contains 11.2 mg of iron per milliliter. In Europe, the same compound is supplied at twice the concentration and is marketed as Endorem™ (Guerbet).[66] Approval, regardless of country, is for the same dose, 0.56 mg of iron per kilogram body weight. The agent is also available in China, Japan, and most of South America.

The compound is a reddish-brown colloid of superparamagnetic iron oxide with dextran. The particles are taken up by the reticuloendothelial system following intravenous administration. The iron then enters the normal body iron metabolism cycle.

The presence of the agent in tissue shortens T2, producing signal loss on T2-weighted scans. Large iron particles also have an effect on T1, although this is substantially less than their T2 effect. The T1 effect is noticeable and can be used for lesion characterization if the agent is given as a bolus injection and early dynamic post-contrast scans are acquired. On delayed scans, tissues with decreased reticuloendothelial function (for example, benign lesions and most tumors) retain their signal intensity, so contrast between normal and abnormal tissue is increased.

In the original clinical trial performed with Ferumoxides, two adverse reactions were seen in 15 patients.[67] One patient developed a rash. Another patient developed transient hypotension, resulting in termination of dose escalation. Subsequent trials employed lower doses and slower infusion.

Approval for the use of this MR contrast agent in the U.S. is for adult patients and liver imaging only. The dose is diluted in 100 ml and given over 30 min. Since the formulation contains iron, a transient increase in serum iron and ferritin and a decrease in iron binding capacity are seen.[68] These laboratory changes are of no clinical significance. Ferumoxides are contraindicated in patients with known allergic or hypersensitivity reactions to parenteral iron or dextran. Anaphylactic-like reactions and hypotension have been noted following administration.

The agent should be used with caution in patients with iron overload disorders (e.g., hemosiderosis and hemochromatosis). In all patients, extreme caution should be exercised during injection to avoid extravasation. Acute severe back, leg, or groin pain can occur within 1 to 15 min following injection, alone or with other symptoms such as hypotension and dyspnea. In clinical trials, this was severe enough to cause interruption or discontinuation of infusion in 2.5% of patients (12.5% of patients with cirrhosis). Low back pain is the most frequent side effect.

In phase III clinical trials conducted in the U.S. (213 doses), 15% of the patients experienced adverse reactions.[69] Reactions in 8% of the patients were classified as possibly or probably related to drug administration. The two most frequently reported adverse reactions were back pain (4%) and flushing (2%). The mechanism for these adverse reactions is unknown.[70]

VI. OFF-LABEL USE

In diagnostic radiology, off-label use is defined as the use in patients of an approved contrast agent for a purpose not contained in product labeling. Off-label use is permitted (and specifically not a violation of U.S. law), providing that it occurs in the course of normal medical practice and is not part of an investigation into safety or effectiveness.

In the U.S., radiologists are free to use approved contrast media in any manner that in their professional judgement would best serve the patient. The FDA specifically does not have the authority to regulate such use. For example, although the gadolinium chelates are approved for specific indications and specific portions of the body, they can be and are commonly used for other purposes. The use of gadolinium chelates for contrast-enhanced MR angiography is a current major example. FDA approval is based on safety and efficacy.

The FDA regulates how a drug may be marketed, but not how a physician may choose to use it once it becomes commercially available. For example, mangafodipir trisodium is only clinically approved for liver use, yet it has other potential applications (for example, in imaging of pancreatic neoplasms) which are by definition off-label.

A. INFANTS

None of the gadolinium chelates are approved for use in patients under the age of 2 years in the U.S. Important differential diagnostic information, as well as improved lesion detection, is provided by post-contrast scans in infants with suspected neoplastic disease or active infection in the central nervous system. Although several small trials have been published, there has been no large-scale examination of clinical safety in this patient population. However, there are no reported problems, and no significant safety concerns have been raised.

B. DOSE

In recent years, the use of contrast doses greater than 0.1 mmol/kg with the gadolinium chelates has become more common. In the U.S., this is an off-label use of gadopentetate dimeglumine since the agent carries approval for only a dose of 0.1 mmol/kg. Although gadoteridol and gadodiamide are approved in the U.S. for use up to 0.3 mmol/kg, the approved labeling is limited. Thus, when used at high doses, particularly for MR angiography or brain perfusion studies, the application of even these agents is considered off-label. However, their safety at these doses has been studied and approved by the FDA. In all such applications, the use of an increased dose is based on the radiologist's clinical judgement regarding risk vs. benefit ratio.

C. RENAL FAILURE

Gadolinium chelates are used in patients with renal dysfunction or failure, despite the lack of specific approval for this application. Clinical indications are many.[71-78] Gadopentetate dimeglumine, gadoteridol, gadodiamide, and gadoterate meglumine are all cleared from the body by glomerular filtration. As indicated in the package inserts for all agents, caution should be exercised in their use in patients with impaired renal function. All four of these gadolinium chelates are dialyzable.[79-87]

A new off-label application of the gadolinium chelates is in X-ray angiography in patients with renal failure. Although not originally developed for such use, the gadolinium chelates can be employed successfully for digital subtraction angiography following intra-arterial injection.[88] Deterioration in renal functin following intra-artenal injectin has, however, been observed.

Mangafodipir trisodium is cleared partially by glomerular filtration and partially by hepatobiliary excretion. Ferumoxides are not renally cleared. No studies have been performed with either mangafodipir trisodium or ferumoxides in patients with renal insufficiency.

D. PREGNANCY

Adverse effects upon the fetus have been documented in animal models with all MR contrast media, to a lesser or greater extent depending upon the agent. Gadopentetate dimeglumine has been shown to slightly retard fetal development in rats (at 2.5 times the human dose, 0.1 mmol/kg) and rabbits (at 7.5 times the human dose). No congenital anomalies were found in either species.

When administered at 10 mmol/kg/day (100 times the typical human dose), gadoteridol doubled the incidence of post-implantation loss in rats. At 60 times the typical dose (and when given for 12 days at this dose), gadoteridol increased the incidence of spontaneous abortion and early delivery in rabbits.

Gadodiamide has been shown to have an adverse effect on embryo-fetal development in animals when given at doses as low as 0.5 mmol/kg/day (five times the typical human dose). Mangafodipir trisodium has been shown to be teratogenic and fetotoxic in animal studies. Ferumoxides have been shown to be teratogenic in animal studies.

Adequate and well-controlled studies in pregnant women have not been conducted with any MR contrast agent. Although clinical indications theoretically exist for intravenous contrast administration in pregnancy, contrast administration should only be performed if the potential benefit justifies the potential risk. Written informed consent should be obtained if a decision is reached to administer intravenous contrast. In my own experience, one reasonable but rare request for contrast enhancement in this population has been made on several occasions — a request for diagnosis (in a pregnant woman with symptoms of subarachnoid and cord hemorrhage) of an underlying spinal cord or canal arteriovenous malformation.

VII. ORAL CONTRAST MEDIA

Opacification of the gastrointestinal tract by oral and rectal contrast administration can be important in MR to distinguish normal bowel from adjacent structures, whether normal or abnormal. A relatively new indication for oral contrast media is the use in MR cholangiopancreatography (MRCP) to negate the signal from overlying bowel. Two general classes of agents exist, those that cause an increase in signal intensity (or positive contrast enhancement) and those that cause a decrease in signal intensity (or negative contrast enhancement).

FerriSeltz® (a formulation of ferric ammonium citrate; Nycomed Inc.) falls within the first class of agents, and GastroMARK® (superparamagnetic iron oxide; Ferumoxsil, Mallinckrodt Inc.) falls within the second class of agents. Agents can also be differentiated by whether they are water soluble (like ferric ammonium citrate) or insoluble (like the particulate iron oxide preparations).

Positive enhancement of the bowel contents can lead to image degradation. Motion of high signal intensity bowel, due to normal peristalsis, produces ghosting artifacts that can obscure normal structures and pathology. This specific problem is not encountered with negative agents. However, delineation of the bowel wall and disease thereof is best obtained following the administration of positive agents.

Susceptibility artifacts from iron oxide particles can degrade visualization of the bowel wall. In addition to the contrast media described in the following paragraphs, limited utility has been described with two other agents. Infant formula has high signal intensity on both Tl- and T2-weighted scans, providing excellent visualization of the gastrointestinal tract in newborns.[89] Certain barium sulfate preparations have also been evaluated as negative agents.[90,91]

A. PARTICULATE AGENTS

GastroMARK is a dark-brown aqueous suspension of superparamagnetic iron oxide.[92,93] This agent was approved by the FDA for clinical use in 1997 and is in active clinical use in the U.S. After oral administration, the bowel lumen appears dark or has low signal intensity regardless of the imaging technique. The agent is not absorbed by the bowel and is excreted within 24 h after administration. The recommended dose is 600 ml (900 ml maximum), administered orally at a rate of 300 ml over 15 min.

For the upper gastrointestinal (GI) tract, imaging is optimal by 30 min, with delayed images (4 to 7 h) useful in delineating the lower GI tract. The approved indication is for oral use in adults to enhance delineation of the upper GI tract. With pancreatic or gastric masses, there was increased confidence in delineating a mass in 44 to 49% of cases.

An important current clinical application of the agent is for improved image quality in MRCP, by removal of the bowel signal intensity within the imaging volume of interest. Although transit time and dilution limit usefulness in the lower GI tract, GastroMARK is the best of all approved agents in this application.

As with other large volume, oral contrast agents, GastroMARK is contraindicated when intestinal perforation or obstruction is known or suspected. GI adverse events were observed in 30% of patients in clinical trials within 2 h of ingestion. These events included abdominal pain, diarrhea, nausea, and vomiting. Diarrhea occurred within 24 h of administration in 24% of patients. Since GastroMARK contains iron, it should be used with caution in patients with iron overload (e.g., hemosiderosis and hemochromatosis).

B. WATER-SOLUBLE IRON FORMULATIONS

The FDA approved Ferriseltz for clinical use in 1999. The recommended dose is two packets (6 g) dissolved in 600 ml of water and administered orally over 15 to 30 min. MR scanning should be initiated within 5 to 20 min after administration. The approved indication is for adult patients, on T1-weighted scans, to enhance bowel delineation in the upper GI tract.[94]

Ferriseltz has high signal intensity on T1-weighted scans. In phase II and III clinical trials, increased intraluminal signal intensity, improved contrast enhancement of the GI tract, distention, and improved signal homogeneity were found in 89 to 98% of patients after ingestion.[95] Ferriseltz provided new or additional radiologic information in 64% of patients and information that changed diagnosis, management, or surgical approach in 15% of patients.

As with other ferric ammonium citrate preparations, some of the iron in Ferriseltz is absorbed following oral ingestion. The iron is then incorporated into hemoglobin or into ferritin for storage. Adverse events associated with Ferriseltz ingestion include nausea (4%), vomiting (3%), diarrhea (17%), and abdominal pain (4%). As with GastroMARK, Ferriseltz (since it contains iron) should be used with caution in patients with iron overload.

C. MANGANESE-BASED AGENTS

A manganese chloride-based oral contrast agent (Lumenhance®, Bracco Diagnostics) has also been evaluated in MR exams.[96] Volunteers were studied before and after oral ingestion of 900 ml using three different concentrations (20, 40, and 60 mg/l Mn^{2+}). Opacification was evaluated at three different anatomic sites: the stomach, the middle of the small bowel, and the ileocecal region. There were no adverse events. A minimal rise in blood levels of manganese was noted at 6 h, with a return to baseline by 24 h.

Good-to-excellent hyperintense bowel marking was noted with all three concentrations on T1-weighted images. On T2-weighted images, the two higher concentrations provided improved hypointense bowel marking relative to the lower concentration. Lumenhance is approved for use by the FDA, but is not marketed to date.

D. GADOLINIUM CHELATES

Gadopentatate dimeglumine has been evaluated in clinical trials in Europe[97,98] as an oral contrast agent. The formulation used was a dilution of gadopentatate dimeglumine in water and mannitol. Bowel opacification permitted ready differentiation between bowel loops and intra-abdominal masses (with specific applicability for study of pancreatic and pelvic lesions). Pathologic thickening of the bowel wall could also be identified.

Prior to contrast use, the bowel and its contents were isointense on T1-weighted images relative to soft tissue and muscle. After gadopentatate dimeglumine ingestion, the bowel contents were of homogeneous high signal intensity and were easily differentiated from fecal material (with intermediate signal intensity) and air (with low signal intensity). In one study, the delineation of abdominal abnormalities was improved following oral gadopentatate dimeglumine ingestion in 19 of 32 MR exams.[99] Diarrhea was reported as a complication, presumably due to the mannitol included in the oral preparation. In a larger series of 150 exams, abdominal distention and diarrhea were noted as side effects in 25% of patients.[100]

It is important to note that for oral contrast use, a different formulation of gadopentatate dimeglumine is used than that approved for intravenous administration. An oral formulation of gadopentatate dimeglumine is neither approved for clinical use in the U.S. nor clinically available.

VIII. CONCLUSIONS

Although theoretical safety concerns exist, gadolinium chelates have been shown in worldwide trials and subsequent clinical use to be safe and well tolerated as intravenous contrast media in both adult and pediatric patients. Administration of a gadolinium chelate to improve lesion detection and differential diagnosis in MR imaging examinations is an accepted and standard practice. These agents were approved in the time frame of the late 1980s and early 1990s and have been in widespread use since that time.

All intravenous agents should be used with caution, as adverse effects are known to occur, although infrequently. However, the gadolinium chelates have proved to be an exceptionally well-tolerated class of contrast media. In particular, this class of agents does not exhibit any nephrotoxicity (at approved doses) in distinction to the iodinated agents. Much less data exist concerning the safety of iron particles and other non-gadolinium containing agents for intravenous injection. However, examples of agents in each of these categories have been approved and in clinical use for a number of years, although for a substantially shorter time period than with the renally excreted gadolinium chelates. Several oral contrast media are approved for clinical use in the U.S. Adverse events with these agents are common but minor. Clinical utilization of oral contrast media is low due to a perception of low utility.

REFERENCES

1. Vogl, T.J., Pegios, W., McMahon, C., et al., Gadobenate dimeglumine — a new contrast agent for MR imaging: preliminary evaluation in healthy volunteers, *Am. J. Roentgenol.*, 158(4):887-1892, 1992.
2. Spinazzi, A., Lorusso, V., Pirovano, G., and Kirchin, M., Safety, tolerance, biodistribution, and MR imaging enhancement of the liver with gadobenate dimeglumine: results of clinical pharmacologic and pilot imaging studies in nonpatient and patient volunteers, *Acad. Radiol.*, 6(5):282-291, 1999.
3. Staks, T., Schuhmann-Giampieri, G., Frenzel, T., et al., Pharmacokinetics, dose proportionality, and tolerability of gadobutrol after single intravenous injection in healthy volunteers, *Invest. Radiol.*, 29(7):709-715, 1994.
4. Hartmann, M., Forsting, M., Jansen, O., et al., Does the administration of a high dose of a paramagnetic contrast medium (Gadovist) improve the diagnostic value of magnetic resonance tomography in glioblastomas?, *Rofo Fortschr. Geb. Rontgenstr. Neuen Bildgeb Verfahr*, 164(2):119-125, 1996.
5. Small, W.C., DeSimone-Macchi, D., Parker, J.R., et al., A multisite phase III study of the safety and efficacy of a new manganese chloride-based gastrointestinal contrast agent for MRI of the abdomen and pelvis, *J. Magn. Reson. Imaging*, 10(1):15-24, 1999.
6. Hamm, B., Staks, T., Muhler, A., et al., Phase I clinical evaluation of Gd-EOB-DTPA as a hepatobiliary MR contrast agent: safety, pharmacokinetics, and MR imaging, *Radiology*, 195(3):785-792, 1995.
7. Reimer, P., Rummeny, E.J., Shamsi, K., et al., Phase II clinical evaluation of Gd-EOB-DTPA: dose, safety aspects, and pulse sequence, *Radiology*, 199(1):177-183, 1996.
8. Giovagnoni, A. and Paci, E., Liver. III: gadolinium-based hepatobiliary contrast agents (Gd-EOB-DTPA and Gd-BOPTA/Dimeg), *Magn. Reson. Imaging Clin. North Am.*, 4(1):61-72, 1996.
9. Ni, Y. and Marchal, G., Enhanced magnetic resonance imaging for tissue characterization of liver abnormalities with hepatobiliary contrast agents: an overview of preclinical animal experiments, *Top. Magn. Reson. Imaging*, 9(3):183-195, 1998.
10. Hamm, B., Staks, T., Taupitz, M., et al., Contrast-enhanced MR imaging of liver and spleen: first experience in humans with a new superparamagnetic iron oxide, *J. Magn. Reson. Imaging*, 4(5):659-668, 1994.
11. Laniado, M., Kopp, A.F., Current status of the clinical development of MR contrast media, *Rofo Fortschr. Geb. Rontgenstr. Neuen Bildgeb Verfahr*, 167(6):541-550, 1997.
12. Chen, F., Ward, J., and Robinson, P.J., MR imaging of the liver and spleen: a comparison of the effects on signal intensity of two superparamagnetic iron oxide agents, *Magn, Reson. Imaging*, 17(4):549-556, 1999.
13. Runge, V.M., Schoerner, W., Niendorf, H.P., et al., Initial clinical evaluation of gadolinium DTPA for contrast-enhanced magnetic resonance imaging, *Magn, Reson. Imaging*, 3(1):27-35, 1985.
14. Goldstein, H.A., Kashanian, F.K., Blumetti, R.F., et al., Safety assessment of gadopentetate dimeglumine in U.S. clinical trials, *Radiology*, 174(1):17-23, 1990.
15. Nelson, K.L., Gifford, L.M., Lauber-Huber, C., et al., Clinical safety of gadopentetate dimeglumine, *Radiology*, 196(2):439-443, 1995.

16. Niendorf, H.P., Alhassan, A., Geens, V.R., and Clauss, W., Safety review of gadopentetate dimeglumine. Extended clinical experience after more than five million applications, *Invest. Radiol.*, 29 (Suppl. 2):S179-S182, 1994.

17. Runge, V.M., Bradley, W.G., Brant-Zawadzki, M.N., et al., Clinical safety and efficacy of gadoteridol: a study in 411 patients with suspected intracranial and spinal disease, *Radiology*, 181(3):701-709, 1991.

18. Seiderer, M., Phase III clinical studies with gadoteridol for the evaluation of neurologic pathology. A European perspective, *Invest. Radiol.*, 27 (Suppl. 1):S33-S38, 1992.

19. Olukotun, A.Y., Parker, J.R., Meeks, M.J., et al., Safety of gadoteridol injection: U.S. clinical trial experience, *J. Magn. Reson. Imaging*, 5(1):17-25, 1995.

20. Yuh, W.T., Fisher, D.J., Runge, V.M., et al., Phase III multicenter trial of high-dose gadoteridol in MR evaluation of brain metastases, *Am. J. Neuroradiol.*, 15(6):1037-1051, 1994.

21. Runge, V.M. and Parker, J.R., Worldwide clinical safety assessment of gadoteridol injection: an update, *Eur. Radiol.*, 7(Suppl. 5):243-245, 1997.

22. Tweedle, M.F., The ProHance story: the making of a novel MRI contrast agent, *Eur. Radiol.*, 7(Suppl. 5):225-230, 1997.

23. Sze, G., Brant-Zawadzki, M., Haughton, V.M., et al., Multicenter study of gadodiamide injection as a contrast agent in MR imaging of the brain and spine, *Radiology*, 181(3):693-699, 1991.

24. Brugieres, P., Gaston, A., Degryse, H.R., et al., Randomised double blind trial of the safety and efficacy of two gadolinium complexes (Gd-DTPA and Gd-DOTA), *Neuroradiology*, 36(1):27-30, 1994.

25. Oudkerk, M., Sijens, P.E., Van Beek, E.J., and Kuijpers, T.J., Safety and efficacy of dotarem (Gd-DOTA) versus magnevist (Gd-DTPA) in magnetic resonance imaging of the central nervous system, *Invest. Radiol.*, 30(2):75-78, 1995.

26. Tweedle, M.F., Nonionic or neutral?, *Radiology*, 178(3):891, 1991.

27. McAlister, W.H., McAlister, V.I., and Kissane, J.M., The effect of Gd-dimeglumine on subcutaneous tissues: a study with rats, *Am. J. Neuroradiol.*, 11(2):325-327,1990.

28. Cohan, R.H., Leder, R.A., Herzberg, A.J., et al., Extravascular toxicity of two magnetic resonance contrast agents. Preliminary experience in the rat, *Invest. Radiol.*, 26(3):224-226, 1991.

29. Vehmas, T. and Markkola, A.T., Gd-DTPA as an alternative contrast agent in conventional and interventional radiology, *Acta Radiol.*, 39(3):223-226, 1998.

30. Tweedle, M.F., Hagan, J.J., Kumar, K., et al., Reaction of gadolinium chelates with endogenously available ions, *Magn. Reson. Imaging*, 9(3):409-415, 1991.

31. Puttagunta, N.R., Gibby, W.A., and Puttagunta, V.L., Comparative transmetallation kinetics and thermodynamic stability of gadolinium-DTPA bis-glucosamide and other magnetic resonance imaging contrast media, *Invest. Radiol.*, 31(10):619-624, 1996.

32. Wedeking, P., Kumar, K., and Tweedle, M.F., Dissociation of gadolinium chelates in mice: relationship to chemical characteristics, *Magn. Reson. Imaging*, 10(4):641-648, 1992.

33. Tweedle, M.F., Wedeking, P., and Kumar, K., Biodistribution of radiolabeled, formulated gadopentetate, gadoteridol, gadoterate, and gadodiamide in mice and rats, *Invest. Radiol.*, 30(6):372-380, 1995.

34. Puttagunta, N.R., Gibby, W.A., and Smith, G.T., Human in vivo comparative study of zinc and copper transmetallation after administration of magnetic resonance imaging contrast agents, *Invest. Radiol.*, 31(12):739-742, 1996.

35. Corot, C., Idee, J.M., Hentsch, A.M., et al., Structure-activity relationship of macrocyclic and linear gadolinium chelates: investigation of transmetallation effect on the zinc-dependent metallopeptidase angiotensin-converting enzyme, *J. Magn. Reson. Imaging*, 8(3):695-702, 1998.

36. Toft, K.G., Hustvedt, S.O., Grant, D., et al., Metabolism and pharmacokinetics of MnDPDP in man, *Acta Radiol.*, 38(4, Pt. 2):677-689, 1997.

37. Toft, K.G., Kindberg, G.M., and Skotland, T., Mangafodipir trisodium injection, a new contrast medium for magnetic resonance imaging: in vitro metabolism and protein binding studies of the active component MnDPDP in human blood, *J. Pharm. Biomed. Anal.*, 15(7):983-988, 1997.

38. Toft, K.G., Hustvedt, S.O., Grant, D., et al., Metabolism of mangafodipir trisodium (MnDPDP), a new contrast medium for magnetic resonance imaging, in beagle dogs, *Eur. J. Drug Metab. Pharmacokinet.*, 22(1):65-72, 1997.

39. Weiss, K.L., Severe anaphylactoid reaction after i.v. Gd-DTPA, *Magn. Reson. Imaging*, 8(6):817-818, 1990.

40. Lufkin, R.B., Severe anaphylactoid reaction to Gd-DTPA, *Radiology*, 176(3):879, 1990.

41. Tishler, S. and Hoffman, J.C., Jr., Anaphylactoid reactions to i.v. gadopentetate dimeglumine, *Am. J. Neuroradiol.*, 11(6):1167, 1990.

42. Salonen, O.L., Case of anaphylaxis and four cases of allergic reaction following Gd-DTPA administration, *J. Comput. Assist. Tomogr.*, 14(6):912-913, 1990.

43. Tardy, B., Guy, C., Barral, G., et al., Anaphylactic shock induced by intravenous gadopentetate dimeglumine, *Lancet*, 339(8791):494, 1992.

44. Katoh, A., Kishikawa, T., Kudo, S., et al., Anaphylactoid reaction after intravenous administration of Gd-DTPA, *Nippon Igaku Hoshasen Gakkai Zasshi*, 53(8):973-975, 1993.

45. Nomura, M., Takeshita, G., Katada, K., et al., A case of anaphylactic shock following the administration of Gd-DTPA, *Nippon Igaku Hoshasen Gakkai Zasshi*, 53(12):1387-1391, 1993.

46. Jordan, R.M. and Mintz, R.D., Fatal reaction to gadopentetate dimeglumine, *Am. J. Roentgenol.*, 164(3):743-744, 1995.

47. Shellock, F.G., Hahn, H.P., Mink, J.H., and Itskovich, E., Adverse reaction to intravenous gadoteridol, *Radiology*, 189(1):151-152, 1993.

48. Witte, R.J. and Anzai, L.L., Life-threatening anaphylactoid reaction after intravenous gadoteridol administration in a patient who had previously received gadopentetate dimeglumine, *Am. J. Neuroradiol.*, 15(3):523-524, 1994.

49. Meuli, R.A. and Maeder, P., Life-threatening anaphylactoid reaction after iv injection of gadoterate meglumine, *Am. J. Roentgenol.*, 166(3):729, 1996.

50. Carr, J.J., Magnetic resonance contrast agents for neuroimaging. Safety issues, *Neuroimaging Clin. North Am.*, 4(1):43-54, 1994.

51. Niendorf, H.P., Dinger, J.C., Haustein, J., et al., Tolerance data of Gd-DTPA: a review, *Eur. J. Radiol.*, 13(1):15-20, 1991.

52. Murphy, K.J., Brunberg, J.A., and Cohan, R.H., Adverse reactions to gadolinium contrast media: a review of 36 cases, *Am. J. Roentgenol.*, 167(4):847-849, 1996.

53. Caro, J.J., Trindade, E., and McGregor, M., The cost-effectiveness of replacing high-osmolality with low-osmolality contrast media, *Am. J. Roentgenol.*, 159(4):869-874, 1992.

54. Hustvedt, S.O., Grant, D., Southon, T.E., and Zech, K., Plasma pharmacokinetics, tissue distribution and excretion of MnDPDP in the rat and dog after intravenous administration, *Acta Radiol.*, 38(4, Pt. 2):690-699, 1997.

55. Lim, K.O., Stark, D.D., Leese, P.T., et al., Hepatobiliary MR imaging: first human experience with MnDPDP, *Radiology*, 178(1):79-82, 1991.

56. Kopp, A.F., Laniado, M., Aicher, K.P., et al., Manganese DPDP as a contrast medium for MR tomography of focal liver lesions. Tolerance and image quality in 20 patients, *Rofo Fortschr. Geb. Rontgenstr. Neuen Bildgeb Verfahr.*, 157(6):539-547, 1992.

57. Rummeny, E., Ehrenheim, C., Gehl, H.B., et al., Manganese-DPDP as a hepatobiliary contrast agent in the magnetic resonance imaging of liver tumors. Results of clinical phase II trials in Germany including 141 patients, *Invest. Radiol.*, 26(Suppl. 1):S142-S145, 1991.

58. Aicher, K.P., Laniado, M., Kopp, A.F., et al., Mn-DPDP-enhanced MR imaging of malignant liver lesions: efficacy and safety in 20 patients, *J. Magn. Reson. Imaging*, 3(5):731-737, 1993.

59. Toft, K.G., Friisk, G.A., and Skotland, T., Mangafodipir trisodium injection, a new contrast medium for magnetic resonance imaging: detection and quantitation of the parent compound MnDPDP and metabolites in human plasma by high performance liquid chromatography, *J. Pharm. Biomed. Anal.*, 15(7):973-981, 1997.

60. Wang, C., Ahlstrom, H., Ekholm, S., et al., Diagnostic efficacy of MnDPDP in MR imaging of the liver. A phase III multicentre study, *Acta Radiol.*, 38(4, Pt. 2):643-649, 1997.

61. Torres, C.G., Lundby, B., Sterud, A.T., et al., MnDPDP for MR imaging of the liver. Results from the European phase III studies, *Acta Radiol.*, 38(4, Pt. 2):631-637, 1997.

62. Mayo-Smith, W.W., Schima, W., Saini, S., et al., Pancreatic enhancement and pulse sequence analysis using low-dose mangafodipir trisodium, *Am. J. Roentgenol.*, 170(3):649-652, 1998.

63. Wang, C., Johansson, L., Western, A., et al., Sequence optimization in mangafodipir trisodium-enhanced liver and pancreas MRI, *J. Magn. Reson. Imaging*, 9(2):280–284, 1999.

64. Ni, Y., Petre, C., Bosmans, H., et al., Comparison of manganese biodistribution and MR contrast enhancement in rats after intravenous injection of MnDPDP and MnCl$_2$, *Acta Radiol.*, 38(4, Pt. 2):700-707, 1997.

65. Schima, W., Petersein, J., Hahn, P.F., et al., Contrast-enhanced MR imaging of the liver: comparison between Gd-BOPTA and Mangafodipir, *J. Magn. Reson. Imaging*, 7(1):130-135, 1997.

66. Laniado, M. and Chachuat, A., The endorem tolerance profile, *Radiologe*, 35(11, Suppl. 2):S266-S270, 1995.

67. Stark, D.D., Weissleder, R., Elizondo, G., et al., Superparamagnetic iron oxide: clinical application as a contrast agent for MR imaging of the liver, *Radiology*, 168(2):297-301, 1988.

68. Yoshikawa, K., Sasaki, Y., Ogawa, N., Sakuma, S., Clinical application of AMI-25 (superparamagnetic iron oxide) for the MR imaging of hepatic tumors: a multicenter clinical phase III study, *Nippon Igaku Hoshasen Gakkai Zasshi*, 54(2):137-153, 1994.

69. Ros, P.R., Freeny, P.C., Harms, S.E., et al., Hepatic MR imaging with ferumoxides: a multicenter clinical trial of the safety and efficacy in the detection of focal hepatic lesions, *Radiology*, 196(2):481-488, 1995.

70. Ferrucci, J.T. and Stark, D.D., Iron oxide-enhanced MR imaging of the liver and spleen: review of the first 5 years, *Am. J. Roentgenol.*, 155(5):943-950, 1990.

71. Rofsky, N.M., Weinreb, J.C., Bosniak, M.A., et al., Renal lesion characterization with gadolinium-enhanced MR imaging: efficacy and safety in patients with renal insufficiency, *Radiology*, 180(1):85-89, 1991.

72. Rominger, M.B., Kenney, P.J., Morgan, D.E., et al., Gadolinium-enhanced MR imaging of renal masses, *Radiographics*, 12(6):1097-1116, 1992.

73. Terens, W.L., Gluck, R., Golimbu, M., and Rofsky, N.M., Use of gadolinium-DTPA-enhanced MRI to characterize renal mass in patient with renal insufficiency, *Urology*, 40(2):152-154, 1992.

74. Brown, E.D. and Semelka, R.C., Magnetic resonance imaging of the adrenal gland and kidney, *Top. Magn. Reson. Imaging*, 7(2):90–101, 1995.

75. Yamashita,Y., Miyazaki, T., Hatanaka, Y., and Takahashi, M., Dynamic MRI of small renal cell carcinoma, *J. Comput. Assist. Tomogr.*, 19(5):759-765, 1995.

76. Kaufman, J.A., Geller, S.C., and Waltman, A.C., Renal insufficiency: gadopentetate dimeglumine as a radiographic contrast agent during peripheral vascular interventional procedures, *Radiology*, 198(2):579-581, 1996.

77. Ghantous, V.E., Eisen, T.D., Sherman, A.H., and Finkelstein, F.O., Evaluating patients with renal failure for renal artery stenosis with gadolinium-enhanced magnetic resonance angiography, *Am. J. Kidney Dis.*, 33(1):36-42, 1999.

78. Cambria, R.P., Kaufman, J.L., Brewster, D.C., et al., Surgical renal artery reconstruction without contrast arteriography: the role of clinical profiling and magnetic resonance angiography, *J. Vasc. Surg.*, 29(6):1012-1021, 1999.

79. Schuhmann-Giampieri, G. and Krestin, G., Pharmacokinetics of Gd-DTPA in patients with chronic renal failure, *Invest. Radiol.*, 26(11):975-979, 1991.

80. Haustein, J., Niendorf, H.P., Krestin, G., et al., Renal tolerance of gadolinium-DTPA/dimeglumine in patients with chronic renal failure, *Invest. Radiol.*, 27(2):153-156, 1992.

81. Bellin, M.F., Deray, G., Assogba, U., et al., Gd-DOTA: evaluation of its renal tolerance in patients with chronic renal failure, *Magn. Reson. Imaging*, 10(1):115-118, 1992.

82. Dorsam, J., Knopp, M.V., Schad, L., et al., Elimination of gadolinium-DTPA by peritoneal dialysis, *Nephrol. Dial. Transplant*, 10(7):1228-1230, 1995.

83. Choyke, P.L., Girton, M.E., Vaughan, E.M., et al., Clearance of gadolinium chelates by hemodialysis: an in vitro study, *J. Magn. Reson. Imaging*, 5(4):470–472, 1995.

84. Niendorf, E.R., Santyr, G.E., Brazy, P.C., and Grist, T.M., Measurement of Gd-DTPA dialysis clearance rates by using a look-locker imaging technique, *Magn. Reson. Med.*, 36(4):571-578, 1996.

85. Arsenault, T.M., King, B.F., Marsh, J.W., Jr., et al., Systemic gadolinium toxicity in patients with renal insufficiency and renal failure: retrospective analysis of an initial experience, *Mayo Clin. Proc.*, 71(12):1150–1154, 1996.

86. Yoshikawa, K. and Davies, A., Safety of ProHance in special populations, *Eur. Radiol.*, 7(Suppl. 5):246-250, 1997.

87. Joffe, P., Thomsen, H.S., and Meusel, M., Pharmacokinetics of gadodiamide injection in patients with severe renal insufficiency and patients undergoing hemodialysis or continuous ambulatory peritoneal dialysis, *Acad. Radiol.*, 5(7):491-502, 1998.

88. Hammer, F.D., Goffette, P.P., Malaise, J., and Mathurin, P., Gadolinium dimeglumine: an alternative contrast agent for digital subtraction angiography, *Eur. Radiol.*, 9(1):128-136, 1999.

89. Gerscovich, E.O., McGahan, J.P., Buonocore, M.H., et al., The rediscovery of infant feeding formula with magnetic resonance imaging, *Pediatr. Radiol.*, 20:147-151, 1990.

90. King, C.P.L., Tart, R.P., Fitzsimmons, J.R., et al. Barium sulfate suspension as a negative oral MRI contrast agent: in vitro and human optimization studies, *Magn, Reson. Imaging*, 9:141-150, 1991.

91. Marti-Bonmati, L., Vilar, J., Paniagua, J.C., and Talens, A., High density barium sulphate as an MRI oral contrast, *Magn, Reson. Imaging*, 19:259-261, 1991.

92. Haldemann Heusler, R.C., Wight, E., and Marincek, B., Oral superparamagnetic contrast agent (ferumoxsil): tolerance and efficacy in MR imaging of gynecologic diseases, *J. Magn. Reson. Imaging*, 5(4):385-391, 1995.

93. Scheidler, J., Heuck, A.F., Meier, W., and Reiser, M.F., MRI of pelvic masses: efficacy of the rectal superparamagnetic contrast agent Ferumoxsil, *J. Magn. Reson. Imaging*, 7(6):1027-1032, 1997.

94. Hirohashi, S., Uchida, H., Yoshikawa, K., et al., Large scale clinical evaluation of bowel contrast agent containing ferric ammonium citrate in MRI, *Magn, Reson. Imaging*, 12(6):837-846, 1994.

95. Patten, R.M., Lo, S.K., Phillips, J.J., et al., Positive bowel contrast agent for MR imaging of the abdomen: phase II and III clinical trials, *Radiology*, 189(1):277-283, 1993.

96. Bernardino, M.E., Weinreb, J.C., Mitchell, D.G., et al., Safety and optimum concentration of a manganese chloride-based oral MR contrast agent, *J. Magn. Reson. Imaging*, 4(6):872-876, 1994.

97. Laniado, M., Kornmesser, W., Hamm, B., et al., MR imaging of the gastrointestinal tract: value of Gd-DTPA, *Am. J. Roentgenol.*, 150:817-821, 1988.

98. Kaminsky, S., Laniado, M., Gogoll, M., et al., Gadopentetate dimeglumine as a bowel contrast agent: safety and efficacy, *Radiology*, 178:503-508, 1991.

99. Claussen, C., Kornmesser, W., Laniado, M., et al., Oral contrast media for magnetic resonance tomography of the abdomen: III. Initial patient research with gadolinium DTPA, *Rofo Fortschr. Geb. Rontgenstr. Neuen Bildgeb Verfahr.*, 148:683-689, 1988.

100. Krahe, T., Dolken, W., Lackner, K., et al., Gadolinium DTPA as an oral contrast medium for MR tomography of the abdomen, *Rofo Fortschr. Geb. Rontgenstr. Neuen Bildgeb Verfahr.*, 153:167-173, 1990.

13 Pre-Magnetic Resonance Procedure Screening

Anne M. Sawyer-Glover and Frank G. Shellock

CONTENTS

I. INTRODUCTION

Maintaining a safe magnetic resonance (MR) environment is a daily challenge for technologists, radiologists, physicians, scientists, nurses, and allied health professionals worldwide. The types of biomedical implants and devices that are encountered in individuals and patients continue to grow, and other unexpected issues such as body piercing and cosmetic trends (tattooed eyebrows, eyeliner, lip-liner, etc.) constantly change. Up-to-date documentation must be obtained for these implants, devices, and conditions to provide the safest possible MR environment.[1-3] The establishment of comprehensive, efficient, and effective pre-MR imaging (MRI) procedure screening policies and procedures is critical for protecting all individuals who need to enter the MR environment.[1-7]

Most reported cases of MR-related injuries have been the direct result of misinformation or deficiencies in screening methods.[1-7] Unfortunately, not all MR healthcare workers conduct rigorous screening procedures. Furthermore, there tends to be a lack of agreement on what constitutes an appropriate or necessary protocol that will ensure the safety of individuals and patients in the clinical MR environment.[1-3,5,7]

In 1994, the Safety Committee of the Society for Magnetic Resonance Imaging (SMRI) published screening recommendations and a screening questionnaire.[4] An international panel of MR experts developed guidelines intended for use as the "standard of care" by all MR facilities.[4] Elster et al.[5] also published screening recommendations in 1994 that were remarkably similar to the content of those provided by the SMRI safety committee (this is not surprising, since many of the same MR clinicians and scientists were involved in the development of both documents). Since then, recommendations and guidelines for pre-MRI procedure screening continue to evolve and have been recently revised in consideration of the present state-of-the-art information on this topic.[1,3]

This chapter presents information on the various critical components of the pre-MRI procedure screening process that should be followed carefully before allowing individuals and patients to enter the MR environment. A comprehensive pre-MRI procedure screening form recommended for use by all MR facilities is also included.

II. PRE-MR SCREENING PROCEDURES

As a standard policy that should be strictly enforced, all individuals and patients that intend to enter the MR environment must be screened thoroughly by a qualified, trained MR healthcare worker using procedures that involve a written form and a verbal interview.[1-3] Any individual accompanying the patient into the MR system room, such as a parent, spouse, or friend, must also undergo the screening procedure prior to being exposed to the MR environment.

A. WRITTEN SCREENING FORM

1. Safety Questions and Information

A comprehensive, two-page, pre-MRI procedure screening form has been specially developed for use by clinical MR facilities in consideration of all the important safety factors[1] (Figure 13.1). Requiring the completion of this written form ensures that health conditions or items that pose potential safety problems will not be missed during the screening procedure.[1] Additionally, the answers to the questions and information provided on this form serve as a means of documenting medical records for the patient preparing to undergo the examination. This tends to be helpful information for the interpreting radiologist and/or MR healthcare worker. For example, the name of the referring physician is requested so that additional information about the patient's condition can be reviewed and verified.

The pre-MRI procedure screening form includes inquiries about previous surgeries and/or medical imaging procedures, including dates and locations. This provides potentially important information for medical implants or devices that may have been implanted during surgery or with respect to special precautions that were taken for previous diagnostic imaging procedures. Notably, previous MR procedures completed without safety incidents do not guarantee the safety of subsequent examinations, especially if a different MR system is used. For example, the field strength of the MR system, the orientation of the patient to the magnetic field, as well as other factors can significantly change the scenario.

A pre-MRI procedure screening form must be completed every time a patient or individual prepares to enter the MR environment. This is not an inconsequential matter, as a surgical intervention or an accident involving a metallic foreign body may have occurred in the interim, the impact of which may not be obvious to the patient.

The pre-MRI procedure screening form includes questions regarding occupations or hobbies involving metal grinding, any previous injury to the eye with a metal object (e.g., metallic slivers or shavings), or any previous injury with a metallic foreign body (e.g., bullet, BB, buckshot, or shrapnel).[1-3,7-14] Even the smallest piece of metal embedded in the eye could move when placed in the MR environment, resulting in serious injury to the patient.[9] Other metallic objects embedded in the body may cause painful sensations in the MR environment.[2,3,8] Therefore, it is essential that the type and composition of foreign bodies be identified, as well as the anatomical location relative to sensitive neural, vascular, or soft tissue structures (see Sections II.3 and II.4).

The pre-MRI procedure screening form has questions regarding potential pregnancy or a late menstrual period. Any possible pregnancy must be identified prior to exposure to the MR environment so that the risks and benefits of the MR procedure may be carefully considered by the referring physician, patient, and radiologist (see Chapter 8, "Magnetic Resonance Procedures and Pregnancy").

IMAGING FACILITY
PRE-MRI SCREENING FORM

Date _____ / _____ / _____   MRI Number _____

Name _____ Height_____ Weight_____
   Last name   First name   M.I.
Birth Date_____   Social Security No._____ / _____ / _____
Address_____ City_____
State_____ Zip Code_____ Phone (H)(_____)_____ (W)(_____)_____
Physician's name & address   _____
                                    _____

1. Have you ever had surgery or any similar invasive procedure?   ❑ No   ❑ Yes
   If yes, please list:
   Type:_____   Date:_____ / _____ / _____
   Type:_____   Date:_____ / _____ / _____

2. Have you had any previous studies?   ❑ No   ❑ Yes
   If yes, please list:.

	Body part	Date	Facility Location
MRI	_____	____ / ____	_____
CT/CAT Scan	_____	____ / ____	_____
X-Ray	_____	____ / ____	_____
Ultrasound	_____	____ / ____	_____
Nuclear Medicine	_____	____ / ____	_____

3. Have you ever worked with metal (grinding, fabricating, etc.) or ever had an injury to the eye involving a
   metallic object (e.g., metallic slivers, shavings, foreign body)?   ❑ No   ❑ Yes
   If yes, please describe:_____

4. Are you pregnant or experiencing a late menstrual period?   ❑ No   ❑ Yes

5. Are you breast feeding?   ❑ No   ❑ Yes   6. Date of last menstrual period:_____ / _____ / _____

7. Are you taking any type of fertility medication or having fertility treatments?   ❑ No   ❑ Yes

8. Are you taking oral contraceptives or receiving hormone treatment?   ❑ No   ❑ Yes

9. Are you currently taking or have you recently taken any medication?   ❑ No   ❑ Yes
   If yes, please list:_____

10. Do you have anemia or any diseases that affect your blood, a history of renal disease or seizures?
                                                                            ❑ No   ❑ Yes
    If yes, please describe:_____

11. Do you have drug allergies?   ❑ No   ❑ Yes
    If yes, please list:_____

12. Have you ever had asthma, allergic reaction, respiratory disease, or other reaction to a contrast medium
    or dye used for an MRI or CT examination?   ❑ No   ❑ Yes
    If yes, please describe:_____

FIGURE 13.1 The pre-MRI screening form used to screen individuals and patients prior to permitting them
into the MR environment. Note that permission is granted by the authors for MRI facilities to copy and use
this form.   (*continued*)

According to the recommendations provided by the SMRI safety committee (later adopted by
the American College of Radiology), MRI procedures may be used in pregnant patients if other
nonionizing forms of diagnostic imaging are inadequate or if the examination provides important
information that would otherwise require exposure to a diagnostic procedure that requires ionizing

Some of the following items may be hazardous to your safety and some can interfere with the MRI examination. Please check the correct answer for each of the following. Do you have any of the following:

❏ Yes ❏ No	Cardiac pacemaker	Please mark on the figure below, the location of any implant or metal inside of or on your body.
❏ Yes ❏ No	Implanted cardiac defibrillator	
❏ Yes ❏ No	Aneurysm clip(s)	
❏ Yes ❏ No	Carotid artery vascular clamp	
❏ Yes ❏ No	Neurostimulator	
❏ Yes ❏ No	Insulin or infusion pump	
❏ Yes ❏ No	Implanted drug infusion device	
❏ Yes ❏ No	Bone growth/fusion stimulator	
❏ Yes ❏ No	Cochlear, otologic, or ear implant	
❏ Yes ❏ No	Any type of prosthesis (eye, penile, etc.)	
❏ Yes ❏ No	Heart valve prosthesis	
❏ Yes ❏ No	Artificial limb or joint	
❏ Yes ❏ No	Electrodes (on body, head, or brain)	
❏ Yes ❏ No	Intravascular stents, filters, or coils	
❏ Yes ❏ No	Shunt (spinal or intraventricular)	
❏ Yes ❏ No	Vascular access port and/or catheter	
❏ Yes ❏ No	Swan-Ganz catheter	
❏ Yes ❏ No	Any implant held in place by a magnet	Right Left
❏ Yes ❏ No	Transdermal delivery system (Nitro)	
❏ Yes ❏ No	IUD or diaphragm	
❏ Yes ❏ No	Tattooed makeup (eyeliner, lips, etc.)	
❏ Yes ❏ No	Body piercing(s)	
❏ Yes ❏ No	Any metal fragments	
❏ Yes ❏ No	Internal pacing wires	
❏ Yes ❏ No	Aortic clip	
❏ Yes ❏ No	Metal or wire mesh implants	
❏ Yes ❏ No	Wire sutures or surgical staples	
❏ Yes ❏ No	Harrington rods (spine)	
❏ Yes ❏ No	Metal rods in bones	
❏ Yes ❏ No	Joint replacement _____	
❏ Yes ❏ No	Bone/joint pin, screw, nail, wire, plate	*Before your MRI, please remove all metallic objects including keys, hair pins, barrettes, jewelry, watch, safety pins, paperclips, money clip, credit cards, coins, pens, belt, metal buttons, pocket knife, & clothing with metal in the material.*
❏ Yes ❏ No	Hearing aid (*Remove before MRI*)	
❏ Yes ❏ No	Dentures (*Remove before MRI*)	
❏ Yes ❏ No	Breathing disorder	
❏ Yes ❏ No	Motion disorder	
❏ Yes ❏ No	Claustrophobia	
❏ Yes ❏ No	Anxiety	

Other, please explain:_____

NOTE: YOU ARE REQUIRED TO WEAR EARPLUGS OR EARPHONES DURING THE MRI EXAMINATION.

_____   Date____/____/____
                Signature of Person Completing Form

Form completed by: ❏ Patient   ❏ Relative:_____
                                                    Name & relationship to patient
                      ❏ Physician or other:_____
                                                    Name & relationship to patient

To be completed by the MRI Facility Medical record number:_____ Completed by:_____
Procedure:_____ Diagnosis:_____
Clinical History:_____

FIGURE 13.1 (CONTINUED) The pre-MRI screening form used to screen individuals and patients prior to permitting them into the MR environment. Note that permission is granted by the authors for MRI facilities to copy and use this form. Alternatively, a copy may be downloaded from www.MRIsafety.com.

radiation (e.g., computed tomography [CT], fluoroscopy, etc.).[4] Therefore, examination of a pregnant patient using MRI is only recommended to address an important clinical question for the patient or fetus and should only be done with written informed consent. The form used for written informed consent for the use of MRI in a pregnant patient should be developed by the MRI facility in conjunction with the risk management group.

Patients undergoing fertility treatments or receiving certain medications should also be closely evaluated for pregnancy and should probably undergo a pregnancy test as part of the MR facility's policy. Certain hormonal and similar medications can alter MR findings. Therefore, for patients undergoing gynecologic or obstetric MR procedures, this information is especially useful to the interpreting radiologist. The MR facility should have a clearly defined procedure to follow in the event of a possible or confirmed pregnancy identified for the patient, MR healthcare worker, or accompanying individual.[1-3]

An inquiry about breast feeding is included on the pre-MRI procedure screening form to address the situation whereby it may be necessary to administer MR contrast media in nursing mothers (see Chapter 12, "Safety of Magnetic Resonance Contrast Agents"). Requesting the date of the last menstrual period and taking of oral contraceptives or hormonal therapy are necessary for MR procedures evaluating breast disease, as these may affect the pattern of enhancement with the administration of contrast media. These inquiries may also assist in the determination of a potential pregnancy.

Questions about current medications and drug allergies are also included on the pre-MRI procedure screening form so that the radiologist and MR healthcare worker are aware of the present medical status of the patient. Additionally, this information may be helpful in case of the need to administer drugs to the patient (e.g., in the event of a life-threatening incident such as a reaction to an MR contrast agent, heart attack, or other similar medical problem). This information is also useful to have on record if the patient experiences any "after effects" that may be misinterpreted as a side effect of the MR examination, but may actually be due to an unrelated incident (such as the recent initiation of drug therapy or a new prescription).

Because of potential issues pertaining to the use of MR contrast agents in patients as well as other possible related problems, a question is posed on the pre-MRI procedure screening form pertaining to the presence of pre-existing anemia, any diseases that affect the blood, a history of renal disease, or a history of seizures. Finally, the first page of the pre-MRI procedure screening form has a question pertaining to health conditions that may impact the MRI examination, such as asthma, previous allergic reaction, the presence of respiratory disease, or a previous reaction to a CT or MR contrast agent.

The second page of the pre-MRI procedure screening form lists biomedical implants, devices, objects, and materials that may be present in patients or individuals and, thus, are important to identify prior to allowing them into the MR environment (see also Chapters 14 and 15). In general, these items are arranged on a checklist in order of the relative safety hazards (e.g., cardiac pacemaker, implantable cardioverter defibrillator, aneurysm clip, etc.), followed by items that may simply produce imaging artifacts that could be problematic for interpretion of the MRI procedure (e.g., IVC, diaphragm, wire suture, etc.).

A diagram of the human body is also included on the second page of the form as a means of showing the location for objects that might be present. This is particularly useful so that the individual or patient may specifically indicate the position of any object that may be hazardous or that would interfere with or confuse the interpretation of the MRI procedure by producing an artifact.[1-3]

Finally, there is a statement at the bottom of the checklist that informs the individual or patient that hearing protection is required during the MRI examination. The use of hearing protection is advisable for all individuals, including those accompanying the patient as well as MR healthcare workers, who must remain in the room during the operation of the MR system (see also Chapter 6, "Acoustic Noise and Magnetic Resonance Procedures").

With the use of any type of written questionnaire, limitations exist related to incomplete or incorrect answers provided by the patient or individual preparing to enter the MR environment.[3] For example, there may be difficulties associated with individuals that are impaired with respect to their vision, fluency, or level of literacy. Therefore, an appropriate accompanying individual should be involved in the screening procedure to clarify or verify any information that may impact the safety of the patient. Versions of the pre-MRI procedure screening form should also be available in other languages for individuals and patients as needed (i.e., specific to the demographics of the MR facility).

In the event that the patient is comatose or unable to communicate, the pre-MRI procedure screening form should be completed by the most qualified individual available (referring physician, spouse, relative, etc.) that has knowledge about the patient. Upon completion of the form, the information should be thoroughly reviewed with the patient by a qualified, trained MR healthcare worker to answer questions or clarify any potential confusion with medical terminology. The person performing this review should be educated to understand all potential hazards and issues pertaining to the MR environment and familiar with all information contained on the pre-MRI procedure screening form.

2. Metallic Implants, Devices, and Materials

A variety of metallic implants, devices, and materials may be encountered in individuals or patients during screening procedures.[1-3] *Ex vivo* testing is required to determine the relative safety of allowing any individual with a metallic object to enter the MR environment.[2,3] Fortunately, a publication that is updated yearly provides information about the metallic objects that have been tested for MR safety.[3] Additionally, the Web site **www.MRIsafety.com** provides this information to MR healthcare workers. For a comprehensive presentation and discussion of metallic implants, devices, and materials, and the implications for individuals and patients in the MR environment, please refer to Chapters 14 and 15.

3. Metallic Foreign Bodies

All patients or other individuals with a history of being injured by a metallic foreign body should be thoroughly evaluated using proper clinical examination and plain film radiograph techniques prior to admission to the MR environment.[1-3] This is particularly important because painful experiences and serious injuries have been reported from movement or dislodgment of metallic foreign bodies as a result of magnetic field interactions with MR systems.[5-9,11]

The relative risk is dependent on the ferromagnetic properties of the foreign body, the geometry and dimensions of the object, the strength of the static magnetic field, and the strength of the spatial gradients of the MR system. Additionally, the potential for injury is dependent on the amount of counterforce acting on the object within the tissue (i.e., retention force) and whether or not it is positioned in or adjacent to a particularly sensitive site of the body.[1-3] Notably, plain film radiography is the technique of choice recommended to detect metallic foreign bodies for individuals and patients prior to admission to the MR environment.[1-3,5,10,12-15] This includes screening individuals and patients for the presence of metallic orbital foreign bodies (see below). The sensitivity of plain film radiography is considered sufficient to identify any metal with a mass large enough to present a hazard to an individual or patient in the MR environment.

4. Orbital Foreign Bodies

In the past, any individual with a suspected metallic foreign body in the ocular region was required to have film radiographs of the orbits to determine the presence of a metallic fragment prior to exposure to the MR environment.[2,3,5,10,13] Thus, screening plain films of the orbit were deemed necessary for every individual with a history of a known intraocular or periorbital foreign body or a history of exposure to potential metallic ocular injury (e.g., welders, grinders, metal workers, sculptors, etc.).[2,3,10] This was considered the standard of care to prevent serious injuries to the eye associated with the MR environment. However, based on a recent investigation by Seidenwurm et al.,[15] new guidelines for radiographic screening of patients with suspected metallic foreign bodies have been proposed and implemented in the clinical MR setting.

a. New Guidelines for Screening

The single case report[9] in 1986 of a patient that sustained an ocular injury from a retained metallic foreign body has led to great controversy regarding the procedure required to screen patients prior to MRI procedures. Notably, this incident is the only serious eye-related injury that has occurred in the MR environment (i.e., based on a review of the peer-reviewed literature).[15] In consideration of this, the standard policy of performing radiographic screening for orbital foreign bodies in patients simply because of a history of occupational or other similar exposure to metal fragments needs to be reconsidered.[15]

A study by Seidenwurm et al.[15] evaluated the cost-effectiveness of using clinical vs. radiographic techniques to screen patients for orbital foreign bodies before MRI procedures. The costs of screening were determined on the basis of published reports, disability rating guides, and a practice survey.[13] A sensitivity analysis was performed for each variable. For this analysis, the benefits of screening were avoidance of immediate, permanent, nonameliorable, or unilateral blindness.

The findings of Seidenwurm et al.[15] support the fact that the use of clinical screening before radiography increases the cost-effectiveness of foreign body screening by an order of magnitude (i.e., assuming base case ocular foreign body removal rates). From a clinical screening standpoint for a metallic foreign body located in the orbit, asking the patient, "Did a doctor get it all out?" serves this purpose.

Seidenwurm et al.[15] have implemented the following policy with regard to screening patients with suspected metallic foreign bodies: "If a patient reports injury from an ocular foreign body that was subsequently removed by a doctor or that resulted in negative findings on any examination, we perform MR imaging ... Those persons with a history of injury and no subsequent negative eye examination are screened radiographically." Of note is that Seidenwurm et al.[15] have performed approximately 100,000 MRI procedures under this protocol without incident.

Thus, an occupational history of exposure to metallic fragments by itself is not sufficient to mandate radiographic orbital screening.[15,16] Therefore, current practice guidelines for foreign body screening should be altered in consideration of this new information and because radiographic screening before MRI procedures on the basis of occupational exposure alone is not cost-effective.[15] Furthermore, it is not clinically necessary.[15]

Clinical Screening Protocol — Basically, the procedure to follow with regard to patients with suspected foreign bodies involves an initial clinical screening protocol, as recommended by Seidenwurm et al.[15] This involves asking patients whether they have a high-risk occupation and whether they have had an ocular injury. If they sustained an ocular injury from a metallic object, they are asked whether they had a medical examination at the time of the injury and whether they were told by the doctor, "It's all out." If they did not have an injury, if they were told their ophthalmologic examination was normal, and/or if the foreign body was removed at the time of the injury, then they proceed to MRI as scheduled.[15]

Radiographic Screening Protocol — Based on the results of the clinical screening protocol, patients are screened radiographically if they sustained an ocular injury related to a metallic foreign object and were not told their post-injury eye examination was normal. In these cases, the MR examination is postponed, and the patient is scheduled for screening radiography.[15]

b. Screening Adolescents

A published case report illustrates that special precautions are needed for screening adolescent patients prior to MRI procedures.[11] This case report described an incident in which a 12-year-old patient accompanied by his parent completed all routine screening procedures prior to preparation for MRI of the lumbar spine. The patient and parent provided negative answers to all questions regarding prior injuries by metallic objects and the presence of metallic foreign bodies.[11]

Upon entering the MR system room, the adolescent patient appeared to be anxious about the examination. He was placed in a feet-first, supine position on the MR system table and prepared for the imaging examination. During this time, the patient became more anxious and restless, shifting his position several times on the table. As the patient was moved slowly toward the opening of the bore of a 1.5-T MR system, he complained of a pressure sensation in his left eye. The MR technologist immediately removed the patient from the MR system and out of the MR environment.[11]

Once again, the patient was questioned regarding any previous eye injuries, and again he denied any history of injury or problems. Despite the patient's response, a metallic foreign body in the orbit was suspected. Therefore, plain film radiographs of the orbits were obtained with the patient performing upward and downward fixed gazes.[11] The plain films revealed a metallic foreign body in the left orbit, curvilinear in shape and approximately 5 mm in size. Fortunately, the patient did not appear to have sustained an injury to the eye during this incident. The patient and parent were counseled regarding the implications of future MRI procedures with respect to the possibility of significant eye injury related to movement or dislodgment of the metallic foreign body.[11]

This case demonstrates that routine guidelines and safety protocols may not always be sufficient for evaluation of potential hazardous situations that may be present, particularly in adolescents referred for MR procedures. There are possible additional risks involved whenever parents or guardians fill out pre-MRI procedure screening forms because children may not be willing to disclose previous injuries or accidents.[11]

In consideration of this incident and to avoid unfortunate accidents related to the electromagnetic fields used for MRI procedures, it is recommended that adolescents be provided additional screening that includes private counseling about the hazards associated with the MR environment. Furthermore, the MR technical staff should be educated about these similarly related issues.

B. Verbal Screening Procedures

Following the completion of the written pre-MRI procedure screening form, a verbal screening procedure should be conducted to obtain additional details before the individual or patient is permitted into the MR environment.[1-3] A thorough, verbal screening procedure optimally includes several discussions with the individual or patient. For example, an interview should be accomplished during the initial communication with the patient. At the very least, questions posed to the patient should include those pertaining to major safety issues such as the presence of aneurysm clips, pacemakers, etc. This verbal screening procedure would occur typically during the scheduling of the MR examination with the patient, the patient's physician, or the referring physician's office to prevent inappropriate scheduling of MR examinations. To further facilitate verbal screening, we recommend reviewing the pre-MRI procedure screening form over the telephone with the patient or having an electronic version of the document available for the patient via electronic mail.[3]

Past experience has demonstrated that a verbal interview conducted before allowing the individual or patient to enter the MR system room is absolutely crucial to ensure safety.[1] For example, it is at this point that individuals and patients remember past accidents involving metal objects, prior surgeries, or metallic objects in their undergarments. Additionally, during this time, a patient that is required to be transferred from a gurney or wheelchair to the MR table (i.e., outside of the MR system room) should be thoroughly checked for metal objects under the sheets or blankets (e.g., a ferromagnetic oxygen tank).

Finally, for patients that are "poor historians," it may be necessary to physically inspect the upper chest, abdomen, or other areas of the body for scars indicating previous surgical procedures. This procedure is particularly helpful for identifying cardiac pacemakers, implantable cardioverter defibrillators, and other potentially hazardous implants and devices.

III. PROTECTION FROM "MISSILE EFFECT" INCIDENTS AND INJURIES

The missile effect refers to the capability of the fringe field associated with the MR system to attract ferromagnetic objects (e.g., oxygen tanks, paper clips, tools, etc.) to the MR system by considerable force. Obviously, the missile effect may pose substantial hazards to individuals and patients in the MR environment.[1-3] Notably, in extreme cases, the magnet may need to be "quenched" in order to remove large ferromagnetic items from the MR system.[2] This problem results in substantial financial loss associated with MR system downtime and the replacement of cryogens. Additionally, small metallic objects may become lodged in difficult to reach positions of the magnet, causing distortion and artifacts on MR images. Therefore, a policy should be established by the MR facility to detect metallic objects prior to allowing individuals or patients to enter the MR environment in order to avoid problems or injuries related to the missile effect.[1-3]

For example, to prevent missile-effect-related incidents, the immediate area around the MR system should be clearly demarcated, labeled with appropriate warning signs, and secured by trained staff aware of MR safety procedures. Additionally, all individuals and patients that need to enter the MR environment should be carefully screened for metallic objects that may be involved in the missile effect. There should be a policy that all individuals and patients remove metallic personal items (i.e., analog watches, hair clips, jewelry, pocket knives, nail clippers, etc.) and clothing items that have metallic fasteners or other metallic components. Obviously, the most effective means of preventing a ferromagnetic object from inadvertently becoming a missile is to require the patient to wear a gown.

Furthermore, all hospital personnel that may need to periodically enter the MR environment (e.g., maintenance workers, housekeeping staff, bioengineers, nurses, etc.) should be educated about the potential problems and hazards associated with the magnetic fringe field of the MR system. Many serious incidents have occurred when individuals who were unaware of the powers of the fringe field entered the MR environment with items such as oxygen tanks, wheelchairs, monitors, and other similar ferromagnetic objects.[1-3,6]

IV. SUMMARY AND CONCLUSIONS

Performance of a comprehensive, efficient, and effective pre-MR screening procedure is crucial to protect individuals and patients from possible incidents or accidents associated with the MR environment. The initial screening process should involve completion of a questionnaire designed to determine any reason the individual or patient may have an adverse reaction to the MR environment. The pre-MRI procedure screening form should also provide a means of determining additional pertinent information related to the safe performance of the MR procedure. For example, questions may be asked concerning previous adverse reactions to contrast media, which should alert the healthcare provider to potential problems. In addition to reviewing the information provided on the pre-MRI procedure screening form, it is recommended that oral interviews be conducted to further ensure the safety of the individual or patient entering the MR environment. This allows a mechanism for clarification or confirmation of the answers to the questions posed to the individual so that there is no miscommunication regarding important MR safety issues.

REFERENCES

1. Sawyer, A. M. and Shellock, F. G., Pre-MRI procedure screening: recommendations and safety considerations for biomedical implants and devices, *J. Magn. Reson. Imaging,* 12, 92, 2000.
2. Shellock, F. G. and Kanal, E., *Magnetic Resonance: Bioeffects, Safety, and Patient Management,* Lippincott-Raven Press, New York, 1996.
3. Shellock, F. G., *Pocket Guide to MR Procedures and Metallic Objects: Update 2000,* Lippincott, William & Wilkins, Philadelphia, 2000.
4. Shellock, F. G. and Kanal, E., SMRI Report. Policies, guidelines and recommendations for MR imaging safety and patient management. Questionnaire for screening patients before MR procedures, *J. Magn. Reson. Imaging,* 4, 749, 1994.

5. Elster, A. D., Link, K. M., and Carr, J. J., Patient screening prior to MR imaging: a practical approach synthesized from protocols at 15 U.S. medical centers, *Am. J. Roentgenol.,* 162, 195, 1994.

6. Gangarosa, R. E., Minnis, J. E., Nobbe, J., Praschan, D., and Genberg, R. W., Operational safety issues in MRI, *Magn. Reson. Imaging,* 5, 287, 1987.

7. Boutin, R. D., Briggs, J. E., and Williamson, M. R., Injuries associated with MR imaging: survey of safety records and methods used to screen patients for metallic foreign bodies before imaging, *Am. J. Roentgenol.,* 162, 189, 1994.

8. Dupuy, D. E., Hartnell, G. C., and Lipsky, M., MR imaging of a patient with a ferromagnetic foreign body, *Am. J. Roentgenol.,* 160, 893, 1993.

9. Kelly, W. M., Pagle, P. G., Pearson, A., San Diego, A. G., and Soloman, M. A., Ferromagnetism of intraocular foreign body causes unilateral blindness after MR study, *Am. J. Neuroradiol.,* 7, 243, 1986.

10. Murphy, K. J. and Brunberg, J. A., Orbital plain film as a prerequisite for MR imaging: is a known history of injury sufficient screening criteria?, *Am. J. Roentgenol.,* 167, 1053, 1996.

11. Elmquist, C., Shellock, F. G., and Stoller, D., Screening adolescents for metallic foreign bodies before MR procedures, *J. Magn. Reson. Imaging,* 5, 784, 1996.

12. Mani, R. L., In search of an effective screening system for intraocular metallic foreign bodies prior to MR — an important issue of patient safety, *Am. J. Neuroradiol.,* 9, 1032, 1988.

13. Williams, S., Char, D. H., Dillon, W. P., Lincoff, N., and Moseley, M., Ferrous intraocular foreign bodies and magnetic resonance imaging, *Am. J. Opthalmol.,* 105, 398, 1988.

14. Shellock, F. G. and Kanal, E., Re: Metallic foreign bodies in the orbits of patients undergoing MR imaging: prevalence and value of pre-MR radiography and CT, *Am. J. Roentgenol.,* 162, 985, 1994.

15. Seidenwurm, D. J., McDonnell, C. H., Raghavan, N., and Breslau, J., Cost utility analysis of radiographic screening for an orbital foreign body before MR imaging, *Am. J. Neuroradiol.,* 21, 426, 2000.

16. Jarvik, J. G., and Ramsey, J.G., Radiographic screening for orbital foreign bodies prior to MR imaging: is it worth it?, *Am. J. Neuroradiol.,* 21, 245, 2000.

14 The Magnetic Resonance Environment and Implants, Devices, and Materials

Frank G. Shellock and Anne M. Sawyer-Glover

CONTENTS

I. INTRODUCTION

The electromagnetic fields associated with the magnetic resonance imaging (MRI) environment may pose serious risks to individuals or patients with certain types of implants, devices, or materials.[1,2] In general, most injuries occur as the result of magnetic field-induced movement or dislodgment of ferromagnetic objects.[1,2] However, other possible hazards can occur from the induction of electrical currents, excessive heating, and/or the misinterpretation of an imaging artifact as an abnormality.[1,2]

For biomedical implants, devices, and material, *ex vivo* testing is typically required to assess magnetic field interactions and heating in order to determine the relative safety of the objects in the magnetic resonance (MR) environment. For certain devices and objects (e.g., cervical fixation devices, catheters with conductive wires, etc.), it is also desirable to determine induced electrical currents. Importantly, this information serves as the basis for determining what objects may be present in a patient or individual prior to admittance into the MR environment.[1,2]

This chapter presents information for the many implants, devices, and materials that have been evaluated for safety in the MR environment. Notably, this represents a compilation of the current data available from assessments of magnetic field interactions (i.e., the mechanism most responsible for injuries to patients and individuals) for these objects and is based primarily on published reports in the peer-reviewed literature. This information also includes unpublished data acquired from the *ex vivo* testing of objects conducted using the most commonly performed and accepted techniques for evaluation of MRI safety.

In addition, other possible hazards associated with the presence of implants, devices, and materials in the MR environment are described. Recommendations and guidelines for the prevention of injuries are also provided.[1,2]

II. SOURCES OF HAZARDS ASSOCIATED WITH MR PROCEDURES

A. INDUCED ELECTRICAL CURRENTS

The potential for MR procedures to injure patients by inducing electrical currents in conductive devices or materials is well documented.[1,2] Various reports have indicated that substantial electrical currents may be generated during MR procedures in electrocardiographic leads, indwelling catheters with metallic components (e.g., thermodilution catheters), guide wires, disconnected or broken surface coils, certain cervical fixation devices, or improperly used physiologic monitors. Recommendations concerning techniques to protect patients from injuries related to induced currents that may develop during an MR procedure will be discussed later in this chapter.

B. Heating

Temperature elevations produced during MR procedures have been studied using *ex vivo* testing techniques to evaluate various implants, devices, and materials of a variety of sizes, shapes, and metallic compositions. In general, reports have indicated that only minor temperature changes occur in association with conventional MR procedures (i.e., those that use standard pulse sequences and techniques) involving metallic objects. Therefore, heat generated during an MR procedure involving a patient with a passive metallic implant (i.e., it does not require operation by means of an electrical or similar mechanism), particularly if it is small, does not appear to be a substantial hazard.

Notably, there has never been a report of a patient being seriously injured as a result of excessive heat developing in a metallic implant or device.[1] Of course, the only exceptions to this are the burns that have occurred in association with conductive devices that were not used according to manufacturer's recommendations (see additional information in Section XXXVI). Nevertheless, MR healthcare workers should remain vigilant in their patient screening procedures, especially for those patients that have relatively large metallic implants or devices made from conductive materials.[1,2]

C. Artifacts

Artifacts caused by the presence of implants, devices, and materials have been described and are well recognized on MR images. Signal loss and distortion of the image by the presence of a metallic object is predominantly caused by the disruption of the local magnetic field that perturbs the relationship between position and frequency, which are crucial for proper image reconstruction.[1,2] For this reason, objects that incorporate magnets produce especially large artifacts on MR images because of the accentuated effect on the local magnetic field.

The relative amount of artifact seen on an MR image is dependent on the magnetic susceptibility, quantity, shape, orientation, and position of the object in the body as well as the technique used for imaging (i.e., the specific pulse sequence parameters) and the image processing method (i.e., two-dimensional Fourier transform reconstruction, back projection, etc.). Of note is that the extent, configuration, and other characteristics of the artifact are frequently unpredictable.

Nonferromagnetic objects tend to produce artifacts that are less severe than ferromagnetic objects for a given set of MRI parameters. Artifacts caused by nonferromagnetic implants usually result from eddy currents generated in the objects by gradient magnetic fields that, in turn, disrupt the local magnetic field and distort the image.

D. Magnetic Field Interactions

Numerous studies have assessed the magnetic field interactions for implants, devices, and materials by measuring deflection forces, attraction, torque, or other interactions associated with the static magnetic fields of MR systems.[1,2] In general, these investigations have demonstrated that MR procedures may be performed safely in patients if the metallic object is nonferromagnetic. Additionally, MRI may be performed safely if the object is ferromagnetic and only minimally attracted by the magnetic field in relation to its *in vivo* application or intended use (i.e., the associated attractive force is insufficient to move or dislodge the object *in situ* or affect its intended function).[1,2]

Accordingly, MR procedures are deemed safe for patients with objects that have been shown to be nonferromagnetic or weakly ferromagnetic. [For the sake of this presentation, the term "weakly ferromagnetic" refers to metal that may demonstrate some extremely low ferromagnetic qualities using highly sensitive measurement techniques (e.g., vibrating sample magnetometer, superconducting quantum interference device or SQUID magnetometer, etc.) and, as such, may not be technically referred to as being "nonferromagnetic."] Understandably, all metals possess some degree of magnetism, such that no metal is considered to be entirely nonferromagnetic.[1-3]

Furthermore, patients with certain implants or devices that have relatively strong ferromagnetic qualities may safely undergo MR procedures because the objects are held in place by sufficient retentive forces that prevent them from being moved or dislodged by magnetic field interactions. For example, a certain highly ferromagnetic interference screw (Perfix Interference Screw, Instrument Makar, Okemos, MI) used for reconstruction of the anterior cruciate ligament is firmly screwed into the patient's bone when implanted. This prevents it from being moved by magnetic field interactions associated with a 1.5-T MR system *in situ*.[1] Additionally, this implant will not heat excessively; however, being ferromagnetic, a rather large signal void is seen on the MRI examination[1] (Figure 14.1).

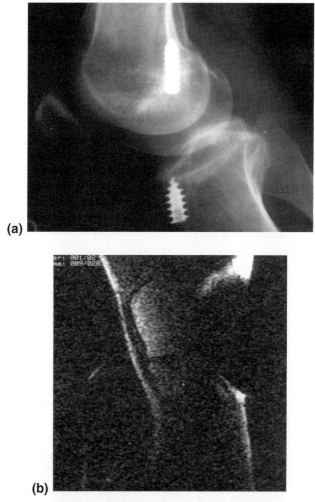

(a)

(b)

FIGURE 14.1 (a) Plain film radiograph of the knee obtained in a patient with two Perfix interference screws. These orthopedic implants are used for reconstruction of the anterior cruciate ligament. (b) T1-weighted, sagittal plane image of the knee obtained in a patient with two Perfix interference screws. Note the substantial artifact and image distortion caused by the presence of these ferromagnetic implants.

Various factors influence the risk of performing an MR procedure in a patient with a metallic object, including the strength of the static and gradient magnetic fields, the degree of ferromagnetism of the object, the mass of the object, the geometry of the object, the location and orientation of the object *in situ*, the presence of retentive mechanisms (i.e., fibrotic tissue, bone, sutures, etc.), and the length of time the object has been in place.[1,2] These factors should be considered carefully before subjecting a patient or individual with a ferromagnetic object to an MR procedure or allowing them entrance into the MR environment. This is particularly important if the object is located in a potentially dangerous area of the body, such as near a vital neural, vascular, or soft tissue structure where movement or dislodgment could injure the patient. Furthermore, in certain cases, there is the possibility of changing the operational or functional aspects of the implant, material, or device as a result of exposure to the electromagnetic fields used by the MR systems.[1,2]

MR systems with very low (0.2 T or less) or very high (2.0 to 8.0 T) static magnetic fields are currently being used for a variety of clinical MR applications.[4-9] Considering that most objects evaluated for magnetic field interactions were assessed using 1.5-T MR systems,[1,2] an appropriate adjustment of the MRI safety information that is provided for certain objects may exist for an MR system with a lower or higher static magnetic field strength used for an MR procedure. For example, it may be acceptable to modify the safety recommendations, perhaps making them more strict, depending on the strength of the MR system's static magnetic field. Obviously, performing an MR procedure using a 0.064-T MR system has different risk implications for a patient with a ferromagnetic object when compared with the use of an 8.0-T MR system. Additional discussion of this issue is provided later in this chapter.

III. ANEURYSM CLIPS

The surgical management of intracranial aneurysms and arteriovenous malformations (AVMs) by the application of aneurysm clips is a well established and, frequently, life-saving procedure[10] (Figure 14.2).

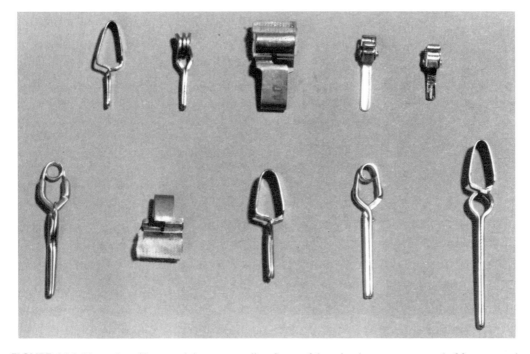

FIGURE 14.2 Examples of intracranial aneurysm clips. Some of these implants are composed of ferromagnetic materials and, thus, are contraindicated for patients undergoing MR procedures using conventional MR systems.

The presence of an intracranial aneurysm clip in an individual that needs to enter the MR environment or in a patient referred for an MR procedure represents a situation that requires the utmost consideration and attention because of the serious problems related to possible movement or dislodgment of the clip. Thus, many investigations have addressed MRI safety for intracranial aneurysm clips.[9,11-23]

A. INDIVIDUALS AND PATIENTS WITH ANEURYSM CLIPS

Certain types of intracranial aneurysm clips (e.g., those made from martensitic stainless steels such as 17-7PH or 405 stainless steel) are an absolute contraindication to the use of MR procedures because excessive magnetic field interactions can displace these clips and cause serious injuries or fatalities.[1,2] By comparison, aneurysm clips classified as nonferromagnetic or weakly ferromagnetic (e.g., those made from Phynox, Elgiloy, austenitic stainless steels, titanium alloy, or commercially pure titanium) are considered safe for patients undergoing MR procedures[3,4,11-22] (Figure 14.3).

It is not uncommon to use MR procedures to evaluate patients with certain types of aneurysm clips. Becker et al.[11] reported using MR systems that ranged from 0.35 to 0.6 T to study three patients with nonferromagnetic aneurysm clips and one patient with a ferromagnetic aneurysm clip without incidents or injuries. Dujovny et al.[12] similarly reported no adverse effects in patients with nonferromagnetic aneurysm clips who underwent procedures using 1.5-T MR systems.

Notably, only a single fatality has occurred due to the presence of a ferromagnetic aneurysm clip in a patient in the MR environment.[23-25] The patient involved in this incident complained of a headache at a distance of approximately 1.2 m from the magnet bore, indicating that the translational forces associated with the inhomogeneous component of the magnetic field were likely responsible for dislodgment of the aneurysm clip.[1,23]

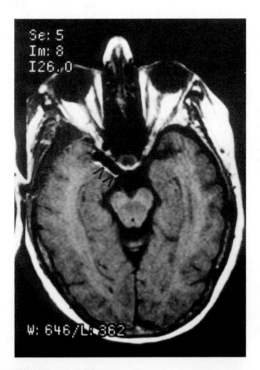
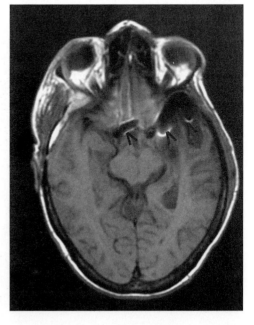

FIGURE 14.3 MRI of the brain in patients with aneurysm clips. These aneurysm clips are made from commercially pure titanium and are considered safe for patients undergoing MR procedures performed using MR systems operating at 8.0 T or less. Relatively small artifacts are seen associated with the aneurysm clips (arrowheads).

This unfortunate incident was the result of erroneous information pertaining to the specific type of aneurysm clip that was used in the patient. That is, the clip was thought to be a nonferromagnetic Yasargil aneurysm clip (Aesculap, Inc., South San Francisco, CA) and turned out to be a ferromagnetic Vari-Angle aneurysm clip (Codman & Shurtleff, Randolf, MA).

There has never been a report of an injury to a patient or individual in the MR environment related to the presence of an aneurysm clip made from a nonferromagnetic or weakly ferromagnetic material. In fact, there have been several cases in which patients with ferromagnetic aneurysm clips (i.e., based on the extent of the artifact seen during MRI or other information) have undergone MR procedures without any incidents or injuries reported (personal communications, D. Kroker, 1995, and E. Kanal, 1996).[1,2] In these cases, the aneurysm clips were exposed to magnetic field-induced translational and torque forces associated with MR systems that had static magnetic fields up to 1.5 T. Although these cases do not prove or suggest safety, they do demonstrate the relative difficulty of predicting the outcome for patients with ferromagnetic aneurysm clips who undergo MR procedures.

B. Evaluation of Aneurysm Clips for MRI Safety

Unfortunately, there is much controversy and confusion regarding the amount of ferromagnetism that needs to be present in an aneurysm clip to constitute a hazard for a patient in the MR environment.[1–3,14,16] Consequently, this issue has not only created problems for MR healthcare workers, but for the manufacturers of aneurysm clips as well.

For example, MR healthcare workers who performed testing on aneurysm clips, similar to testing reported by Kanal et al.,[16] supposedly identified magnetic field interactions and returned several clips made from Phynox to the manufacturer (personal communication, Aesculap, Inc., 1997). However, the testing method used by Kanal et al.[16] was admittedly crude. This simple test procedure was primarily developed to obtain rapid, qualitative screening data for large numbers of aneurysm clips to determine if more sophisticated testing was necessary.

Furthermore, this particular test technique may be problematic and yield spurious results, especially if the aneurysm clips have configurations that are somewhat "unstable" (unpublished observations, F.G. Shellock, 1997). For example, aneurysm clips with blades that are bayonet, curved, or angled configurations are less stable on a piece of plate glass (i.e., using the test method described by Kanal et al.[16]) when placed in certain orientations compared to aneurysm clips that have blades with straight configurations. Thus, movement of the aneurysm clips due to shape-related instability during the test procedure may be misconstrued as being magnet related.

A variety of more sophisticated and appropriate testing techniques have been developed and utilized over the years to evaluate the relative amount of ferromagnetism present for objects in association with the MR environment. For example, the "deflection angle test," originally described by New et al.,[17] has been indicated for the specific evaluation of aneurysm clips by the U.S. Food and Drug Administration (FDA). The FDA suggests that an evaluation of torque be performed as well. Obviously, procedures such as the deflection angle test and some form of evaluation of torque force are the most appropriate means of determining which specific intracranial aneurysm clip may present a hazard to a patient or individual in the MR environment.

The deflection angle test is considered to be useful, reliable, and reproducible and has been utilized for over 15 years to assess magnetic-induced translational forces for many metallic objects. In 1994, a standard issued from the American Society for Testing and Materials (ASTM) for the requirements and disclosure of aneurysm clips indicated that the deflection angle test should be used to specifically evaluate aneurysm clips.[26] (Note that the ASTM document is currently undergoing revision, and a new document will be published in the near future pertaining to the recommended test procedures to assess magnetic field interactions for passive implants.) This document was intended for use by manufacturers, users, engineers, government agencies, and designers of aneurysm clips to provide uniformity in reporting performance characteristics and test methodology.

The ASTM report states that the operational definition of a nonferromagnetic aneurysm clip is met only if the clip passes the following test: "The clip is suspended at the end of a string and held stationary in the vertical direction (that is, perpendicular to the ground) while it is placed in position at the portal of the imaging magnet. Following release of the clip, the deflection of the string from the vertical is then observed. The magnetic force is less than the gravitational force (that is, the clip's weight) if the deflection of the string with respect to the vertical is less than 45 degrees. The clip is then judged to be nonferromagnetic and suitable for implantation."[26] According to the ASTM, the deflection angle test as described above must be conducted such that the procedure is performed on a "finished" aneurysm clip using a 1.5-T MR system at the point where the highest spatial gradient field exists for that specific MR system.

Although not specified by the ASTM, for most MR systems with a conventional design, the highest spatial gradient is likely to exist somewhere between 30 to 45 cm inside the bore of the magnet. Therefore, it is at this position that the deflection angle test should be conducted. Additionally, it is recommended that a specific length (e.g., 30 cm) of 4.0 silk or similar low weight string be used for the test procedure.

Basically, the deflection angle test allows aneurysm clips made from weakly ferromagnetic materials to be used safely in patients undergoing MR procedures (i.e., those aneurysm clips that display deflection angles between 1° and 44°). Other testing methods, if they are more subjective or insensitive than the deflection angle test, will not yield the type of information required to adequately determine if an aneurysm clip will present a risk to an individual or patient in the MR environment.

An example of a test that may be performed to qualitatively determine the presence of magnetic field interactions for an aneurysm clip is the "Petri dish test." This test procedure involves the use of a plastic Petri dish with a millimeter etching on the bottom (alternatively, any see-through, enclosed device with a flat, relatively frictionless surface can be used to perform this test).

The aneurysm clip is placed in the Petri dish in an orientation that is perpendicular to the static magnetic field. Preferably, a 1.5-T MR system should be used for this evaluation. The Petri dish with the aneurysm clip is then positioned in the center of the MR system, where the effect of torque force from the static magnetic field is known to be the greatest.

The aneurysm clip should be directly observed for any type of possible motions with respect to movement, alignment, or rotation to the magnetic field. The observation process is facilitated by being inside the bore of the magnet during the test procedure. Using this simple test procedure, the presence of magnetic field interactions may be quickly ascertained. If a positive result is noted, deflection angle testing should be performed along with an evaluation of torque as needed.[1]

C. ANEURYSM CLIPS AND MRI SAFETY AT 1.5 T AND LESS

In a 1.5-T MR environment or less, aneurysm clips that have been reported to be acceptable for patients or others include those made from commercially pure titanium, titanium alloy, Elgiloy, Phynox, and austenitic stainless steels.[1,3,11-13,15,17,18,21,22] Those aneurysm clips were deemed safe because none of them, when tested in association with a 1.5-T MR system, displayed greater than a 2° deflection angle and there was either minor or no torque present.[1] Thus, the magnetic field interactions were relatively nonsignificant.

D. ANEURYSM CLIPS AND MRI SAFETY AT 8.0 T

Currently, the most powerful whole-body MR system in existence operates at a static magnetic field strength of 8.0 T.[8,9] Obviously, it is necessary to conduct *ex vivo* testing to identify potentially hazardous bioimplants, devices, and materials prior to subjecting individuals or patients with these objects to this ultra-high-field-strength MR environment. Therefore, the first investigation to determine magnetic field interactions for aneurysm clips exposed to an 8.0-T MR system was recently conducted by Kangarlu and Shellock.[9]

Twenty-six different aneurysm clips were tested for magnetic field interactions using previously described techniques.[9] These clips were specifically selected for this investigation because they represent various types of clips made from nonferromagnetic or weakly ferromagnetic materials used for temporary or permanent treatment of aneurysms or AVMs. Additionally, these aneurysm clips were previously reported to be safe for patients undergoing MR procedures using MR systems with static magnetic field strengths of 1.5 T or less.[1,3,4,13,17,18,20–22]

According to the test results, six aneurysm clips (i.e., type, model, blade length) made from stainless steel alloy (Perneczky, Zepplin Chirurgishe Instrumente, Pullach, Germany) and Phynox (Yasargil, Models FE 748 and FE 750, Aesculap, Inc.) displayed deflection angles above 45° and relatively high torque qualitative measurements. These findings indicated that those aneurysm clips may be unsafe for individuals or patients in an 8.0-T MR environment.

Aneurysm clips made from commercially pure titanium (Spetzler, Elekta Instruments, Inc., Atlanta, GA), Elgiloy (Sugita, Mizuho American, Inc., Beverly, MA), titanium alloy (Yasargil, Model FE 750T), and MP35N (Sundt) displayed deflection angles less than 45° and relatively minor torque. Accordingly, those aneurysm clips are likely to be safe for patients or individuals exposed to an 8.0-T MR system.

As previously indicated, at 1.5 T, aneurysm clips that are considered to be acceptable for patients or others in the MR environment include those made from commercially pure titanium, titanium alloy, Elgiloy, Phynox, and austenitic stainless steel. By comparison, findings from the 8.0-T study indicated that deflection angles for the aneurysm clips made from commercially pure titanium and titanium alloy ranged from 5° to 6°, suggesting that those aneurysm clips would be safe for patients or individuals in the 8.0-T MR environment. However, deflection angles for aneurysm clips made from Elgiloy ranged from 36° to 42°, such that consideration must be given to the specific type of Elgiloy clip that is present. For example, an Elgiloy clip that has a greater mass than those tested in this study may exceed a deflection angle of 45° in association with an 8.0-T MR system.

Notably, depending on the actual dimensions and mass, an aneurysm clip made from Elgiloy may or may not be acceptable for a patient or individual in the 8.0-T MR environment. Thus, the results of this investigation are highly specific to the types of intracranial aneurysm clips that underwent testing (i.e., with regard to model, shape, size, blade length, material, etc.).

E. EFFECTS OF LONG-TERM AND MULTIPLE EXPOSURES TO THE MR SYSTEM

Of note is that aneurysm clip testing procedures that have been recommended may result in the potential for reintroduction of aneurysm clips (prior to implantation) into strong MR system-related magnetic fields several times prior to ultimate patient implantation.[1,15] Furthermore, there are patients with implanted aneurysm clips previously tested as "MR compatible" or "MR safe" that have undergone repeated exposure to follow-up MR examinations and exposures to the strong magnetic fields of the systems.[1,15]

A safety concern for aneurysm clips is that there may be possible alterations in the magnetic properties of pre- or post-implanted aneurysm clips as a result of long-term or multiple exposures to strong magnetic fields.[1,15] It has been suggested that long-term or multiple exposures to strong magnetic fields (such as those associated with MR systems) may "magnetize" aneurysm clips, even if they are made from nonferromagnetic or weakly ferromagnetic materials.

Obviously, this scenario would present a significant hazard to an individual with an aneurysm clip in the MR environment. Therefore, an investigation was conducted to study intracranial aneurysm clips *in vitro* prior to and following long-term and multiple exposures to the magnetic fields associated with a 1.5-T MR system.[15] This was done to characterize possible changes in the magnetic properties of the aneurysm clips.

Aneurysm clips made from Elgiloy, Phynox, titanium alloy, commercially pure titanium, and austenitic stainless steel were tested in association with long-term and multiple exposures to 1.5-T

MR systems.[15] The findings of this research conducted by Kanal and Shellock[15] indicated that there was a lack of response to the various magnetic field exposure conditions that were used. Thus, long-term and/or multiple exposures to diagnostic MR examinations or *in vitro* clips to MR systems for testing purposes should not result in clinically significant changes in their magnetic properties or related MRI safety aspects.

F. ARTIFACTS ASSOCIATED WITH ANEURYSM CLIPS

An additional problem related to aneurysm clips is that artifacts produced by these metallic implants may substantially detract from the diagnostic aspects of MR procedures.[19-21] It is often necessary to evaluate the brain or cerebral vasculature of patients with aneurysm clips using MRI or MR angiography. For example, to reduce morbidity and mortality after sub-arachnoid hemorrhage, it is imperative to assess the results of the surgical treatment of cerebral aneurysms.

The extent of the artifact produced by a given aneurysm clip will have a direct effect on the diagnostic aspects of MR procedures.[19-21] Therefore, an investigation was conducted to characterize and compare the artifacts associated with aneurysm clips made from nonferromagnetic or weakly ferromagnetic materials.[19] Five different aneurysm clips made from five different materials were evaluated in this investigation, as follows:

1. Yasargil, Phynox
2. Yasargil, titanium alloy
3. Sugita, Elgiloy
4. Spetzler Titanium Aneurysm Clip, commercially pure titanium
5. Perneczky, cobalt alloy

These aneurysm clips were selected for testing because they are made from nonferromagnetic or weakly ferromagnetic materials and represent the most frequently used aneurysm clips and the latest versions of aneurysm clips that are commercially available in the U.S. Furthermore, these aneurysm clips have been previously reported to be safe for patients in the MR environment and, as such, are often found in patients referred for MR procedures.[1,3,4,11-18,20,21]

The MRI artifact test procedure revealed that the sizes of the signal voids were directly related to the type of material used to make the particular aneurysm clip. Arranged in decreasing order of artifact size, the materials responsible for the artifacts associated with the aneurysm clips were Elgiloy (Sugita), cobalt alloy (Perneczky), Phynox (Yasargil), titanium alloy (Yasargil), and commercially pure titanium (Spetzler) (Figure 14.4). These results have implications when one considers the various critical factors that are responsible for the decision to use a particular type of aneurysm clip (e.g., size, shape, closing force, biocompatibility, corrosion resistance, material-related effects on diagnostic imaging examinations, etc.).

An aneurysm clip that causes a relatively large artifact is less desirable because it can reduce the diagnostic power of MRI if the area of interest is in the immediate location of where the aneurysm clip was placed (Figure 14.4). Fortunately, newly developed aneurysm clips exist that are made from materials (i.e., commercially pure titanium and titanium alloy) that minimize artifacts produced by aneurysm clips.[19-21]

G. ANEURYSM CLIP GUIDELINES

In view of the current knowledge pertaining to aneurysm clips, the following guidelines are recommended for careful consideration prior to permitting an individual or patient with an aneurysm clip into the MR environment.[1,3]

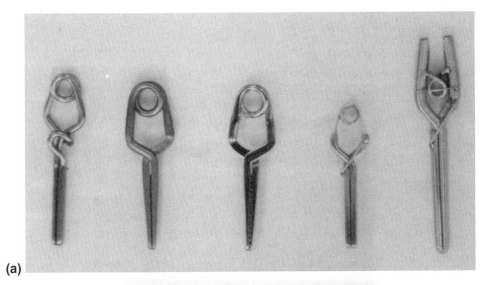

(a)

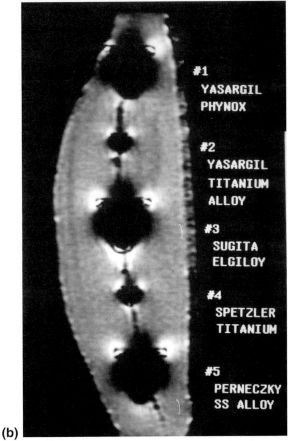

(b)

FIGURE 14.4 (a) Aneurysm clips evaluated for MRI artifacts (#1, Yasargil, Phynox; #2, Yasargil, titanium alloy; #3, Sugita, Elgiloy; #4, Spetzler, commercially pure titanium; #5, Perneczky, stainless steel alloy). (b) MR image (fast gradient echo) obtained through the blade portions of the aneurysm clips showing artifacts for the clips in (a). Note that the smallest artifacts are seen for the aneurysm clips made from titanium alloy and commercially pure titanium.   *(continued)*

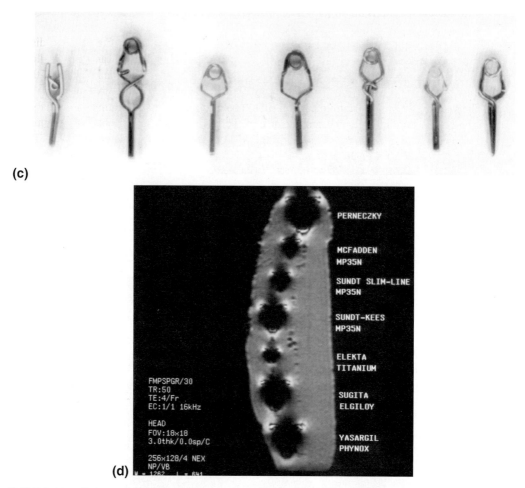

(c)

(d)

FIGURE 14.4 (CONTINUED) (c) Aneurysm clips evaluated for MRI artifacts (Top to bottom: #1, Pernec-zky, stainless steel alloy; #2, McFadden, MP35N; #3, Sundt Slim Line, MP35N; #4, Sundt-Kees, MP35N; #5, Elekta (Spetzler), commercially pure titanium; #6, Sugita, Elgiloy; #7, Yasargil, Phynox). (d) MR image (fast gradient echo) obtained through the blade portions of the aneurysm clips showing artifacts for the clips in (c). Note that the smallest artifact is seen for the aneurysm clip made from commercially pure titanium.

1. Specific information (i.e., manufacturer, type or model, material, lot, and serial numbers) about the aneurysm clip must be known, especially with respect to the material used to make the aneurysm clip, so that only patients or individuals with nonferromagnetic or weakly ferromagnetic clips are allowed into the MR environment. This information is provided by the manufacturer in the labeling of the aneurysm clip. The implanting surgeon is responsible for properly communicating this information in the patient's or individual's records.

2. An aneurysm clip that is in its original package and made from Phynox, Elgiloy, MP35N, titanium alloy, commercially pure titanium, or other material known to be nonferromag-netic or weakly ferromagnetic at 1.5 T or less does not need to be evaluated for ferro-magnetism. Aneurysm clips made from nonferrromagnetic or weakly ferromagnetic materials in original packages do not require testing of ferromagnetism because the manufacturers ensure the pertinent MR safety aspects of these clips and, therefore, should be held responsible for the accuracy of the labeling.

3. If the aneurysm clip is not in its original package and properly labeled, it should undergo testing for magnetic field interactions.

4. Testing for magnetic field interactions should first involve a procedure like the Petri dish test (i.e., for one or a few aneurysm clips) or the procedure described by Kanal et al.[16] (i.e., for screening large numbers of aneurysm clips). If a positive test result is noted, then the deflection angle test should be conducted following the guidelines of the ASTM.[26]

5. The radiologist and implanting surgeon should be responsible for evaluating the available information pertaining to the aneurysm clip, verifying its accuracy, obtaining written documentation, and deciding to perform the MR procedure after considering the risk vs. benefit aspects for a given patient.

IV. BIOPSY NEEDLES, MARKERS, AND DEVICES

MRI has been used to guide tissue biopsies and apply tissue markers with excellent results.[27,28] Obviously, the performance of these specialized procedures requires instruments and tools that are compatible with MR systems. Many commercially available biopsy needles, markers, and devices (i.e., guide wires, stylets, marking wires, marking clips, biopsy guns, etc.) have been evaluated with respect to compatibility with MR procedures, not only to determine ferromagnetic qualities, but also to characterize imaging artifacts. The results have indicated that most of the commercially available biopsy needles, markers, and devices are not useful for MR-guided biopsy procedures due to the presence of excessive ferromagnetism and the associated imaging artifacts that limit or obscure the area of interest.[1,2,29]

For many of the commercially available devices, MRI findings showed that the presence of the ferromagnetic biopsy needles and lesion marking wires in the tissue phantom used for testing produced such substantial artifacts that they would not be useful for MR-guided procedures.[29] Needles or devices containing any type of ferromagnetic material tend to have too much associated magnetic susceptibility to allow effective use for MR-guided procedures.

Fortunately, several needles, markers, and devices have been constructed out of nonferromagnetic materials specifically for use in MR-guided procedures.[1,2,27-30] Certain nonferromagnetic materials, such as titanium, do not appear to have the same properties, which should be carefully considered whenever selecting an MR-compatible biopsy needle for an MR-guided procedure.

Although most of the biopsy guns tested for magnetic field interactions were found to be ferromagnetic, since they are not used in the immediate area of the sampled tissue, artifacts associated with these devices are unlikely to affect the resulting images during MR-guided biopsy procedures.[1,2,29] Nevertheless, the presence of ferromagnetism is likely to preclude the optimal use of most biopsy guns in the MR environment. Currently, there is at least one commercially available biopsy gun that has been developed specifically for use in MR-guided procedures that does not have ferromagnetic components.[1]

A metallic marking clip, the Micromark™ made from 316L stainless steel (Biopsys Medical, Irvine, CA), has been developed for percutaneous placement after a stereotactic breast biopsy procedure.[31] The placement of a marking clip is of obvious benefit, especially in cases where mammographic findings may not be readily apparent or visible. The use of a marking clip enables the accurate localization of the surgical excision site. Furthermore, it is a useful surrogate target, even when the entire lesion is removed and there is a subsequent need for wire localization prior to surgery.

A current limitation of an MR-guided needle localization procedure is that there is an inability to document lesion retrieval because it is not possible to perform contrast enhancement (i.e., the MRI technique used to identify and characterize breast lesions) of the resected specimen. A Micromark clip placed during MR-guided biopsy or localization can permit radiography to be performed on the surgical specimen to confirm retrieval of the clip and, thus, document retrieval of the lesion.[31]

Tests conducted to assess magnetic field interaction, heating, and artifacts indicated that the presence of the Micromark clip presents no risk to a patient undergoing an MR procedure using an MR system with a static magnetic field of 1.5 T or less.[31] Unfortunately, the probe used with the Micromark is strongly attracted by a 1.5-T MR system, preventing its use in this specific MR environment. However, the marking clip could be placed outside of the influence of the magnetic field after placement of an MR-compatible introducer.[31]

V. BONE FUSION STIMULATOR/SPINAL FUSION STIMULATOR

The bone fusion stimulator or, more precisely, the implantable spinal fusion stimulator (Electro-Biology, Inc., Parsippany, NJ) is designed for use as an adjunct therapy to a spinal fusion procedure[32] (Figure 14.5). This device consists of a direct current (DC) generator with a lithium iodine battery and solid-state electronics encased in a titanium shell that acts as an anode.[32]

The generator weighs 10 g and has the following dimensions: $45 \times 22 \times 6$ mm. Two nonmagnetic, silver/stainless steel leads insulated with silastic provide a connection to two titanium electrodes that serve as the cathodes. A continuous 20-μA current is produced by this device. The cathodes are comprised of insulated wire leads that terminate as bare wire leads, which are

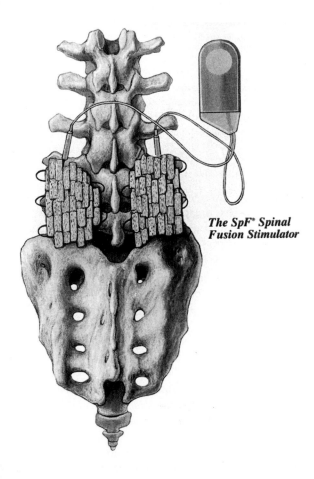

The SpF® Spinal Fusion Stimulator

FIGURE 14.5 Drawing of a bone fusion stimulator shows electrodes implanted at the L4-L5 level embedded in pieces of bone grafted onto lateral aspects of fusion sites.

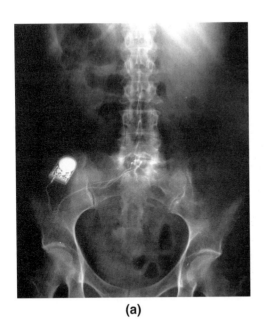

(a)

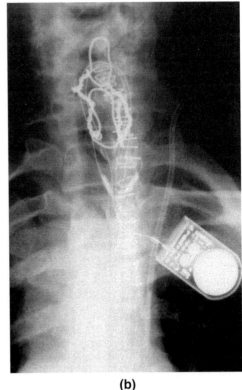

(b)

FIGURE 14.6 Examples of plain film radiographs showing the implanted bone fusion stimulators implanted in (a) the lumbar spine and (b) cervical spine.

embedded in pieces of bone grafted onto the lateral aspects of fusion sites (Figure 14.6). The generator is implanted beneath the skin and muscle near the vertebral column and provides the full-rated current for approximately 24 to 26 weeks.[32]

The use of this implantable spinal fusion stimulator provides a faster consolidation of the bone grafts, leading to higher fusion rates and improved surgical outcomes, along with a reduced need for orthopedic instrumentation.[32] To date, the implantable spinal fusion device has been utilized successfully to increase the probability of bone fusion in more than 70,000 patients.[32]

Recent studies using excessively high electromagnetic fields under highly specific experimental conditions and modeling scenarios for the lumbar/torso area (i.e., high-field-strength MR system, excessive exposures to RF fields, excessive exposures to gradient magnetic fields, etc.) have demonstrated that the implantable spinal fusion stimulator will not present a hazard to a patient undergoing MRI with respect to movement, heating, or induced electric fields during the use of conventional MR techniques.[32,33] Additionally, there was no evidence of malfunction of the implantable spinal fusion stimulator based on *in vitro* and *in vivo* experimental findings.[32] These studies addressed the use of conventional pulse sequences and parameters with an acknowledgement that echo planar techniques or imaging parameters that require excessive radiofrequency (RF) power will have different implications and consequences for the patient with an implantable spinal fusion stimulator.[32,33]

More than 120 patients with implantable spinal fusion stimulators have undergone MRI examinations (conceivably, using MRI conditions that involved a wide variety of imaging parameters and conditions) with no reports of substantial adverse events. Furthermore, the manufacturer of this implant and the FDA have not received complaints of injuries associated with the presence of this device in patients undergoing MR procedures.

In an *in vivo* study, there were no reports of immediate or delayed (minimum of 1 month follow-up) adverse events from patients with implantable spinal fusion stimulators who underwent MR imaging at 1.5 T.[32] Each patient was visually inspected following the MRI examination, and there was no evidence of excessive heating (i.e., change in skin color or other similar response). One patient indicated a sensation of "warming" felt at the site of the stimulator; however, this feeling was described as minor and the MR examination was completed without further indication of unusual sensations or problems.[32] Of further note is that there were no reports of excessive heating or neuromuscular stimulation in association with the presence of the implantable spinal fusion stimulators in patients that underwent MRI.[32]

Chou et al.[33] conducted a thorough investigation of the effect of heating of the implantable spinal fusion stimulator associated with MRI. This work was performed using a full-sized human phantom during MR procedures involving a relatively high exposure to RF energy (i.e., at whole-body-averaged specific absorption rates of approximately 1.0 W/kg).[33] Fiber-optic thermometry probes were placed at various positions on and near the cathodes, leads, and stimulator for each experiment to record temperature changes.

The phantom used by Chou et al.[33] did not include the effects of blood flow, which obviously would help dissipate heating that may occur during MRI, and, therefore, it further represents an excessive RF exposure condition. With the implantable spinal fusion stimulator in place and the leads intact, the maximum temperature rise after 25 min of scanning occurred at the center of the stimulator and was less than 2°C.[33]

The temperature rise at the cathodes was less than 1°C. When the simulator and leads were removed, the maximum temperature rise was less than 1.5°C, recorded at the tip of the electrode with insignificant temperature changes occurring at the cathode.[33] These temperature changes are within physiologically acceptable ranges for the tissues where the implantable spinal fusion stimulator is implanted, especially considering that the temperatures for muscle and subcutaneous tissues are at levels that are known to be several degrees below the normal core temperature of 37°C.[33]

Chou et al.[33] also investigated heating of the tips of broken leads of the implantable spinal fusion stimulator (this device was the same as that which underwent testing in the present study). Temperature changes occurred in localized regions that were within a few millimeters of the cut ends of the leads, with maximum temperature increases that ranged from 11° to 14°C.

If these levels of temperatures occurred during MRI, the amount of possible tissue damage would be comparable in characteristics and clinical significance to a small electrosurgical lesion and would likely occur in the scar tissue that typically forms around the implanted leads.[32,33] Additionally, the potential for tissue damage is only theoretical, and a brief temperature elevation around a broken lead, over an approximated volume of 2 to 3 mm radius, may not be clinically worse than the scar tissue that forms over the leads during implantation. Fortunately, broken leads are rare, occurring in approximately 10 out of the 70,000 devices implanted over the last 10 years (personal communication, Bruce J. Simon, Ph.D, Electro-Biology, Inc., 1999).[32]

Based on the available findings from the various investigations that have been conducted, RF energy-induced heating during MRI does not appear to present a major problem for a patient with the implantable spinal fusion stimulator, as long as there is no broken lead. The integrity of the leads should be assessed using a radiograph prior to the MR procedure. In general, it is believed that the implantable spinal fusion stimulator is safe for patients undergoing MR procedures following specific guidelines.[32] Recommended guidelines for conducting an MR examination in a patient with an implantable spinal fusion stimulator are as follows:

1. The cathodes of the implantable spinal fusion stimulator should be positioned a minimum of 1 cm from nerve roots to reduce the possibility of nerve excitation during an MR procedure.
2. Plain films should be obtained prior to MRI to verify that there are no broken leads present for the implantable spinal fusion stimulator. If this cannot be reliably determined, then the potential risks and benefits to the patient requiring MRI must be carefully

assessed in consideration of the possibility of the potential for excessive heating to develop in the leads of the stimulator.

3. MRI should be performed using MR systems with static magnetic fields of 1.5 T or less and conventional techniques including spin echo, fast spin echo, and gradient echo pulse sequences. Pulse sequences (e.g., echo planar techniques) or conditions that produce exposures to high levels of RF energy (i.e., exceeding a whole-body-averaged specific absorption rate of 1.0 W/kg) or exposure to gradient fields that exceed 20 T/s, or any other unconventional MR technique should be avoided.

4. Patients should be continuously observed during MRI and instructed to report any unusual sensations, including any feelings of warming, burning, or neuromuscular excitation or stimulation.

5. The implantable spinal fusion stimulator should be placed as far as possible from the spinal canal and bone graft, since this will decrease the likelihood that artifacts will affect the area of interest on MR images.

6. Special consideration should be given to selecting an imaging strategy that minimizes artifacts if the area of interest for MRI is in close proximity to the implantable spinal fusion stimulator. The use of fast spin echo pulse sequences will minimize the amount of artifact associated with the presence of the implantable spinal fusion stimulator (Figure 14.7).

VI. BREAST TISSUE EXPANDERS AND IMPLANTS

Adjustable breast tissue expanders and mammary implants are utilized for breast reconstruction following mastectomy, for the correction of breast and chest-wall deformities and underdevelopment, for tissue defect procedures, and for cosmetic augmentation.[1,2,34] These devices are equipped with either an integrated injection site or a remote injection dome that is utilized to accept a needle for placement of saline for expansion of the prosthesis intraoperatively and/or post-operatively.

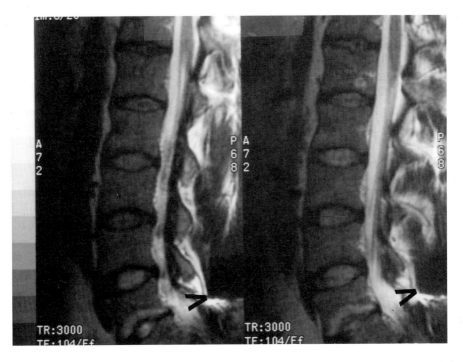

FIGURE 14.7 An MR image of the lumbar spine (sagittal, T2-weighted, fast spin echo) shows a relative lack of artifacts (arrowheads) for the bone fusion stimulator.

The Becker and the Siltex prostheses are additionally equipped with the choice of a standard injection dome or a microinjection dome.[1,2] The Radovan expander is indicated for temporary implantation only. The injection ports contain 316L stainless steel to guard against piercing the injection port by the needle.

There are two different breast tissue expanders that are constructed with magnetic ports to allow for a more accurate detection of the injection site.[1,2,34] These devices are substantially attracted to the static magnetic field of MR systems. Therefore, these breast tissue expanders may be uncomfortable or injurious to a patient undergoing an MR procedure. Notably, breast tissue expanders with magnetic ports produce relatively large artifacts on MR images.

The relative amount of image distortion caused by the metallic components of these devices should not greatly affect the diagnostic quality of an MRI examination, unless the imaging area of interest is at the same location as the metallic portion of the breast tissue expander. For example, there may be a situation during which a patient is referred for MRI for the determination of breast cancer or a breast implant rupture, such that the presence of the metallic artifact could obscure the precise location of the abnormality. In view of this possibility, it is recommended that patients with breast tissue expanders that have metallic components be identified so that the individual interpreting the MR images is aware of the potential problems related to the generation of artifacts.

VII. CARDIAC PACEMAKERS AND IMPLANTABLE CARDIOVERTER DEFIBRILLATORS

A. CARDIAC PACEMAKERS

Cardiac pacemakers (i.e., pulse generators) are crucial implanted devices for patients with heart conditions and have served to maintain the quality of life and substantially reduce morbidity for these individuals. The first cardiac pacemaker was implanted in 1958. Since then, more than 2 million patients have had cardiac pacemakers implanted. Each year, over 100,000 patients in the U.S. and an additional 100,000 in other parts of the world receive pacemakers for treatment of heart rhythm disturbances.[1,2]

Cardiac pacemakers are the most common electrically activated implants found in patients that may be referred for MR procedures. Unfortunately, the presence of a cardiac pacemaker is considered a strict contraindication for patients referred for MR procedures using conventional MR systems [with the exception of musculoskeletal MRI examinations performed using a dedicated extremity MR system (Artoscan, Lunar Corporation, Madison, WI). Several patients with cardiac pacemakers have died as a result of being in the MR environment or while undergoing MR procedures.[1,2,40]

The effects of the MR system on the function of a cardiac pacemaker are variable and dependent on several factors, including the type of cardiac pacemaker, the static magnetic field strength of the MR system, and the specific type of imaging conditions used (i.e., the anatomic region imaged, the type of surface coil used, the pulse sequence, etc.).[1,2,35-47] Cardiac pacemakers present potential problems to patients undergoing MR procedures from several mechanisms, including:

1. Movement of the pacemaker due to interaction with the strong static magnetic field of the MR system;
2. Modification of the function of the pacemaker, temporarily and/or permanently, by the static magnetic field of the MR system;
3. Heating induced in the pacemaker leads due to the time-varying (RF) magnetic fields of the MR system during imaging; and
4. Voltages and currents induced in the pacemaker leads and/or myocardium during MRI by the time-varying RF and/or the gradient magnetic fields.

There has been much discussion concerning the ability of the static magnetic fields of MR systems to close the reed switches of cardiac pacemakers.[1,2,42-47] Cardiac pacemaker switches may close in static fields as low as 15 gauss. However, all this accomplishes is to place the cardiac pacemaker into an asynchronous mode of operation. A predetermined fixed pacing rate takes over during the time period that the reed switch is activated. Patients with cardiac pacemakers may have these devices placed into asynchronous mode during evaluation by cardiologists, as the pacemakers are interrogated as part of their routine maintenance program.[2] Thus, it would appear that this often-quoted reed switch activation by the static magnetic field of the MR system may not be the causative factor for adverse problems with regard to cardiac pacemakers in the MR environment.

Studies conducted in laboratory animals and human subjects with cardiac pacemakers have reported a rapid acceleration in heart rate (i.e., tachyarrhythmia) and/or hypotension during MR procedures.[42-44] Conceivably, the cause of this may be the induction of voltages or currents within the pacemaker-lead-myocardial loop sufficient to induce action potentials or contraction of the myocardium that results in unwanted physiological responses. Notably, at least one study reported cardiac pacing at the selected repetition time (TR) of the MR procedure.[44] Rapid pacing rates yield cardiac outputs that are not compatible with sustaining life and, thus, may be the cause of death in some of the cardiac pacemaker patients that underwent MR procedures.

Heating the leads of the cardiac pacemaker pacing leads during MRI is also potentially problematic, and thermal injury to the endocardium or myocardium must be considered as a possible adverse outcome if electromagnetic fields are transmitted in the vicinity of the cardiac pacemaker and/or its leads. An investigation by Achenbach et al.[35] reported that it was possible for cardiac pacemaker electrodes exposed to MRI under certain conditions in a 1.5-T MR system to generate temperature increases of up to 63.1°C within 90 sec of scanning.

In consideration of the above, it should be considered a contraindication to permit any patient with a cardiac pacemaker to enter the MR environment. However, it is possible that this policy will change as more information is acquired about this issue and as more information becomes available defining which patients may be safely imaged with MR systems and under what specific conditions. Various theories do suggest that it may be possible to perform MR procedures safely in certain patients (such as patients who are not pacemaker dependent) with certain pacemakers under certain conditions. In fact, currently, there are several cardiac pacemaker companies investigating the possibility of developing MR-compatible devices because of the ubiquitous use of this important diagnostic imaging modality.

Despite the obvious substantial issues related to the MR environment and patients with cardiac pacemakers, several patients have intentionally undergone MRI with special precautionary measures in place. In one case, a patient who was not pacemaker dependent was examined by MRI after having his cardiac pacemaker "disabled" during the procedure.[36] Although this patient did not experience any apparent discomfort and the cardiac pacemaker was not damaged, it is inadvisable to perform this type of maneuver routinely in patients with cardiac pacemakers because of the potential to encounter the various aforementioned hazards.

Garcia-Bolao et al.[41] reported a case of a patient with a dual-chamber pacemaker that underwent two MRI examinations of the head without any sequelae. Both procedures were performed using a 1.0-T MR system. Notably, the reed switch was activated, probably due to the static magnetic field, resulting in asynchronous pacing.[41] This is an example whereby MRI may be used in certain carefully selected patients.

Sommer et al.[46] prospectively studied, using *in vivo* and *in vitro* techniques, 21 different models of "new generation" cardiac pacemakers and 51 patients implanted with these devices. The patients underwent MRI examinations using standard spin echo, fast spin echo, and gradient echo sequences and were continuously monitored during the procedures. The cardiac pacemakers were interrogated before and after the MRI examinations, including assessment of stimulation thresholds.[46]

The results indicated that the static magnetic field caused all of the cardiac pacemakers to be switched to the asynchronous mode of operation due to activation of the reed switches. The MRI exposures produced no program changes, damage to pacemaker components, dislocation or torque of the pacemaker, or rapid pacing under the conditions used for this investigation.

Thus, Sommer et al.[46] concluded that MRI at 0.5 T should not be regarded as absolutely contraindicated in patients with implanted new-generation cardiac pacemakers. This group indicated that MRI at 0.5 T can be safely performed in patients with implanted pacemakers in carefully selected circumstances when appropriate strategies (e.g., programming to the asynchronous mode, adequate monitoring techniques, and limited exposure to RF energy) are used.

Gimbel et al.[39] studied five patients with permanent cardiac pacemakers that underwent MRI at 1.5 T. Only one patient (underlying rhythm asystole) was pacemaker dependent. A variety of pacing configurations (single and dual chamber, unipolar and bipolar, sensor and nonsensor driven) were scanned. A thorough evaluation of each pacing system was performed before and after MRI, including determination of pacing and sensing thresholds. During MRI, the patients were monitored using either electrocardiogram (ECG), pulse oximetry, or direct voice contact. In four patients, heavy dressings were applied over the pacemaker pocket site to minimize or prevent movement. According to the findings of Gimbel et al.,[39] the four nonpacemaker-dependent patients remained in sinus rhythm throughout the MRI examinations. During and after the MRI, all cardiac pacemakers continued to function normally except for one transient pause of approximately 2 sec (noted by pulse oximetry) toward the end of the scan. This occurred in a pacemaker-dependent patient with a unipolar dual chamber device. None of the patients experienced any pacemaker movement torque or heat sensations.

Gimbel et al.[39] concluded that when appropriate strategies are used, MRI may be performed in patients with cardiac pacemakers when necessary, with an acceptable risk-benefit ratio to the patient. Appropriate patient selection, close monitoring during the scan, and follow-up after MRI are of paramount importance. Further study is necessary to refine the appropriate strategies that could be used to consistently perform MRI safely in a selected cardiac pacemaker patient population.

B. IMPLANTABLE CARDIOVERTER DEFIBRILLATORS (ICDs)

Implantable cardioverter defibrillators (ICDs) are medical devices designed to automatically detect and treat episodes of ventricular fibrillation, ventricular tachycardias, and bradycardia. When an arrhythmia is detected, the device can deliver defibrillation, cardioversion, antitachycardia pacing, or bradycardia pacing therapy. Each year, over 35,000 ICDs are implanted in patients throughout the world. ICDs are often used to treat patients with sustained arrhythmias that are refractory to antiarrhythmic pharmacologic treatment.

An ICD typically uses a programmer that has an external magnet to test the battery charger and to activate and deactivate the system. Deactivation of an ICD is usually accomplished by holding a magnet over the device for approximately 30 sec. Deactivations of ICDs have occurred accidentally as a result of patients encountering magnetic fields in home and workplace environments. For example, deactivations of ICDs have occurred in patients from exposures to the magnetic fields found in stereo speakers, bingo wands, and 12 volt battery starters.[37]

Obviously, MR systems would have a similar effect on ICDs as on pacemakers since the components are comparable. Therefore, patients with these devices should avoid exposure to the MR environment. In addition, since ICDs also have electrodes placed in the myocardium, patients should not undergo MR procedures because of risks related to the presence of these conductive materials.

In consideration of the potential hazardous situations related to the presence of cardiac pacemakers and ICDs, it is advisable to double-check all patients and individuals, particularly those that may have communication difficulties, before letting them into the MR environment. In the event that the exposure (inadvertent or intentional) of a patient with a cardiac pacemaker or implantable cardioverter defibrillator to the MR environment occurs, it would be prudent to have the functionality of the device assessed by a cardiologist or cardiac nurse specialist.

VIII. CARDIOVASCULAR CATHETERS AND ACCESSORIES

Cardiovascular catheters and accessories are indicated for use in the assessment and management of critically ill or high risk patients including those with acute heart failure, cardiogenic shock, severe hypovolemia, complex circulatory abnormalities, acute respiratory distress syndrome, pulmonary hypertension, certain types of arrhythmias, and other various medical emergencies.[1,2,48] In these cases, cardiovascular catheters are used to measure intravascular pressures, intracardiac pressures, cardiac output, and oxyhemoglobin saturation. Secondary indications include venous blood sampling and therapeutic infusion of solutions or medications. In addition, some cardiovascular catheters are designed for temporary cardiac pacing and intra-atrial or intraventricular electrocardiographic monitoring.[48]

Because patients with cardiovascular catheters and associated accessories may require evaluation using MR procedures, or these devices may be used during MR-guided procedures, it is imperative that a thorough *ex vivo* assessment of MR safety be conducted for these devices to ascertain the potential risks of their use in the MR environment. For example, MR imaging, angiography, and spectroscopy procedures may play an important role in the diagnostic evaluation of these patients. Furthermore, the performance of certain MR-guided interventional procedures may require the utilization of cardiovascular catheters and accessories to monitor patients during biopsies, interventions, or treatments.

There is at least one report of a cardiovascular catheter that melted in a patient undergoing MRI.[1,2] Obviously, there are realistic concerns pertaining to the use of similar devices during MRI examinations. Therefore, an investigation was conducted using *ex vivo* testing techniques to evaluate cardiovascular catheters and accessories with regard to magnetic field attraction, heating, and artifacts associated with MRI.[48]

A total of 15 different cardiovascular catheters and accessories (Abbott Laboratories, Morgan Hill, CA) were selected for evaluation because they represent a wide variety of the styles and types of devices that are commonly used in the critical care setting (i.e., the basic structures of these devices are comparble to those made by other manufacturers). Of these devices, the 3-Lumen CVP Catheter, CVP-PVC Catheter (used for central venous pressure monitoring, administration of fluids, and venous blood sampling; polyurethane and polyvinyl chloride, respectively), Thermoset-Iced and Thermoset-Room (used as accessories for determination of cardiac output using the thermodilution method; plastic), and Safe-set with In-Line Reservoir (used for in-line blood sampling; plastic) were determined to have no metallic components. Therefore, these devices were deemed safe for patients undergoing MR procedures and were not included in the overall *ex vivo* tests for MR safety. The remaining ten devices were evaluated for the presence of potential problems in the MR environment.

Excessive heating of implants or devices made from conductive materials has been reported to be a hazard for patients who undergo MR procedures. This is particularly a problem for devices that are in the form of a loop or coil because current can be induced in this shape during operation of the MR system, to the extent that a first, second, or third-degree burn can be produced.[1,2]

The additional physical factors responsible for this hazard have not been identified or well-characterized (i.e., the imaging parameters, specific gradient field effects, size of the loop associated with excessive heating, etc.). For this reason, the previously published study[48] examining cardiovascular catheters and accessories did not attempt to investigate the effect of various "coiled" catheter shapes on the development of substantial heating during an MR procedure, particularly since there are many factors in addition to the shape of the catheter with a conductive component that can also influence the amount of heating that occurs during an MR procedure.

Although a thermodilution Swan-Ganz catheter (specific manufacturer unknown) is constructed of nonferromagnetic materials that include a conductive wire, a report indicated that a portion of this catheter that was outside a patient melted during MRI. It was postulated that the high-frequency electromagnetic fields generated by the MR system caused eddy current-induced heating of either the wires within the thermodilution catheter or the radiopaque material used in the construction of the catheter. This incident suggests that patients with this catheter or a similar device that has conductive wires or other component parts could be potentially injured during an MR procedure.

Because of the obvious deleterious and unpredictable effects, patients referred for MR procedures with cardiovascular catheters and accessories that have internally or externally positioned conductive wires or similar components should not undergo examinations because of the possible associated risks. Further support of this recommendation is based on the fact that inappropriate use of monitoring devices during MR procedures is often the cause of patient injuries. For example, burns have primarily resulted in the MR environment in association with the use of devices that utilize a conductive wire interface to the patient.[1,2]

The cardiovascular catheters and accessories evaluated contained metallic materials that are good electrical conductors, which, in turn, could potentially present a hazard for a patient undergoing an MR procedure. Therefore, in general, cardiovascular catheters and accessories with conductive metallic components should not be present in patients undergoing MR procedures, unless *ex vivo* testing demonstrates MR safety. Additionally, catheters and accessories from various manufacturers made from a similar design as the devices that were previously tested (i.e., with conductive wire components, etc.) are also likely to present problems to patients in the MR environment.

IX. CAROTID ARTERY VASCULAR CLAMPS

Various types of carotid artery vascular clamps have been evaluated for MR safety by Teitelbaum et al.[49] in association with a 1.5-T MR system. Each carotid artery vascular clamp tested for magnetic field interactions displayed attraction to the magnetic field. However, only the Poppen-Blaylock carotid artery vascular clamp was reported to be contraindicated for patients undergoing MR procedures due to the existence of substantial ferromagnetism.[49] The other carotid artery clamps were considered safe for patients exposed to the magnetic fields of MR systems because they were only "weakly" ferromagnetic.[49] With the exception of the Poppen-Blaylock clamp, patients with metallic carotid artery vascular clamps have been imaged by MR systems with static magnetic fields ranging up to 1.5 T without experiencing any discomfort or neurologic sequelae.

X. COCHLEAR IMPLANTS

Some types of cochlear implants employ a relatively strong magnet used in conjunction with an external component to align and retain an RF transmitter coil on the patient's head.[50-54] The magnet may also be used to provide sufficient transmission quality between the external transmitter and the internal receiver.

Typically, cochlear implants are electronically activated devices. Consequently, MR procedures are typically contraindicated for patients with this type of implant because of the possibility of injuring the patient and/or damaging or altering the function of the cochlear implant. In general, visitors or other individuals should also be prevented from entering the MR environment if they have a cochlear implant.

Investigations have been conducted to determine if there are any situations during which a patient with a cochlear implant could safely undergo an MR procedure.[50-54] Two studies were conducted to evaluate the safety of performing MR procedures in patients with specially modified devices: the Nucleaus Mini-22 Cochlear Implant (Cochlear Corporation, Engelwood, CO) and the Multichannel Auditory Brainstem Implant.

Tests were conducted to assess the operation of these cochlear implants in the MR environment, as well as to determine magnetic field interactions, artifacts, induced current, and heating during MRI. The reports indicated that a large margin of safety exists with regard to the MR environment and these devices, as long as specific recommendations contained within the product labeling are adhered to.

In vitro experiments were conducted to determine MR safety for the cochlear implant, the Combi 40/40+ Multichannel System (MedEl, Innsbruck, Austria).[53,54] This cochlear implant underwent testing associated with 0.2- and 1.5-T MR systems. According to the results of the experiments, partial demagnetization of the cochlear implant occurred within the 1.5-T MR system, while the 0.2-T MR system produced no alteration in the magnetic component of this implant. Partial demagnetization could be avoided by orienting the patient's head parallel to the magnetic field of the 1.5-T MR system.

In general, electromagnetic interference related to the use of the 1.5-T MR system remained within acceptable limits. Of greatest concern were the relative amounts of magnetic field translational attraction and torque acting on the cochlear implant, which have important implications for the safe performance of MR procedures using the 1.5-T MR system. By comparison, MR safety issues were minimal with the use of the 0.2-T MR system. The authors recommended that MRI may be performed in a patient with the Combi 40/40+ Multichannel System only if there are strong medical indications.

Additional *in vitro* work was conducted on the Combi 40/40+ cochlear implant to determine MRI safety within a wide range of clinical applications using a 1.5-T MR system. Torque, translational force, demagnetization, artifacts, induced voltages, and heating were assessed under extreme MRI conditions. Of the MRI safety issues evaluated for this implant, only the torque on the internal magnet of this cochlear implant was deemed problematic. Thus, some form of external stabilization is required (e.g., tape, support bandage, etc.) for the Combi 40/40+ cochlear implant for a patient undergoing an MR procedure. The overall test findings for the Combi 40/40+ cochlear implant indicated that an MR procedure should only be performed in a patient with this device if there is a strong medical necessity. An assessment of the relative risks involved vs. the risk of not providing the diagnostic information from an MR procedure for the specific patient is required.

XI. COILS, STENTS, AND FILTERS

Various types of intravascular coils, stents, and filters have been evaluated for safety with MR systems[1,2,55-65] (Figure 14.8). Several of these studies reported positive findings for magnetic field interactions associated with exposures to MR systems. Fortunately, these particular devices typically become incorporated securely into the vessel wall primarily due to tissue ingrowth within approximately 6 weeks after their introduction.[62-64] Therefore, it is unlikely that any of them would become moved or dislodged as a result of being attracted by static magnetic fields of MR systems up to 1.5 T. However, it should be noted that because new coils, stents, and filters continue to be developed, there may be certain devices that prove hazardous for individuals and patients in the MR environment (Figure 14.9).

Other similar devices made from nonferromagnetic materials, such as the LGM IVC filter (Vena Tech) used for caval interruption or the Wallstent biliary endoprosthesis [Schneider (USA) Inc., Minneapolis, MN] used for treatment of biliary obstruction, are considered safe for patients undergoing MR procedures. Notably, it is unnecessary to wait any period of time after surgery to perform an MR procedure in a patient with a metallic implant that is made from a nonferromagnetic, albeit weakly ferromagnetic, material.

The Guglielmi detachable coil (GDC) (Target Therapeutics, San Jose, CA) used for endovascular embolization, was evaluated for MRI safety by Shellock et al.[59] Importantly, because of the coiled shape of the GDC, excessive heating from induced current may occur during MRI. Therefore, a study was performed using *ex vivo* testing techniques to determine the MR safety for the GDC with respect to magnetic field interactions, heating, and artifacts (Figure 14.10).

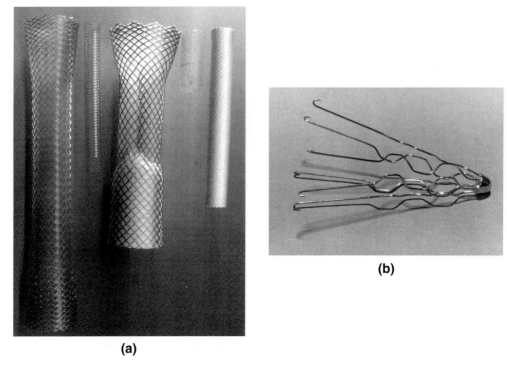

(a)

(b)

FIGURE 14.8 Examples of stents (a) and the Greenfield filter, stainless steel version (b).

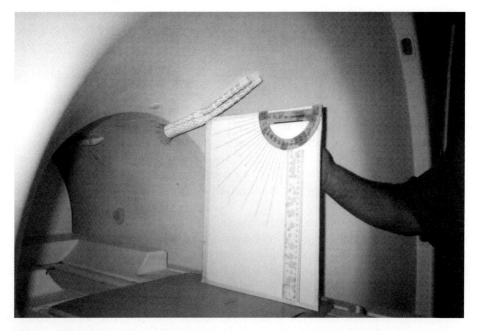

FIGURE 14.9 Assessment of the deflection angle for a prototype stent. This measurement was performed using a 1.5-T MR system. Note the 90° deflection angle, indicating that this stent could pose a hazard to an individual or patient in the MR environment.

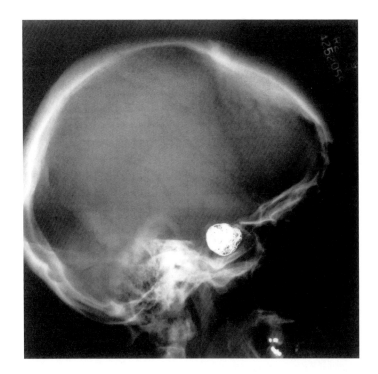

FIGURE 14.10 Plain film radiograph of the skull showing the GDC.

The results indicated that there was no magnetic field attraction, the temperature increase was minimal during "worst case" or extreme MR procedure, and the artifacts involved a mild signal void relative to the size and shape of the GDC.[49] Subsequently, more than 100 patients with GDCs have undergone MRI without incident. Similarly, other embolization coils made from nitinol, platinum, or platinum and iridium have been evaluated and found to be safe for patients undergoing MR procedures.

Patients with specific intravascular coils, filters, and stents that have been evaluated for MR safety[1,2,55-65] had procedures using MR systems with static magnetic fields up to 1.5 T without reports of injuries or other problems. An MR procedure should not be performed if there is any possibility that the intravascular coil, stent, or filter is not positioned properly or firmly in place.

XII. CRANIAL FLAP FIXATION CLAMPS

After performing a craniotomy, bone flaps are typically fixed with wire, suture material, or small plates and screws. Problems related to cranial bone flap fixation after craniotomy are more common with the trend for performing smaller craniotomies that are frequently utilized for minimally invasive surgical procedures. The use of small plates and screws for fixation of cranial bone flaps has improved the overall attachment process and end result. However, this technique requires a considerable amount of time and expense compared to using wire and suture techniques.

In consideration of the various problems with bone flap fixation, a special metallic implant system, named the Craniofix (Aesculap, Inc.) was developed for fixation of cranial bone flaps after craniotomy[66] (Figure 14.11). MR safety tests conducted to assess magnetic field interaction, heating, and artifacts indicated that the clamps used for the cranial bone flap fixation system present no risk to the patient in the MR environment of MR systems operating at 1.5 T or less.[66] Furthermore, the quality of the diagnostic MR images is more than acceptable, particularly if conventional spin echo or fast spin echo pulse sequences are used for imaging.[66]

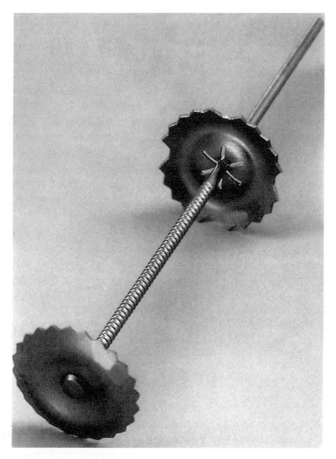

FIGURE 14.11 The Craniofix developed for fixation of cranial bone flaps after craniotomy.

XIII. DENTAL IMPLANTS, DEVICES, AND MATERIALS

Many of the dental implants, devices, and materials evaluated for magnetic field interactions exhibited measurable positive results, but only the ones with magnetically activated components present a potential problem for patients and individuals in the MR environment.[1,2,17,67-69] The other dental implants, devices, and materials are held in place with sufficient counterforces to prevent them from causing problems for patients by being moved or dislodged by magnetic fields of MR systems[1,2,17,67-69] (Figure 14.12).

XIV. DIAPHRAGMS

Contraceptive diaphragms have metallic rings that serve to maintain them in position during use (Figure 14.13). The contraceptive diaphragms were shown to be attracted by the 1.5-T static magnetic field used to test these objects.[1,2] However, MR procedures have been performed in patients with these devices and the patients did not complain of any sensation related to movement of the diaphragms. Furthermore, there is no danger of heating a contraceptive diaphragm during an MR procedure. Therefore, the presence of a diaphragm is not a contraindication for a patient undergoing an MRI examination using an MR system operating at 1.5 T or less. Notably, the presence of a diaphragm during MR imaging produces a substantial artifact that can impair the diagnostic aspects of the examination if the area of interest is located near the position of the diaphragm (Figure 14.14).

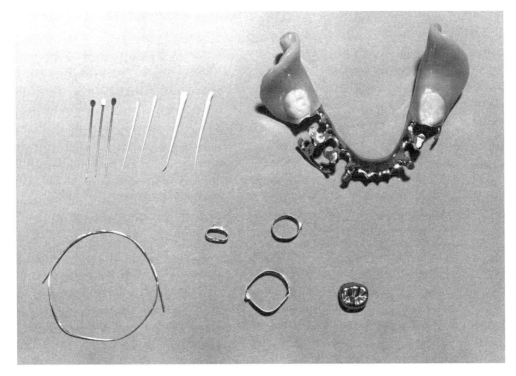

FIGURE 14.12 Examples of various dental implants and materials tested for MR safety.

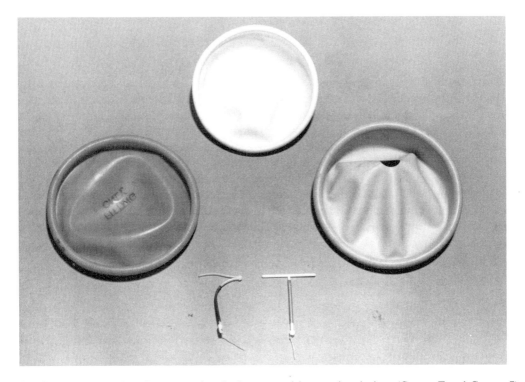

FIGURE 14.13 Examples of contraceptive diaphragms and intrauterine devices (Copper T and Copper 7) tested for MR safety.

298298298298
298

298

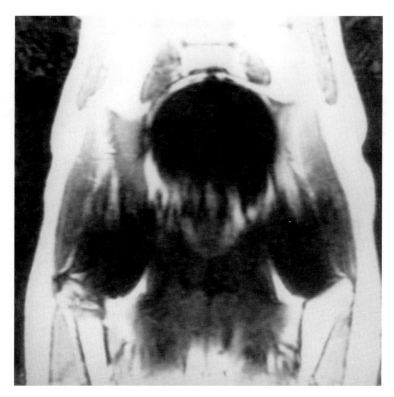

FIGURE 14.14 T1-weighted, coronal plane image of the hips and pelvis obtained from a patient with a contraceptive diaphragm in place. Note the presence of the substantial artifacts and image distortion.

XV. ECG ELECTRODES

Patients should be monitored routinely if the potential exists for a change of physiologic status during the MR procedure.[2] With the advent of newer types of MRI applications such as MR-guided therapy, there is also an increased need to monitor patients in these MR settings. Studies that need to record the ECG for the purpose of gating also require the proper acquisition of the appropriate physiologic signal for accurate and timely representation of the desired MR images.[1,2,70]

The use of MR-safe ECG electrodes is strongly recommended to ensure patient safety and proper recording of the ECG in the MR environment. Accordingly, ECG electrodes that have been specially developed for use during MR procedures protect the patient from these potentially hazardous conditions and produce minimal MRI-related artifacts.[70] Many different types of commercially available ECG electrodes have been evaluated for MR safety.[70]

XVI. FOLEY CATHETERS WITH TEMPERATURE SENSORS

Certain Foley catheters have temperature sensors to permit recording of the temperature of the urine in the bladder, which is a sensitive means of determining "deep" body or core temperature.[1] This type of Foley catheter typically has a thermistor or thermocouple located on or near the tip of the device and a wire that runs the length of the catheter to a connector that plugs into a temperature monitor. A Foley catheter with a temperature sensor should never be connected to the temperature monitor during the MR procedure because this equipment is not compatible or safe in the MR environment.[1]

Several Foley catheters with temperature sensors have been evaluated for safety in the MR environment by determining magnetic field interactions, artifacts, and heating.[1] In general, the findings of this assessment indicated that it would be safe to perform MR procedures in patients with the particular Foley catheters with temperature sensors that have been tested as long as highly specific recommendations are followed.[1]

Similar to any device with a wire component, the position of the wire of the Foley catheter with a temperature sensor has an important effect on the amount of heating that develops during an MR procedure. Accordingly, the Foley catheter with a temperature sensor must be positioned in a straight configuration without any loop(s) to prevent possible excessive heating associated with an MR procedure. Furthermore, only conventional pulse sequences should be used (e.g., no echo planar techniques, magnetization transfer contrast, etc.) while imaging with an MR system with a static magnetic field of 1.5 T or less.[1] Additional recommendations include the following:

1. If the Foley catheter with a temperature sensor has a removable catheter connector cable, it should be disconnected prior to the MR procedure.
2. Remove all electrically conductive material from the bore of the MR system that is not required for the procedure (i.e., unused surface coils, cables, etc.).
3. Keep electrically conductive material that must remain in the bore of the MR system from directly contacting the patient by placing thermal and/or electrical insulation (including air) between the conductive material and the patient.
4. Position the Foley catheter with a temperature sensor in a straight configuration to prevent cross points and conductive loops.
5. MRI should be performed using MR systems with static magnetic fields of 1.5 T or less and conventional magnetic fields. Pulse sequences, techniques (e.g., echo planar techniques) or conditions that produce exposures to high levels of RF energy (i.e., exceeding a whole-body-averaged specific absorption rate of 1.0 W/kg) or exposure to gradient fields that exceed 20 T/s, or any other unconventional MR technique should be avoided.
6. If the patient reports feeling warm or hot in association with the presence of the Foley catheter with a temperature sensor, discontinue the MR procedure immediately.

XVII. HALO VESTS AND CERVICAL FIXATION DEVICES

Halo vests or cervical fixation devices may be constructed from either ferromagnetic, nonferromagnetic, or a combination of metallic components and other materials[1,2,71-77] (Figure 14.15). Although some commercially available halo vests or cervical fixation devices are composed entirely of nonferromagnetic materials, there is a theoretical hazard of inducing electrical current in the ring portion of any halo device made from conductive materials according to Faraday's law of electromagnetic induction that presents potential risks to the patient during an MR procedure. Additionally, there is a potential for the patient's tissue to be involved in part of this current loop, so there would be the possibility of a burn or electrical injury to the patient.

The induced current within such a ring or conductive loop is of additional concern because of eddy current induction and potential image degradation effects.[75-77] Artifacts associated with the production of eddy currents during MRI may be substantially reduced by adjusting the phase encoding direction of the pulse sequences so that it is parallel to the axis of the halo vest.

At present, there are no reports of injuries associated with MR procedures performed in patients with halo vests or cervical fixation devices. However, one incident of "electrical arcing" without injury was reported in the 1988 Society for Magnetic Resonance Imaging Safety Survey (Phase I Study; personal communication, E. Kanal, M.D., 1988). Because of safety and image quality issues, MR procedures should only be performed on patients with specially designed halo vests or cervical fixation devices made from nonferromagnetic and nonconductive materials that have little or no interaction with the electromagnetic fields generated by MR systems.

There have been anecdotal reports of patients with halo vests or cervical fixation devices experiencing sensations of heat during MRI procedures. This has also been presumed to be a

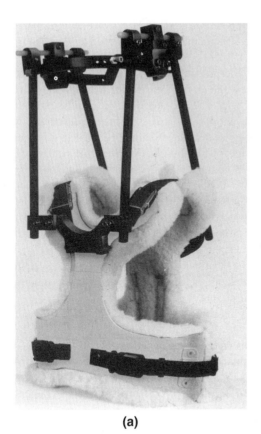

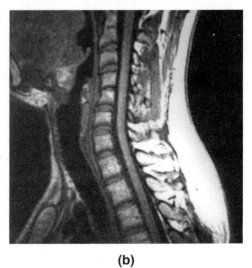

(b)

(a)

FIGURE 14.15 (a) Example of a nonconductive, nonferromagnetic halo vest designed for use during MR procedures. (b) T1-weighted, sagittal plane image of the cervical spine obtained from a patient wearing an MR-compatible halo vest.

problem for certain stereotactic headframes used in the MR environment. However, experiments using MR safety test methods demonstrated that there is no heating for at least one such device (unpublished observations, F. G. Shellock, 1996).

A study was conducted by Shellock and Slimp[77] to assess the possible heating of halo vests and cervical fixation devices during MRI performed using a 1.5-T MR system and various pulse sequences typically used to image the cervical spine. The data indicated that no substantial heating was detected. Of interest is that there appeared to be subtle motions of the halo ring associated with the use of a magnetization transfer contrast (MTC) pulse sequence, as shown by recordings obtained using a motion-sensitive, laser-Doppler flow monitor.[77]

Apparently, the specific imaging parameters used for the MTC pulse sequence produced sufficient vibration of the halo ring to create the sensation of heating. These rapid vibrations may have been felt by the subject and interpreted as a "heating" sensation. This is likely to occur when the frequency and/or amount of vibration at a certain level stimulates nerve receptors located in the subcutaneous region that detect sensations of pain and temperature changes. The aforementioned is merely a hypothesis based on the available experimental data and requires further investigation to substantiate this theory. However, additional support to this premise comes from a report by Hartwell and Shellock.[73]

In this case, a halo ring and vest (removed from a patient who complained of severe "burning" in a front skull pin during MRI) was evaluated for heating or other potential problems associated with MRI by the neurosurgeon who applied the device.[73] The halo ring and vest were connected in a manner similar to the way it was used on the patient, and a fluid-filled Plexiglas phantom was placed within the vest.

The device was then placed within a 1.5-T MR system, and MRI was performed using the same parameters that were associated with the burning sensation experienced by the patient. The neurosurgeon remained within the MR system to visually observe and touch the cervical fixation device during the MR procedure.[73]

No perceivable temperature change was noted for any of the metallic components during MRI. However, the metallic components of this device (e.g., halo ring, vertical supports, vest bolts, etc.) vibrated substantially during MRI.[73] Furthermore, when the skull pins were held firmly during MRI, there was a so-called "drilling" sensation, which could have been interpreted as a burning effect by the patient. Nevertheless, the skull pins remained cool to the touch throughout the MR procedure.

In consideration of the above information, it is inadvisable to permit patients with certain cervical fixation devices to undergo MR procedures using an MTC pulse sequence until this problem can be further characterized to avoid other similar patient responses, regardless of the lack of safety concern related to excessive heating. Other comparable pulse sequences should likewise be avoided when performing MRI on patients with halo vests and cervical fixation devices until the precise cause of this problem is determined. Additionally, all instructions for use and patient application provided by the halo vest and cervical fixation device manufacturers should be followed, without exception.

XVIII. HEARING AIDS

External hearing aids are included in the category of electrically activated implants or devices that may be found in patients referred for MR procedures. Understandably, the magnetic fields used for MRI examinations can easily damage these devices. Therefore, a patient or other individual with an external hearing aid must not enter the MR environment due to the possible risk of damage to the device. Fortunately, an external hearing aid can be readily identified and removed from the patient or individual prior to entering the MR environment to prevent damage to the device.

XIX. HEART VALVE PROSTHESES

Many heart valve prostheses have been evaluated for the presence of attraction to static magnetic fields of MR systems at field strengths as high as 2.35 T[1,2,17,78-84] (Figure 14.16). Of these, the majority displayed measurable, yet relatively minor, magnetic field interactions to the static magnetic field of the MR systems that were used for testing.

Because the actual attractive forces exerted on these heart valves were minimal compared to the force exerted by the beating heart (i.e., approximately 7.2 N), an MR procedure is not considered hazardous for a patient that has any of the heart valve prostheses that have been tested.[81,82] This recommendation includes the Starr-Edwards Model Pre-6000 heart valve prosthesis (Baxter Healthcare Corporation, Santa Ana, CA) that was previously suggested to be a potential risk for a patient undergoing an MR procedure.[1,2] With respect to clinical MR procedures, there has never been a report of a patient incident or injury related to the presence of a heart valve prosthesis.

XX. HEMOSTATIC CLIPS

To date, none of the various hemostatic vascular clips that have been evaluated have displayed magnetic field interactions in association with MR systems operating at 1.5 T.[1,2,13,17,85,86] These hemostatic clips are made from nonferromagnetic materials such as tantalum and nonferromagnetic forms of stainless steel (Figure 14.17). Therefore, patients that have these particular hemostatic vascular clips are not at risk for injury during MR procedures. Additionally, patients or individuals may be immediately exposed to the MR environment after placement of nonmagnetic hemostatic clips without concern for hazards. There has never been a report of injury to a patient in association with the presence of a hemostatic vascular clip in the MR environment.

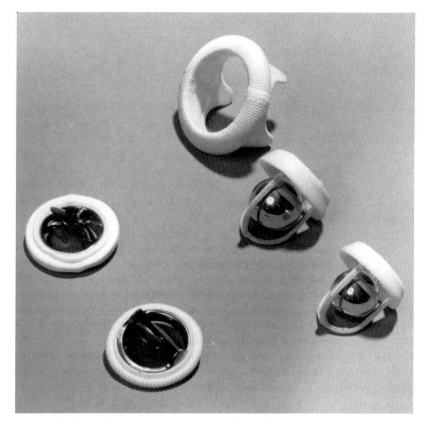

FIGURE 14.16 Examples of prosthetic heart valves. Each heart valve has a metallic component. Some of these valves are made from materials that are "mildly" ferromagnetic. However, all of these prosthetic heart valves were shown to be safe for patients undergoing MR procedures at 1.5 T or less because the associated deflection forces were less than the *in vivo* forces.

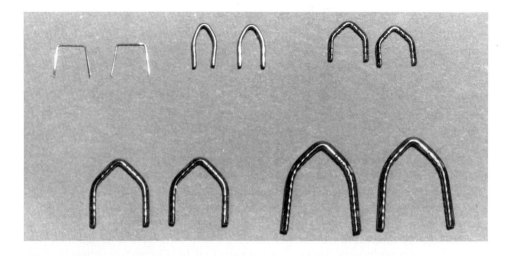

FIGURE 14.17 Examples of metallic hemostatic clips.

XXI. INTRAUTERINE CONTRACEPTIVE DEVICES

Contraceptive intrauterine devices (IUDs) may be made from nonmetallic materials (e.g., plastic) or a combination of nonmetallic and metallic materials.[1,2,87,88] Copper is typically the metal used in an IUD.

The Copper T and Copper 7 both have a fine copper coil wound around a portion of the IUD (Figure 14.13). Testing conducted to determine the MRI safety aspects of IUDs with metal indicated that these objects are safe for patients in the MR environment using MR systems operating at 1.5 T or less.[1,2,87,88] This includes the Multiload Cu375, the Nova T (containing copper and silver), and the Gyne T IUDs. An artifact may be seen for the metallic component of the IUD, however, the extent of this artifact is relatively small because of the low mass of the metal present and the low magnetic susceptibility of copper.

XXII. MAGNETICALLY ACTIVATED IMPLANTS AND DEVICES

Various types of implants incorporate magnets as a means of activating or operating the devices. The magnet may be used to keep the implant in place (e.g., certain prosthetic devices), to change the operation of the implant, to program the device, or to guide a ferromagnetic object into a specific position.[1,2,89-98] With regard to the MR environment, because there is a high likelihood of perturbing the function of magnetically activated implants, demagnetizing the implants, or displacing the implants, MR procedures typically should not be performed in patients with these implants or devices.[1,2,89-98]

However, in some cases, patients with magnetically activated implants and devices may undergo MR procedures as long as certain precautions are followed. Knowledge of the specific aspects of the magnetically activated implant or device is essential to recognize potential problems and to guarantee that an MR procedure may be performed on a patient without problems or injuries.[1,2]

Implants and devices that use magnets (e.g., certain types of dental implants, magnetic sphincters, magnetic stoma plugs, magnetic ocular implants, otologic implants, and other similar prosthetic devices) may be damaged by the magnetic fields of the MR systems, which, in turn, may necessitate surgery to replace or reposition them. For example, Schneider et al.[93] reported that the MRI procedure is capable of demagnetizing the permanent magnet associated with an otologic implant (i.e., the Audiant implant). Obviously, this has important implications for the patient with this device if there is a need for an MR procedure.

Whenever possible, and if this can be done without risk to the patient (i.e., from the retained magnetic "keeper" or similar component), a magnetically activated implant or device (e.g., an externally applied prosthesis or magnetic stoma plug) should be removed from the patient prior to entrance into the MR environment. This will typically permit the examination to be performed safely.

Extrusion of an eye socket magnetic implant in a patient imaged with a 0.5-T MR system has been described by Yuh et al.[96] This paticular type of magnetic ocular prosthesis is used in a patient after enucleation. The removable eye prosthesis adheres with a magnet of opposite polarity to a permanent implant sutured to the rectus muscles and conjunctiva by magnetic attraction through the conjunctiva. This "magnetic linkage" enables the eye prosthesis to move in a coordinated fashion with the normal eye movement. In the reported incident,[96] the static magnetic field of the MR system produced sufficient attraction of the ferromagnetic portion of the magnetic prosthesis to cause it to extrude through the tissue, thus injuring the patient.

Certain dental prosthetic appliances utilize magnetic forces to hold the implant in place.[95] The magnet may be contained within the prosthesis and attached to a ferromagnetic post implanted in the mandible or vise versa. An MR procedure may be performed safely in a patient with this type of dental magnetic appliance as long as it has been determined that it is properly attached to supporting tissue.[1,2]

Patients with hydrocephalus or other disorders, who are often treated with a percutaneous adjustable pressure valve, may have a magnetically activated component that allows a change to be made to the resistance required to open the valve.[1,2,88,91] This is accomplished by using an externally applied magnet. Pressure adjustable valves permit noninvasive readjustment of the opening pressure of an implanted shunt to cerebrospinal fluid hydrodynamics.

Changing the resistance of this type of valve by MR-induced dysfunction of this implant without recognizing it could cause problems, including acute hydrocephalus, for the patient. Currently, it is recommended that patients with the percutaneous adjustable pressure valves [e.g., the Sophy (Sophysa, Orsay, France) or Codman-Medos (Medos S.A., LeCocle, Switzerland) programmable valves] have the specific valve checked immediately before and after the MR procedure to determine if exposure to the MR system caused a change in the valve setting.

If a change occurred as a result of the MR procedure, the neurosurgeon or other individual responsible for the medical management of the patient and familiar with the operation of this type of device should be notified to reset the percutaneous adjustable pressure valve to its original setting. Fortunately, there are no known risks or hazards associated with the Sophy or Codman-Medos programmable valves with respect to movement, torque, or heating in the MR environment.[1,2,91]

An *in vitro* study conduced by Hunyadi et al.[97] assessed a new electromagnetic, semi-implantable, middle ear hearing device for MR safety in a 1.5-T environment. Five small, titanium-encased magnets and four solid titanium cylinders were cemented onto the incus of five preserved human temporal bones and two cadaver heads. They were all inserted into an MR system and evaluated for possible disruption.[97] The findings indicated that as a result of magnetic torque, three of the magnets on the temporal bone were disrupted from the incus. The two cylinders on the temporal bones and the two cylinders and two magnets on the whole heads were not affected.[97] Thus, the large torque associated with a 1.5-T MR system may disrupt the magnet–cement and cement–incus interfaces, causing dislodgement, such that MR procedures would be contraindicated in patients with this particular hearing device.[97]

XXIII. MISCELLANEOUS OBJECTS

Many different miscellaneous implants, materials, devices, and objects have been tested for safety in the MR environment.[1,2,98-104] Kanal and Shabaini[98] tested various types of firearms in the MR environment. Each firearm exhibited strong ferromagnetism, and two of the six discharged reproducibly. The authors concluded that a firearm in the MR environment should be unloaded before removal or any other manipulation of the firearm is attempted.[98]

Conventional surgical techniques that rely on direct viewing of the surgical field have several limitations, including the fact that the surgical exposures are typically larger than necessary (i.e., to provide the surgeon adequate room to assess the involved anatomy). Additionally, there may be the need to remove normal tissue to have access to deep targets.

Whereas the implementation of endoscopy has resulted in the ability to perform minimally invasive surgery, there are also limitations associated with this technique. The limitations are primarily due to the reduced visibility afforded by the relatively small field of view of the endoscope, such that there is impaired depth perception and an inability of the endoscopist to relate the visual field of the endoscope to the surrounding anatomy.

The performance of endoscopy in combination with MR guidance has been proposed to offer several advantages, including a dramatic improvement in the visualization and orientation of the endoscope, an ability to appreciate complex three-dimensional anatomy in immediate and remote anatomic areas, and a reduction in procedure-related morbidity. The lack of commercially available, MR-compatible medical devices and instruments has obviously hindered the widespread implementation of MR-guided procedures, particularly those involving the use of somewhat complicated instruments like endoscopes.

Commercially available endoscopes are constructed from materials that are ferromagnetic. Therefore, the use of these devices is restricted in the MR environment, primarily due to the associated substantial magnetic field attraction and production of large imaging artifacts (unpublished observations, F. G. Shellock, 1997). Obviously, the presence of a metallic medical device not only creates possible hazards for the patient undergoing the procedure, but also may produce problems for the physician using the instrument in the MR environment.

Recently, endoscopes and other support devices (Greatbatch Scientific, Clarence, NY) have been specially designed for use in the MR environment.[100] *Ex vivo* testing indicated that there were no apparent concerns of movement, excessive heating, or substantial artifacts that would prevent the safe and successful use of these devices for MR-guided endoscopic procedures.[100]

MR-guided biopsy, therapeutic, and minimally invasive surgical procedures are important clinical applications that are performed on conventional, open-architecture, or "double-donut" MR systems specially designed for this work. These procedures present challenges with regard to the instruments and devices that are needed to support these interventions. Metallic surgical instruments and other devices potentially pose hazards (e.g., "missile effects") or other problems (i.e., image distortion that can obscure the area of interest and either affect adequate visualization of the abnormality or prevent performance of the procedure) that must be addressed to apply MR-guided techniques effectively. Various manufacturers have used weakly ferromagnetic, nonferromagnetic, or nonmetallic materials to make special instruments for interventional MR procedures.[102] At least one manufacturer has used ceramic material as a means of constructing prototype devices that include scalpels, cranial drill bits, scissors, and tweezers which have been determined to be MR compatible.[101] Other manufacturers have developed surgical instruments made from a titanium alloy that are intended for use in MR-guided surgical procedures (Figure 14.18).

Ceramic instruments were shown to have particularly good qualities for the MR environment, insofar as there was no magnetic field attraction, negligible heating, and no substantial image distortion determined by the *ex vivo* testing techniques for this material.[101] Other medical products and devices have been developed with metallic components that are either entirely nonferromagnetic (e.g., stereotactic headframe, Compass International, Inc., Rochester, MN) or made from metals that are minimally attracted to the magnetic fields of MR systems.

XXIV. NEUROSTIMULATORS

The incidence of patients receiving implanted neurostimulators for treatment of various forms of neurological disorders is increasing. There are two basic types of neurostimulators:

1. *Passive receivers* — Neurostimulators that receive RF energy that is magnetically coupled from an external device by means of a coil placed over the implanted device.
2. *Hermetically encased pulsed generators* — Neurostimulators that contain a battery and are programmed by an external device to produce the various stimulus parameters.

Because of the specific design and intended function of neurostimulators, the electromagnetic fields used for MR procedures may produce problems with the operation of these devices.[1,2,105-107] Malfunction of a neurostimulator that results from exposure to the electromagnetic fields of an MR system may cause discomfort, pain, or injury to the patient. In extreme cases, damage to the nerve fibers at the site of the implanted electrodes of the neurostimulator may also occur. Therefore, the present policy regarding a patient with a neurostimulator is that the individual should not undergo an MR procedure unless testing has been conducted to define parameters and guidelines for the safe use of an MRI procedure for a given neurostimulator device.[1,2]

Currently, implantable pulse generators/neurostimulators are being used for suppression of upper extremity tremors in patients who are diagnosed with essential tremor or Parkinsonian tremor not adequately controlled by medications, or where the tremor constitutes a significant functional

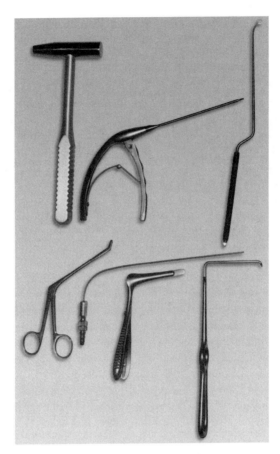

FIGURE 14.18 Examples of surgical instruments made from titanium alloy for use in MR-guided surgical procedures.

disability. For example, the Medtronic Activa Tremor Control System (Medtronic, Minneapolis, MN) is an implantable, multiprogrammable, quadripolar system that delivers electrical stimulation to the thalamus to control tremor. It is comprised of the Itrel II Model 7424 Implantable Pulse Generator (Medtronic) that has electronic circuitry and a battery, which are hermetically sealed in a titanium case. The operation of this device is supported by a console programmer and a control magnet (product information, Medtronic Neurological, Minneapolis, MN, 1997).

The product insert information for the Medtronic Activa Tremor Control System indicates that patients with this system should not be exposed to the electromagnetic fields produced by MRI. Besides possible dislodgment, heating, and induced voltages in the pulse generator and/or lead, an induced voltage through the pulse generator or lead may cause uncomfortable "jolting" or "shocking" levels of stimulation for the patient in the MR environment.[1]

There have been anecdotal reports from patients using deep brain stimulation for the treatment of chronic pain who have experienced speech problems, temporary sensation of visual light, dizziness, and nausea when exposed to MRI (product information, Medtronic Neurological, 1997). Due to the obvious associated problems, it is not recommended to perform MR procedures in patients with this or similar devices.

The neurostimulators ITREL II and ITREL III (Medtronic) underwent safety testing during MRI at 0.2, 0.25, and 1.5 T. While no apparent heating occurred, the reed switches of those devices were activated, altering the functional aspects of the neurostimulators. Furthermore, local electrical effects were not determined for those particular neurostimulators, indicating that additional MRI

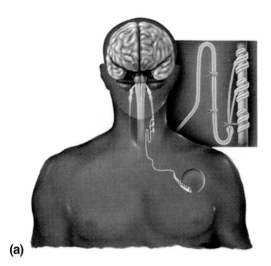
(a)

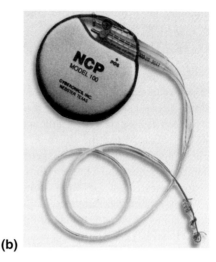
(b)

FIGURE 14.19 (a) VNS with the NCP system sends signals from the vagus nerve in the neck to the brain. (b) The NCP device is implanted in the chest and neck.

safety work remains to be conducted to assess other potential problems that may pose a risk to the patient undergoing MRI.

Vagus nerve stimulation (VNS) with the Cyberonics NeuroCybernetic Prosthesis System (NCP®, NeuroCybernetic Prosthesis System, Cyberonics, Houston, TX) is the first new approach to the treatment of epilepsy in over 100 years (Figure 14.19). After 15 years of research and clinical studies, VNS was approved by the FDA as an add-on therapy. This therapy reduces the frequency of seizures in adults and adolescents over 12 years of age with partial onset seizures that are refractory to antiepileptic medications. To date, over 3000 patients of all ages with a variety of seizure types have been treated by physicians at over 300 centers in the U.S. and Europe.

VNS consists of electrical signals that are applied to the vagus nerve in the neck for transmission to the brain. The vagus nerve averages 22 in. in length in adults and is located in the upper body. It is one of the primary communication lines from the major organs of the body to the brain. It has proven to be a good way for VNS to communicate with the brain because (1) there are few if any pain fibers in the vagus nerve, (2) over 80% of the electrical signals are applied to the vagus, (3) nerves in the neck are sent upwards to the brain, and (4) the stimulation lead may be attached to the vagus nerve in a surgical procedure which does not involve the brain and is not brain surgery.

The Model 100 NCP Pulse Generator is an implantable, multiprogrammable pulse generator that delivers electrical signals to the vagus nerve. Constant current, charge-balanced signals are transmitted from the generator to the vagus nerve via the NCP lead (Model 300 Series). The Model 100 NCP Pulse Generator is housed in a hermetically sealed titanium case. Feedthrough capacitors are used to filter electromagnetic interference from the pulse generator circuitry.

The major components and functions of the generator for this device are as follows: a microprocessor, a voltage regulator, a 76.8-kHz crystal oscillator, one antenna to transmit information and another antenna to receive information, communication circuitry, DC-DC voltage generation and control circuitry, constant-current control circuitry, a dual-pole magnetic reed switch for manual activation of the generator and for inhibition of the output pulses, and a lithium thionyl chloride cell to provide power for stimulation and circuit operation.

The lithium thionyl chloride battery chemistry has the low impedance and high energy density characteristics required for the rapid pulsing needed in peripheral nerve stimulation, and similar batteries have been previously used in cardiac pacemakers, implantable spinal cord stimulators, and implantable drug pumps. The implantable lead delivers electrical signals from the generator to the vagus nerve. The lead has two helical electrodes with a helical anchor tether for placement around the nerve and two 5-mm connectors for attachment to the generator.

The helix of the lead is available in two sizes of inner diameter (2 and 3 mm) to allow for an appropriate fit on different-sized nerves. The helical design is soft, pliable, and expands or contracts with changes in nerve diameter, which may occur immediately post-implant. These design features allow the 2-mm inside diameter helical electrode to fit most vagus nerves. The Model 300 NCP Bipolar Lead is insulated with silicone rubber and is bifurcated at each end. The lead wire is quadrifilar MP-35N, and the electrode is a platinum ribbon.

The Model 100 NCP Pulse Generator has a number of programmable settings that allow the physician to optimize the treatment for a patient. Those settings include pulse width, output current, signal frequency, signal ON time, signal OFF time, magnet-activated ON time, magnet-activated pulse width, and magnet-activated output current. Cyberonics provides a magnet that may be used to either manually initiate stimulation or to turn OFF the device.

The Model 100 NCP Pulse Generator has telemetry capability which supplies information about its operating characteristics, such as parameter settings, lead impedance, and history of magnet use. The generator has a number of characteristics intended to enhance operational reliability and safety, such as electromagnetic interference (EMI) filter capacitors, a series battery resistor to limit temperature rise in the event of short circuit, defibrillation protection diodes, DC-blocking capacitors on both leads that prevent DC from being applied to the patient, a software watchdog timer to prevent continuous stimulation, and protection against voltage dips on the battery that could disrupt microprocessor memory.

The neurostimulator, Model 100 NCP Pulse Generator, has received approval of an MR-safe labeling claim from the FDA, allowing MR procedures to be conducted in a patient with this device, as long as strict guidelines are followed. These guidelines are as follows (note: this information is from the product label, NeuroCybernetic Prosthesis, NCP Pulse Generator, Model 100, Cyberonics, Houston, TX, 1999):*

Magnetic resonance imaging (MRI) should not be performed with a magnetic resonance body coil in the transmit mode. The heat induced in the bipolar lead by an MRI body scan can cause injury.

If an MRI should be done, use only a transmit and receive type of head coil. Magnetic and radiofrequency (RF) fields produced by MRI may change the pulse generator settings (change to reset parameters) or activate the device. Stimulation has been shown to cause the adverse events reported in the "Adverse Events" section of this manual. MRI compatibility was demonstrated using a 1.5 T General Electric Signa Imager only. Testing on this imager as performed on a phantom indicated that the following pulse generator and MRI settings can be used safely without adverse events:

- Pulse Generator output programmed to 0 mA for the MR procedure, and afterward, retested by performing the Lead Test diagnostics and reprogrammed to the original settings.

- Head coil type: transmit and receive only

- Static magnetic field strength: ≤ 2.0 Tesla

- Specific-rate absorption (SAR): < 1.3 W/kg for a 154.5-lb (70-kg) patient

- Time-varying intensity: < 10 Tesla/sec

---

* The information for the NCP was provided by Gayle Nesom of Cyberonics and obtained from the Cyberonics Web site, 1999, www.cyberonics.com.

Use caution when other MRI systems are used, since adverse events may occur because of different magnetic field distributions.

No scan in which the radiofrequency (RF) is transmitted by the body coil should be done on a patient who has the NCP System. Thus, protocols must not be used which utilize local coils that are RF-receive only, with RF-transmit performed by the body coil. Note that some RF head coils are receive only, and that most other local coils, such as knee and spinal coils, are also RF-receive only. These coils must not be used in patients with the NCP System.

XXV. OCULAR IMPLANTS AND DEVICES

Of the different ocular implants and devices tested,[1,2,108-114] the Fatio eyelid spring, the retinal tack made from martensitic (i.e., ferromagnetic) stainless steel (Western European), the Troutman magnetic ocular implant, and the Unitek round wire eyelid spring exhibited magnetic field interactions in association with a 1.5-T MR system. The clips that have been tested for scleral buckling procedures have been shown to be safe for patients undergoing MR procedures at 1.5 T or less[114] (Figure 14.20).

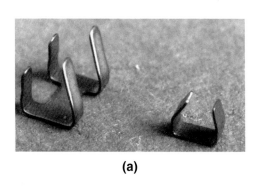

(a)

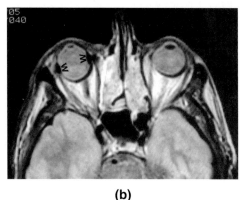

(b)

FIGURE 14.20 (a) Example of clips used for scleral buckling. These clips are made from nonferromagnetic materials and, therefore, are safe for patients undergoing MR procedures at 1.5 T or less. (b) MR image of the ocular area showing the presence of clips used for the scleral buckling procedure (arrowheads).

A patient with a Fatio eyelid spring or round wire eyelid spring may experience discomfort, but would probably not be injured as a result of exposure to the magnetic fields of an MR system (Figure 14.21). Patients have undergone MR procedures with eyelid wires after having a protective plastic covering placed around the globe along with a firmly applied eye patch. The retinal tack made from martensitic stainless steel and the Troutman magnetic ocular implant may injure a patient undergoing an MR procedure, although no such case has ever been reported.

XXVI. ORTHOPEDIC IMPLANTS, MATERIALS, AND DEVICES

Most of the orthopedic implants, materials, and devices evaluated for magnetic field interactions are made from nonferromagnetic materials and have been demonstrated to be safe for patients undergoing MR procedures[1,2,115-119] (Figure 14.22). Only the Perfix interference screw used for reconstruction of the anterior cruciate ligament has been found to be highly ferromagnetic.[119] Because this interference screw is firmly imbedded in bone for its specific application, it is held in place with sufficient force to prevent it from being moved or dislodged by magnetic field interactions.

The presence of the Perfix interference screw causes extensive image distortion during MRI of the knee. Therefore, one of the other nonferromagnetic interference screws that are commercially

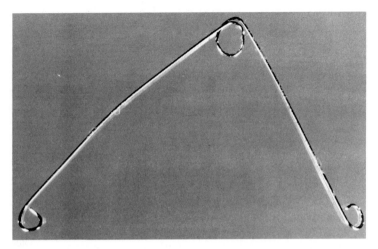

FIGURE 14.21 The Fatio eyelid wire. These implants may be composed of either gold or a ferromagnetic material. Patients with the Fatio eyelid spring made from ferromagnetic material should not undergo MR procedures because they may experience discomfort due to the attraction of this implant by the magnetic field.

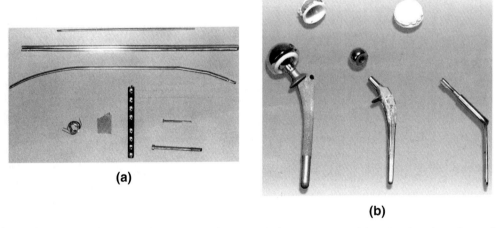

(a)

(b)

FIGURE 14.22 Examples of various metallic orthopedic implants and materials: (a) rods, wire, wire mesh, screws, and plate; (b) hip prostheses.

available should be used for reconstruction of the anterior cruciate ligament if MRI is to be utilized for subsequent evaluation of the knee.[119]

XXVII. OTOLOGIC IMPLANTS

The MR safety aspects of cochlear implants were discussed earlier in this chapter. For the remaining otologic implants that have been evaluated for MR safety,[120-124] the McGee stapedectomy piston prosthesis (Richards Medical Co., Memphis, TN), made from platinum and a stainless steel alloy, is ferromagnetic. This particular otologic implant has been recalled by the manufacturer, and any patient that has received this device has been issued a warning to avoid the MR environment. The specific item and lot numbers of the McGee implants that were recalled and considered to be contraindicated for MR procedures are as follows (personal communication, Winston Geer, Smith & Nephew Richards Inc., Barlett, TN, 1995):

Item No.	Lot No:
14-0330	1W91100, 4U09690
14-0331	4U09700
14-0332	1W91110, 4U58540, 4U86300
14-0333	4U09710, 1W34390, 2WR4073
14-0334	4U09720, 1W34390, 2WR4073
14-0335	1W34400, 4U09730
14-0336	3U18350, 3U50470, 4UR2889
14-0337	3U18370, 4UR2889
14-0338	3U18390, 4U02900, 4UR1453
14-0339	3U18400, 3U50500
14-0340	3U18410, 3U50500
14-0341	3U41200, 4UR2889

In consideration of the fact that there is at least one otologic implant that is potentially hazardous for individuals in the MR environment, it is proper to screen all patients with regard to otologic implants.[1,2]

XXVIII. PATENT DUCTUS ARTERIOSUS (PDA), ATRIAL SEPTAL DEFECT (ASD), AND VENTRICULAR SEPTAL DEFECT (VSD) OCCLUDERS

Metallic cardiac occluders are implants used to treat patients with PDA, ASD, or VSD heart conditions. As long as the proper size of the occluder is used, the amount of retention provided by the folded-back, hinged arms of the device is sufficient to keep it in place, acutely. Eventually, tissue growth covers the cardiac occluder and facilitates retention.

The metallic PDA, ASD, and VSD occluders that have been tested for MR safety were made from either 304V stainless steel or MP35N.[125] The occluders made from 304V stainless steel were weakly ferromagnetic, whereas those made from MP35N were nonferromagnetic in association with a 1.5-T MR system.[125] Thus, patients with cardiac occluders made from MP35N (i.e., a nonferromagnetic alloy) may undergo MR procedures any time after placement of these implants. Patients with cardiac occluders made from 304V stainless steel may undergo MR procedures approximately 6 weeks after placement of these devices to allow tissue ingrowth to provide additional retentive force.

XXIX. PELLETS AND BULLETS

The majority of pellets and bullets tested for MR safety are composed of nonferromagnetic materials.[1,126-128] Ammunition that proved to be ferromagnetic tended to be manufactured in foreign countries and/or used for military applications. Because pellets, bullets, and shrapnel may be contaminated with ferromagnetic materials, the risk vs. the benefit of performing an MR procedure in a patient should be carefully considered. Additional consideration should be given as to whether or not the metallic object is located near a vital anatomic structure, with the assumption that the object is likely to be ferromagnetic.[1,2] Shrapnel typically contains steel and, therefore, presents a potential hazard for patients undergoing MR procedures.

In an effort to reduce lead poisoning in puddling type ducks, the federal government requires many areas of the eastern U.S. to use steel shotgun pellets instead of lead. The presence of steel shotgun pellets presents a potential hazard to patients undergoing MR procedures and causes severe imaging artifacts at the immediate position of these metallic objects.

In one case, a small metallic BB located in a subcutaneous site caused painful symptoms in a patient exposed to the magnetic fields of the MR system. In consideration of this information, MR users should exercise caution whenever deciding to perform MR procedures in patients with pellets, bullets, shrapnel, or any other similar ballistic objects.

An investigation by Smugar et al.[126] was conducted to determine whether neurologic problems developed in patients with intraspinal bullets or bullet fragments in association with MRI performed at 1.5 T. Patients were queried during scanning for symptoms of discomfort or pain or for changes in neurologic status. Additionally, detailed neurologic examinations were performed prior to MRI, post-MRI, and at the patients' discharge. Based on the findings, Smugar et al.[126] concluded that patients with a complete spinal chord injury may undergo MRI if they have intraspinal bullets or fragments without concern for affecting their physical or neurological status. Thus, metallic fragments in the spinal canals of paralyzed patients represent only a relative contraindication to MR procedures.

XXX. PENILE IMPLANTS

Several different types of penile implants and prostheses have been evaluated for MR safety[1,2,129] (Figure 14.23). Of these, two of them [i.e., the Duraphase and OmniPhase models (Dacomed Corp., Minneapolis, MN)] demonstrated substantial magnetic field interactions when exposed to a 1.5-T static magnetic field of an MR system. Nevertheless, it is unlikely that a penile implant would severely injure a patient undergoing an MR procedure because of the relative strength of the magnetic field interactions associated with a 1.5-T MR system. This is especially the case considering the manner in which this type of device is utilized. However, it would undoubtedly be uncomfortable for the patient to undergo an examination using an MR system. For this reason, subjecting a patient with one of these penile implants to an MR procedure is inadvisable.[1,2]

XXXI. RETAINED CARDIAC PACING WIRES AND TEMPORARY CARDIAC PACING WIRES

A patient referred for an MR procedure may have temporary cardiac pacing wires retained after cardiac surgery or may have cardiac pacing wires that are not permanently connected to a pulse generator (e.g., for periodic treatment of bradycardia)[1,2] (Figure 14.24). Careful consideration must be given to these cases prior to performance of an MR procedure.[1,2,130,131] A study by Hartnell et al.[130] reported that patients with retained temporary epicardial pacing wires cut short at the skin (i.e., after they were no longer used post-surgically) did not experience any changes in baseline electrocardiographic rhythms or any symptoms during MR procedures.

The investigation by Hartnell et al.[130] is of particular importance because the presence of retained pacing wires was previously considered to be a relative contraindication for MR procedures due to the theoretical risk of inducing current which, in turn, could produce arrhythmias in patients. Notably, the study by Hartnell et al.[130] utilized 1.0- and 1.5-T MR systems operating with conventional pulse sequences. Therefore, it would be prudent to use similar MR techniques and parameters as this investigation for patients with temporary pacing wires until additional investigations are conducted.

XXXII. TATTOOS, PERMANENT COSMETICS, AND EYE MAKEUP

Before undergoing an MR procedure, the patient should be asked if he or she has ever had any type of permanent coloring technique (i.e., tattooing) applied to any part of the body.[1,2] This includes cosmetic applications such as eyeliner, lip-liner, lip coloring, as well as decorative designs.[1,2,132-137] This question is necessary because of the associated imaging artifacts and, more importantly, because a small number of patients (fewer than ten) have experienced transient skin irritation, cutaneous swelling, or heating sensations at the site of the permanent colorings in

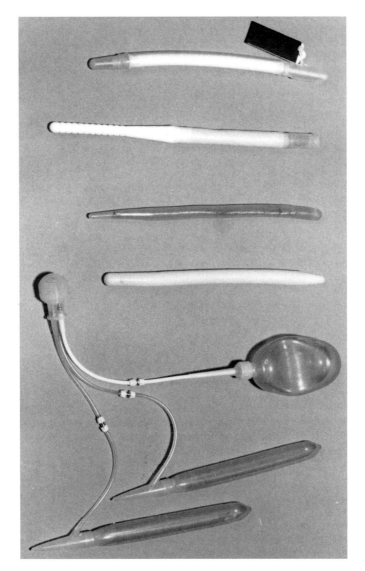

FIGURE 14.23 Examples of penile implants.

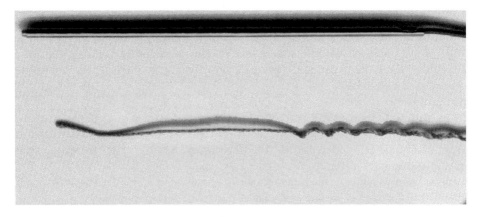

FIGURE 14.24 Examples of temporary pacing wires.

association with MR procedures. With regard to permanent cosmetics, when one considers the many millions of clinical MR procedures that have been conducted in patients over the past 18 years, and that only a few individuals have had difficulties related to the presence of permanent coloring, it is apparent that tattoo-related problems have an extremely low rate of occurrence and relatively minor consequences.

More recently, there has been one anecdotal report of a patient undergoing MRI who complained of a burning sensation at the site where a large tattoo had been applied on his arm using a black pigment. Additionally, Vahlensieck[133] reported tattoo-related cutaneous inflammation (first degree burn) in a patient in association with an MR procedure performed in a 0.5-T MR system.

Investigation of the incidents revealed that there was a tendency for the problem to occur whenever pigments that contained iron oxide or other similar ferromagnetic substance(s) were used. This includes those pigments that are especially black or blue in color. Supposedly, certain ferrous pigments used for the tattooing process can interact with the electromagnetic fields used for MR procedures, producing the reported problems.

A recent case report by Kreidstein et al.[134] indicated that a 24-year-old patient experienced a sudden burning pain at the site of a decorative tattoo while undergoing an MR procedure on the lumbar spine using a 1.5-T MR system. Swelling and erythema was resolved within 12 h, with no evident permanent sequela. To permit completion of the MR examination, an excision of the tattooed skin with primary closure of the site was performed (134). Apparently, the tattoo pigment used in this case was ferromagnetic, accounting for the symptoms experienced by the patient.

Of note is that the authors of this report wrote, "Theoretically, the application of a pressure dressing of the tattoo may prevent any tissue distortion due to ferromagnetic pull."[134] However, this was not attempted for this patient. They also indicated, "In some cases, removal of the tattoo may be the most practical means of allowing MRI."[134] In response to this unfortunate incident, Kanal and Shellock[135] commented in a letter to the editor that the reaction to this problem was "rather aggressive." Clearly, the trauma, expense, and morbidity associated with excision of the tattoo far exceed those that may be associated with ferromagnetic tattoo interactions.

The demonstration of grossly detectable ferromagnetic characteristics of a tattoo is not new and has been well known for over a decade. Certainly, the painful sensation experienced by the patient could not be considered a serious adverse event nor warrant the excision of the tattoo, particularly in consideration of the existence of other imaging modalities that could be used to assess the lumbar spine (computed tomography, myelography, etc.).

Kanal and Shellock[135] further recommended the following procedures to prevent potential problems associated with a similar incident:

1. Bandage the area with a pressure dressing and immobilize the tattooed skin with sufficient force to prevent motion of the skin upon exposure to the static magnetic field of the MR system.
2. In the very rare instance where a patient reports ferromagnetic discomfort or pain, have the patient approach the MR system in a manner to minimize both translational and rotational forces by orienting the patient's tattoo parallel to the magnetic lines of force associated with the MR system.

Any problem performing an MR procedure in a patient that has a tattoo is unlikely to prevent the examination, since the important diagnostic information that is provided by this imaging modality is typically critical to the care of the patient. If a patient with a tattoo requires an MR procedure, the individual should be informed of the relatively minor risk associated with the site of the permanent coloring application. In addition, the patient should be requested to advise the MR operator regarding any unusual sensations felt at the site of the tattoo during the MR examination.

Patients with tattoos located on extremities or peripheral sites should be positioned in the MR system to avoid direct contact with the body coil or surface coils (e.g., foam rubber pads may be placed in between the site of the tattoo and the coil) to minimize the potential problem. Similar to other patients undergoing MR procedures, patients with tattoos should be closely monitored using visual and auditory means throughout the entire operation of the MR system to ensure their safety.

With respect to eye makeup, patients may develop eye irritation if the makeup, which may contain ferromagnetic particles, becomes displaced from the eyelid into the eye during exposure to the MR system. Therefore, it is necessary to inform individuals with certain types of eye makeup about the potential problems related to the presence of eye makeup and request that they remove it (if appropriate) before undergoing the MR procedure.

XXXIII. TRANSDERMAL PATCHES

There have been several anecdotal reports pertaining to patients undergoing MR procedures who experienced heating in association with wearing drug delivery systems that involve transdermal "patch" techniques (e.g., for administration of nitroglycerine, nicotine, or other similar medication). Apparently, the metallic components of these devices can be heated during MR procedures.

In one reported case, a Deponit (nitroglycerin transdermal delivery system; Shwarz Pharma, Milwaukee, WI) patch, which contains an aluminum component, was worn by a patient during MRI. The metallic component of this patch is nonferromagnetic and, therefore, not attracted to the static magnetic field of an MR system. However, the patient wearing this patch received a second-degree burn during MRI performed using standard pulse sequences and conventional imaging procedures (personal communication, Robert E. Mucha, Schwarz Pharma, 1995). This potentially occurred due to the conductive qualities of the metal component of this transdermal patch.

In consideration of the above, it is recommended that any patient using the Deponit or similar transdermal delivery system with a metallic component have the patch removed prior to the MR procedure. A new patch should be applied after the examination is completed (personal communication, Robert E. Mucha, Schwarz Pharma, 1995). The patient's physician should be contacted prior to removing the transdermal patch to obtain proper information related to the proper administration of any transdermal patch medication that is dispensed by a prescription.

XXXIV. VASCULAR ACCESS PORTS AND CATHETERS

Vascular access ports and catheters are devices that are commonly used to provide long-term vascular administration of chemotherapeutic agents, antibiotics, analgesics, and other medications. Vascular access ports are implanted typically in a subcutaneous pocket over the upper chest wall, with the catheters inserted either in the jugular, subclavian, or cephalic vein. Smaller vascular access ports, which are less obtrusive and tend to be tolerated better, have also been designed for implantation in the arms of children or adults, with vascular access via an antecubital vein.

Vascular access ports have a variety of inherent features (e.g., a reservoir, central septum, and catheter) and are constructed from various types of materials, including stainless steel, titanium, silicone, and various forms of plastic. Because of the widespread use of vascular access ports and associated catheters and the high probability that patients with these devices may require MR procedures, it was necessary to determine the MR safety aspects of these implants.[1,2,138,139]

Three of the implantable vascular access ports and catheters evaluated for safety with the MR environment showed measurable attraction to the static magnetic fields of the MR systems used for testing, but the forces were considered to be minor relative to the *in vivo* application of these implants.[138,139] Therefore, an MR procedure may be performed safely in a patient that has one of the vascular access ports that has been tested and reported in the peer-reviewed literature.

With respect to MRI and artifacts, vascular access ports will generally produce the least amount of artifact in association with MRI if made entirely from nonmetallic materials. Alternatively, the ones that produce the greatest amount of artifact are composed of metal(s) or have metal in an unusual shape.

Some manufacturers of vascular access ports have decided to make devices entirely from nonmetallic materials under the assumption that this is required for the device to be MRI compatible. In fact, several manufacturers have produced brochures that state that their devices allow "distortion free imaging" or "will not obscure important structures" during MRI.

In one marketing brochure, an MR image is shown that is color-enhanced such that the artifact caused by a "competitors" metallic vascular access port appears to be inordinately large, whereas the manufacturer's plastic vascular access port caused essentially no distortion of the image (unpublished observations, F.G. Shellock, 1994).

This misrepresents the actual MRI compatibility issue and promotes a marketing claim that is without support from a diagnostic MRI standpoint. Even the so-called MRI compatible or "MRI ports" made entirely from nonmetallic materials are, in fact, seen on the MR images because they contain silicone. The septum portion of each of the vascular access ports typically is made from silicone. Using MRI, the Larmor precessional frequency of fat is close to that of silicone (i.e., 100 Hz at 1.5 T). Therefore, silicone used in the construction of vascular access ports may be observed on MR images with varying degrees of signal intensity depending on the pulse sequence selected for imaging.

Manufacturers of nonmetallic vascular access ports have not addressed this finding during advertising and marketing of their products. On the contrary, vascular access ports made from nonmetallic materials are claimed to be MRI compatible and "invisible" on MR images. However, if a radiologist did not know that this type of vascular access port was present in a patient, the MR signal produced by the silicone component of the device could be considered an abnormality or, at the very least, present a confusing image.[138,139] For example, this may present a diagnostic problem in a patient being evaluated for a rupture of a silicone breast implant, because silicone from the vascular access port may be misread as an "extracapsular silicone implant rupture."

In more general terms, it is improbable that an artifact produced by the presence of a metallic vascular access port will detract from the diagnostic capabilities of MRI. Notably, the extent of the artifact is relatively minor and, as such, is unlikely to obscure any important anatomical structures by its presence. MRI examinations of the chest, where most vascular access ports are typically implanted in a subcutaneous pocket, account for less than 5% of diagnostic studies performed using this imaging modality.

Finally, an important issue related to the construction of vascular access ports should be discussed. Metal typically is used to make these devices to guard against piercing of the injection site by repetitive insertions of needles used to refill the reservoir. Additionally, repeated needle access of a plastic reservoir compared to a metal reservoir may perturb the functional integrity and long-term durability of the vascular access port. This could result in embolization by fragmented plastic pieces or a reduced ability to properly flush the vascular access port. Therefore, vascular access ports with reservoirs made from metal or other similar hard material may, in fact, be more acceptable for use in a patient compared to those made from plastic.

XXXV. IMPLANTABLE, PROGRAMMABLE INFUSION PUMP

The implantable, programmable infusion pump (SynchroMed® Infusion System, SynchroMed EL Infusion System, Medtronic Inc., Minneapolis, MN) is an important therapeutic device. This implant has two parts that are both placed in the body during a surgical procedure: the catheter and the pump (Figure 14.25). The catheter is a small, soft tube. One end is connected to the pump, and the other is placed in the intrathecal space (where fluid flows around the spinal cord).

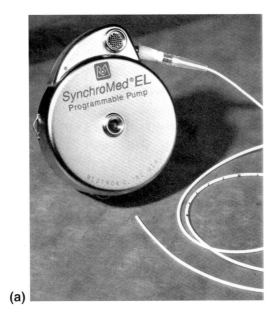

(a)

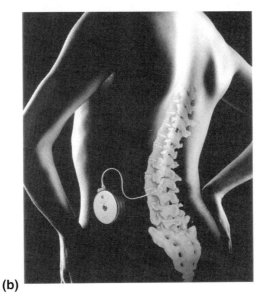

(b)

FIGURE 14.25 The programmable, implantable infusion pump (SynchroMed EL Infusion System), used for automatic delivery of drug therapy (a). This device is surgically placed under the skin of the abdomen to deliver medication directly into the intrathecal space (b).

The pump is a round metal device that stores and releases prescribed amounts of medication directly into the intrathecal space. It is about 1 in. (2.5 cm) thick, 3 in. (8.5 cm) in diameter, and weighs about 6 oz (205 g). This device is made of titanium, a light-weight, medical-grade metal.

The reservoir is the space inside the pump that holds the medication. The fill port is a raised center portion of the pump through which the pump is refilled. The physician or nurse inserts a needle through the patient's skin and through the fill port to fill the pump. Some pumps have a side catheter access port that allows the physician to inject other medications or sterile solutions directly into the catheter, bypassing the pump.

A. MRI SAFETY INFORMATION

Exposure to the MR system and MRI procedure will temporarily stop the rotor of the pump motor due to the magnetic field of the MR system and suspend drug infusion for the duration of the MRI exposure. The pump should resume normal operation upon termination of the MRI exposure.

Prior to MRI, the physician should determine if the patient can safely be deprived of drug delivery. If the patient cannot be safely deprived of drug delivery, alternative delivery methods for the drug can be utilized during the time required for the MRI scan.

If there is concern that depriving the patient of drug delivery may be unsafe for the patient during the MRI procedure, medical supervision should be provided while the MRI procedure is conducted. Prior to scheduling an MRI scan and upon completion of the MRI scan, or shortly thereafter, the pump status should be confirmed using the SynchroMed programmer. In the unlikely event that any change to the pump status has occurred, a "pump memory error" message will be displayed and the pump will sound a pump memory error alarm (double tone).

Testing conducted on the SynchroMed pump has established the following with regard to other MR safety issues.

Tissue Heating Adjacent to Implant During MRI Scans — Specific Absorption Rate (SAR): The presence of the pump can potentially cause a twofold increase of the local temperature rise in tissues near the pump.

During a 20-min pulse sequence in a 1.5-T GE Signa Scanner with a whole-body average SAR of 1.0 W/kg, a temperature rise of 1°C in a static phantom was observed near the pump implanted in the "abdomen" of the phantom. The temperature rise in a static phantom represents a worst case for physiological temperature rise, and the 20-min scan time is representative of a typical imaging session. FDA MRI guidance allows a physiological temperature rise of up to 2°C in the torso; therefore, the local temperature rise in the phantom is considered by FDA guidance to be below the level of concern. Implanting the pump more lateral to the midline of the abdomen may result in higher temperature rises in tissues near the pump. In the unlikely event that the patient experiences uncomfortable warmth near the pump, the MRI scan should be stopped and the scan parameters adjusted to reduce the SAR to comfortable levels.

Peripheral Nerve Stimulation During MRI Scans — Time-Varying Gradient Magnetic Fields: The presence of the pump may potentially cause a twofold increase of the induced electric field in tissues near the pump. With the pump implanted in the abdomen, using pulse sequences that have dB/dt up to 20 T/s, the measured induced electric field near the pump is below the threshold necessary to cause stimulation.

In the unlikely event that the patient reports stimulation during the scan, the proper procedure is the same as for patients without implants: stop the MRI scan and adjust the scan parameters to reduce the potential for nerve stimulation.

Static Magnetic Field: For magnetic fields up to 1.5 T, the magnetic force and torque on the SynchroMed pump will be less than the force and torque due to gravity.

For magnetic fields of 2.0 T, the patient may experience a slight tugging sensation at the pump implant site. An elastic garment or wrap will prevent the pump from moving and reduce the sensation the patient may experience. SynchroMed pump performance has not been established in >2.0-T MR scanners, and it is not recommended that patients have MRI using these scanners.

Image Distortion: The SynchroMed pump contains ferromagnetic components that will cause image distortion and image dropout in areas around the pump. The severity of image artifact is dependent on the MR pulse sequence used. For spin echo pulse sequences, the area of significant image artifact may be 20 to 25 cm across. Images of the head or lower extremities should be largely unaffected.

Minimizing Image Distortion: MR image artifacts may be minimized by careful choice of pulse sequence parameters and location of the angle and the imaging plane. However, the reduction in image distortion obtained by adjustment of pulse sequence parameters will usually be at a cost in the signal-to-noise ratio. The following general principles should be followed.

1. Use imaging sequences with stronger gradients for both slice and read encoding directions. Employ higher bandwidth for both RF pulse and data sampling.
2. Choose an orientation for read-out axis that minimizes the appearance of in-plane distortion.
3. Use spin echo (SE) or gradient echo (GE) MRI sequences with a relatively high data sampling bandwidth.
4. Use shorter echo time (TE) for GE techniques whenever possible.
5. Be aware that the actual imaging slice shape can be curved in space due to the presence of the field disturbance of the pump (as stated above, this is image distortion).
6. Identify the location of the implant in the patient, and when possible, orient all imaging slices away from the implanted pump.

XXXVI. IMPLANTS AND DEVICES: THE PREVENTION OF BURNS

Various types of devices or objects (e.g., monitoring devices, surface coils, etc.) may present a risk or hazard to the patient in the MR environment as a result of excessive heat that may develop in the object during the MR procedure.[1,2,140–149] Notably, first-, second-, and third-degree burns have occurred in patients undergoing MR procedures as a result of misinformation, misuse of implants or devices (including monitoring systems and surface RF coils), and defective devices. Recommendations for protection of the patient from excessive heating or burns related to induced current or other conditions that may develop during an MR procedure include the following:[1,2,142]

1. Only perform MR procedures in patients with implants that have been thoroughly assessed for heating associated with the MR environment.
2. Use only devices and monitoring equipment that have been thoroughly tested and determined to be safe for patients during MR procedures.
3. Allow only properly trained individuals to operate devices and monitoring equipment and to be responsible for the patient in the MR environment.
4. Before using the device or equipment, check the integrity of the electrical insulation of the components or accessories of the device, including monitoring leads, cables, and wires. Preventive maintenance should be practiced routinely.
5. Remove all electrically conductive material that is not required for the procedure (i.e., unused surface coils, cables, etc.) from the bore of the MR system.
6. Keep electrically conductive material that must remain in the bore of the MR system from directly contacting the patient by placing thermal and/or electrical insulation (including air) between the conductive material and the patient.
7. Keep the electrically conductive material(s) (e.g., ECG leads, cables, wires, etc.) that must remain within the bore of the MR system from forming large diameter, conductive loops. Remember, the patient's tissue is conductive and, therefore, may be involved in the formation of the conductive loop.
8. Position all cables to prevent "cross points." A cross point is the point where a cable crosses another cable, where a cable loops across itself, or where a cable touches either the patient or sides of the magnet bore more than once. Note that loops can be closed, U shaped, or S shaped.
9. Position all cables and wires so that they exit as close as possible to the center of the table of the MR system.

28. Lufkin, R., Teresi, L., and Hanafee, W., New needle for MR-guided aspiration cytology of the head and neck, *Am. J. Roentgenol.*, 149, 380, 1987.
29. Moscatel, M., Shellock, F. G., and Morisoli, S., Biopsy needles and devices: assessment of ferromagnetism and artifacts during exposure to a 1.5 Tesla MR system, *J. Magn. Reson. Imaging*, 5, 369, 1995.
30. Shellock, F. G. and Shellock, V. J., Additional information pertaining to the MR-compatibility of biopsy needles and devices, *J. Magn. Reson. Imaging*, 6, 411, 1996.
31. Shellock, F. G. and Shellock, V. J., Metallic marking clips used after stereotactic breast biopsy: ex vivo testing of ferromagnetism, heating, and artifacts associated with MRI, *Am. J. Roentgenol.*, 172, 1417, 1999.
32. Shellock, F. G., Hatfield, M., Simon, B. J., Block, S., Wamboldt, J., Starewicz, P. M., and Punchard, W. F. B., Implantable spinal fusion stimulator: assessment of MRI safety, *J. Magn. Reson. Imaging*, 12, 214, 2000.
33. Chou, C.-K., McDougall, J. A., and Chan, K. W., RF heating of implanted spinal fusion stimulator during magnetic resonance imaging, *IEEE Trans. Biomed. Eng.*, 44, 357, 1997.
34. Liang, M. D., Narayanan, K., and Kanal, E., Magnetic ports in tissue expanders: a caution for MRI, *Magn. Reson. Imaging*, 7, 541, 1989.
35. Achenbach, S., Moshage, W., Diem, B., Bieberle, T., Schibgilla, V., and Bachmann, K., Effects of magnetic resonance imaging on cardiac pacemakers and electrodes, *Am. Heart J.*, 134, 467, 1997.
36. Alagona, P., Toole, J., C., Maniscalco, B. S., et al., Nuclear magnetic resonance imaging in a patient with a DDD pacemaker [Letter], *Pacing Clin. Electrophysiol.*, 12, 619, 1989.
37. Bonnet, C. A., Elson, J. J., and Fogoros, R. N., Accidental deactivation of the automatic implantable cardioverter defibrillator, *Am. Heart J.*, 3, 696, 1990.
38. Erlebacher, J. A., Cahill, P. T., Pannizzo, F., et al., Effect of magnetic resonance imaging on DDD pacemakers, *Am. J. Cardiol.*, 57, 437, 1986.
39. Gimbel, J. R., Johnson, D., Levine, P. A., and Wilkoff, B. L., Safe performance of magnetic resonance imaging on five patients with permanent cardiac pacemakers, *Pacing Clin. Electrophysiol.*, 19, 913, 1996.
40. Gangarosa, R. E., Minnis, J. E., Nobbe, J., et al., Operational safety issues in MRI, *Magn. Reson. Imaging*, 5, 287, 1987.
41. Garcia-Bolao, I., Albaladejo, V., Benito, A., Alegria, E., and Zubieta, J. L., Magnetic resonance imaging in a patients with a dual-chamber pacemaker, *Acta Cardiol.*, 53, 33, 1998.
42. Hayes, D. L., Holmes, D. R., and Gray, J. E., Effect of a 1.5 Tesla magnetic resonance imaging scanner on implanted permanent pacemakers, *J. Am. Coll. Cardiol.*, 10, 782, 1987.
43. Holmes, D. R., Hayes, D. L, Gray, J. E., et al., The effects of magnetic resonance imaging on implantable pulse generators, *Pacing Clin. Electrophysiol.*, 9, 360, 1986.
44. Pavlicek, W., Geisinger, M., Castle, L., et al., The effects of nuclear magnetic resonance on patients with cardiac pacemakers, *Radiology*, 147, 49, 1983.
45. Shellock, F. G., O'Neil, M., Ivans, V., Kelly, D., O'Connor, M., Toay, L., and Crues, J. V., Cardiac pacemakers and implantable cardiac defibrillators are unaffected by operation of an extremity MR system, *Am. J. Roentgenol.*, 72, 165, 1999.
46. Sommer, T., Valhous, C., Lauck, G., von Smekal, A., Reinke, M., Hofer, U., Block, W., et al., MR imaging and cardiac pacemakers: in vitro evaluation and in vivo studies in 51 patients at 0.5 T, *Radiology*, 215, 869, 2000.
47. Zimmermann, B. H. and Faul, D. D., Artifacts and hazards in NMR imaging due to metal implants and cardiac pacemakers, *Diagn. Imaging Clin. Med.*, 53, 53, 1984.
48. Shellock, F. G. and Shellock, V. J., Cardiovascular catheters and accessories: ex vivo testing of ferromagnetism, heating, and artifacts associated with MRI, *J. Magn. Reson. Imaging*, 8, 1338, 1998.
49. Teitelbaum, G. P., Lin, M. C. W., Watanabe, A. T., et al., Ferromagnetism and MR imaging: safety of cartoid vascular clamps, *Am. J. Neuroradiol.*, 11, 267, 1990.
50. Chou, H.-K., McDougall, J. A., and Can, K. W., Absence of radiofrequency heating from auditory implants during magnetic resonance imaging, *Bioelectromagnetics*, 16, 307, 1995.
51. Heller, J. W., Brackmann, D. E., Tucci, D. L., Nyenhuis, J. A., and Chou, H.-K., Evaluation of MRI compatibility of the modified nucleus multi-channel auditory brainstem and cochlear implants, *Am. J. Otol.*, 17, 724, 1996.

52. Ouayoun, M., Dupuch, K., Aitbenamou, C., and Chouard, C. H., Nuclear magnetic resonance and cochlear implant, *Ann. Oto-Laryngol. Chir. Cervico-Fac.*, 114, 65, 1997.

53. Teissl, C., Kremser, C., Hochmair, E. S., and Hochmair-Desoyer, I. J., Cochlear implants: in vitro investigation of electromagnetic interference at MR imaging-compatibility and safety aspects, *Radiology*, 208, 700, 1998.

54. Teissl, C., Kremser, C., Hochmair, E. S., and Hochmair-Desoyer, I. J., Magnetic resonance imaging and cochlear implants: compatibility and safety aspects, *J. Magn. Reson. Imaging*, 9, 26, 1999.

55. Girard, M. J., Hahn, P., Saini, S., Dawson, S. L., Goldberg, M. A., and Mueller, P. R., Wallstent metallic biliary endoprosthesis: MR imaging characteristics, *Radiology*, 184, 874, 1992.

56. Kiproff, P. M., Deeb, D. L., Contractor, F. M., and Khoury, M. B., Magnetic resonance characteristics of the LGM vena cava filter: technical note, *Cardiovasc. Intervent. Radiol.*, 14, 254, 1991.

57. Leibman, C. E., Messersmith, R. N., Levin, D. N., et al., MR imaging of inferior vena caval filter: safety and artifacts, *Am. J. Roentgenol.*, 150, 1174, 1988.

58. Marshall, M. W., Teitelbaum, G. P., Kim, H. S., et al., Ferromagnetism and magnetic resonance artifacts of platinum embolization microcoils, *Cardiovasc. Intervent. Radiol.*, 14, 163, 1991.

59. Shellock, F. G., Detrick, M. S., and Brant-Zawadski, M., MR-compatibility of the Guglielmi detachable coils, *Radiology*, 203, 568, 1997.

60. Shellock, F. G. and Shellock, V. J., Stents: evaluation of MRI safety, *Am. J. Roentgenol.*, 173, 543, 1999.

61. Teitelbaum, G. P., Bradley, W. G., and Klein, B. D., MR imaging artifacts, ferromagnetism, and magnetic torque of intravascular filters, stents, and coils, *Radiology*, 166, 657, 1988.

62. Teitelbaum, G. P., Lin, M. C. W., Watanabe, A. T., et al., Ferromagnetism and MR imaging: safety of cartoid vascular clamps, *Am. J. Neuroradiol.*, 11, 267, 1990.

63. Teitelbaum, G. P., Ortega, H. V., Vinitski, S., et al., Low artifact intravascular devices: MR imaging evaluation, *Radiology*, 168, 713, 1988.

64. Teitelbaum, G. P., Raney, M., Carvlin, M. J., et al., Evaluation of ferromagnetism and magnetic resonance imaging artifacts of the Strecker tantalum vascular stent, *Cardiovasc. Intervent. Radiol.*, 12, 125, 1989.

65. Watanabe, A. T., Teitelbaum, G.P., Gomes, A. S., et al., MR imaging of the bird's nest filter, *Radiology*, 177, 578, 1990.

66. Shellock, F. G. and Shellock, V. J., Evaluation of cranial flap fixation clamps for compatibility with MR imaging, *Radiology*, 207, 822, 1998.

67. Gegauff, A., Laurell, K. A., Thavendrarajah, A., et al., A potential MRI hazard: forces on dental magnet keepers, *J. Oral Rehabil.*, 17, 403, 1990.

68. Lissac, M. I., Metrop, D., Brugigrad, B., et al., Dental materials and magnetic resonance imaging, *Invest. Radiol.*, 26, 40, 1991.

69. Shellock, F. G., Ex vivo assessment of deflection forces and artifacts associated with high-field strength MRI of "mini-magnet" dental prostheses, *Magn. Reson. Imaging*, 7(Suppl. 1), 38, 1989.

70. Shellock, F. G., MRI and ECG electrodes, *Signals*, 29, 10, 1999.

71. Ballock, R. T., Hajed, P. C., Byrne, T. P., et al., The quality of magnetic resonance imaging, as affected by the composition of the halo orthosis, *J. Bone Joint Surg.*, 71-A, 431, 1989.

72. Clayman, D. A., Murakami, M. E., and Vines, F. S., Compatibility of cervical spine braces with MR imaging. A study of nine nonferrous devices, *Am. J. Neuroradiol.*, 11, 385, 1990.

73. Hartwell, C. G. and Shellock, F. G., MRI of cervical fixation devices: sensation of heating caused by vibration of metallic components, *J. Magn. Reson. Imaging*, 7, 771, 1997.

74. Hua, J. and Fox, R. A., Magnetic resonance imaging of patients wearing a surgical traction halo, *J. Magn. Reson. Imaging*, 1, 264, 1996.

75. Malko, J. A., Hoffman, J. C., and Jarrett, P. J., Eddy-current-induced artifacts caused by an "MR-compatible" halo device, *Radiology*, 173, 563, 1989.

76. Shellock, F. G., MR imaging and cervical fixation devices: assessment of ferromagnetism, heating, and artifacts, *Magn. Reson. Imaging*, 14, 1093, 1996.

77. Shellock, F. G. and Slimp, G., Halo vest for cervical spine fixation during MR imaging, *Am. J. Roentgenol.*, 154, 631, 1990.

78. Frank, H., Buxbaum, P., Huber, L., et al., In vitro behavior of mechanical heart valves in 1.5 T superconducting magnet, *Eur. J. Radiol.*, 2, 555, 1992.

79. Hassler, M., Le Bas, J. F., Wolf, J. E., et al., Effects of magnetic fields used in MRI on 15 prosthetic heart valves, *J. Radiol.,* 67, 661, 1986.
80. Randall, P. A., Kohman, L. J., Scalzetti, E. M., et al., Magnetic resonance imaging of prosthestic cardiac valves in vitro and in vivo, *Am. J. Cardiol.,* 62, 973, 1988.
81. Soulen, R. L., Budinger, T. F., and Higgins, C. B., Magnetic resonance imaging of prosthetic heart valves, *Radiology,* 154, 705, 1985.
82. Soulen, R. L., Magnetic resonance imaging of prosthetic heart valves [Letter]. *Radiology,* 158, 279, 1986.
83. Shellock, F. G. and Morisoli, S. M., Ex vivo evaluation of ferromagnetism, heating, and artifacts for heart valve prostheses exposed to a 1.5 Tesla MR system, *J. Magn. Reson. Imaging,* 4, 756, 1994.
84. Edwards, M.-B., Taylor, K. M., and Shellock, F. G., Prosthetic heart valves: evaluation of magnetic field interactions, heating, and artifacts at 1.5 Tesla, *J. Magn. Reson. Imaging,* 12, 363, 2000.
85. Brown, M. A., Carden, J. A., Coleman, R. E., et al., Magnetic field effects on surgical ligation clips, *Magn. Reson. Imaging,* 5, 443, 1987.
86. Hess, T., Stepanow, B., and Knopp, M. V., Safety of intrauterine contraceptive devices during MR imaging, *Eur. Radiol.,* 6, 66, 1996.
87. Mark, A. S. and Hricak, H., Intrauterine contraceptive devices: MR imaging, *Radiology,* 162, 311, 1987.
88. Fransen, P., Dooms, G., and Thauvoy, C., Safety of the adjustable pressure ventricular valve in magnetic resonance imaging: problems and solutions, *Neuroradiology,* 34, 508, 1992.
89. Gaston, A., Marsault, C., Lacaze, A., et al., External magnetic guidance of endovascular catheters with a superconducting magnet: preliminary trials, *J. Neuroradiol.,* 15, 137, 1988.
90. Grady, M. S., Howard, M. A., Molloy, J. A., et al., Nonlinear magnetic stereotaxis: three dimensional in vivo remote magnetic manipulation of a small object in canine brain, *Med. Phys.,* 17, 405, 1990.
91. Ortler, M., Kostron, H., and Felber, S., Transcutaneous pressure-adjustable valves and magnetic resonance imaging: an ex vivo examination of the Codman-Medos programmable valve and the Sophy adjustable pressure valve, *Neurosurgery,* 40, 1050, 1997.
92. Ranney, D. F. and Huffaker, H. H., Magnetic microspheres for the targeted controlled release of drugs and diagnostic agents, *Ann. N.Y. Acad. Sci.,* 507, 104, 1987.
93. Schneider, M. L., Walker, G. B., and Dormer, K. J., Effects of magnetic resonance imaging on implantable permanent magnets, *Am. J. Otol.,* 16, 687, 1995.
94. Shellock, F. G., Ex vivo assessment of deflection forces and artifacts associated with high-field strength MRI of "mini-magnet" dental prostheses, *Magn. Reson. Imaging,* 7(Suppl. 1), 38, 1989.
95. Young, D. B. and Pawlak, A. M., An electromagnetically controllable heart valve suitable for chronic implantation, *ASAIO Trans.,* 36, M421, 1990.
96. Yuh, W. T. C., Hanigan, M. T., Nerad, J. A., et al., Extrusion of a eye socket magnetic implant after MR imaging examination: potential hazard to a patient with eye prosthesis, *J. Magn. Reson. Imaging,* 1, 711, 1991.
97. Hunyadi, S., Werning, J. W., Lewin, J. S., and Maniglia, A. J., Effect of magnetic resonance imaging on a new electromagnetic implantable middle ear hearing device, *Am. J. Otol.,* 18, 328, 1997.
98. Kanal, E. and Shabaini, A., Firearm safety in the MR imaging environment, *Radiology,* 193, 875, 1994.
99. Lufkin, R., Jordan, S., Lylyck, P., et al., MR imaging with topographic EEG electrodes in place, *Am. J. Neuroradiol.,* 9, 953, 1988.
100. Shellock, F. G., MR-compatibility of an endoscope designed for use in interventional MR procedures, *Am. J. Roentgenol.,* 71, 1297, 1998.
101. Shellock, F. G. and Shellock, V. J., Ceramic surgical instruments: evaluation of MR-compatibility at 1.5 Tesla, *J. Magn. Reson. Imaging,* 6, 954, 1996.
102. Shellock, F. G. and Shellock, V. J., Evaluation of MR compatibility of 38 implants and devices, *Radiology,* 197, 174, 1995.
103. To, S. Y. C., Lufkin, R. B., and Chiu, L., MR-compatible winged infusion set, *Comput. Med. Imaging Graphics,* 13, 469, 1989.
104. Zhang, J., Wilson, C. L., Levesque, M. F., Behnke, E. J., and Lufkin, R. B., Temperature changes in nickel-chromium intracranial depth electrodes during MR scanning, *Am. J. Neuroradiol.,* 14, 497, 1993.

105. Gleason, C. A., Kaula, N. F., Hricak, H., et al., The effect of magnetic resonance imagers on implanted neurostimulators, *Pacing Clin. Electrophysiol.,* 15, 81, 1992.
106. Liem, L. A. and van Dongen, V. C., Magnetic resonance imaging and spinal cord stimulation systems, *Pain,* 70, 95, 1997.
107. Tronnier, V. M., Stauber, A., Hahnel, S., and Sarem-Aslani, A., Magnetic resonance imaging with implanted neurostimulators: an in vitro and in vivo study, *Neurosurgery,* 44, 118, 1999.
108. Albert, D. W., Olson, K. R., Parel, J. M., et al., Magnetic resonance imaging and retinal tacks, *Arch. Ophthalmol.,* 108, 320, 1990.
109. de Keizer, R. J. and Te Strake, L., Intraocular lens implants (pseudophakoi) and steelwire sutures: a contraindication for MRI?, *Doc. Ophthalmol.,* 61, 281, 1984.
110. Joondeph, B. C., Peyman, G. A., Mafee, M. F., et al., Magnetic resonance imaging and retinal tacks [Letter], *Arch. Ophthalmol.,* 105, 1479, 1987.
111. Marra, S., Leonetti, J. P., Konior, R. J., and Raslan, W., Effect of magnetic resonance imaging on implantable eyelid weights, *Ann. Otol. Rhinol. Laryngol.,* 104, 448, 1995.
112. Roberts, C. W., Haik, B. G., and Cahill, P., Magnetic resonance imaging of metal loop intraocular lenses, *Arch. Ophthalmol.,* 108, 320, 1990.
113. Seiff, S. R., Vestel, K. P., and Truwit, C. L., Eyelid palpebral springs in patients undergoing magnetic resonance imaging: an area of possible concern [Letter], *Arch. Ophthalmol.,* 109, 319, 1991.
114. Shellock, F.G., Myers, S.M., and Schatz, C.J., Ex vivo evaluation of ferromagnetism determined for metallic scleral "buckles" exposed to a 1.5 T MR scanner, *Radiology,* 185, 288, 1992.
115. Lyons, C. J., Betz, R. R., Mesgarzadeh, M., et al., The effect of magnetic resonance imaging on metal spine implants, *Spine,* 14, 670, 1989.
116. Mechlin, M., Thickman, D., Kressel, H. Y., et al., Magnetic resonance imaging of postoperative patients with metallic implants, *Am. J. Roentgenol.,* 143, 1281, 1984.
117. Mesgarzadeh, M., Revesz, G., Bonakdarpour, A., et al., The effect on medical metal implants by magnetic fields of magnetic resonance imaging, *Skeletal Radiol.,* 14, 205, 1985.
118. Shellock, F. G. and Crues, J. V., High-field-strength MR imaging and metallic implants: an in vitro evaluation of deflection forces and temperature changes induced in large prostheses, *Radiology,* 165, 150, 1987.
119. Shellock, F. G., Mink, J. H., Curtin, S., et al., MRI and orthopedic implants used for anterior cruciate ligament reconstruction: assessment of ferromagnetism and artifacts, *J. Magn. Reson. Imaging,* 2, 225, 1992.
120. Applebaum, E. L. and Valvassori, G. E., Effects of magnetic resonance imaging fields on stapedectomy prostheses, *Arch. Otolaryngol.,* 11, 820, 1985..
121. Applebaum, E. L. and Valvassori, G. E., Further studies on the effects of magnetic resonance fields on middle ear implants, *Ann. Otol. Rhinol. Laryngol.,* 99, 801, 1990.
122. Leon, J. A. and Gabriele, O. F., Middle ear prothesis: significance in magnetic resonance imaging, *Magn. Reson. Imaging,* 5, 405, 1987.
123. Nogueira, M. and Shellock, F. G., Otologic implants: ex vivo assessment of ferromagnetism and artifacts at 1.5 Tesla, *Am. J. Roentgenol.,* 163, 1472, 1995.
124. White, D. W., Interaction between magnetic fields and metallic ossicular prostheses, *Am. J. Otol.,* 8, 290, 1987.
125. Shellock, F. G. and Morisoli, S. M., Ex vivo evaluation of ferromagnetism and artifacts for cardiac occluders exposed to a 1.5 Tesla MR system, *J. Magn. Reson. Imaging,* 4, 213, 1994.
126. Smugar, S. S., Schweitzer, M. E., and Hume, E., MRI in patients with intraspinal bullets, *J. Magn. Reson. Imaging,* 9, 151, 1999.
127. Teitelbaum, G. P., Metallic ballistic fragments: MR imaging safety and artifacts [Letter], *Radiology,* 177, 883, 1990.
128. Teitelbaum, G. P., Yee, C. A., Van Horn, D. D., et al., Metallic ballistic fragments: MR imaging safety and artifacts, *Radiology,* 175, 855, 1990.
129. Shellock, F. G., Crues, J. V., and Sacks, S. A., High-field magnetic resonance imaging of penile prostheses: in vitro evaluation of deflection forces and imaging artifacts [Abstract], in *Book of Abstracts,* Vol. 3, Society of Magnetic Resonance in Medicine, Berkeley, CA, 1987, 915.
130. Hartnell, G. G., et al., Safety of MR imaging in patients who have retained metallic materials after cardiac surgery, *Am. J. Roentgenol.,* 168, 1157, 1997.

131. Murphy, K. J., Cohan, R. H., and Ellis, J. H., MR imaging in patients with epicardial pacing wires, *Am. J. Roentgenol.,* 172, 727, 1999.

132. Jackson, J. G. and Acker, J. D., Permanent eyeliner and MR imaging, *Am. J. Roentgenol.,* 49, 1080, 1987.

133. Vahlensieck, M., Tattoo-related cutaneous inflammation (burn grade I) in a mid-field MR scanner, *Eur. Radiol.,* 10, 197, 2000.

134. Kreidstein, M. L., Giguere, D., and Friedberg, A., MRI interaction with tattoo pigments: case report, pathophysiology, and management, *Plast. Reconstr. Surg.,* 99, 1717, 1997.

135. Kanal, E. and Shellock, F. G., MRI interaction with tattoo pigments, *Plast. Reconstr. Surg.,* 101, 1150, 1998.

136. Lund, G., Nelson, J. D., Wirtschafter, J. D., and Williams, P. A., Tattooing of eyelids: magnetic resonance imaging artifacts, *Ophthalmic Surg.,* 17, 550, 1986.

137. Sacco, D., Artifacts caused by cosmetics in MR imaging of the head, *Am. J. Roentgenol.,* 148, 1001, 1987.

138. Shellock, F. G., Nogueira, M., and Morisoli, S., MR imaging and vascular access ports: ex vivo evaluation of ferromagnetism, heating, and artifacts at 1.5 T, *J. Magn. Reson. Imaging,* 4, 481, 1995.

139. Shellock, F. G. and Shellock, V. J., Vascular access ports and catheters tested for ferromagnetism, heating, and artifacts associated with MR imaging, *Magn. Reson. Imaging,* 14, 443, 1996.

140. ECRI, Health Devices Alert, A new MRI complication?, *Health Devices Alert,* May 27, 1, 1988.

141. ECRI, Thermal injuries and patient monitoring during MRI studies, *Health Devices Alert,* 20, 362, 1991.

142. Kanal, E. and Shellock, F. G., Burns associated with clinical MR examinations, *Radiology,* 175, 585, 1990.

143. Kanal, E. and Shellock, F. G., Policies, guidelines, and recommendations for MR imaging safety and patient management, *J. Magn. Reson. Imaging,* 2, 247, 1992.

144. Kanal, E. and Shellock, F. G., Patient monitoring during clinical MR imaging, *Radiology,* 185, 623, 1992.

145. Knopp, M. V., Essig, M., Debus, J., Zabel, H. J., and van Kaick, G., Unusual burns of the lower extremities caused by a closed conducting loop in a patient at MR imaging, *Radiology,* 200, 572, 1996.

146. Keens, S. J. and Laurence, A. S., Burns caused by ECG monitoring during MRI imaging, *Anesthesiology,* 51, 1188, 1996.

147. Brown, T. R., Goldstein, B., and Little, J., Severe burns resulting from magnetic resonance imaging with cardiopulmonary monitoring. Risks and relevant safety precautions, *Am. J. Phys. Med. Rehabil.,* 72, 166, 1993.

148. Bashein, G. and Syrory, G., Burns associated with pulse oximetry during magnetic resonance imaging, *Anesthesiology,* 75, 382, 1991.

149. Heinz, W., Frohlich, E., and Stork, L., Burns following magnetic resonance tomography, *Z. Gastroenterol.,* 37, 31, 1999.

15 The List of Implants, Devices, and Materials Tested in the Magnetic Resonance Imaging Environment*

Frank G. Shellock

CONTENTS

I. INTRODUCTION

To date, over 700 different biomedical implants, devices, and materials have been tested for various aspects of safety in the magnetic resonance imaging (MRI) environment. Over the years, various lists have summarized this important information for magnetic resonance (MR) healthcare workers and patients.[1-9] The safety information for the objects tested in the MRI environment is typically compiled and organized once a year, appearing as a publication commonly referred to by MR healthcare workers as "The List."[4-9]

The List continues to be an indispensable reference for ascertaining the relative safety of exposing patients or individuals with implants, devices, or materials to the MRI environment.[1-9] This information is required to properly screen patients and individuals prior to permitting them into the MRI environment. In general, if an object has not been previously evaluated for safety in the MRI environment, the patient or individual with a questionable object or an object made from a metallic or conductive material is not allowed near or inside the MR system because of the potential risk of injury.[1-9]

This chapter discusses the information and terminology used to describe and characterize the objects contained in *The List* and presents comprehensive data for over 700 implants, devices, and materials (Table 15.1).

---

* Portions of this chapter are reprinted with permission from Shellock, F. G., *Pocket Guide to MR Procedures and Metallic Objects: Update 2000*, Lippincott, Williams & Wilkins, Philadelphia, 2000. This information is also provided in a searchable format on the Internet at www.MRIsafety.com

II. INFORMATION AND TERMINOLOGY

The content of *The List* continues to be revised and reorganized in an effort to make the information more "user friendly." The current version was designed to make the information less confusing or subject to interpretation and, thus, readily useful to MR healthcare workers and understood by patients.

The objects compiled in *The List* (Table 15.1) are divided into general categories to facilitate the access and review of information (see additional information in Chapter 16). To properly utilize *The List*, particular attention must be given to the information indicated for the highest static magnetic **field strength** used for testing and the **status** information indicated for each **object** (note these specific terms correspond to the column headings for *The List*) (Table 15.1). The relevant terminology for *The List* is as follows:

Object — This is the implant, device, material, or product that underwent an evaluation for MRI safety. Information is also provided for the material(s) used to make the object and the manufacturer of the object, if this information is known.

Status — This information pertains to the results of the tests that were conducted for the object in the MRI environment. These tests typically included an assessment of magnetic field interactions (i.e., deflection and/or torque) and heating. In certain cases, an assessment of induced electrical fields was also performed.

The resulting safety information for each object has been specially categorized using a *status* designation. This categorizes the object as *safe, conditional,* or *unsafe* as follows:

Safe — The object is considered safe for the patient or individual in the MRI environment, with special reference to the highest static magnetic field strength that was used for the MRI safety test. The object has undergone testing to demonstrate that it is safe or it is made from materials that are considered safe with regard to the MRI environment. (Please refer to additional information in Chapter 14 for the particular object indicated.)

Conditional — The object may or may not be safe for the patient or individual in the MRI environment, depending on the specific MRI conditions that are present for the patient or individual under consideration. This information has been subcategorized to indicate specific recommendations for the particular object as follows:

Conditional 1 — The object is considered safe for the patient or individual in the MRI environment, despite the fact that it showed magnetic field interaction during testing. Notably, the object is considered to be only "weakly ferromagnetic."

In general, the object is safe because the magnetic interaction was characterized as "mild" relative to the *in vivo* forces that are present for the object. For example, certain prosthetic heart valves were attracted to the magnetic fields of MR systems used for testing, but the attractive forces were less than the forces exerted on the heart valves by the beating heart.[1-9]

Additionally, there may be substantial "retentive" or counterforces present provided by tissue ingrowth, scarring, or granulation that serve to prevent the object from presenting a risk or hazard to the patient or individual in the MRI environment.

For a device or product that is used for an MR-guided procedure (e.g., laryngoscope, endoscope, etc.), there may be minor magnetic interactions in association with MR systems. However, the device or product is considered to be "MRI safe" if it is used in its "intended" manner, as indicated by the manufacturer of the device or product.

Conditional 2 — These "weakly" ferromagnetic intravascular coils, filters, stents, and cardiac occluders typically become firmly incorporated into the tissue 6 to 8 weeks following placement. Therefore, it is unlikely that these objects will be moved or dislodged by interactions with magnetic fields of the MR systems operating at the static magnetic field strength used for testing.

Furthermore, there has never been a report of an injury to a patient or individual in association with an MR procedure for one of these coils, stents, filters, and cardiac occluders. ***Special Note:*** **If there is any concern regarding the integrity of the tissue with regard to its ability to retain the object in place, the patient or individual should not be allowed into the MRI environment.**

Also, if the coil, stent, filter, or occluder is made from a nonmagnetic material (e.g., Phynox, Elgiloy, titanium, titanium alloy, MP35N, etc.), it is unnecessary to wait 6 to 8 weeks before performing the MR procedure using an MR system operating at 1.5 T or less.

Conditional 3 — The Deponit, nitroglycerin transdermal delivery system (Schwarz Pharma, Milwaukee, WI), although not attracted to an MR system, has been found to heat excessively during MRI. This excessive heating may produce discomfort or burn a patient or individual wearing this patch. Therefore, it is recommended that the patch be removed prior to the MR procedure. A new patch should be applied immediately after the examination. Notably, this procedure should only be done in consultation with the patient or individual's personal physician.

Conditional 4 — This halo vest or cervical fixation device is known to have ferromagnetic components. However, the relative amount of magnetic field interaction has not been determined. Nevertheless, there has been no report of patient injury in association with the presence of this device in the MRI environment.

Conditional 5 — This object is considered safe for a patient or individual in the MRI environment as long as specific guidelines and recommendations are followed. Please refer to the specific criteria for performing a safe MR procedure by reviewing the information for the object in the text of this book (i.e., please refer to the information in Chapter 14 for the object in question).

Unsafe 1 — The object is considered to pose a potential risk or hazard to a patient or individual in the MRI environment, primarily as the result of movement or dislodgment of the object. The presence of this object is considered to be a contraindication for an MRI procedure.

Unsafe 2 — This object displays only minor magnetic field interactions that, in consideration of the *in vivo* application of this object, are unlikely to pose a hazard or risk in association with movement or dislodgment. Nevertheless, the presence of this object is considered a contraindication for an MR procedure. Notably, the potential risk to performing an MR procedure in a patient or individual with this object is related to induced electrical current, excessive heating, or other potentially hazardous conditions. Therefore, it is inadvisable to perform an MR procedure in a patient or individual with this object.

For example, although certain cardiovascular catheters and accessories typically do not exhibit magnetic field interactions, there are other mechanisms whereby these devices may pose a hazard to the patient or individual in the MRI environment.

The triple-lumen, thermodilution, Swan-Ganz catheter displays no attraction to the MR system. However, there has been a report that a Swan-Ganz catheter "melted" in a patient during an MRI procedure. Therefore, the presence of this cardiovascular catheter and any other similar device is considered to be a contraindication for a patient or individual in the MRI environment.

Field Strength — This is the highest strength of the static magnetic field of the MR system that was used for safety testing an object. In most cases, a 1.5-T MR system was used for testing. However, there are some objects that were tested at field strengths lower (e.g., 0.15 T) or higher (e.g., 2.35 T) than 1.5 T.

Notably, there are MR systems with static magnetic fields that exceed 2.0 T (e.g., 3.0-, 4.0-, and 8.0-T MR systems are used for clinical and research MR procedures). Very few objects have been assessed to determine the magnetic field interactions in association with those very high static magnetic field strengths. Thus, extra precautionary measures should be taken for patients and others with metallic implants and objects in consideration of the potential risks.

Note that it is conceivable that an object that exhibited only mild or weak ferromagnetism or magnetic field interactions in association with a 1.5-T MR system is attracted with sufficient force by a higher field strength MR system (i.e., >2.0 T) to pose a hazard to the patient or individual. Therefore, careful consideration must be given to each object relative to the particular MR system used for testing as well as the conditions that are present for the patient or individual prior to exposure to the MRI environment.

Reference – This is the publication used for the MRI safety information indicated for the particular object (see the reference list following Table 15.1).

TABLE 15.1
The List

Object	Status	Field Strength (T)	Reference
Aneurysm Clips			
Downs multi-positional, aneurysm clip (17-7PH)	Unsafe 1	1.39	1
Drake (301 SS), aneurysm clip Edward Weck Triangle Park, NJ	Unsafe 1	1.5	2
Drake (DR 14, DR 21), aneurysm clip Edward Weck Triangle Park, NJ	Unsafe 1	1.39	1
Drake (DR 16), aneurysm clip Edward Weck Triangle Park, NJ	Unsafe 1	0.147	1
Heifetz (17-7PH), aneurysm clip Edward Weck Triangle Park, NJ	Unsafe 1	1.89	4
Heifetz (Elgiloy), aneurysm clip Edward Weck Triangle Park, NJ	Safe	1.89	2
Housepian, aneurysm clip	Unsafe 1	0.147	1
Kapp (405 SS), aneurysm clip V. Mueller	Unsafe 1	1.89	2
Kapp, curved (404 SS), aneurysm clip V. Mueller	Unsafe 1	1.39	1
Kapp, straight (404 SS), aneurysm clip V. Mueller	Unsafe 1	1.39	1
Mayfield (301 SS), aneurysm clip Codman Randolf, MA	Unsafe 1	1.5	3
Mayfield (304 SS), aneurysm clip Codman Randolf, MA	Unsafe 1	1.89	5

TABLE 15.1 (CONTINUED)
The List

Object	Status	Field Strength (T)	Reference
McFadden (301 SS), aneurysm clip Codman Randolf, MA	Unsafe 1	1.5	2
McFadden Vari-Angle, aneurysm clip micro clip, straight, fenestrated, 9 mm blade (MP35N) Codman Johnson & Johnson Professional, Inc. Raynham, MA	Safe	1.5	
McFadden Vari-Angle, aneurysm clip micro clip, straight, 9 mm blade (MP35N) Codman Johnson & Johnson Professional, Inc. Raynham, MA	Safe	1.5	
Olivercrona, aneurysm clip	Safe	1.39	1
Perneczky Aneurysm Clip 20 mm, curved Zeppelin Chirurgische Instruments Germany	Safe	1.5	
Perneczky Aneurysm Clip 3 mm, straight Zeppelin Chirurgische Instruments Germany	Safe	1.5	
Perneczky Aneurysm Clip 9 mm, curved Zeppelin Chirurgische Instruments Germany	Safe	1.5	
Perneczky Aneurysm Clip 9 mm, straight Zeppelin Chirurgische Instruments Germany	Safe	1.5	
Pivot (17-7PH) aneurysm clip	Unsafe 1	1.89	5
Scoville (EN58J), aneurysm clip Downs Surgical, Inc. Decatur, GA	Safe	1.89	2
Spetzler Titanium Aneurysm Clip straight, 13 mm blade, double turn (C.P. titanium) Elekta Instruments, Inc. Atlanta, GA	Safe	1.5	68
Spetzler Titanium Aneurysm Clip straight, 13 mm blade, single turn (C.P. titanium) Elekta Instruments, Inc. Atlanta, GA	Safe	1.5	68

TABLE 15.1 (CONTINUED)
The List

Object	Status	Field Strength (T)	Reference
Spetzler Titanium Aneurysm Clip straight, 9 mm blade, single turn (C.P. titanium) Elekta Instruments, Inc. Atlanta, GA	Safe	1.5	68
Spetzler Titanium Aneurysm Clip straight, 9 mm blade, double turn (C.P. titanium) Elekta Instruments, Inc. Atlanta, GA	Safe	1.5	68
Stevens (silver alloy) aneurysm clip	Safe	0.15	6
Sugita (Elgiloy) aneurysm clip Downs Surgical, Inc. Decatur, GA	Safe	1.89	2
Sugita AVM Micro Clip (Elgiloy) aneurysm clip Mizuho America, Inc. Beverly, MA	Safe	1.5	
Sugita, bent, fenestrated large aneurysm clip for permanent occlusion (Elgiloy) Mizuho America, Inc. Beverly, MA	Safe	1.5	
Sugita, bent, mini aneurysm clip for temporary occlusion (Elgiloy) Mizuho America, Inc. Beverly, MA	Safe	1.5	
Sugita, bent, standard aneurysm clip for temporary occlusion (Elgiloy) Mizuho America, Inc. Beverly, MA	Safe	1.5	
Sugita, sideward CVD bayonet, standard aneurysm clip for permanent occlusion Mizuho America, Inc. Beverly, MA	Safe	1.5	
Sugita, straight, large Aneurysm clip for permanent occlusion (Elgiloy) Mizuho America, Inc. Beverly, MA	Safe	1.5	
Sundt AVM, Micro Clip (MP35N), aneurysm clip Codman Johnson & Johnson Professional, Inc. Raynham, MA	Safe	1.5	
Sundt Slim-Line, Graft Clip (MP35N), aneurysm clip Codman Johnson & Johnson Professional, Inc. Raynham, MA	Safe	1.5	

TABLE 15.1 (CONTINUED)
The List

Object	Status	Field Strength (T)	Reference
Sundt Slim-Line, Temporary Aneurysm Clip 10 mm blade (MP35N) Codman Johnson & Johnson Professional, Inc. Raynham, MA	Safe	1.5	
Sundt-Kees Multi-Angle (17-7PH) aneurysm clip Downs Surgical, Inc. Decatur, GA	Unsafe 1	1.89	2
Sundt-Kees Slim-Line, fenestrated, aneurysm clip 9 mm blade (MP35N) Codman Johnson & Johnson Professional, Inc. Raynham, MA	Safe	1.5	
Sundt-Kees, Slim-Line 9 mm blade, (MP35N) aneurysm clip Codman Johnson & Johnson Professional, Inc. Raynham, MA	Safe	1.5	
Vari-Angle (17-7PH) aneurysm clip Codman Randolf, MA	Unsafe 1	1.89	5
Vari-Angle McFadden (MP35N) aneurysm clip Codman Randolf, MA	Safe	1.89	2
Vari-Angle Micro (17-7PH) aneurysm clip Codman Randolf, MA	Unsafe 1	0.15	2
Vari-Angle Spring (17-7PH) aneurysm clip Codman Randolf, MA	Unsafe 1	0.15	2
Yasargil (316 SS), aneurysm clip Aesculap, Inc. South San Francisco, CA	Safe	1.89	5
Yasargil, Model FD, aneurysm clip Aesculap, Inc. South San Francisco, CA	Unsafe 1	1.5	
Yasargil, Model FE 720T, aneurysm clip mini, permanent, 7 mm blade, (titanium alloy) Aesculap, Inc. South San Francisco, CA	Safe	1.5	
Yasargil, Model FE 740T, aneurysm clip standard, permanent, 7 mm blade, (titanium alloy) Aesculap, Inc. South San Francisco, CA	Safe	1.5	

TABLE 15.1 (CONTINUED)
The List

Object	Status	Field Strength (T)	Reference
Yasargil, Model FE 748, aneurysm clip standard, 9 mm blade, bayonet (Phynox) Aesculap, Inc. South San Francisco, CA	Safe	1.5	
Yasargil, Model FE 750, aneurysm clip 9 mm blade, straight (Phynox) Aesculap, Inc. South Francisco, CA	Safe	1.5	
Yasargil, Model FE 750T, aneursym clip standard, permanent, 9 mm blade (titanium alloy) Aesculap, Inc. South San Francisco, CA	Safe	1.5	
Yasargil, Model FE, aneurysm clip Aesculap, Inc. South San Francisco, CA	Safe	1.5	
Biopsy Needles, Markers, and Devices			
Adjustable, Automated Aspiration Biopsy Gun 10, 15, and 20 mm (304 SS) MD Tech Watertown, MA	Unsafe 1	1.5	7
Adjustable, Automated Biopsy Gun 6, 13, and 19 mm (304 SS) MD Tech Watertown, MA	Unsafe 1	1.5	7
ASAP 16, Automatic 16 G Core Biopsy System 19 cm length (304 SS)	Unsafe 1	1.5	7
Automatic Cutting Needle with Dept Markings 14 G, 10 cm length (304 SS), biopsy needle Manan Northbrook, IL	Unsafe 1	1.5	7
Automatic Cutting Needle with Ultrasound Tip & Depth Markings 18 G, 16 cm length (304 SS), biopsy needle Manan Northbrook, IL	Unsafe 1	1.5	7
Automatic Cutting Needle with Ultrasound Tip & Depth Markings 18 G, 20 cm length (304 SS), biopsy needle Manan Northbrook, IL	Unsafe 1	1.5	7
Basic II Hookwire Breast Localization Needle (304 SS) MD Tech Watertown, MA	Unsafe 1	1.5	7
Beaded Breast Localization Wire Set 19 G, 3-1/2 inch needle with 7-7/8 inch wire (304 SS) Inrad Grand Rapids, MI	Unsafe 1	1.5	7

TABLE 15.1 (CONTINUED)
The List

Object	Status	Field Strength (T)	Reference
Beaded Breast Localization Wire Set 20 G, 2 inch needle with 5-7/8 inch wire (304 SS) Inrad Grand Rapids, MI	Unsafe 1	1.5	7
Biopsy Gun 13 mm, biopsy needle Meadox Oakland, NJ	Unsafe 1	1.5	7
Biopsy Gun 25 mm, biopsy needle Meadox Oakland, NJ	Unsafe 1	1.5	7
Biopsy Needle 17 G, 10 cm length Meadox Oakland, NJ	Unsafe 1	1.5	7
Biopsy Needle 20 G, 15 cm length Meadox Oakland, NJ	Unsafe 1	1.5	7
Biopsy Needle 22 G, 15 cm length Cook, Inc. Bloomington, IN	Unsafe 1	1.5	7
Biopsy Needle 22 G, 15 cm length Meadox Oakland, NJ	Unsafe 1	1.5	7
Biopty-Cut Biopsy Needle 14 G, 10 cm length (304 SS) C.R. Bard, Inc. Covington, GA	Unsafe 1	1.5	7
Biopty-Cut Biopsy Needle 16 G, 16 cm length (304 SS) C.R. Bard, Inc. Covington, GA	Unsafe 1	1.5	7
Biopty-Cut Biopsy Needle 18 G, 18 cm length (304 SS) C.R. Bard, Inc. Covington, GA	Unsafe 1	1.5	7
Biopty-Cut Biopsy Needle 18 G, 20 cm length (304 SS) C.R. Bard, Inc. Covington, GA	Unsafe 1	1.5	7
Breast Localization Needle 20 G, 5 cm length (304 SS) Manan Northbrook, IL	Unsafe 1	1.5	7

TABLE 15.1 (CONTINUED)
The List

Object	Status	Field Strength (T)	Reference
Breast Localization Needle 20 G, 7 cm length (304 SS) Manan Northbrook, IL	Unsafe 1	1.5	7
Chiba Needle and HiLiter Ultrasound Enhancement 22 G, 3-7/8 inch biopsy needle (304 SS) Inrad Grand Rapids, MI	Unsafe 1	1.5	7
Coaxial Needle Set Chiba-type 22 G, 5-7/8 inch biopsy needle (304 SS) Inrad Grand Rapids, MI	Unsafe 1	1.5	7
Coaxial Needle Set Introducer 19 G, 2-15/16 inch biopsy needle (304 SS) Inrad Grand Rapids, MI	Unsafe 1	1.5	7
Cutting Needle & Gun 18 G, 155 mm length, biopsy needle Meadox Oakland, NJ	Unsafe 1	1.5	7
Cutting Needle 14 G, 9 cm length biopsy needle West Coast Medical Laguna Beach, CA	Unsafe 1	1.5	7
Cutting Needle 16 G, 17 mm length (304 SS) biopsy needle BIP USA, Inc. Niagara Falls, NY	Unsafe 1	1.5	7
Cutting Needle 16 G, 19 mm length (304 SS) biopsy needle BIP USA, Inc. Niagara Falls, NY	Unsafe 1	1.5	7
Cutting Needle 18 G, 100 mm length biopsy needle Meadox Oakland, NJ	Unsafe 1	1.5	7
Cutting Needle 18 G, 15 cm length biopsy needle West Coast Medical Laguna Beach, CA	Unsafe 1	1.5	7

TABLE 15.1 (CONTINUED)
The List

Object	Status	Field Strength (T)	Reference
Cutting Needle 18 G, 150 mm length biopsy needle Meadox Oakland, NJ	Unsafe 1	1.5	7
Cutting Needle 18 G, 9 cm length biopsy needle West Coast Medical Laguna Beach, CA	Unsafe 1	1.5	7
Cutting Needle 19 G, 15 cm length biopsy needle West Coast Medical Laguna Beach, CA	Unsafe 1	1.5	7
Cutting Needle 19 G, 6 cm length biopsy needle West Coast Medical Laguna Beach, CA	Unsafe 1	1.5	7
Cutting Needle 19 G, 9 cm length biopsy needle West Coast Medical Laguna Beach, CA	Unsafe 1	1.5	7
Cutting Needle 20 G, 15 cm length biopsy needle West Coast Medical Laguna Beach, CA	Unsafe 1	1.5	7
Cutting Needle 20 G, 20 cm length biopsy needle West Coast Medical Laguna Beach, CA	Unsafe 1	1.5	7
Cutting Needle 20 G, 9 cm length biopsy needle West Coast Medical Laguna Beach, CA	Unsafe 1	1.5	7
Hawkins Blunt Needle (304 SS) biopsy needle MD Tech Watertown, MA	Unsafe 1	1.5	7
Hawkins III Breast Localization Needle MD Tech Watertown, MA	Unsafe 1	1.5	7

TABLE 15.1 (CONTINUED)
The List

Object	Status	Field Strength (T)	Reference
Lufkin Aspiration Cytology Needle 20 G, 5 cm length, biopsy needle (high nickel alloy) E-Z-Em, Inc. Westbury, NY	Safe	1.5	9
Lufkin Biopsy Needle 18 G, 15 cm length (high nickel alloy) E-Z-Em, Inc. Westbury, NY	Safe	1.5	8
Lufkin Biopsy Needle 18 G, 5 cm length (high nickel alloy) E-Z-Em, Inc. Westbury, NY	Safe	1.5	8
Lufkin Biopsy Needle 22 G, 10 cm length (high nickel alloy) E-Z-Em, Inc. Westbury, NY	Safe	1.5	8
Lufkin Biopsy Needle 22 G, 15 cm length (high nickel alloy) E-Z-Em, Inc. Westbury, NY	Safe	1.5	8
Lufkin Biopsy Needle 22 G, 5 cm length (high nickel alloy) E-Z-Em, Inc. Westbury, NY	Safe	1.5	8
Micromark Clip, marking clip (316L SS) Biopsys Medical Irvine, CA	Safe	1.5	61
MReye Chiba Biopsy Needle William Cook Europe A/S Bjaeverskov, Denmark	Safe	1.5	
MReye Franseen Lung Biopsy Needle William Cook Europe A/S Bjaeverskov, Denmark	Safe	1.5	
MReye Interventional Needle biopsy needle William Cook Europe A/S Bjaeverskov, Denmark	Safe	1.5	
MReye Kopans Breast Lesion Localization Needles (21, 20, 19 gauges; 5.0, 9.0, 15.0 lengths) William Cook Europe A/S Bjaeverskov, Denmark	Safe	1.5	

TABLE 15.1 (CONTINUED)
The List

Object	Status	Field Strength (T)	Reference
MRI BioGun	Safe	1.5	8
18 G, 10 cm length (high nickel alloy)			
biopsy needle			
E-Z-Em, Inc.			
Westbury, NY			
MRI Histology Needle	Safe	1.5	7
18 G, 15 cm length (high nickel alloy)			
biopsy needle			
E-Z-Em, Inc.			
Westbury, NY			
MRI Histology Needle	Safe	1.5	8
18 G, 5 cm length (high nickel alloy)			
biopsy needle			
E-Z-Em, Inc.			
Westbury, NY			
MRI Histology Needle	Safe	1.5	8
20 G, 10 cm length (high nickel alloy)			
biopsy needle			
E-Z-Em, Inc.			
Westbury, NY			
MRI Histology Needle	Safe	1.5	8
20 G, 15 cm length (high nickel alloy)			
biopsy needle			
E-Z-Em, Inc.			
Westbury, NY			
MRI Histology Needle	Safe	1.5	7
20 G, 5 cm length (high nickel alloy)			
biopsy needle			
E-Z-Em, Inc.			
Westbury, NY			
MRI Histology Needle	Safe	1.5	8
20 G, 7.5 cm length (high nickel alloy)			
biopsy needle			
E-Z-Em, Inc.			
Westbury, NY			
MRI Lesion Marking System	Safe	1.5	8
20 G, 7.5 cm length (high nickel alloy)			
E-Z-Em, Inc.			
Westbury, NY			
MRI Needle (surgical grade SS) biopsy needle	Safe	1.5	7
Cook, Inc.			
Bloomington, IN			
mrt Biopsy Needle	Safe	1.5	
all sizes			
(titanium alloy)			
Daum Medical			
Baltimore, MD and			
Schwerin, Germany			

TABLE 15.1 (CONTINUED)
The List

Object	Status	Field Strength (T)	Reference
Percucut Biopsy Needle and Stylet 19.5 gauge × 10 cm (316L SS) E-Z-Em, Inc. Westbury, NY	Unsafe 1	1.5	7
Percucut Biopsy Needle and Stylet 21 gauge × 10 cm (316L SS) E-Z-Em, Inc. Westbury, NY	Unsafe 1	1.5	7
Sadowsky Breast Marking System 20 G, 5 cm length needle and 7 inch hook wire (316 L SS) Ranfac Corporation Avon, MA	Unsafe 1	1.5	7
Soft Tissue Biopsy Needle Gun & biopsy needle (304 SS) Anchor Procducts Co. Addison, IL	Unsafe 1	1.5	7
Trocar Needle (304 SS) biopsy needle BIP USA, Inc. Niagara Falls, NY	Unsafe 1	1.5	7
Trocar Needle, Disposable (SS) biopsy needle Cook, Inc. Bloomington, IN	Unsafe 1	1.5	7
Ultra-Core, biopsy needle 16 G, 16 cm length (304 SS)	Unsafe 1	1.5	7
Breast Tissue Expanders and Implants			
Becker Expander/Mammary Mentor H/S Prosthesis (316L SS), breast implant Santa Barbara, CA	Safe	1.5	10
Infall, breast implant (inflatable with magnetic port) 3101198 Model, breast implant Heyerschultzz	Unsafe 1	1.5	
Radovan Tissue Expander (316L SS) Mentor H/S Santa Barbara, CA	Safe	1.5	10
Siltex Spectrum Post-Operatively Adjustable Saline-Filled Mammary Prosthesis (316L SS) Mentor H/S Santa Barbara, CA	Safe	1.5	10
Tissue expander with magnetic port breast implant McGhan Medical Corporation Santa Barbara, CA	Unsafe 1	1.5	
Opti-Q SvO2/CCO catheter Abbott Laboratories Morgan Hill, CA	Unsafe 2	1.5	60

TABLE 15.1 (CONTINUED)
The List

Object	Status	Field Strength (T)	Reference

Opticath Catheter, Model U400, catheter
  Abbott Laboratories
  Morgan Hill, CA
	Unsafe 2	1.5	60

Opticath PA Catheter with extra port
  Abbott Laboratories
  Morgan Hill, CA
	Unsafe 2	1.5	60

Opticath PA Catheter with RV Pacing Port
  Abbott Laboratories
  Morgan Hill, CA
	Unsafe 2	1.5	60

Oximetric 3, SO2
  Optical Module
  Abbott Laboratories
  Morgan Hill, CA
	Unsafe 2	1.5	60

RV Pacing Lead
  Abbott Laboratories
  Morgan Hill, CA
	Unsafe 2	1.5	60

Swan-Ganz thermodilution catheter
  American Edwards
  Laboratories
  Irvine, CA
	Unsafe 2	1.5	57

Swan-Ganz triple-lumen thermodilution catheter
  American Edwards Laboratories
  Irvine, CA
	Unsafe 2	1.5	60

TD Thermodilution Catheter
  Flow-directed thermodilution pulmonary artery catheter
  Abbott Laboratories
  Morgan Hill, CA
	Unsafe 2	1.5	60

TDQ CCO Catheter
  Flow-directed thermodilution continuous
  cardiac output pulmonary artery catheter
  Abbott Laboratories
  Morgan Hill, CA
	Unsafe 2	1.5	60

Torque-Line Flow-directed
  thermodilution pulmonary artery catheter
  Abbott Laboratories
  Morgan Hill, CA
	Unsafe 2	1.5	60

Transpac IV
  Abbott Laboratories
  Morgan Hill, CA
	Safe	1.5	60

Carotid Artery Vascular Clamps			

Crutchfield (SS)
  carotid artery vascular clamp
  Codman
  Randolf, MA
	Conditional 1	1.5	11

Kindt (SS)
  carotid artery vascular clamp
  V. Mueller
	Conditional 1	1.5	11

TABLE 15.1 (CONTINUED)
The List

Object	Status	Field Strength (T)	Reference
Poppen-Blaylock (SS)	Unsafe 1	1.5	11
carotid artery vascular clamp			
Codman			
Randolf, MA			
Salibi (SS)	Conditional 1	1.5	11
carotid artery vascular clamp			
Codman			
Randolf, MA			
Selverstone (SS)	Conditional 1	1.5	11
carotid artery vascular clamp			
Codman			
Randolf, MA			
Coils, Stents, and Filters			
ACS Stent	Safe	1.5	
316L SS			
Guidant			
Menlo Park, CA			
Amplatz IVC filter	Safe	4.7	21
Cook, Inc.			
Bloomington, IN			
AneuRX Graft Stent	Safe	1.5	
Medtronic AneuRx			
Sunnyvale, CA			
AneuRx Stent Graft	Safe	1.5	70
Medtronic AneuRx			
Sunnyvale, CA			
Angiomed Memotherm Femoral	Safe	1.5	
4 mm × 120 mm (Nitinol)			
C.R. Bard, Inc.			
Billerica, MA			
Angiomed Memotherm Femoral	Safe	1.5	
5 mm × 20 mm (Nitinol)			
C.R. Bard, Inc.			
Billerica, MA			
Angiomed Memotherm Iliac	Safe	1.5	
12 mm × 110 mm (Nitinol)			
C.R. Bard, Inc.			
Billerica, MA			
Angiomed Memotherm Iliac	Safe	1.5	
8 mm × 20 mm (Nitinol)			
C.R. Bard, Inc.			
Billerica, MA			
AngioStent	Safe	1.5	
15 mm (platinum, iridium)			
Angiodynamics			
Queensbury, NY			
AngioStent	Safe	1.5	
stent			

TABLE 15.1 (CONTINUED)
The List

Object	Status	Field Strength (T)	Reference
AVE GFX Stent	Safe	1.5	69
316L SS			
Arterial Vascular Engineering			
Santa Rosa, CA			
AVE Micro I Stent	Safe	1.5	69
316L SS			
Arterial Vascular Engineering			
Santa Rosa, CA			
AVE Micro II Stent	Safe	1.5	69
316L SS			
Arterial Vascular Engineering			
Santa Rosa, CA			
Bard Stent, bifurcated	Safe	1.5	70
36 × 20 mm			
nitinol			
Bard XT Stent	Safe	1.5	69
316 LVM			
Bard Limited			
Ireland			
Bestent	Safe	1.5	69
MR-safe SS			
Medtronic			
Minneapolis, MN			
BX Stent	Safe	1.5	69
316L SS			
Cordis			
Miami, FL			
Cook occluding spring embolization coil	Conditional 2	1.5	
MWCE- 338-5-10			
Cook, Inc.			
Bloomington, IN			
Cook-Z Stent	Conditional 2	1.5	
Gianturco-Rosch Biliary Design			
10 mm x 3 cm			
Cook, Inc.			
Bloomington, IN			
Cook-Z Stent	Conditional 2	1.5	
Gianturco-Rosch Tracheobronchial Design			
20 mm x 5 cm			
Cook, Inc.			
Bloomington, IN			
Corvita Endoluminal	Safe	1.5	64
Graft for Abdominal			
Aortic Aneurysm			
27 × 120			
Schneider (USA) Inc.			
Pfizer Medical Technology Group			
Minneapolis, MN			
Cragg Nitinol spiral filter	Safe	4.7	21

TABLE 15.1 (CONTINUED)
The List

Object	Status	Field Strength (T)	Reference
Crossflex Stent	Safe	1.5	69
316L SS			
Cordis			
Miami, FL			
Crown Stent	Safe	1.5	69
316L SS			
Cordis			
Miami, FL			
Flower embolization microcoil (platinum)	Safe	1.5	22
Target Therapeutics			
San Jose, CA			
GDC 3D Shape	Safe	1.5	
various sizes			
platinum			
Boston Scientific/Target			
Wayne, NJ			
GDC SR Coil	Safe	1.5	
"stretch resistant"			
various sizes			
platinum			
Boston Scientific/Target			
Wayne, NJ			
Gianturco bird nest IVC filter	Conditional 2	1.5	21
Cook, Inc.			
Bloomington, IN			
Gianturco embolization coil	Conditional 2	1.5	21
Cook, Inc.			
Bloomington, IN			
Gianturco zig-zag stent	Conditional 2	1.5	21
Cook, Inc.			
Bloomington, IN			
Gianturco-Roubin Stent	Safe	1.5	69
316L SS			
Cook			
Bloomington, IN			
Greenfield vena cava filter (SS)	Conditional 2	1.5	21
MD Tech			
Watertown, MA			
Greenfield vena cava filter (titanium alloy)	Safe	1.5	21
Ormco			
Glendora, CA			
Guglielmi detachable coil (platinum)	Safe	1.5	25
Target Therapeutics			
San Jose, CA			
Gunther IVC filter	Conditional 2	1.5	21
William Cook			
Europe			

TABLE 15.1 (CONTINUED)
The List

Object	Status	Field Strength (T)	Reference
Hilal embolization microcoil Cook, Inc. Bloomington, IN	Safe	1.5	23
Iliac Wallgraft Endoprosthesis 12 × 90 Schneider (USA) Inc. Pfizer Medical Technology Group Minneapolis, MN	Safe	1.5	64
Iliac Wallstent Endoprosthesis 12 × 90 Schneider (USA) Inc. Pfizer Medical Technology Group Minneapolis, MN	Safe	1.5	64
Iliac Wallstent Endoprosthesis 5 × 80 Schneider (USA) Inc. Pfizer Medical Technology Group Minneapolis, MN	Safe	1.5	64
Iliac Wallstent Endoprosthesis 6 × 90 Schneider (USA) Inc. Pfizer Medical Technology Group Minneapolis, MN	Safe	1.5	64
Inflow Stent 316L SS Inflow Dynamics Munich, Germany	Safe	1.5	69
IVC venous clip (Teflon) Pilling Weck Co.	Safe	1.5	
Jostent 316L SS Jomed Helsingborg, Sweden	Safe	1.5	69
LGM IVC filter (Phynox) B. Braun Vena Tech Evanston, IL	Safe	1.5	26
LPS Stent, bifurcated 36 × 20 mm nitinol World Medical Manufacturing Corp. Sunrise, FL	Safe	1.5	70
LPS Thoracic Stent 46 mm nitinol World Medical Manufacturing Corp. Sunrise, FL	Safe	1.5	70

TABLE 15.1 (CONTINUED)
The List

Object	Status	Field Strength (T)	Reference
Maas helical endovascular stent	Safe	4.7	21
Medinvent			
Lausanne, Switzerland			
Maas helical IVC filter	Safe	4.7	21
Medinvent			
Lausanne, Switzerland			
Magic Wallstent	Safe	1.5	69
platinum and cobalt alloy			
Schneider			
Bulach, Switzerland			
Medtronic AVE Stent	Safe	1.5	70
316 L SS, gold			
Medtronic AVE			
Ireland			
Mini-Crown Stent	Safe	1.5	69
316L SS			
Cordis			
Miami, FL			
Mobin-Uddin IVC/umbrella filter	Safe	4.7	21
American Edwards			
Santa Ana, CA			
MReye Embolization Coil	Safe	1.5	
William Cook Europe A/S			
Bjaeverskov, Denmark			
Multi-Link Stent	Safe	1.5	69
316L SS			
Guidant			
Santa Clara, CA			
New retrievable IVC filter	Conditional 2	1.5	21
Thomas Jefferson University			
Philadelphia, PA			
NIR Stent	Safe	1.5	69
MR-safe metal			
Medinol Ltd.			
Boston Scientific			
Tel Aviv, Israel			
Palmaz endovascular stent	Conditional 2	1.5	21
Ethicon			
Palmaz endovascular stent	Safe	1.5	
Johnson & Johnson Interventional			
Warren, NJ			
Palmaz-Schatz Stent	Safe	1.5	69
P-S 153			
316L SS			
Cordis			
Miami, FL			

TABLE 15.1 (CONTINUED)
The List

Object	Status	Field Strength (T)	Reference
Palmaz-Schatz Stent	Safe	1.5	69
P-S 154			
316L SS			
Cordis			
Miami, FL			
Palmaz-Shatz balloon-expandable stent	Conditional 2	1.5	
Johnson & Johnson Interventional			
Warren, NJ			
Passager Stent (tantalum)	Safe	1.5	
10 mm × 30 mm, coil, stent, filter			
Meadox Surgimed			
Oakland, NJ			
Passager Stent (tantalum)	Safe	1.5	
4 mm × 30 mm, coil, stent, filter			
Meadox Surgimed			
Oakland, NJ			
PowerLink	Safe	1.5	70
cobalt alloy			
Endologix, Inc.			
Irvine, CA			
PowerWeb, Model 1	Safe	1.5	70
cobalt alloy			
Endologix, Inc.			
Irvine, CA			
PowerWeb	Safe	1.5	70
cobalt alloy			
Endologix, Inc.			
Irvine, CA			
Precedent Stent	Safe	1.5	70
nitinol, platinum			
Boston Scientific			
Wayne, NJ			
Precise-TM Microvascular Anastomotic Device (MACD)	Safe	1.5	71
316 L SS			
R Stent	Safe	1.5	
316 LVM SS			
Spectranetics Corporation			
Colorado Springs, CO			
Radius	Safe	1.5	69
nitinol			
Scimed			
Maple Grove, MN			
Strecker stent (tantalum)	Safe	1.5	27
MD Tech			
Watertown, MA			

TABLE 15.1   (CONTINUED)
The List

Object	Status	Field Strength (T)	Reference
Talent Graft Stent bare spring model 16 × 8 mm (Nitinol) World Medical Manufacturing Corp. Sunrise, FL	Safe	1.5	
Talent Graft Stent bare spring model 36 × 20 mm (Nitinol) World Medical Manufacturing Corp. Sunrise, FL	Safe	1.5	
Talent Graft Stent open web model 16 × 8 mm (Nitinol) World Medical Manufacturing Corp. Sunrise, FL	Safe	1.5	
Talent Graft Stent open web model 36 × 20 mm (Nitinol) World Medical Manufacturing Corp. Sunrise, FL	Safe	1.5	
Tracheobronchial Wallstent Endoprosthesis 14 × 80, stent Schneider (USA) Inc. Pfizer Medical Technology Group Minneapolis, MN	Safe	1.5	64
Tracheobronchial Wallstent Endoprosthesis 24 × 70, stent Schneider (USA) Inc. Pfizer Medical Technology Group Minneapolis, MN	Safe	1.5	64
Ureteral stent	Safe	1.5	
Vanguard Stent nitinol, platinum Boston Scientific Wayne, NJ	Safe	1.5	70
Wallstent biliary endoprosthesis (high nickle stainless steel) Schneider USA Plymouth, MN	Safe	1.5	28
Wallstent Endoprosthesis Magic Wallstent 3.5 × 25, stent Schneider (USA) Inc. Pfizer Medical Technology Group Minneapolis, MN	Safe	1.5	64

TABLE 15.1 (CONTINUED)
The List

Object	Status	Field Strength (T)	Reference
Wallstent Endoprosthesis	Safe	1.5	64
With Permalume covering			
8 × 80, stent			
Schneider (USA) Inc.			
Pfizer Medical Technology Group			
Minneapolis, MN			
Wallstent Esophageal II Endoprosthesis	Safe	1.5	64
20 × 130, stent			
Schneider (USA) Inc.			
Pfizer Medical Technology Group			
Minneapolis, MN			
Wallstent	Safe	1.5	69
platinum and cobalt alloy			
Schneider			
Bulach, Switzerland			
Wiktor coronary artery stent	Safe	1.5	
Medtronic Inverventional Vascular, Inc.			
X-Trode, 3 segment (316 SS), stent	Safe	1.5	
C.R. Bard, Inc.			
Billerica, MA			
X-Trode, 9 segment (316 SS), stent	Safe	1.5	
C.R. Bard, Inc.			
Billerica, MA			
Dental Implants, Devices, and Materials			
Brace band (SS), dental	Conditional 1	1.5	3
American Dental			
Missoula, MT			
Brace wire (chrome alloy), dental	Conditional 1	1.5	3
Ormco Corp.			
San Marcos, CA			
Castable alloy, dental	Conditional 1	1.5	12
Golden Dental Products, Inc.			
Golden, CO			
Cement-in keeper, dental	Conditional 1	1.5	12
Solid State Innovations, Inc.			
Mt. Airy, NC			
Dental amalgam, dental	Safe	1.39	1
GDP Direct Keeper, Pre-formed post, dental	Conditional 1	1.5	12
Golden Dental Products, Inc.			
Golden, CO			
Gutta Percha Points, dental	Safe	1.5	
Indian Head Real Silver Points, dental	Safe	1.5	
Union Broach Co., Inc.			
New York, NY			
Keeper, pre-formed post, dental	Conditional 1	1.5	1
Parkell Products, Inc.			
Farmingdale, NY			

TABLE 15.1 (CONTINUED)
The List

Object	Status	Field Strength (T)	Reference
Magna-Dent, large indirect keeper, dental Dental Ventures of America Yorba Linda, CA	Conditional 1	1.5	1
Palladium clad magnet, dental Parkell Products, Inc. Farmingdale, NY	Unsafe 1	1.5	13
Palladium/palladium keeper, dental Parkell Products, Inc. Farmingdale, NY	Conditional 1	1.5	13
Palladium/platinum casting alloy, dental Parkell Products, Inc. Farmingdale, NY	Conditional 1	1.5	13
Permanent crown (amalgam), dental Ormco Corp.	Safe	1.5	3
Silver point, dental Union Broach Co., Inc. New York, NY	Safe	1.5	3
Stainless steel clad magnet, dental Parkell Products, Inc. Farmingdale, NY	Unsafe 1	1.5	13
Stainless steel keeper, dental Parkell Products, Inc. Farmingdale, NY	Conditional 1	1.5	13
Titanium clad magnet, dental Parkell Products, Inc. Farmingdale, NY	Unsafe 1	1.5	13
ECG Electrodes			
Accutac, ECG electrode ConMed Corp. Utica, NY	Safe	1.5	
Accutac, ECG electrode Diaphoretic ConMed Corp. Utica, NY	Safe	1.5	
Adult Cloth, ECG electrode ConMed Corp. Utica, NY	Safe	1.5	
Adult ECG, ECG electrode Electrode 3-Pack ConMed Corp. Utica, NY	Safe	1.5	
Adult Foam, ECG electrode ConMed Corp. Utica, NY	Safe	1.5	
Cleartrace 2, ECG electrode ConMed Corp. Utica, NY	Safe	1.5	

TABLE 15.1 (CONTINUED)
The List

Object	Status	Field Strength (T)	Reference
Dyna/Trace Diagnostic ECG Electrode ConMed Corp. Utica, NY	Safe	1.5	
Dyna/Trace Mini, ECG electrode ConMed Corp. Utica, NY	Safe	1.5	
Dyna/Trace Stress, ECG electrode ConMed Corp. Utica, NY	Safe	1.5	
Dyna/Trace, ECG electrode ConMed Corp. Utica, NY	Safe	1.5	
High Demand, ECG electrode ConMed Corp. Utica, NY	Safe	1.5	
Holtrode, ECG electrode ConMed Corp. Utica, NY	Safe	1.5	
HP M2202A Radio-lucent, ECG electrode Monitoring Electrode, Ag/AgCL Hewlett-Packard Medical Supplies Andover, MA	Safe	1.5	
Invisatrace Adult, ECG electrode ConMed Corp. Utica, NY	Safe	1.5	
Pediatric Foam, ECG electrode ConMed Corp. Utica, NY	Safe	1.5	
Plia Cell Diagnostic, ECG electrode ConMed Corp. Utica, NY	Safe	1.5	
Plia-Cell Diaphoretic, ECG electrode ConMed Corp. Utica, NY	Safe	1.5	
Plia-Cell, ECG electrode ConMed Corp. Utica, NY	Safe	1.5	
Quadtrode MRI, ECG electrode InVivo Research, Inc. Orlando, FL	Safe	1.5	
Silvon Adult ECG Electrode ConMed Corp. Utica, NY	Safe	1.5	
Silvon Diaphoretic, ECG electrode ConMed Corp. Utica, NY	Safe	1.5	

TABLE 15.1 (CONTINUED)
The List

Object	Status	Field Strength (T)	Reference
Silvon Stress, ECG electrode ConMed Corp. Utica, NY	Safe	1.5	
Silvon, ECG electrode ConMed Corp. Utica, NY	Safe	1.5	
Snaptrace, ECG electrode ConMed Corp. Utica, NY	Safe	1.5	
SSE Radiotransparent ECG Electrode ConMed Corp. Utica, NY	Safe	1.5	
SSE, ECG electrode ConMed Corp. Utica, NY	Safe	1.5	
Foley Catheters with Temperature Sensors			
Bardex I.C. Foley Catheter with silver and hydrogel coating, 16 Fr. Bard Medical Division Covington, GA	Conditional 5	1.5	
Bardex I.C. Temp. Sensing Foley Catheter with a 6 foot cable, 16 Fr. Bard Medical Division Covington, GA	Conditional 5	1.5	
Bardex Lubricath Temp. Sensing Urotrack Plus Foley Catheter with a 6 foot cable, 16 Fr Bard Medical Division Covington, GA	Conditional 5	1.5	
Bardex Pediatric Temp. Sensing 400-Series Urotrack Foley Catheter with a detachable cable, 12 Fr. Bard Medical Division Covington, GA	Conditional 5	1.5	
Extension cable for Foley Catheter with temperature sensor, 10 feet RSP Respiratory Support Products, Inc. SIMS Smiths Industries Irvine, CA	Conditional 5	1.5	

TABLE 15.1 (CONTINUED)
The List

Object	Status	Field Strength (T)	Reference
Foley Catheter with temperature sensor, 10 Fr. RSP Respiratory Support Products, Inc. SIMS Smiths Industries Irvine, CA	Conditional 5	1.5	
Foley Catheter with temperature sensor, 18 Fr. RSP Respiratory Support Products, Inc. SIMS Smiths Industries Irvine, CA	Conditional 5	1.5	
Halo Vests and Cervical Fixation Devices			
Ambulatory Halo System halo and cervical fixation	Conditional 4	1.5	14
Bremer standard halo crown and vest halo and cervical fixation Bremmer Medical Co. Jacksonville, FL	Safe	1.0	15
Bremmer halo system MR-compatible halo and cervical fixation Bremmer Medical Co. Jacksonville, FL	Safe	1.0	15
Closed-back halo (titanium) halo and cervical fixation DePuy ACE Medical Co. El Segundo, CA	Safe	1.5	16
EXO adjustable coller halo and cervical fixation Florida Manufacturing Co. Daytona, FL	Conditional 4	1.0	15
Guilford cervical orthosis, modified halo and cervical fixation Guilford & Son, Ltd. Cleveland, OH	Safe	1.0	15
Guilford cervical orthosis halo and cervical fixation Guilford & Son, Ltd. Cleveland, OH	Conditional 4	1.0	15
Mark III halo vest (aluminum superstructure, stainless steel rivets, titanium bolts) DePuy ACE Medical Co. El Segundo, CA	Safe	1.5	16

TABLE 15.1 (CONTINUED)
The List

Object	Status	Field Strength (T)	Reference
Mark IV halo vest	Safe	1.5	16
(aluminum superstructure and titanium bolts)			
DePuy ACE Medical Co.			
El Segundo, CA			
MR-compatible	Safe	1.5	
halo vest and cervical fixation			
Lerman & Son Co.			
Beverly Hills, CA			
Open-back halo (aluminum)	Safe	1.5	16
DePuy ACE Medical Co.			
El Segundo, CA			
Open-back halo	Safe	1.5	16
with Delrin inserts for skull pins			
(aluminum and Delrin)			
DePuy ACE Medical Co.			
El Segundo, CA			
Philadelphia coller	Safe	1.0	15
Philadelphia Coller Co.			
Westville, NJ			
PMT halo cervical orthosis	Safe	1.0	15
PMT Corp.			
Chanhassen, MN			
PMT halo cervical orthosis	Safe	1.0	15
with graphite rods and halo ring			
PMT Corp.			
Chanhassen, MN			
S.O.M.I. cervical orthosis	Conditional 4	1.0	15
U.S. Manufacturing Co.			
Pasadena, CA			
Trippi-Wells tong (titanium)	Safe	1.5	16
DePuy ACE Medical Co.			
El Segundo, CA			
Heart Valve Protheses			
Beall	Conditional 1	2.35	17
heart valve			
Coratomic Inc.			
Indiana, PA			
Bileaflet	Safe	1.5	
Model A7760, 29 mm			
heart valve			
Medtronic Heart Valve Division			
Minneapolis, MN			
Bjork-Shiley (convexo/concave)	Safe	1.5	3
heart valve			
Shiley Inc.			
Irvine, CA			

TABLE 15.1 (CONTINUED)
The List

Object	Status	Field Strength (T)	Reference
Bjork-Shiley (universal/spherical) heart valve Shiley Inc. Irvine, CA	Conditional 1	1.5	3
Bjork-Shiley, Model 22 MBRC 11030 heart valve Shiley Inc. Irvine, CA	Conditional 1	2.35	18
Bjork-Shiley, Model MBC heart valve Shiley Inc. Irvine, CA	Conditional 1	2.35	18
CarboMedics Heart Valve Prosthesis Annuloflo Annuloplasty Ring, Size 26 CarboMedics Austin, TX	Safe	1.5	
CarboMedics Heart Valve Prosthesis Annuloflo Annuloplasty Ring, Size 36 CarboMedics Austin, TX	Safe	1.5	
CarboMedics Heart Valve Prosthesis Aortic Reduced, Model R500, Size 19 CarboMedics Austin, TX	Safe	1.5	19
CarboMedics Heart Valve Prosthesis Aortic Reduced, Model R500, Size 21 CarboMedics Austin, TX	Safe	1.5	19
CarboMedics Heart Valve Prosthesis Aortic Reduced, Model R500, Size 23 CarboMedics Austin, TX	Safe	1.5	19
CarboMedics Heart Valve Prosthesis Aortic Reduced, Model R500, Size 25 CarboMedics Austin, TX	Safe	1.5	19
CarboMedics Heart Valve Prosthesis Aortic Reduced, Model R500, Size 27 CarboMedics Austin, TX	Safe	1.5	19
CarboMedics Heart Valve Prosthesis Aortic Reduced, Model R500, Size 29 CarboMedics Austin, TX	Safe	1.5	19
CarboMedics Heart Valve Prosthesis Aortic Standard, Model 500, Size 31 CarboMedics Austin, TX	Safe	1.5	19

TABLE 15.1 (CONTINUED)
The List

Object	Status	Field Strength (T)	Reference
CarboMedics Heart Valve Prosthesis	Safe	1.5	
Aortic Valve, Size 16			
CarboMedics			
Austin, TX			
CarboMedics Heart Valve Prosthesis	Safe	1.5	
Carboseal, Size 31			
CarboMedics			
Austin, TX			
CarboMedics Heart Valve Prosthesis	Safe	1.5	19
Mitral Standard, Model 700, Size 23			
CarboMedics			
Austin, TX			
CarboMedics Heart Valve Prosthesis	Safe	1.5	19
Mitral Standard, Model 700, Size 25			
CarboMedics			
Austin, TX			
CarboMedics Heart Valve Prosthesis	Safe	1.5	19
Mitral Standard, Model 700, Size 27			
CarboMedics			
Austin, TX			
CarboMedics Heart Valve Prosthesis	Safe	1.5	19
Mitral Standard, Model 700, Size 29			
CarboMedics			
Austin, TX			
CarboMedics Heart Valve Prosthesis	Safe	1.5	19
Mitral Standard, Model 700, Size 31			
CarboMedics			
Austin, TX			
CarboMedics Heart Valve Prosthesis	Safe	1.5	19
Mitral Standard, Model 700, Size 33			
CarboMedics			
Austin, TX			
CarboMedics Heart Valve Prosthesis	Safe	1.5	
Mitral Valve, Size 33			
CarboMedics			
Austin, TX			
Carpentier-Edwards (porcine)	Conditional 1	2.35	18
heart valve			
American Edwards Laboratories			
Santa Ana, CA			
Carpentier-Edwards Annuloplasty Ring	Safe	1.5	
Model 4400, heart valve			
Baxter Healthcare Corporation			
Santa Ana, CA			
Carpentier-Edwards Annuloplasty Ring	Safe	1.5	
Model 4500, heart valve			
Baxter Healthcare Corporation			
Santa Ana, CA			

TABLE 15.1 (CONTINUED)
The List

Object	Status	Field Strength (T)	Reference
Carpentier-Edwards Annuloplasty Ring	Safe	1.5	
Model 4600, heart valve			
Baxter Healthcare Corporation Santa Ana, CA			
Carpentier-Edwards Bioprosthesis	Safe	1.5	
Model 2625, heart valve			
Baxter Healthcare Corporation			
Santa Ana, CA			
Carpentier-Edwards Bioprosthesis	Safe	1.5	
Model 6625, heart valve			
Baxter Healthcare Corporation			
Santa Ana, CA			
Carpentier-Edwards Pericardial Bioprosthesis	Safe	1.5	
Model 2700, heart valve			
Baxter Healthcare Corporation			
Santa Ana, CA			
Carpentier-Edwards Physio Annuloplasty Ring	Safe	1.5	
Model 4450, heart valve			
Baxter Healthcare Corporation			
Santa Ana, CA			
Carpentier-Edwards	Conditional 1	2.35	18
Model 2650, heart valve			
American Edwards Laboratories			
Santa Ana, CA			
Cosgrove-Edwards Annuloplasty Ring	Safe	1.5	
Model 4600, heart valve			
Baxter Healthcare Corporation			
Santa Ana, CA			
Duraflex Low Pressure Bioprosthesis	Safe	1.5	
Model 6625E6R-LP, heart valve			
Baxter Healthcare Corporation			
Santa Ana, CA			
Duraflex Low Pressure Bioprosthesis	Safe	1.5	
Model 6625LP, heart valve			
Baxter Healthcare Corporation			
Santa Ana, CA			
Duran Annuloplasty Ring	Safe	1.5	
Model H601H, 35 mm, heart valve			
Medtronic Heart Valve Division			
Minneapolis, MN			
Edwards TEKNA Bileaflet Valve	Safe	1.5	
Model 3200, heart valve			
Baxter Healthcare Corporation			
Santa Ana, CA			
Edwards TEKNA Bileaflet Valve	Safe	1.5	
Model 9200, heart valve			
Baxter Healthcare Corporation			
Santa Ana, CA			

TABLE 15.1 (CONTINUED)
The List

Object	Status	Field Strength (T)	Reference
Edwards-Duromedics Bileaflet Valve Model 3160, heart valve Baxter Healthcare Corporation Santa Ana, CA	Safe	1.5	
Edwards-Duromedics Bileaflet Valve Model 9120, heart valve Baxter Healthcare Corporation Santa Ana, CA	Safe	1.5	
Freestyle Model 995, 27 mm heart valve Medtronic Heart Valve Division Minneapolis, MN	Safe	1.5	
Hall-Kaster, Model A7700 heart valve Medtronic Heart Valve Division Minneapolis, MN	Conditional 1	1.5	3
Hancock 342 35 mm, Model 342, heart valve Medtronic Heart Valve Division Minneapolis, MN	Safe	1.5	
Hancock Conduit Model 100, 30 mm heart valve Medtronic Heart Valve Division Minneapolis, MN	Safe	1.5	
Hancock extracorporeal Model 242R heart valve Johnson & Johnson Anaheim, CA	Conditional 1	2.35	19
Hancock extracorporeal Model M 4365-33 heart valve Johnson & Johnson Anaheim, CA	Conditional 1	2.35	19
Hancock I (porcine) heart valve Johnson & Johnson Anaheim, CA	Conditional 1	1.5	3
Hancock II (porcine) heart valve Johnson & Johnson Anaheim, CA	Conditional 1	1.5	3
Hancock II Model T510, 33 mm heart valve Medtronic Heart Valve Division Minneapolis, MN	Safe	1.5	

TABLE 15.1 (CONTINUED)
The List

Object	Status	Field Strength (T)	Reference
Hancock Vascor, Model 505 heart valve Johnson & Johnson Anaheim, CA	Safe	2.35	19
Inonescu-Shiley, Universal ISM heart valve	Conditional 1	2.35	19
Lillehi-Kaster Model 300S, heart valve Medical Inc. Inver Grove Heights, MN	Conditional 1	2.35	17
Lillehi-Kaster Model 5009, heart valve Medical Inc. Inver Grove Heights, MN	Conditional 1	2.35	19
Med Hall Conduit Model R7700, 33 mm heart valve Medtronic Heart Valve Division Minneapolis, MN	Safe	1.5	
Medtronic Hall heart valve Medtronic Heart Valve Division Minneapolis, MN	Conditional 1	2.35	18
Medtronic Hall Model 7700, 33 mm heart valve Medtronic Heart Valve Division Minneapolis, MN	Safe	1.5	
Medtronic Hall Model A7700-D-16 heart valve Medtronic Heart Valve Division Minneapolis, MN	Conditional 1	2.35	18
Mitral Prosthetic Heart Valve Model 2100, heart valve TRI Technologies Brazil	Safe	1.5	70
Mitroflow Pericardial Heart Valve Model 12, heart valve Sulza-Medica and Mitroflow International Richmond, B.C. Canada	Safe	1.5	70
Mosaic Model 310, 33 mm, heart valve Medtronic Heart Valve Division Minneapolis, MN	Safe	1.5	

TABLE 15.1 (CONTINUED)
The List

Object	Status	Field Strength (T)	Reference
Omnicarbon	Conditional 1	2.35	18
Model 35231029, heart valve			
Medical Inc.			
Inver Grove Heights, MN			
Omniscience	Conditional 1	2.35	18
Model 6522, heart valve			
Medical Inc.			
Inver Grove Heights, MN			
On-X Valve	Safe	1.5	
Model 6816, heart valve			
Medical Carbon Research Institute			
Austin, TX			
Sculptor Annuloplasty Ring	Safe	1.5	
Model 605M, 35 mm			
heart valve			
Medtronic Heart Valve Division			
Minneapolis, MN			
Smeloff-Cutter	Conditional 1	2.35	18
Cutter Laboratories			
Berkeley, CA			
Sorin, No. 23	Conditional 1	1.5	20
heart valve			
St. Jude, Model A 10O	Conditional 1	2.35	19
heart valve			
St. Jude Medical Inc.			
St. Paul, MN			
St. Jude, Model M 101	Conditional 1	2.35	19
heart valve			
St. Jude Medical Inc.			
St. Paul, MN			
St. Jude	Safe	1.5	3
heart valve			
St. Jude Medical Inc.			
St. Paul, MN			
Starr-Edwards, Model 1000	Conditional 1	1.5	
heart valve			
Baxter Healthcare Corporation			
Santa Ana, CA			
Starr-Edwards, Model 1200	Conditional 1	1.5	
heart valve			
Baxter Healthcare Corporation			
Santa Ana, CA			
Starr-Edwards, Model 1260	Conditional 1	2.35	17
heart valve			
American Edwards Laboratories			
Baxter Healthcare Corporation			
Santa Ana, CA			

TABLE 15.1 (CONTINUED)
The List

Object	Status	Field Strength (T)	Reference
Starr-Edwards, Model 2300 heart valve Baxter Healthcare Corporation Santa Ana, CA	Conditional 1	1.5	
Starr-Edwards, Model 2310 heart valve Baxter Healthcare Corporation Santa Ana, CA	Conditional 1	1.5	
Starr-Edwards, Model 2320 heart valve American Edwards Laboratories Baxter Healthcare Corporation Santa Ana, CA	Conditional 1	2.35	17
Starr-Edwards, Model 2400 heart valve American Edwards Laboratories Baxter Healthcare Corporation Santa Ana, CA	Safe	1.5	3
Starr-Edwards, Model 6000 heart valve Baxter Healthcare Corporation Santa Ana, CA	Conditional 1	1.5	
Starr-Edwards, Model 6120 heart valve Baxter Healthcare Corporation Santa Ana, CA	Conditional 1	1.5	
Starr-Edwards, Model 6300 heart valve Baxter Healthcare Corporation Santa Ana, CA	Conditional 1	1.5	
Starr-Edwards, Model 6310 heart valve Baxter Healthcare Corporation Santa Ana, CA	Conditional 1	1.5	
Starr-Edwards, Model 6320 heart valve Baxter Healthcare Corporation Santa Ana, CA	Conditional 1	1.5	
Starr-Edwards, Model 6400 heart valve Baxter Healthcare Corporation Santa Ana, CA	Conditional 1	1.5	
Starr-Edwards, Model 6520 heart valve Baxter Healthcare Corporation Santa Ana, CA	Conditional 1	2.35	19

TABLE 15.1 (CONTINUED)
The List

Object	Status	Field Strength (T)	Reference
Starr-Edwards, Model Pre 6000 heart valve American Edwards Laboratories Baxter Healthcare Corporation Santa Ana, CA	Conditional 1	2.35	17
Sulzer/Carbomedics Synergy PC Pericardial Heart Valve Sulza-Medica and Mitroflow International Richmond, B.C. Canada	Safe	1.5	70
Hemostatic Clips			
Gastrointestinal anastomosis clip Auto Suture SGIA, (SS) hemostatic clip United States Surgical Corp. Norwalk, CT	Safe	1.5	3
Hemoclip, #10, (316L SS) Edward Weck Triangle Park, NJ	Safe	1.5	3
Hemoclip (tantalum) hemostatic clip Edward Weck Triangle Park, NJ	Safe	1.5	3
Ligaclip (tantalum) hemostatic clip Ethicon, Inc. Sommerville, NJ	Safe	1.5	3
Ligaclip, #6 (316L SS) hemostatic clip Ethicon, Inc. Sommerville, NJ	Safe	1.5	3
Surgiclip, Auto Suture M-9.5 (SS) hemostatic clip United States Surgical Corp. Norwalk, CT	Safe	1.5	3
Miscellaneous			
357 Magnum Revolver Model 66-3 Smith and Wesson Springfield, MA	Unsafe 1	1.5	46
Accusite pH Enteral Feeding System pH Site Locator 10 Fr. Zinetics Medical Salt Lake City, UT	Unsafe 2	1.5	

TABLE 15.1 (CONTINUED)
The List

Object	Status	Field Strength (T)	Reference
Adson Tissue Forcep (Ti6Al-4V) Johnson & Johnson Professional, Inc. Raynham, MA	Safe	1.5	62
AMS Artificial Bowel Sphincter Prosthesis American Medical Systems Minnetonka, MN	Safe	1.5	
AMS Artificial Urinary Sphincter 791 American Medical Systems Minnetonka, MN	Safe	1.5	
AMS Mainstay Soft-Tissue Anchor American Medical Systems Minnetonka, MN	Safe	1.5	
Artificial urinary sphincter AMS 800 American Medical Systems Minnetonka, MN	Safe	1.5	3
Battery, lithium, 3.9 Volt (304 SS and 316L SS, nickle) Greatbatch Scientific Clarence, NY	Conditional 1	1.5	
Biosearch endo-feeding tube	Safe	1.5	
Cerebral ventricular shunt tube connector (type unknown)	Unsafe 1	0.147	1
Cerebral ventricular shunt tube connector, Accu-flow right angle Codman Randolf, MA	Safe	1.5	3
Cerebral ventricular shunt tube connector, Accu-Flow, straight Codman Randolf, MA	Safe	1.5	3
Cerebral ventricular shunt tube connector, Accu-flow, T-connector Codman Randolf, MA	Safe	1.5	3
Codman-Medos Programmable Valve Medos S.A., LeLocle, Switzerland	Conditional 5	1.5	67
Contraceptive diaphragm All Flex Ortho Pharmaceutical Raritan, NJ	Conditional 1	1.5	3
Contraceptive diaphragm Flat Spring Ortho Pharmaceutical Raritan, NJ	Conditional 1	1.5	3
Contraceptive diaphragm Gyne T	Safe	1.5	47

TABLE 15.1 (CONTINUED)
The List

Object	Status	Field Strength (T)	Reference
Contraceptive diaphragm	Conditional 1	1.5	3
Koroflex			
Young Drug Products			
Piscataway, NJ			
Contraceptive IUD	Safe	1.5	47
Multiload Cu375 (copper, silver)			
Contraceptive IUD	Safe	1.5	47
Nova T (copper, silver)			
Cranial Ceramic Drill bit (ceramic)	Safe	1.5	48
MicroSurgical Techniques Inc.			
Fort Collins, CO			
Craniofix, bone flap fixation system (titanium alloy)	Safe	1.5	50
Aesculap, Inc.			
South San Francisco, CA			
CT-MRI Topographic Marker	Safe	1.5	
E-Z-Em			
Westbury, NY			
Deponit, nitroglycerin	Conditional 3	1.5	
transdermal delivery system (aluminized plastic)			
Schwarz Pharma			
Milwaukee, WI			
EEG electrodes, Adult E-6-GH (gold plated silver)	Safe	0.3	51
Grass Co.			
Quincy, MA			
EEG electrodes, Pediatric E-5-GH (gold plated silver)	Safe	0.3	51
Grass Co.			
Quincy, MA			
Endoscope, rigid, 2.7 mm (Sinuscope)	Safe	1.5	59
Greatbatch Scientific			
Clarence, NY			
Endoscope, rigid, 8.0 mm (Laryngoscope)	Safe	1.5	59
Greatbatch Scientific			
Clarence, NY			
Endotracheal tube with metal ring marker	Safe	1.5	
Trachmate			
Eyelid weight (gold)	Safe	1.5	52
Fiber-optic Intubating	Safe	1.5	
Laryngoscope Blade			
Greatbatch Scientific			
Clarence, NY			
Fiber-optic Intubating	Safe	1.5	
Laryngoscope Handle			
Greatbatch Scientific			
Clarence, NY			
Firestar	Unsafe 1	1.5	46
9-mm semiautomatic			
Star Bonifacio Echeverria			
Eibar, Spain			

TABLE 15.1 (CONTINUED)
The List

Object	Status	Field Strength (T)	Reference
Flex-tip Plus Epidural Catheter (304V SS) Arrow International Inc. Reading, PA	Unsafe 2	1.5	
Forceps (ceramic) MicroSurgical Techniques Inc. Fort Collins, CO	Safe	1.5	48
Forceps (titanium)	Safe	1.39	1
Hakim valve and pump	Safe	1.39	1
Implantable Spinal Fusion Stimulator bone fusion stimulator Electro-Biology, Inc. (EBI) Parsippany, NJ	Conditional 5	1.5	63
Intracranial depth electrodes for EEG recordings (nickle- chromium alloy) Superior Tube Company Norristown, NY	Safe	1.5	53
Intraflex Feeding Tube tungsten weight, plastic	Safe	1.5	
Intrauterine contraceptive device (IUD), Copper T (copper) Searle Pharmaceuticals Chicago, IL	Safe	1.5	54
Intrauterine contraceptive device (IUD) Lippey loop, plastic	Safe	1.5	
Intrauterine contraceptive device (IUD) Perigard Gyne Pharmaceuticals	Safe	1.5	
Langenbeck Periosteal Elevator (304 SS) Johnson & Johnson Professional, Inc. Raynham, MA	Safe	1.5	62
Laparoscopic Graspers Greatbatch Scientific Clarence, NY	Safe	1.5	
LMA Fastrach Endotracheal Tube size 8 mm endotracheal tube LMA North America, Inc. San Diego, CA	Conditional 5	1.5	
LMA-Classic size 5, large adult laryngeal mask airway LMA North America, Inc. San Diego, CA	Conditional 5	1.5	
LMA-Flexible size 2 larygeal mask airway LMA North America, Inc. San Diego, CA	Conditional 5	1.5	

TABLE 15.1   (CONTINUED)
The List

Object	Status	Field Strength (T)	Reference
Low Magnetic Signature Lithium Battery (C size) Greatbatch Scientific Clarence, NY	Safe	1.5	
May Hegar Needle Holder (Ti6Al-4V) Johnson & Johnson Professional, Inc. Raynham, MA	Safe	1.5	62
Mercury Duotube-feeding, feeding tube	Safe	1.5	
Micro Needle Holder Greatbatch Scientific Clarence, NY	Safe	1.5	
Micro Round Handled Scissors Greatbatch Scientific Clarence, NY	Safe	1.5	
Micro Tissue Forceps Greatbatch Scientific Clarence, NY	Safe	1.5	
Micro Tying Forceps Greatbatch Scientific Clarence, NY	Safe	1.5	
Mitek anchor Miteck Products Westood, MA	Safe	1.5	
Penfield Dissector (304 SS) Johnson & Johnson Professional, Inc. Raynham, MA	Safe	1.5	62
Peripheral Nerve Stimulator MR-STIM, Model GN-013 Greatbatch Scientific Clarence, NY	Safe	1.5	
Scalpel (SS)	Unsafe 1	1.5	
Scalpel, Microsharp Ceramic Scalpels, sizes #10, #11, #11c, #15 (ceramic) MicroSurgical Techniques, Inc. Fort Collins, CO	Safe	1.5	48
Scissors, Ceramic (prototype, ceramic) Microsurgical Techniques, Inc. Fort Collins, CO	Safe	1.5	48
Shunt valve, Holter-Hausner type Holter-Hausner, Inc. Bridgeport, PA	Safe	1.5	55
Shunt valve, Holtertype The Holter Co. Bridgeport, PA	Unsafe 1	1.5	55
Sophy adjustable pressure valve	Unsafe 1	1.5	56

TABLE 15.1 (CONTINUED)
The List

Object	Status	Field Strength (T)	Reference
Sophy programmable pressure valve Model SM8 Sophysa Orsay, France	Unsafe 1	1.5	67
Sophy programmable pressure valve Model SP3 Sophysa Orsay, France	Unsafe 1	1.5	67
Sophy programmable pressure valve Model SU8 Sophysa Orsay, France	Unsafe 1	1.5	67
Sponge Forcep (Ti6Al-4V) Johnson & Johnson Professional, Inc. Raynham, MA	Safe	1.5	62
Stereotactic headframe with removable mouthpiece (aluminum, 8-18 SS Delrin, titanium) Compass International, Inc. Rochester, MN	Safe	1.5	
Suction/Irrigation Handle for Sinuscope Greatbatch Scientific Clarence, NY	Safe	1.5	
Super ArrowFlex PSI 10 Fr. × 65 cm (304V SS) Arrow International Inc. Reading, PA	Unsafe 2	1.5	
Super ArrowFlex PSI 9 Fr. × 11 cm (304 V SS) Arrow International Inc. Reading, PA	Unsafe 2	1.5	
SynchroMed, implantable drug infusion device Medtronic Inc. Minneapolis, MN	Conditional 5	1.5	
Tantalum powder	Safe	1.39	1
TheraCath (304 V SS) Arrow International Inc. Reading, PA	Unsafe 2	1.5	
Tweezers, Ceramic (prototype, ceramic) MicroSurgical Techniques, Inc. Fort Collins, CO	Safe	1.5	48
UroLume Endoprosthesis (titanium) American Medical Systems Minnetonka, MN	Safe	1.5	
Vascular marker, O-ring washer (302 SS) PIC Design Middlebury, CT	Conditional 1	1.5	
Vitallium implant	Safe	1.5	

TABLE 15.1 (CONTINUED)
The List

Object	Status	Field Strength (T)	Reference
Winged infusion set	Safe	1.5	58
MRI compatible			
E-Z-EM, Inc.			
Westbury, NY			
Woodson Elevator	Safe	1.5	62
(304 SS)			
Johnson & Johnson Professional, Inc.			
Raynham, MA			
Ocular Implants, Materials, and Devices			
Clip 250, double tantalum clip (tantalum)	Safe	1.5	29
ocular			
Mira Inc.			
Clip 50, double tantalum clip (tantalum)	Safe	1.5	29
ocular			
Mira Inc.			
Clip 51, single tantalum clip (tantalum)	Safe	1.5	29
ocular			
Mira Inc.			
Clip 52, single tantalum clip (tantalum)	Safe	1.5	29
ocular			
Mira Inc.			
Double tantalum clip (tantalum)	Safe	1.5	29
ocular			
Storz Instrument Co.			
Double tantalum clip style 250 (tantalum)	Safe	1.5	29
ocular			
Storz Instrument Co.			
Fatio eyelid spring/wire	Unsafe 1	1.5	30
ocular			
Gold eyelid spring	Safe	1.5	
ocular			
Intraocular lens implant	Safe	1.0	31
Binkhorst, iridocapsular lense			
platinum-iridium loop (platinum, iridium)			
ocular			
Intraocular lens implant	Safe	1.5	31
Binkhorst, iridocapsular lense			
platinum-iridium loop			
ocular			
Intraocular lens implant	Safe	1.0	31
Binkhorst, iridocapsular lense			
titanium loop (titanium)			
ocular			
Intraocular lens implant	Safe	1.0	31
Worst, platinum clip lense			
ocular			

TABLE 15.1 (CONTINUED)
The List

Object	Status	Field Strength (T)	Reference
Retinal tack (303 SS) ocular Bascom Palmer Eye Institute	Safe	1.5	32
Retinal tack (303 SS) ocular Duke	Safe	1.5	32
Retinal tack (aluminum textraoxide) ocular Ruby	Safe	1.5	32
Retinal tack (cobalt, nickel) ocular Greishaber Fallsington, PA	Safe	1.5	32
Retinal tack (martensitic SS) ocular Western European	Unsafe 1	1.5	32
Retinal tack (titanium alloy) ocular Coopervision Irvine, CA	Safe	1.5	32
Retinal tack, Norton staple (platinum, rhodium) ocular Norton	Safe	1.5	32
Single tantalum clip (tantalum) ocular	Safe	1.5	29
Troutman magnetic ocular implant ocular	Unsafe 1	1.5	
Unitech round wire eye spring ocular	Unsafe 1	1.5	
Orthopedic Implants, Materials, and Devices			
AML femoral component bipolar hip prothesis orthopedic implant Zimmer Warsaw, IN	Safe	1.5	3
Cannulated cancellous screw 6.5 × 50 mm (titanium alloy) orthopedic implant DePuy ACE Medical Co. El Segundo, CA	Safe	1.5	
Captured screw assembly, 100 mm (titanium alloy) orthopedic implant DePuy ACE Medical Co. El Segundo, CA	Safe	1.5	
Cervical wire, 18 gauge (316L SS) orthopedic implant	Safe	0.3	33
Charnley-Muller hip prosthesis (Protasyl-10 alloy) orthopedic implant	Safe	0.3	

TABLE 15.1 (CONTINUED)
The List

Object	Status	Field Strength (T)	Reference
Cortical bone screw 4.5 × 36 mm (titanium alloy) orthopedic implant DePuy ACE Medical Co. El Segundo, CA	Safe	1.5	
Cortical bone screw large (titanium alloy) orthopedic implant Zimmer Warsaw, IN	Safe	1.5	34
Cortical bone screw small (titanium alloy) orthopedic implant Zimmer Warsaw, IN	Safe	1.5	34
Cotrel rod (SS-ASTM, grade 2) orthopedic implant	Safe	1.5	
Cotrel rods with hooks (316L SS) orthopedic implant	Safe	0.3	33
Drummond wire (316L SS) orthopedic implant	Safe	0.3	33
DTT, device for transverse traction (316L SS) orthopedic implant	Safe	0.3	33
Endoscopic noncannulated interference screw (titanium) orthopedic implant Acufex Microsurgical Norwood, MA	Safe	1.5	34
Fixation staple (cobalt–chromium alloy) orthopedic implant Richards Medical Co. Memphis, TN	Safe	1.5	34
Halifax clamps orthopedic implant American Medical Electronics Richardson, TX	Safe	1.5	
Harrington compression rod with hooks and nuts (316L SS) orthopedic implant	Safe	0.3	33
Harrington distraction rod with hooks (316L SS) orthopedic implant	Safe	0.3	33
Harris hip prosthesis orthopedic implant Zimmer Warsaw, IN	Safe	1.5	3

TABLE 15.1 (CONTINUED)
The List

Object	Status	Field Strength (T)	Reference
Hip implant (austenitic SS) orthopedic implant DePuy Inc. Warsaw, IN	Safe	1.5	
Jewett nail orthopedic implant Zimmer Warsaw, IN	Safe	1.5	3
Kirschner intermedullary rod orthopedic implant Kirschner Medical Timonium, MD	Safe	1.5	3
L plate, 6-hole (titanium alloy) orthopedic implant DePuy ACE Medical Co. El Segundo, CA	Safe	1.5	
L Rod (cobalt–nickel alloy) orthopedic implant Richards Medical Co. Memphis, TN	Safe	1.5	
Luque Wire orthopedic implant	Safe	0.3	33
Moe spinal instrumentation orthopedic implant Zimmer Warsaw, IN	Safe	1.5	
Perfix interence screw (17-4 SS) orthopedic implant Instrument Makar Okemos, MI	Conditional 1	1.5	34
Rusch Rod orthopedic implant	Safe	1.5	
Side plate, 6-hole (titanium alloy) orthopedic implant DePuy ACE Co. El Segundo, CA	Safe	1.5	
Spinal L-Rod orthopedic implant DePuy Warsaw, IN	Safe	1.5	
Stainless steel mesh orthopedic implant Zimmer Warsaw, IN	Safe	1.5	3
Stainless steel plate orthopedic implant Zimmer Warsaw, IN	Safe	1.5	3

TABLE 15.1 (CONTINUED)
The List

Object	Status	Field Strength (T)	Reference

Stainless steel screw
  orthopedic implant
  Zimmer
  Warsaw, IN
	Safe	1.5	3

Stainless steel wire
  orthopedic implant
  Zimmer
  Warsaw, IN
	Safe	1.5	3

Staple plate, large (Zimaloy)
  orthopedic implant
  Zimmer
  Warsaw, IN
	Safe	1.5	3

Synthes AO DCP 2, 3, 4, 5 hole plate orthopedic implant	Safe	1.5	

Tibial nail, 9 mm (titanium alloy)
  orthopedic implant
  DePuy ACE Medical Co.
  El Segundo, CA
	Safe	1.5	

Universal Reconstruction Ribbon (titanium)
  orthopedic implant
  DePuy ACE Medical Co.
  El Segundo, CA
	Safe	1.5	

Zielke rod with screw
  washer and nut (316L SS)
  orthopedic implant
	Safe	0.3	33

Otologic Implants			

Austin tytan piston (titanium)
  otologic implant
  Treace Medical
  Nashville, TN
	Safe	1.5	35

Berger V bobbin ventilation tube (titanium)
  otologic implant
  Richards Medical Co.
  Memphis, TN
	Safe	1.5	35

Causse Flex H/A
  partial ossicular prosthesis (titanium)
  otologic implant
  Microtek Medical, Inc.
  Memphis, TN
	Safe	1.5	36

Causse Flex H/A
  total ossicular prosthesis (titanium)
  otologic implant
  Microtek Medical Inc.
  Memphis, TN
	Safe	1.5	36

TABLE 15.1 (CONTINUED)
The List

Object	Status	Field Strength (T)	Reference
Cochlear implant, Combi 40/40+ Multichannel system otologic implant MedEl Innsbrook, Austria	Unsafe 2	0.2 and 1.5	65
Cochlear implant Nucleus Mini 20-channel otologic implant Cochlear Corporation Engelwood, CO	Unsafe 1	1.5	38
Cochlear implant otologic implant 3M/House	Unsafe 1	0.6	37
Cochlear implant otologic implant 3M/Vienna	Unsafe 1	0.6	37
Cody tack otologic implant	Safe	0.6	37
Ehmke hook stapes prosthesis (platinum) otologic implant Richards Medical Co. Memphis, TN	Safe	1.5	35
Fisch piston (Teflon, SS) otologic implant Richards Medical Co. Memphis, TN	Safe	1.5	38
Flex H/A notched offset total ossicular prosthesis (316L SS) otologic implant Microtek Medical, Inc. Memphis, TN	Safe	1.5	36
Flex H/A offset partial ossicular prosthesis (316L SS) Microtek Medical, Inc. Memphis, TN	Safe	1.5	36
House double loop (ASTM-318-76 Grade 2 SS) otologic implant Storz St. Louis, MO	Safe	1.5	35
House double loop (tantalum) otologic implant Storz St. Louis, MO	Safe	1.5	35
House single loop (ASTM-318-76, Grade 2 SS) otologic implant Storz St. Louis, MO	Safe	1.5	31

TABLE 15.1 (CONTINUED)
The List

Object	Status	Field Strength (T)	Reference
House single loop (tantalum)	Safe	1.5	35
otologic implant			
Storz			
St. Louis, MO			
House wire (SS)	Safe	0.5	39
otologic implant			
Otomed			
House wire (tantalum)	Safe	0.5	39
otologic implant			
Otomed			
House-type incus prosthesis	Safe	0.6	
otologic implant			
House-type stainless steel	Safe	1.5	35
piston and wire (ASTM-318-76 Grade 2 SS)			
otologic implant			
Xomed-Treace Inc.			
A Bristol-Myers Squibb Co.			
House-type wire loop stapes prosthesis (316L SS)	Safe	1.5	35
otologic implant			
Richards Medical Co.			
Memphis, TN			
McGee piston stapes prosthesis (316L, SS)	Safe	1.5	35
otologic implant			
Richards Medical Co.			
Memphis, TN			
McGee piston stapes prosthesis (platinum, 316L SS)	Safe	1.5	35
otologic implant			
Richards Medical Co.			
Memphis, TN			
McGee piston stapes prosthesis	Unsafe 1	1.5	38
(platinum, chromium-nickel alloy SS)			
otologic implant			
Richards Medical Co.			
Memphis, TN			
McGee Sheperd's Cook stapes prosthesis (316L SS)	Safe	1.5	35
otologic implant			
Richards Medical Co.			
Memphis, TN			
Plasti-pore piston (316L SS/ Plasti-pore material)	Safe	1.5	35
otologic implant			
Richards Medical Co.			
Memphis, TN			
Platinum ribbon loop stapes prosthesis (platinum)	Safe	1.5	35
otologic implant			
Richards Medical Co.			
Memphis, TN			

TABLE 15.1 (CONTINUED)
The List

Object	Status	Field Strength (T)	Reference
Reuter bobbin ventilation tube (316L SS) otologic implant Richards Medical Co. Memphis, TN	Safe	1.5	35
Reuter drain tube otologic implant	Safe	1.5	35
Richards bucket handle stapes prosthesis (316L SS) otologic implant Richards Medical Co. Memphis, TN	Safe	1.5	35
Richards piston stapes prosthesis (platinum, fluoroplastic) otologic implant Richards Medical Co. Memphis, TN	Safe	1.5	35
Richards Plasti-pore with Armstrong-style platinum ribbon (platinum) otologic implant Richards Medical Co. Memphis, TN	Safe	1.5	35
Richards platinum Teflon piston 0.6 mm (Teflon, platinum) otologic implant Richards Medical Co. Memphis, TN	Safe	1.5	38
Richards platinum Teflon piston 0.8 mm (Teflon, platinum) otologic implant Richards Medical Co. Memphis, TN	Safe	1.5	38
Richards Shepherd's crook (platinum) otologic implant Richards Medical Co. Memphis, TN	Safe	0.5	39
Richards Teflon piston (Teflon) otologic implant Richards Medical Co. Memphis, TN	Safe	1.5	38
Robinson incus replacement prosthesis (ASTM-318-76 Grade 2 SS) otologic implant Storz St. Louis, MO	Safe	1.5	35
Robinson stapes prosthesis (ASTM-318-76 Grade 2 SS) otologic implant Storz St. Louis, MO	Safe	1.5	35

TABLE 15.1 (CONTINUED)
The List

Object	Status	Field Strength (T)	Reference
Robinson-Moon offset stapes prosthesis (ASTM-318-76 Grade 2 SS) otologic implant Storz St. Louis, MO	Safe	1.5	35
Robinson-Moon-Lippy offset stapes prosthesis (ASTM- 318-76 Grade 2 SS) otologic implant Storz St. Louis, MO	Safe	1.5	35
Ronis piston stapes prosthesis (316L SS, fluoroplastic) otologic implant Richards Medical Co. Memphis, TN	Safe	1.5	35
Schea cup piston stapes prosthesis (platinum, fluoroplastic) otologic implant Richards Medical Co. Memphis, TN	Safe	1.5	35
Schea malleus attachment piston (Teflon) otologic implant Richards Medical Co. Memphis, TN	Safe	1.5	38
Schea stainless steel and Teflon wire prosthesis (Teflon, 316 L SS) otologic implant Richards Medical Co. Memphis, TN	Safe	1.5	38
Scheer piston (Teflon, 316L SS) otologic implant Richards Medical Co. Memphis, TN	Safe	1.5	33
Scheer piston stapes prosthesis (316L SS, fluoroplastic) otologic implant Richards Medical Co. Memphis, TN	Safe	1.5	35
Schuknecht gelfoam and wire prosthesis, Armstrong style (316L SS) otologic implant Richards Medical Co. Memphis, TN	Safe	1.5	40
Schuknecht piston stapes prosthesis (316L SS, fluoroplastic) otologic implant Richards Medical Co. Memphis, TN	Safe	1.5	35

TABLE 15.1   (CONTINUED)
The List

Object	Status	Field Strength (T)	Reference
Schuknecht Tef-wire incus attachment (ASTM-318-76 Grade 2 SS) otologic implant Storz St. Louis, MO	Safe	1.5	35
Schuknecht Tef-wire malleus attachment (ASTM-318-76 Grade 2 SS) otologic implant Storz St. Louis, MO	Safe	1.5	35
Schuknecht Teflon wire piston 0.6 mm (Teflon, 316L SS) otologic implant Richards Medical Co. Memphis, TN	Safe	1.5	38
Schuknecht Teflon wire piston 0.8 mm (Teflon, 316L SS) otologic implant Richards Medical Co. Memphis, TN	Safe	1.5	38
Sheehy incus replacement (ASTM-318-76 Grade 2 SS) otologic implant Storz St. Louis, MO	Safe	1.5	35
Sheehy incus strut (316L SS) otologic implant Richards Medical Co. Memphis, TN	Safe	1.5	38
Sheehy-type incus replacement strut (Teflon, 316L SS) otologic implant Richards Medical Co. Memphis, TN	Safe	1.5	35
Silverstein malleus clip, ventilation tube (Teflon, 316L SS) otologic implant Richards Medical Co. Memphis, TN	Safe	1.5	38
Spoon bobbin ventilation tube (316L SS) otologic implant Richards Medical Co. Memphis, TN	Safe	1.5	35
Stapes, fluoroplastic/platinum, piston otologic implant Microtek Medical, Inc. Memphis, TN	Safe	1.5	36
Stapes, fluoroplastic/stainless steel piston (316L SS) otologic implant Microtek Medical, Inc. Memphis, TN	Safe	1.5	36

TABLE 15.1 (CONTINUED)
The List

Object	Status	Field Strength (T)	Reference
Tantalum wire loop stages prosthesis (tantalum) otologic implant Richards Medical Co. Memphis, TN	Safe	1.5	35
Tef-platinum piston (platinum) otologic implant Xomed-Treace Inc. A Bristol-Myers Squibb Co.	Safe	1.5	35
Total ossibular replacement prosthesis (TORP) (316L SS) otologic implant Richards Medical Co. Memphis, TN	Safe	1.5	38
Trapeze ribbon loop stapes prosthesis (platinum) otologic implant Richards Medical Co. Memphis, TN	Safe	1.5	35
Williams microclip (316L SS) otologic implant Richards Medical Co. Memphis, TN	Safe	1.5	35
Xomed Baily stapes implant otologic implant	Safe	1.5	35
Xomed ceravital partial ossicular prosthesis otologic implant	Safe	1.5	
Xomed stapes prosthesis Robinson-style otologic implant Richard's Co. Nashville, TN	Safe	1.5	35
Xomed stapes (ASTM-318-76 Grade 2 SS) otologic implant Xomed-Treace Inc. A Bristol-Myers Squibb Co.	Safe	1.5	35
Patent Ductus Arteriosus (PDA), Atrial Septal Defect (ASD), and Ventricular Septal Detect (VSD) Occluders			
Bard Clamshell Septal Umbrella 17 mm, occluder (MP35N) C.R. Bard, Inc. Billerica, MA	Safe	1.5	41
Bard Clamshell Septal Umbrella 23 mm, occluder (MP35N) C.R. Bard, Inc. Billerica, MA	Safe	1.5	41

TABLE 15.1 (CONTINUED)
The List

Object	Status	Field Strength (T)	Reference
Bard Clamshell Septal Umbrella 28 mm, occluder (MP35N) C.R. Bard, Inc. Billerica, MA	Safe	1.5	41
Bard Clamshell Septal Umbrella 33 mm, occluder (MP35N) C.R. Bard, Inc. Billerica, MA	Safe	1.5	41
Bard Clamshell Septal Umbrella 40 mm, occluder (MP35N) C.R. Bard, Inc. Bellerica, MA	Safe	1.5	41
Lock Clamshell Septal Occlusion Implant 17 mm, occluder (304 V SS) C.R. Bard, Inc. Billerica, MA	Conditional 2	1.5	41
Lock Clamshell Septal Occlusion Implant 23 mm, occluder (304 V SS) C.R. Bard, Inc. Billerica, MA	Conditional 2	1.5	41
Lock Clamshell Septal Occlusion Implant 28 mm, occluder (304 V SS) C.R. Bard, Inc. Billerica, MA	Conditional 2	1.5	41
Lock Clamshell Septal Occlusion Implant 33 mm, occluder (304 V SS) C.R. Bard, Inc. Billerica, MA	Conditional 2	1.5	41
Lock Clamshell Septal Occlusion Implant 40 mm, occluder (304 V SS) C.R. Bard, Inc. Billerica, MA	Conditional 2	1.5	41
Rashkind PDA Occlusion Implant 12 mm, occluder (304V SS) C.R. Bard, Inc. Billerica, MA	Conditional 2	1.5	41
Rashkind PDA Occlusion Implant 17 mm, occluder (304 V SS) C.R. Bard, Inc. Billerica, MA	Conditional 2	1.5	41
Pellets and Bullets			
BBs (Crosman)	Unsafe 1	1.5	
BBs (Daisy)	Unsafe 1	1.5	
Bullet, .357 inch (aluminum, lead) pellets and bullets Winchester	Safe	1.5	42

TABLE 15.1 (CONTINUED)
The List

Object	Status	Field Strength (T)	Reference
Bullet, .357 inch (bronze, plastic) pellets and bullets Patton-Morgan	Safe	1.5	42
Bullet, .357 inch (copper, lead) pellets and bullets Cascade	Safe	1.5	42
Bullet, .357 inch (copper, lead) pellets and bullets Hornady	Safe	1.5	42
Bullet, .357 inch (copper, lead) pellets and bullets Patton-Morgan	Safe	1.5	42
Bullet, .357 inch (lead) pellets and bullets Remington	Safe	1.5	42
Bullet, .357 inch (nickel, copper, lead) pellets and bullets Winchester	Safe	1.5	42
Bullet, .357 inch (nylon, lead) pellets and bullets Smith & Wesson	Safe	1.5	42
Bullet, .357 inch (steel, lead) pellets and bullets Fiocchi	Safe	1.5	42
Bullet, .380 inch (copper, nickel, lead) pellets and bullets Winchester	Unsafe 1	1.5	42
Bullet, .380 inch (copper, plastic, lead) pellets and bullets Glaser	Safe	1.5	42
Bullet, .44 inch (Teflon, bronze) pellets and bullets North American Ordinance	Safe	1.5	42
Bullet, .45 inch (copper, lead) pellets and bullets Samson	Safe	1.5	42
Bullet, .45 inch (steel, lead) pellets and bullets Evansville Ordinance	Unsafe 1	1.5	42
Bullet, 7.62 × 39 mm (copper, steel) pellets and bullets Norinco	Unsafe 1	1.5	42
Bullet, 9 mm (copper, lead) pellets and bullets Norma	Unsafe 1	1.5	42
Bullet, 9 mm (copper, lead) pellets and bullets Remington	Safe	1.5	42

TABLE 15.1 (CONTINUED)
The List

Object	Status	Field Strength (T)	Reference
Shot, 00 buckshot (lead)	Safe	1.5	42
pellets and bullets			
Shot, 12 gauge, size: 00 (copper, lead)	Safe	1.5	42
pellets and bullets			
Federal			
Shot, 4 (lead)	Safe	1.5	42
pellets and bullets			
Shot, 7 1/2 (lead)	Safe	1.5	42
pellets and bullets			
Penile Implants			
Penile implant, 700 Ultrex Plus	Safe	1.5	
American Medical Systems			
Minnetonka, MN			
Penile implant, AMS 700 CX Inflatable	Safe	1.5	43
American Medical Systems			
Minnetonka, MN			
Penile implant, AMS 700 CX/CXM	Safe	1.5	
American Medical Systems			
Minnetonka, MN			
Penile implant, AMS 700 Ultrex	Safe	1.5	
American Medical Systems			
Minnetonka, MN			
Penile implant, AMS Ambicor	Safe	1.5	
American Medical Systems			
Minnetonka, MN			
Penile implant, AMS Dynaflex	Safe	1.5	
American Medical Systems			
Minnetonka, MN			
Penile implant, AMS Hydroflex self-contained	Safe	1.5	
American Medical Systems			
Minnetonka, MN			
Penile implant, AMS Malleable 600	Safe	1.5	43
American Medical Systems			
Minnetonka, MN			
Penile implant, AMS Malleable 600M	Safe	1.5	
American Medical Systems			
Minnetonka, MN			
Penile implant, AMS Malleable 650	Safe	1.5	
American Medical Systems			
Minnetonka, MN			
Penile implant, Duraphase	Unsafe 1	1.5	
Penile implant, Flex-Rod II (Firm)	Safe	1.5	43
Surgitek, Medical Engineering Corp.			
Racine, WI			
Penile implant, Flexi-Flate	Safe	1.5	43
Surgitek, Medical Engineering Corp.			
Racine, WI			

TABLE 15.1 (CONTINUED)
The List

Object	Status	Field Strength (T)	Reference
Penile implant, Flexi-Rod (Standard) Surgitek, Medical Engineering Corp. Racine, WI	Safe	1.5	43
Penile implant, Jonas Dacomed Corp. Minneapolis, MN	Safe	1.5	43
Penile implant, Mentor Flexible Mentor Corp Minneapolis, MN	Safe	1.5	43
Penile implant, Mentor Inflatable Mentor Corp. Minneapolis, MN	Safe	1.5	43
Penile implant, OmniPhase Dacomed Corp. Minneapolis, MN	Unsafe 1	1.5	43
Penile implant, Osmond, external	Safe	1.5	
Penile implant, Uniflex 1000	Safe	1.5	
Vascular Access Ports, Infusion Pumps, and Catheters			
A Port Implantable Access System (titanium) vascular access port Therex Corporation Walpole, MA	Safe	1.5	44
Access Implantable (titanium, plastic) vascular access port Celsa Cedex, France	Safe	1.5	44
Broviac catheter single lumen (silicone, barium sulfate) Bard Access Systems Salt Lake City, UT	Safe	1.5	45
Button (polysulfone polymer, silicone) vascular access port Infusaid Inc. Norwood, MA	Safe	1.5	44
CathLink LP (titanium) Bard Access Systems Salt Lake City, UT	Safe	1.5	45
CathLink SP (titanium) Bard Access Systems Salt Lake City, UT	Safe	1.5	45
Celsite Port and Catheter (titanium) B. Braun Medical Bethlehem, PA	Safe	1.5	44
Dome Port (titanium) vascular access port Davol Inc., Subsidiary of C.R. Bard, Inc. Salt Lake City, UT	Safe	1.5	44

TABLE 15.1 (CONTINUED)
The List

Object	Status	Field Strength (T)	Reference
Dual MacroPort (polysulfone polymer, silicone) vascular access port Infusaid Inc. Norwood, MA	Safe	1.5	44
Dual MicroPort (polysulfone polymer, silicone) vascular access port Infusaid Inc. Norwood, MA	Safe	1.5	44
Groshong Catheter, dual lumen, 9.5 Fr. (silicone, barium sulfate, tungsten) Bard Access Systems Salt Lake City, UT	Safe	1.5	45
Groshong Catheter, single lumen, 8 Fr. (silicone, barium sulfate, tungsten) Bard Access Systems Salt Lake City, UT	Safe	1.5	45
Groshong Catheter	Conditional 1	1.5	
Hickman Catheter, dual lumen, 10.0 Fr. (silicone, barium sulfate) Bard Access Systems Salt Lake City, UT	Safe	1.5	45
Hickman Catheter, single lumen, 3.0 Fr. Bard Access Systems Salt Lake City, UT	Safe	1.5	45
Hickman Port (316L SS) vascular access port Davol Inc., Subsidiary of C.R. Bard, Inc. Salt Lake City, UT	Conditional 1	1.5	44
Hickman Port, Pediatric (titanium) vascular access port Davol, Inc., Subsidiary of C.R. Bard, Inc. Salt Lake City, UT	Safe	1.5	44
Hickman subcutaneous port (SS, titanium, plastic) vascular access port Davol, Inc., Subsidiary of C.R. Bard, Inc. Salt Lake City, UT	Safe	1.5	45
Hickman subcutaneous port attachable catheter (titanium) vascular access port Davol, Inc., Subsidiary of C.R. Bard, Inc. Salt Lake City, UT	Safe	1.5	45
Hickman subcutaneous port venous catheter (titanium) vascular access port Davol Inc., Subsidiary of C.R. Bard, Inc. Salt Lake City, UT	Safe	1.5	44

TABLE 15.1 (CONTINUED)
The List

Object	Status	Field Strength (T)	Reference
HMP-Port (plastic) vascular access port Horizon Medical Products Atlanta, GA	Safe	1.5	44
Implantofix II (polysulfone) vascular access port Burron Medical Inc. Bethlehem, PA	Safe	1.5	44
Infusaid, Model 400 (titanium) vascular access port Infusaid Inc. Norwood, MA	Safe	1.5	44
Infusaid, Model 600 (titanium) vascular access port Infusaid Inc. Norwood, MA	Safe	1.5	44
Infuse-A-Kit (plastic) Infusaid Norwood, MA	Safe	1.5	44
LifePort Vascular Access System attachable catheter (plastic) Strato Medical Group Beverly, MA	Safe	1.5	44
LifePort Vascular Access System attachable catheter and bayonet lock ring (plastic) Strato Medical Group Beverly, MA	Safe	1.5	44
Lifeport, Model 1013 (titanium) vascular access port Strato Medical Corp. Beverly, MA	Safe	1.5	44
LifePort, Model 6013 (Delrin) vascular access port Strato Medical Corporation Beverly, MA	Safe	1.5	44
Low Profile MRI Port (Delrin) vascular access port Davol, Inc., Subsidiary of C.R. Bard, Inc. Salt Lake City, UT	Safe	1.5	45
Low Profile MRI Port (titanium) vascular access port Davol, Inc. Subsidiary of C.R. Bard, Inc. Salt Lake City, UT	Safe	1.5	45
Macroport (polysulfone, titanium) vascular access port Infusaid Inc. Norwood, MA	Safe	1.5	

TABLE 15.1 (CONTINUED)
The List

Object	Status	Field Strength (T)	Reference
Mediport vascular access port Cormed	Safe	1.5	
MicroPort (polysulfone, polymersilicone) vascular access port Infusaid Inc. Norwood, MA	Safe	1.5	44
MRI Dual Port (Delrin, titanium) vascular access port Davol, Inc., Subsidiary of C.R. Bard, Inc. Salt Lake City, UT	Safe	1.5	45
MRI Hard Base Implanted Port (plastic) vascular access port Davol, Inc., Subsidiary of C.R. Bard, Inc. Salt Lake City, UT	Safe	1.5	44
MRI Port (Delrin, silicone) vascular access port Davol, Inc., Subsidiary of C.R. Bard, Inc. Salt Lake City, UT	Safe	1.5	44
Norport-AC (titanium) vascular access port Norfolk Medical Skokie, IL	Safe	1.5	44
Norport-DL (316L SS) vascular access port Norfolk Medical Skokie, IL	Safe	1.5	44
Norport-LS (316L SS) vascular access port Norfolk Medical Skokie, IL	Safe	1.5	44
Norport-LS (polysulfone) vascular access port Norfolk Medical Skokie, IL	Safe	1.5	44
Norport-LS (titanium) vascular access port Norfolk Medical Skokie, IL	Safe	1.5	44
Norport-PT (titanium) vascular access port Norfolk Medical Skokie, IL	Safe	1.5	44
Norport-SP (polysulfone, silicone rubber, Dacron) vascular access port Norfolk Medical Skokie, IL	Safe	1.5	44

TABLE 15.1 (CONTINUED)
The List

Object	Status	Field Strength (T)	Reference
OmegaPort Access System (titanium, 316L SS)	Safe	1.5	44
vascular access port			
Norfolk Medical			
Skokie, IL			
OmegaPort-SR Access System (titanium, 316L SS)	Safe	1.5	44
vascular access port			
Norfolk Medical			
Skokie, IL			
Open-ended catheter, single lumen, 6 Fr. (ChronoFlex)	Safe	1.5	45
Davol, Inc., Subsidiary of C.R. Bard, Inc.			
Salt Lake City, UT			
Open-ended catheter, single lumen, 8 Fr. (ChronoFlex)	Safe	1.5	45
Davol, Inc., Subsidiary of C.R. Bard, Inc.			
Salt Lake City, UT			
OptiPort catheter, single lumen (silicone)	Safe	1.5	45
Simms-Deltec			
St. Paul, MN			
PeriPort (polysulfone, titanium)	Safe	1.5	44
vascular access port			
Infusaid, Inc.			
Norwood, MA			
Phantom	Safe	1.5	44
vascular access port			
Norfolk Medical			
Skokie, IL			
Plastic Port (polysulfone, titanium)	Safe	1.5	45
vascular access port			
Cardial			
Saint-Etienne, France			
Port-A-Cath Titanium Dual Lumen Portal (titanium)	Safe	1.5	44
Pharmacia Deltec			
St. Paul, MN			
Port-A-Cath Titanium Peritoneal Portal (titanium)	Safe	1.5	44
Pharmacia Deltec			
St. Paul, MN			
Port-A-Cath Titanium	Safe	1.5	44
Venous Low Profile Portal (titanium)			
Pharmacia Deltec			
St. Paul, MN			
Port-A-Cath Titanium	Safe	1.5	44
Venous Portal (titanium)			
Pharmacia Deltec			
St. Paul, MN			
Port-A-Cath, P.S.A. Port Portal (titanium)	Safe	1.5	44
Pharmacia Deltec			
St. Paul, MN			
Porto-cath	Safe	1.5	44
Pharmacin, NUTECH Pharmacia Deltec			
St. Paul, MN			

TABLE 15.1 (CONTINUED)
The List

Object	Status	Field Strength (T)	Reference
Q-Port (316L SS) vascular access port Quinton Instrument Co. Seattle, WA	Conditional 1	1.5	44
R-Port Premier (silicone, plastic, SS) vascular access port Medi-tech Boston Scientific Corp. Watertown, MA	Safe	1.5	
S.E.A. (titanium) vascular access port Harbor Medical Devices, Inc. Boston, MA	Safe	1.5	44
Snap-Lock (titanium, polysulfone polymer, silicone) vascular access port Infusaid Inc. Norwood, MA	Safe	1.5	44
Synchromed, Model 8500 (titanium, thermoplastic, silicone) Medtronic, Inc. Minneapolis, MN	Conditional 5	1.5	44
TitanPort (titanium) vascular access port Norfolk Medical Skokie, IL	Safe	1.5	
Triple Lumen Arrow International, Inc. Reading, PA	Safe	1.5	
Vascular Access Catheter With Repair Kit	Safe	1.5	
Vasport (titanium, fluoropolymer) Gish Biomedical, Inc. Santa Ana, CA	Safe	1.5	44
Vaxess, plastic (plastic, polyurethane) Medi-tech Boston Scientific Corp. Watertown, MA	Safe	1.5	
Vaxess, titanium (titanium, polyurethane) Medi-tech Boston Scientific Corp. Watertown, MA	Safe	1.5	
Vaxess, titanium mini-port with silicone catheter (titanium, silicone) Medi-tech Boston Scientific Corp. Watertown, MA	Safe	1.5	

TABLE 15.1 (CONTINUED)
The List

Object	Status	Field Strength (T)	Reference
Vital-Port (polysulfone, titanium) vascular access port Cook Pacemaker Corp. Leechburg, PA	Safe	1.5	45
Vital-Port, Dual (polysulfone, titanium) vascular access port Cook Pacemaker Corp. Leechburg, PA	Safe	1.5	45

REFERENCES

1. Shellock, F.G., MR imaging of metallic implants and materials: a compilation of the literature, *Am. J. Roentgenol.*, 151:811, 1988.
2. Shellock, F.G. and Curtis, J.S., MR imaging and biomedical implants, materials, and devices: an updated review, *Radiology*, 180:541, 1991.
3. Shellock, F.G. and Kanal, E., *Magnetic Resonance: Bioeffects, Safety, and Patient Management*, Lippincott-Raven Press, New York, 1996.
4. Shellock, F.G., *Pocket Guide to MR Procedures and Metallic Objects: Update 1994,* First Edition, Raven Press, New York, 1994.
5. Shellock, F.G., *Pocket Guide to MR Procedures and Metallic Objects: Update 1996,* Second Edition, Lippincott-Raven Press, New York, 1996.
6. Shellock, F.G., *Pocket Guide to MR Procedures and Metallic Objects: Update 1997,* Third Edition, Lippincott-Raven Press, New York, 1997.
7. Shellock, F.G., *Pocket Guide to MR Procedures and Metallic Objects: Update 1998,* Fourth Edition, Lippincott-Raven Press, New York, 1998.
8. Shellock, F.G., *Pocket Guide to MR Procedures and Metallic Objects: Update 1999,* Fifth Edition, Lippincott, Williams & Wilkins Healthcare, Philadelphia, 1999.
9. Shellock, F.G., *Pocket Guide to MR Procedures and Metallic Objects: Update 2000,* Sixth Edition, Lippincott, Williams & Wilkins, Philadelphia, 2000.

REFERENCES FOR TABLE 15.1

1. New, P.F.J., Rosen, B.R., Brady, T.J., et al., Potential hazards and artifacts of ferromagnetic and nonferromagnetic surgical and dental materials and devices in nuclear magnetic resonance imaging, *Radiology,* 147:139-148, 1983.
2. Becker, R.L., Norfray, J.F., Teitelbaum, G.P., et al., MR imaging in patients with intracranial aneurysm clips, *Am. J. Roentgenol.,* 9:885-889, 1988.
3. Shellock, F.G. and Crues, J.V., High-field strength MR imaging and metallic biomedical implants: an ex vivo evaluation of deflection forces, *Am. J. Roentgenol.,* 151:389-392, 1988.
4. Brown, M.A., Carden, J.A., Coleman, R.E., et al., Magnetic field effects on surgical ligation clips, *Magn. Reson. Imaging,* 5:443-453, 1987.
5. Dujovny, M., Kossovsky, N., Kossowsky, R., et al., Aneurysm clip motion during magnetic resonance imaging: in vivo experimental study with metallurgical factor analysis, *Neurosurgery,* 17:543-548, 1985.
6. Barrafato, D. and Henkelman, R.M., Magnetic resonance imaging and surgical clips, *Can. J. Surg.,* 27:509-512, 1984.

7. Moscatel, M., Shellock, F.G., and Morisoli, S., Biopsy needles and devices: assessment of ferromagnetism and artifacts during exposure to a 1.5 Tesla MR system, *J. Magn. Reson. Imaging*, 5:369-372, 1995.

8. Shellock, F.G. and Shellock, V.J., Additional information pertaining to the MR-compatibility of biopsy needles and devices, *J. Magn. Reson. Imaging*, 6:441, 1996.

9. Hathout, G., Lufkin, R.B., Jabour, B., et al., MR-guided aspiration cytology in the head and neck at high field strength, *J. Magn. Reson. Imaging*, 2:93-94, 1992.

10. Fagan, L.L., Shellock, F.G., Brenner, R.J., and Rothman, B., Ex vivo evaluation of ferromagnetism, heating, and artifacts of breast tissue expanders exposed to a 1.5 T MR system, *J. Magn. Reson. Imaging*, 5:614-616, 1995.

11. Teitelbaum, G.P., Lin, M.C.W., Watanabe, A.T., et al., Ferromagnetism and MR imaging: safety of cartoid vascular clamps, *Am. J. Neuroradiol.*, 11:267-272, 1990.

12. Gegauff, A., Laurell, K.A., Thavendrarajah, A., et al., A potential MRI hazard: forces on dental magnet keepers, *J. Oral Rehabil.*, 17:403-410, 1990.

13. Shellock, F.G. Ex vivo assessment of deflection forces and artifacts associated with high-field strength MRI of "mini-magnet" dental prostheses, *Magn. Reson. Imaging*, 7(Suppl. 1):38, 1989.

14. Shellock, F.G. and Slimp, G., Halo vest for cervical spine fixation during MR imaging, *Am. J. Roentgenol.*, 154:631-632, 1990.

15. Clayman, D.A., Murakami, M.E., and Vines, F.S., Compatibility of cervical spine braces with MR imaging. A study of nine nonferrous devices, *Am. J. Neuroradiol.*, 11:385-390, 1990.

16. Shellock, F.G., MR imaging and cervical fixation devices: assessment of ferromagnetism, heating, and artifacts, *Magn. Reson. Imaging*, 14:1093–1098, 1996.

17. Soulen, R.L., Budinger, T.F., and Higgins, C.B., Magnetic resonance imaging of prosthetic heart valves, *Radiology*, 154:705-707, 1985.

18. Shellock, F.G., and Morisoli, S.M., Ex vivo evaluation of ferromagnetism, heating, and artifacts for heart valve prostheses exposed to a 1.5 Tesla MR system, *J. Magn. Reson. Imaging*, 4:756-758, 1994.

19. Hassler, M., Le Bas, J.F., Wolf, J.E., et al., Effects of magnetic fields used in MRI on 15 prosthetic heart valves, *J. Radiol.*, 67:661-666, 1986.

20. Frank, H., Buxbaum, P., Huber, L., et al., In vitro behavior of mechanical heart valves in 1.5 T superconducting magnet, *Eur. J. Radiol.*, 2:555-558, 1992.

21. Teitelbaum, G.P., Bradley, W.G., and Klein, B.D. MR imaging artifacts, ferromagnetism, and magnetic torque of intravascular filters, stents, and coils, *Radiology*, 166:657-664, 1988.

22. Marshall, M.W., Teitelbaum, G.P., Kim, H.S., et al., Ferromagnetism and magnetic resonance artifacts of platinum embolization microcoils, *Cardiovasc. Intervent. Radiol.*, 14:163–166, 1991.

23. Watanabe, A.T., Teitelbaum, G.P., Gomes, A.S., et al., MR imaging of the bird's nest filter, *Radiology*, 177:578-579, 1990.

24. Leibman, C.E., Messersmith, R.N., Levin, D.N., et al., MR imaging of inferior vena caval filter: safety and artifacts, *Am. J. Roentgenol.*, 150:1174-1176, 1988.

25. Shellock, F.G., Detrick, M.S., and Brant-Zawadski, M., MR-compatibility of the Guglielmi detachable coils, *Radiology*, 203:568-570, 1997.

26. Kiproff, P.M., Deeb, D.L., Contractor, F.M., and Khoury, M.B., Magnetic resonance characteristics of the LGM vena cava filter: technical note, *Cardiovasc. Intervent. Radiol.*, 14:254-255, 1991.

27. Teitelbaum, G.P., Raney, M., Carvlin, M.J., et al., Evaluation of ferromagnetism and magnetic resonance imaging artifacts of the Strecker tantalum vascular stent, *Cardiovasc. Intervent. Radiol.*, 12:125-127, 1989.

28. Girard, M.J., Hahn, P., Saini, S., Dawson, S.L., Goldberg, M.A., and Mueller, P.R., Wallstent metallic biliary endoprosthesis: MR imaging characteristics, *Radiology*, 184:874-876, 1992.

29. Shellock, F.G., Myers, S.M., and Schatz, C.J., Ex vivo evaluation of ferromagnetism determined for metallic scleral "buckles" exposed to a 1.5 T MR scanner, *Radiology*, 185:288-289, 1992.

30. de Keizer, R.J. and Te Strake, L., Intraocular lens implants (pseudophakoi) and steelwire sutures: a contraindication for MRI?, *Doc. Ophthalmol.*, 61:281-284, 1984.

31. Albert, D.W., Olson, K.R., Parel, J.M., et al., Magnetic resonance imaging and retinal tacks, *Arch. Ophthalmol.*, 108:320–321, 1990.

32. Joondeph, B.C., Peyman, G.A., Mafee, M.F., et al., Magnetic resonance imaging and retinal tacks [Letter], *Arch. Ophthalmol.*, 105:1479-1480, 1987.

33. Lyons, C.J., Betz, R.R., Mesgarzadeh, M., et al., The effect of magnetic resonance imaging on metal spine implants, *Spine*, 14:670-672, 1989.

34. Shellock, F.G., Mink, J.H., Curtin, S., et al., MRI and orthopedic implants used for anterior cruciate ligament reconstruction: assessment of ferromagnetism and artifacts, *J. Magn. Reson. Imaging*, 2:225-228, 1992.

35. Shellock, F.G. and Schatz, C.J., High-field strength MR imaging and metallic otologic implants, *Am. J. Neuroradiol.*, 12:279-281, 1991.

36. Nogueira, M., and Shellock, F.G., Otologic bioimplants: ex vivo assessment of ferromagnetism and artifacts at 1.5 Tesla, *Am. J. Roentgenol.*, 163:1472-1473, 1995.

37. Mattucci, K.F., Setzen, M., Hyman, R., et al., The effect of nuclear magnetic resonance imaging on metallic middle ear protheses, *Otolaryngol. Head Neck Surg.*, 94:441-443, 1986.

38. Applebaum, E.L. and Valvassori, G.E., Further studies on the effects of magnetic resonance fields on middle ear implants, *Ann. Otol. Rhinol. Laryngol.*, 99:801-804, 1990.

39. White, D.W., Interaction between magnetic fields and metallic ossicular prostheses, *Am. J. Otol.*, 8:290–292, 1987.

40. Leon, J.A. and Gabriele, O.F., Middle ear prothesis: significance in magnetic resonance imaging, *Magn. Reson. Imaging*, 5:405-406, 1987.

41. Shellock, F.G. and Morisoli, S.M., Ex vivo evaluation of ferromagnetism and artifacts for cardiac occluders exposed to a 1.5 Tesla MR system, *J. Magn. Reson. Imaging*, 4:213-215, 1994.

42. Teitelbaum, G.P., Yee, C.A., Van Horn, D.D., et al., Metallic ballistic fragments: MR imaging safety and artifacts, *Radiology*, 175:855-859, 1990.

43. Shellock, F.G., Crues, J.V., and Sacks, S.A., High-field magnetic resonance imaging of penile prostheses: in vitro evaluation of deflection forces and imaging artifacts [Abstract], in *Book of Abstracts*, Society of Magnetic Resonance in Medicine. Berkeley, CA, 3:915, 1987.

44. Shellock, F.G., Nogueira, M., and Morisoli, S., MR imaging and vascular access ports: ex vivo evaluation of ferromagnetism, heating, and artifacts at 1.5 T, *J. Magn. Reson. Imaging*, 4:481-484, 1995.

45. Shellock, F.G. and Shellock, V.J., Vascular access ports and catheters tested for ferromagnetism, heating, and artifacts associated with MR imaging, *Magn. Reson. Imaging*, 14:443-447, 1996.

46. Kanal, E. and Shaibani, A., Firearm safety in the MR imaging environment, *Radiology*, 193:875-876, 1994.

47. Hess, T., Stepanow, B., and Knopp, M.V., Safety of intrauterine contraceptive devices during MR imaging, *Eur. Radiol.*, 6:66-68, 1996.

48. Shellock, F.G. and Shellock, V.J., Evaluation of MR compatibility of 38 bioimplants and devices, *Radiology*, 197:174, 1995.

49. Shellock, F.G. and Shellock, V.J., Ceramic surgical instruments: ex vivo evaluation of compatibility with MR imaging, *J. Magn. Reson. Imaging*, 6:954-956, 1996.

50. Shellock, F.G. and Shellock, V.J., Evaluation of cranial flap fixation clamps for compatibility with MR imaging, *Radiology*, 207:822-825, 1998.

51. Lufkin, R., Jordan, S., and Lylcyk, M., MR imaging with topographic EEG electrodes in place, *Am. J. Neuroradiol.*, 9:953-954, 1988.

52. Marra, S., Leonetti, J.P., Konior, R.J., and Raslan, W., Effect of magnetic resonance imaging on implantable eyelid weights, *Ann. Otol. Rhinol. Laryngol.*, 104:448-452, 1995.

53. Zhang, J., Wilson, C.L., Levesque, M.F., Behnke, E.J., and Lufkin, R.B., Temperature changes in nickel-chromium intracranial depth electrodes during MR scanning, *Am. J. Neuroradiol.*, 14:497-500, 1993.

54. Mark, A.S. and Hricak, H., Intrauterine contraceptive devices: MR imaging, *Radiology*, 162:311-314, 1987.

55. Go, K.G., Kamman, R.L., and Mooyaart, E.L., Interaction of metallic neurosurgical implants with magnetic resonance imaging at 1.5 Tesla as a cause of image distortion and of hazardous movement of the implant, *Clin. Neurosurg.*, 91:109-115, 1989.

56. Fransen, P., Dooms, G., and Thauvoy, T., Safety of the adjustable pressure ventricular valve in magnetic resonance imaging: problems and solutions, *Neuroradiology*, 34:508-509, 1992.

57. ECRI, Health devices alert. A new MRI complication? May 27, 1988.

58. To, S.Y.C., Lufkin, R.B., and Chiu, L., MR-compatible winged infusion set, *Comput. Med. Imaging Graphics*, 13:469-472, 1989.

59. Shellock, F.G., MR-compatibility of an endoscope designed for use in interventional MRI procedures, *Am. J. Roentgen.*, 71:1297-1300, 1998.

60. Shellock, F.G. and Shellock, V.J., Cardiovascular catheters and accessories: Ex vivo testing of ferromagnetism, heating, and artifacts associated with MRI, *J. Magn. Reson. Imaging*, 8:1338-1342, 1998.

61. Shellock, F.G. and Shellock, V.J., Metallic marking clips used after stereotactic breast biopsy: ex vivo testing of ferromagnetism, heating, and artifacts associated with MRI, *Am. J. Roentgen.*, 172:1417-1419, 1999.

62. Shellock, F.G., MRI safety of instruments designed for interventional MRI: assessment of ferromagnetism, heating, and artifacts. Workshop on New Insights into Safety and Compatibility Issues Affecting In Vivo MR, *Syllabus*, International Society for Magnetic Resonance in Medicine, Berkeley, CA, p. 39, 1998.

63. Shellock, F.G., Hatfield, M., Simon, B.J., Block, S., Wamboldt, J., Starewicz, P.M., and Punchard, W.F.B., Implantable spinal fusion stimulator: assessment of MRI safety, *J. Magn. Reson. Imaging*, 12:214–223, 2000.

64. Shellock, F.G. and Shellock, V.J., Stents: Evaluation of MRI safety, *Am. J. Roentgen.*, 173:543-546, 1999.

65. Teissl, C., Kremser, C., Hochmair, E.S., and Hochmair-Desoyer, I.J., Cochlear implants: in vitro investigation of electromagnetic interference at MR imaging-compatibility and safety aspects, *Radiology*, 208:700-708, 1998.

66. Teissl, C., Kremser, C., Hochmair, E.S., and Hochmair-Desoyer, I.J., Magnetic resonance imaging and cochlear implants: compatibility and safety aspects, *J. Magn. Reson. Imaging*, 9:26-38, 1999.

67. Ortler, M., Kostron, H., and Felber, S., Transcutaneous pressure-adjustable valves and magnetic resonance imaging: an ex vivo examination of the Codman-Medos programmable valve and the Sophy adjustable pressure valve, *Neurosurgery*, 40:1050–1057, 1997.

68. Shellock, F.G. and Shellock, V.J., MR-compatibility evaluation of the Spetzler titanium aneurysm clip, *Radiology*, 206:838-841, 1998.

69. Jost, C. and Kuman, V., Are current cardiovascular stents MRI safe, *J. Invasive Cardiol.*, 10:477-479, 1998.

70. Shellock, F.G. and Shellock, V.J., MRI Safety of cardiovascular implants: evaluation of ferromagnetism, heating, and artifacts, *Radiology*, 214:P19H, 2000.

71. DeLacure, M.D. and Wang, H.Z., Magnetic resonance imaging assessment of microvascular anastomotic device for ferromagnetism, *J. Reconstr. Microsurg.*, 13:571-574, 1997.

16 Health Effects of Induced Electric Fields: Implications for Metallic Implants

Chris D. Smith, John A. Nyenhuis, and Alexander V. Kildishev

CONTENTS

I. INTRODUCTION

The radio frequency (RF) and pulsed gradient magnetic fields in magnetic resonance imaging (MRI) induce currents in the body, and the principal potential adverse health effects are tissue heating by RF-induced currents and nerve stimulation by the gradient currents. Electrically conducting implants can locally increase these currents, resulting in greater heating and increased possibility for nerve stimulation. The RF field may interfere with the operation of active implants, particularly cardiac pacemakers with sensing leads. The purpose of this chapter is to review the interaction of medical implants with the RF and pulsed gradient fields, with the emphasis being placed on the RF field, since the RF field is more likely to create safety concerns.

The RF field is used for flipping of the nuclear spins, is transverse to the static field B_0, and is typically circularly polarized in an imager with a cylindrical bore. The frequency of the RF field is proportional to B_0 and is approximately 64 MHz in a 1.5-T system. When a time-varying magnetic field acts on a conductive medium, such as the body of a subject, an electric field is generated, per Faraday's law. In a manner resembling that of a microwave oven, the RF field deposits energy in the subject as quantified by the specific absorption rate (SAR), which is a mass normalized measure of the rate at which energy is deposited in the subject.[1] There is a regulatory limit of 4.0 W/kg for patients with normal thermoregulatory systems and 1.5 W/kg for all others.[2] The U.S. Food and Drug Administration (FDA) has also set guidelines according to temperature rise: 1°C in the head, 2°C in the torso, and 3°C in the extremities.[3] The SAR is related to temperature rise by

$$dT/dt = SAR/C \qquad (16.1)$$

where dT/dt is the initial rate of temperature (T) increase per unit time (t) and C is the specific heat.

The electric field can be focused by metallic implants, creating an increased current density in tissues near the implant. The greater currents result in increased heating and can be an important safety issue, especially for those patients with elongated implants.[4,5] Furthermore, the RF field can induce voltages in device leads which, if large enough, may result in improper operation of or damage to the device.

This chapter begins by describing experimental procedures for evaluation of RF-induced heating and then moves on to a survey of the literature. Next, electromagnetic field theory is used to provide an understanding of how and why extreme heating may occur in the presence of a conductive implant. A model is then developed for RF heating, and the heat equation is used to predict the temperature rise for a localized heat source. Finally, the interaction of metallic implants with the pulsed gradient fields is considered.

II. METHODS FOR EVALUATING RF INTERACTIONS WITH MEDICAL IMPLANTS

To quantify the temperature rise that occurs in the presence of a conducting implant, one must perform experiments that duplicate situations actually present in patients. Because the evaluation of device safety *in vivo* is difficult, especially in humans, heating is generally measured using a phantom, which consists of conducting material in an appropriate container.

The composition of the phantom material is chosen to represent the region of the body in which the device is to be implanted and may consist of liquid saline only,[6-8] a combination of saline and a gelling material,[4,9-11] or a meat product such as turkey.[12] With the phantom material chosen, the device to be tested is placed in the phantom in an appropriate anatomical orientation, and then the phantom and the device are placed within the magnetic resonance (MR) system. The temperature rise within the phantom is monitored by equipment that is not affected by the fields developed by an MR system, e.g., a device using fiber-optic temperature probes or a thermographic camera.

Testing of MR safety for implanted devices can be performed in an MR system or an apparatus that creates an RF environment similar to that present in an MR system. An experimental apparatus for evaluating heating due to the RF field is shown in Figure 16.1, and the corresponding block diagram is shown in Figure 16.2. This equipment delivers RF energy in a continuous-wave fashion, in contrast to an MR system which delivers RF energy in the form of short-duration, high-intensity RF pulses. Shown on the table on the left side of Figure 16.1 are an oscilloscope, which is used to measure reflection from the RF body coil, an RF generator, and an RF amplifier. On the right side of Figure 16.1, a flat plastic phantom pan, an MR patient table, and an RF gradient body coil are shown. The numbers shown in the phantom in Figure 16.2 correspond to the locations of the fiber-optic temperature probes. These probes are placed where the greatest increase in temperature is expected, which for an elongated implant is near the ends.

For adequate sensitivity, the applied RF field should produce an average SAR in excess of 1.0 W/kg. This level is SAR corresponds to an average temperature increase of approximately 0.9°C/h, as calculated from Equation 16.1 using the specific heat of water $C = 4184$ J/(kg K). For testing heating in an imager, a suitable protocol is a fast spin-echo (FSE) sequence with a 25-ms echo time (TE) and a 134-ms repetition time (TR) for a 15- to 20-min examination period; the predicted SAR is about 1.0 W/kg for a 70-kg subject.[5] Since many (about 40) RF pulses are applied each

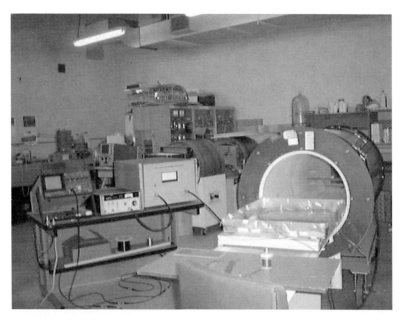

FIGURE 16.1 Photograph of the experimental apparatus used by Smith et al.[4] to evaluate RF-induced heating of elongated conductive implants.

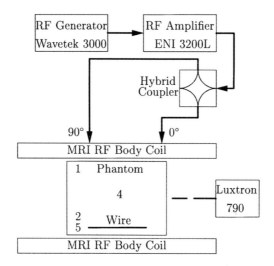

FIGURE 16.2 System block diagram and experimental equipment showing temperature probe position, as used by Smith et al.[4] to evaluate RF-induced heating for elongated conductive implants. Numbers represent locations of fiber-optic temperature probes. Probe 5 is next to the wire end, Probe 2 is 1 cm lateral to the end, Probe 4 is at the center, and Probe 1 is a reference probe contralateral to Probe 5.

second, the heating effects of an RF pulse sequence will be accurately modeled by application of the same average power continuous wave, such as is done with the apparatus of Figure 16.2.

Important physical properties of the phantom material are the electrical conductivity, σ, or resistivity $\rho = 1/\sigma$; relative electrical permittivity, ε_r; thermal conductivity; and viscosity. All of these properties, in particular the electrical properties, may be altered to the accepted values listed in Reference 13 by following the recommendations in References 4 and 9–11. The phantom materials described herein are summarized in Table 16.1, along with the phantom material vendor information.

TABLE 16.1
Summary of Phantom Materials Used to Evaluate MR Safety
and Their Respective Vendors as Described Herein

Ref.	Material	Vendor
4	Polyacrylic Acid	Aldrich Chemical, Milwaukee, WI
9	Hydroxyethylcellulose	BP Chemicals
	Microspheres	Emerson and Coming, Canton, MA
	TWEEN	Sargent-Welch, Skokie, IL
	N-Amyl alcohol	Sargent-Welch, Skokie, IL
	Paraffin oil	Sargent-Welch, Skokie, IL
10	TX-150	Oil Center Research, Lafayette, LA
	Polyethylene powder	Wadco CA, Long Beach CA

Chou et al.[10] recommend phantom materials for muscle tissue for RF frequencies from 13.56 to 2450 MHz. For a phantom to be used at 70 MHz, the recommended weight percents are 10.36% TX-150, 2.72% aluminum powder, 87.59% water, and 0.424% sodium chloride (NaCl). This preparation gives a phantom material having a dielectric constant of 84.7 and a conductivity of 0.76 S/m at 70 MHz; proper viscosity is set by TX-150, which serves as a gelling agent. On a related note, a discrepancy in the literature has been found, in that the gelling agent TX-150 is sometimes incorrectly referred to as TX-151.

Hartsgrove et al.[9] provided recipes for muscle, brain, lung, solid castable bone, and liquid pourable bone. Formulations for muscle and brain tissue are listed in Table 16.2. Saline was used to establish σ; sugar was used to lower ε_r; hydroxyethylcellulose (HEC), also known as Natrosol®, was used to increase viscosity; and a bacteriacide was used to prevent bacteria growth. This yields a phantom with measured permittivity of 70.5 and conductivity of 0.68 S/m at 100 MHz. To create lung tissue, microspheres (Ecospheres SI) were added to the phantom muscle in a ratio of 47:53 by volume, muscle to microspheres. Hartsgrove et al. also provided two recipes for bone material. Their recipe for hard, castable material included two ton epoxy, two ton epoxy hardener, and potassium chloride (KCl) solution. The recipe for liquid bone material contained TWEEN, n-amyl alcohol, paraffin oil, water, and NaCl.

Recommendations for muscle-equivalent phantom materials in the 10- to 100-MHz range were published by Hagmann et al.[11] They specified a saline and glycine phantom for use at frequencies of 13.56, 27.12, and 40.68 MHz.

Recently, a saline and a gel-based phantom were compared at Purdue University in West Lafayette, IN. First, a saline phantom and a polyacrylic acid (PAA) gel-based phantom were compared to evaluate induced heating. One phantom was composed solely of 0.3% saline, and the other was composed of 0.3% saline and 11 g/l PAA. In these experiments, a resistor was placed in the phantom, a current

TABLE 16.2
Muscle and Brain Phantom Composition
as Recommended by Hartsgrove et al.[9]

Material	Percentage by Weight	
	Muscle	Brain
Water	52.4	40.4
NaCl	1.4	2.5
Sugar	45.0	56.0
HEC	1.0	1.0
Bacteriacide	0.1	0.1

was applied to the resistor, and the induced temperature rise in the phantom was measured at the resistor. The temperature rise in the gel phantom, about 10°C, was significantly greater than that in the saline phantom, about 2°C. A gel-based phantom with significantly higher viscosity exhibited a greater temperature increase than saline, but less than the gel phantom of lower viscosity.

One important factor to remember when preparing phantom material is that electrical properties of the phantom are temperature and frequency dependent. For example, data compiled in Reference 13 showed that ε_r for human muscle varied from 73.5 at 50 MHz to 52 at 900 MHz. Similarly, σ varied from 0.61 to 0.92 S/m for 50 to 900 MHz, respectively. As for temperature dependence, electrical properties in the 13.56 to 200 MHz range varied –0.5 to –1.2% per degree Celsius for permittivity and 1.7 to 2.7% per degree Celsius for conductivity with increasing temperature.[10] Additional references which tabulate electrical properties of human and animal tissues can be found in References 14 to 17.

III. REPORTED INTERACTIONS BETWEEN MR FIELDS AND METALLIC IMPLANTS

This section is a summary of the literature, describing device interactions with MRI time-varying fields that have been found in phantoms and experimental subjects. Table 16.3 lists the devices tested and described herein, and Table 16.4 summarizes the imaging sequences used. Sections III.A and III.B describe experiments that have investigated induced heating, and experiments that have investigated device functionality when exposed to the MRI RF field are described in Section III.C.

TABLE 16.3
Summary of Pulse Generators Tested for MR Safety by the Various Investigators

Device Tested	Active/Passive	Phantom Material	Device Type	Ref.
Auditory Brainstem Implant	Active	Phantom head	BI	22
Avery I 110A	Passive	Air	CP	39
Biotronik Ergos 03	Active	Porcine heart	CP	18
Biotronik Ergos 03	Active	Saline	CP	6
Biotronik Physios 01	Active	Porcine heart	CP	18
Biotronik Pikos	Active	Porcine heart	CP	18
Cochlear Implant	Active	Phantom head	CI	22
Cordis 233F	Active	Saline	CP	8
Cordis 233F	Active	Dog, *in vivo*	CP	38
Cordis 240G	Active	Dog, *in vivo*	CP	38
Cordis 334A	Active	Dog, *in vivo*	CP	38
Cordis 402B	Active	Dog, *in vivo*	CP	38
Cordis 415A	Active	Dog, *in vivo*	CP	38
Cordis MKII 904A	Active	Air	INS	39
CPI Command P5 0530	Active	Air	CP	37
CPI Delta T	Active	Porcine heart	CP	18
CPI Vigor 460	Active	Porcine heart	CP	18
CPI Vigor 1130	Active	Porcine heart	CP	18
Cyberonics 100 NCP	Active	Gel	INS	23
Intermedics 283-01	Active	Saline	CP	8
Electro-Biology Spinal Fusion Stimulator	Active	See text	SPF	5
Intermedics Cosmos II 283-01	Active	Saline	CP	6
Intermedics Cosmos II 284-05	Active	Saline	CP	6
Intermedics Cyberlith IV, C-MDS 259-01	Active	Air	CP	37
Medtronic 3360A	Passive	Air	INS	39

continued

TABLE 16.3 (CONTINUED)
Summary of Pulse Generators Tested for MR Safety by the Various Investigators

Device Tested	Active/Passive	Phantom Material	Device Type	Ref.
Medtronic 3464	Passive	Air	INS	39
Medtronic 5375	Active	Saline	EPG	7
Medtronic 5330	Active	Saline	EPG	7
Medtronic 5992	Active	Air	CP	37
Medtronic 8420	Active	Saline	IPG	7
Medtronic 8423	Active	Saline	IPG	7
Medtronic 7000A	Active	Saline	IPG	7
Medtronic 7000A	Active	Saline	CP	8
Medtronic 7100	Active	Saline	IPG	7
Medtronic 7560A	Passive	Air	INS	39
Medtronic Itrel I 7421	Active	Air	INS	39
Medtronic Itrel II	Active	Saline	INS	36
Medtronic Itrel 3	Active	Saline	INS	36
Medtronic Minix 8341	Active	Saline	CP	6
Medtronic Synergist II 7071	Active	Saline	CP	6
Medtronic Elite 7075	Active	Saline	CP	6
Pacesetter 283	Active	Saline	CP	8
Pacesetter 261	Active	Human, *in vivo*	CP	41
Pacesetter 285	Active	Human, *in vivo*	CP	41
Pacesetter 2016T	Active	Human, *in vivo*	CP	41
Pacesetter 2020T	Active	Human, *in vivo*	CP	41
Pacesetter Demand Type Demo 2481	Active	Air	CP	37
Pacesetter Paragon II	Active	Porcine heart	CP	18
Pacesetter Programmable 221	Active	Air	CP	37
Pacesetter Synchrony 2020	Active	Saline	CP	6
Pacesetter Synchrony III	Active	Porcine heart	CP	18
Telectronics 155	Active	Dog, *in vivo*	CP	38
Telectronics 2251	Active	Air	CP	37
Telectronics 2291	Active	Dog, *in vivo*	CP	38
Telectronics 5281	Active	Dog, *in vivo*	CP	38
Telectronics Meta 1206	Active	Porcine heart	CP	18
Telectronics Meta 1254	Active	Porcine heart	CP	18
Telectronics Meta II 1204	Active	Saline	CP	6
Telectronics Meta II 1250	Active	Saline	CP	6
Telectronics Simplex	Active	Porcine heart	CP	18

Note: Abbreviations used are cardiac pacemaker (CP), implantable pulse generator (IPG), external pulse generator (EPG), brainstem implant (BI), spinal fusion stimulator (SPF), cochlear implant (CI), and implanted neurostimulator (INS).

A. HEATING OF ELONGATED DEVICES AND PULSE GENERATORS WITH LEADS

Achenbach et al.[18] examined induced heating when various pacing electrodes, listed in Table 16.5, were present in an MR environment. Theses studies were conducted in a 1.5-T Siemens Magnetom MR system (Siemens, Erlangen, Germany), and the electrodes were inserted into a porcine heart. The electrodes were placed in a 16-cm diameter circular formation, and the opposite end of the lead was either in air or in a saline phantom. The electrodes were examined both when connected to and when disconnected from a cardiac pacemaker.

The average increase in temperature for monopolar electrodes was $13.7 \pm 12.0°C$ in air and not connected to a pacemaker, $2.9 \pm 1.5°C$ in air and connected to a pacemaker, and $1.4 \pm 1.3°C$ in saline

TABLE 16.4
Summary of MRI Sequences Used in the Various Investigations to Assess MR Safety of Devices

Ref.	B_o	Sequence	Trigger	TE (ms)	TR (ms)
5	1.5	N/A	N/A	25	134
6	0.5	SE/GE/FFE	ECG	N/A	N/A
8	0.5	N/A	N/A	30–40	75–600
12	1.5	SPGR	N/A	4	50
	1.5	SE	N/A	20	300
	1.5	FSE	N/A	17	300
18	1.5	SE	None	20	300
	1.5	SE	ECG	10	700
	1.5	GE	ECG	10	700
20	1.5	FSE	N/A	N/A	N/A
21	1.5	FSE	N/A	N/A	N/A
22	1.5	N/A	N/A	25	134
23	1.5	SE	N/A	15	83.3
32	1.5	SE	N/A	25	134
34	1.5	SE	N/A	12	300
35	1.5	FSE	N/A	15	83.3
36	0.2	SE	N/A	15	638
	0.2	GE	N/A	12	34
	1.5	SE	N/A	20	674
	1.5	GE	N/A	4.4	30
	0.25	GE	N/A	7.5	23
37	0.5	N/A	N/A	See text	See text
38	1.5	N/A	N/A	N/A	200–1000
39	0.35	N/A	N/A	See text	37–143
	1.5	N/A	N/A	See text	37–143

Note: Abbreviations used in this table are spin-echo (SE), gradient-echo (GE), fast field-echo (FFE), spoiled gradient-recalled echo (SPGR), fast spin-echo (FSE), electrocardiograph (ECG), and not available (N/A).

and connected to a pacemaker. For bipolar electrodes, the average increase in temperature was $9.0 \pm 23.2°C$ in air and not connected to a pacemaker, $0.9 \pm 1.1°C$ in air and connected to a pacemaker, and $2.2 \pm 2.5°C$ in saline and connected to a pacemaker. One electrode with a length of approximately 1 m exhibited a massive temperature rise on the order of 90°C in a very short imaging time.

Smith et al.[4] examined heating in a gel phantom for wires, which simulate leads, of various lengths and insulation thicknesses using the apparatus shown in Figure 16.2. A 64-MHz RF field was generated in a continuous-wave fashion with a body coil of the birdcage configuration (General Electric Medical Systems, Milwaukee, WI). The phantom was prepared by adding 11 g/*l* of PAA to 0.3% saline, resulting in material with a consistency resembling that of applesauce and having a resistivity of 125 Ω cm.

Copper wires with thin varnish insulation (magnet wires), 1.6 and 2 mm in diameter, with lengths ranging from 5 to 40 cm were examined to evaluate the effect of wire length on induced heating.[4] Figure 16.3 shows a representative heating profile from these experiments. The temperature rise after 20 min near the tip (Probe 5) of a 26-cm-long wire is nearly 7°C, about ten times greater than the background temperature rise (Probe 1).

Figure 16.4 shows the temperature rise at the tip as a function of wire length. The maximal rise of approximately 7°C occurs for wires in the 20- to 26-cm range of lengths; longer and shorter

TABLE 16.5
**Summary of Cardiac Pacemaker Leads Examined
by Achenbach et al.[18]**

Manufacturer and Model	Bi/Monopolar	Length (cm)
Baxter 97-130-5F	Bi	116
Biotronik 385139	Bi	59.5
Biotronik EL 004128	Mono	60
Biotronik Multicath 3	Bi	114
Biotronik SD 60-BP	Bi	59
Biotronik SD 60-UP (V126)	Mono	59.5
Biotronik TIJ 53-BP	Bi	51.5
Biotronik TIJ 53-UP	Mono	51.5
Biotronik TIR 60-BP	Bi	58.5
Biotronik TIR 60-UP	Mono	59
CPI 4161	Mono	59
CPI 4185	Mono	59
CPI 4268	Bi	52.5
CPI 4270	Bi	52.5
Medtronic AJ 049896V	Bi	58
Medtronic Capsure SO4024	Bi	58
Medtronic Capsure SP 4023	Mono	58
Medtronic Capsure SP 4524	Bi	53
Medtronic Target Tip 4081	Mono	65
Medtronic Target Tip 4581	Mono	53
Medtronic Target Tip 4582	Bi	53
Pacesetter 1188T	Bi	52.5
Siemens-Pacesetter 1450T	Bi	58
Telectronics 033-301	Bi	58
Telectronics 033-856	Bi	48

Note: Shown are the manufacturer and model, whether the lead was
bipolar or monopolar, and the length of the lead.

wires exhibit less heating. The half-wavelength in the phantom, $\lambda_{1/2}$, using $\varepsilon_r = 84$, is about 26 cm, and thus, increased heating for wires in the 20- to 26-cm range may be due to resonance effects, which were similarly described in Reference 19.

The effect of insulation thickness on induced heating was also examined by Smith et al.[4] Heat shrink tubing was added to magnet wires, of lengths identical to those mentioned above, to give an overall insulation thickness of 0.6 mm, an increase of about 0.55 mm. For these experiments, the temperature rise for a 5-cm wire was 2.9°C, and for a 40-cm wire, the temperature rise was 16.82°C. Figure 16.5 presents a summary of these results. For the case of thickly insulated wires, the critical length has been increased due to the dielectric loading caused by the additional wire insulation.

Smith et al.[4] also conducted computer simulations of heating at the ends of wires using ANSYS, a finite element modeling program. The simulation results were in reasonable agreement with the experiments, especially for short wires, where the quasistatic assumptions are expected to be most valid.

Ladd et al.[20] described the heating that occurs for catheters and guidewires that are used during vascular interventions under MR guidance. Tests were done in air and 0.9% saline using a 1.5-T General Electric (GE) Signa EchoSpeed and a 0.5-T GE Signa SP MR system. Their results show resonance effects similar to those seen in Reference 4. When only the coil of the lead was placed in saline and the connecting coaxial cable in air, the resonant length was found to be 140 cm. If

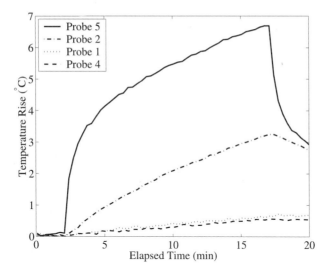

FIGURE 16.3 Representative sample of a temperature rise in a phantom in degrees Celsius as a function of time for a 1.6-mm diameter, 26-cm-long magnet wire during a 15-min period of RF application. Numbers are probe locations as referred to in Figure 16.2.

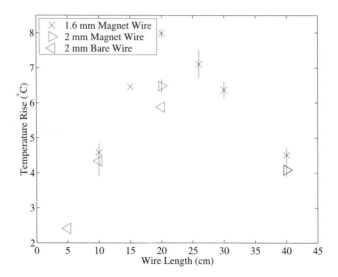

FIGURE 16.4 Summary of experimental results showing temperature changes in degrees Celsius as functions of wire length for 1.6- and 2-mm diameter wires after a 15-min period of RF application. The temperature is measured at the end of the wire corresponding to Probe 5 in Figure 16.2.

the coil and coaxial cable were both in saline, the resonant length was reduced to 45 cm. In both cases, the maximum temperature rise at the resonant length was nearly 20°C for the 1.5-T system.

In a related publication, Ladd and Quick described a method of reducing the heating that occurs when catheters are used in interventional MR.[21] The authors propose a Belden 9222 triaxial cable (Belden Wire and Cable, Richmond, IN), with the addition of a one-quarter wavelength, coaxial choke. This was confirmed with a phantom study using 0.9% saline and a 1.5-T GE Signa LX MR system. The maximum temperature rise at the coil was greatest at the resonant length, 140 cm. Without the choke, the temperature rise was nearly 10°C, but the addition of the choke reduced the temperature rise to about 1°C.

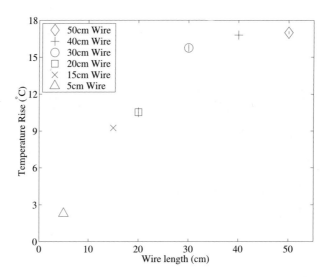

FIGURE 16.5 Summary of experimental results showing temperature change in a phantom in degrees Celsius as a function of wire length for 1.6-mm diameter wires with thick insulation after a 15-min period of RF application. The temperature is measured at the end of the wire corresponding to Probe 5 in Figure 16.2.

The Cochlear (Cochlear Corporation, Englewood, CO) auditory brainstem implant (ABI) and the cochlear implant (CI), each consisting of a pulse generator and a lead with electrodes, were evaluated for possible RF heating by Chou et al.[22] This study used five human head models with appropriate phantom tissues and a 1.5-T GE Signa 4X MR system. These experiments found no appreciable RF heating in either device.[22]

Chou et al.[5] examined a spinal infusion stimulator (Electro-Biology, Parsippany, NJ) in a 1.5-T GE Signa 4X MR system. This was a phantom study using phantom bone, brain, lungs, and muscle, and the conditions simulated were an intact implant, one wire broken, electrodes only, and no implant as a reference. An intact implant produced a maximum temperature rise at the center of the implant of less than 2°C and at the electrodes of less than 1°C. When one wire was broken, the maximum temperature rise was 11°C at the point where the broken lead connects to the stimulator, but the opposite end of the same lead experienced only a 3°C temperature rise.[5] With only the electrodes remaining, the temperature rise was about 1.5°C at one of the electrode pins. Finally, with all parts of the device removed, the maximal increase in temperature was 0.5°C.[5]

Nyenhuis et al.[23] tested the MRI safety of the Cyberonics 100 NCP Generator and 300 series lead (Cyberonics, Webster, TX) in a saline phantom using a 1.5-T GE Signa MR system. The NCP system was tested with a 20-min imaging period, using both a body coil and a head coil. For the RF field applied by the body coil, the temperature rise in the presence of the device was nearly 3°C. With the RF field applied by the head coil, the temperature rise was approximately 0.2°C. It was concluded that patients with this device could be imaged safely, provided that the RF field was applied by the head coil.

B. HEATING OF OTHER IMPLANTS AND DEVICES

In a number of studies, Shellock and colleagues[24-31] examined numerous passive devices, including aneurysm clips, cardiovascular catheters, ceramic surgical instruments, breast tissue expanders, cervical fixation devices, a halo vest for cervical spine fixation, vascular access ports, and heart valve prostheses. No device tested exhibited a temperature rise greater than 1.1°C.

Cranial bone flap fixation clamps were evaluated by Shellock and Shellock[12] in a 1.5-T GE Signa MR system with a turkey meat phantom. In these experiments, the maximum temperature rise seen was 0.4°C. In another article, Shellock[32] examined an endoscope which was designed for use during an MR-guided procedure. In this experiment, a 1.5-T MR system and a phantom filled with physiologic saline were used. The maximum measured temperature rise was 1.1°C.

Shellock et al.[33] also examined the Guglielmi Detachable Coil. Experiments were conducted using a 1.5-T GE Signa MR system and deploying the coil in a fluid-filled phantom. The maximum temperature rise measured in the deployed coil was 0.2°C, after an imaging time of 60 min.

Heating under small electrocardiogram (ECG) electrodes was examined by Felmlee et al.[34] using a human volunteer and three 1.5-T MR systems. With an electrode area of 0.79 cm^2, the temperature beneath the electrode increased 12°C in a time of about 25 s. When the electrode area was increased to 4 cm^2, the temperature increase was neither as rapid nor as great: 8°C in 150 s.

Nyenhuis et al.[35] examined the Medtronic IsoMed 8472-60 infusion pump and Medtronic SynchroMed 8617L-18 (Medtronic, Minneapolis, MN) in a gelled saline phantom using a 1.5-T GE Signa MR system. The maximum temperature rise in the presence of either device was about 0.7°C. It was concluded that the presence of neither the IsoMed nor the SynchroMed pumps would cause increased risk to patients undergoing an MR procedure.

C. Impact of MRI on the Functionality of Pulse Generators

This section discusses reports on the effects of the RF field developed during MRI on the functionality of pulse generators. These may be described as devices which use electrical pulses to cause stimulation and include neurostimulators, cardiac pacemakers, implants to improve hearing, and stimulators for the treatment of pain. Issues that weigh heavily on the functionality of these devices are asynchronous vs. synchronous modes, sensing in synchronous mode, and voltages induced in the leads. Note that pacemakers and other pulse generators often contain a magnetic relay switch; this switch is strongly influenced by the static field.

Tronnier et al.[36] conducted an *in vivo* and an *in vitro* study on the Medtronic ITREL II and 3 which were used in connection with Medtronic percutaneous leads, models 3387, 3388, and 3389, and Medtronic Resume II 3587A.[36] No induced heating of devices or leads was detected in any of these experiments, i.e., less than 0.15°C, but induced voltages were detected. Voltages between 2.4 and 5.5 V were measured during the experiments, but did not appear to harm the patients.

Tronnier et al.[36] concluded that patients with deep brain stimulating leads and pulse generators for the treatment of movement disorders or chronic pain can be examined using MRI. Another conclusion was that MRI of patients with spinal cord stimulation and percutaneous leads is possible. Notably, two of four patients in the study did experience discomfort during MRI from their spinal cord stimulation systems, which used a large plate electrode.

Pavlicek et al.[37] evaluated the Pacesetter Demand Type Demo Unit No. 2481 (Pacesetter, Sylmar, CA), the Telectronics 2251 (Telectronics Pacing Systems, Englewood, CO), the Intermedics Cyberlith IV 259-01 (Intermedics, Freeport, TX), the Pacesetter 221, the CPI Command P5 0530 (CPI, St. Paul, MN), and the Medtronic 5992 in 0.15-, 0.35-, and 0.5-T nuclear magnetic resonance (NMR) systems (Technicare, Solon, OH). During imaging, the peak applied power was 5 to 10 kW. The authors concluded that induced voltages might inhibit the devices and that further investigation was necessary.[37]

Fetter et al.[7] tested external and implantable pulse generators in a 1500-G (0.15-T) NMR system (Picker International, Highland Heights, OH). The RF field was applied at 6.4 MHz, with a peak applied power of 1000 W and a duty cycle of 5%. The external pulse generators examined were the single-chamber Medtronic 5375 and the dual-chamber Medtronic 5330. The Medtronic 8420, 8423, 7100, and 7000A implantable pulse generators (IPG) were also examined. The pacing rate of the Medtronic 8423 changed to a multiple of the RF pulsed field when placed in the center of the coil. For an RF pulse period of 700 ms, the pacing period changed to 1400 ms, and for an RF pulse period of 400 ms, the pacing period changed to 1600 ms.

When the Medtronic 7100 was placed in the RF field, with a 700-ms period, the pacing rate was unaffected, but the pacing period changed to 800 ms when the RF pulse period was changed to 400 ms. Induced RF voltages at the electrodes were measured between 10 and 22 V, depending on the device and leads used.[7]

Erlebacher et al.[8] examined cardiac pacemakers placed in a saline phantom using a 0.5-T Technicare Teslacon MR system (Johnson & Johnson, Anaheim, CA). Devices tested were the Cordis 233F (Cordis, Miami, FL), the Intermedic 283-01, the Medtronic 7000A, and the Pacesetter 283. All pacemakers in this study exhibited malfunctions when exposed to the 10-kW peak, 20.91-MHz RF field.

Erlebacher et al.[8] reported that the Pacesetter, Intermedic, and Medtronic pacemakers were completely inhibited by the application of the RF field. Furthermore, the Cordis model produced an atrial output which appeared to be triggered by the initial pulse of the RF pulse train. This atrial rate was affected by a TR in the 75- to 600-ms range. Ventricular pacing resumed as the TR was shortened to the 300- to 400-ms range.[8] By separate application of the fields, they showed that the RF field, and not the pulsed gradient fields, induced the malfunctions.

Implanted permanent cardiac pacemakers were examined by Hayes et al.[38] in a 1.5-T GE MR system. The devices tested were the Cordis 415A, 240G, 334A, 402B, and 233F and the Telectronics 2291, 155, and 5281, in connection with Medtronic 4011 and 4511 pacing leads. These devices were examined as implanted in an anesthetized 20-kg mongrel dog. When the laboratory animal and the Cordis 415A dual-chamber pulse generator underwent MRI, the measured arterial pressure decreased significantly.[38] This occurred for an RF field pulse period of 200 ms. The ventricular lead was removed, and the experiment was repeated with no adverse effects noted. The Cordis 240G showed no adverse reaction to RF pulse periods of 200 and 1000 ms.[38]

Examination of the Cordis 334A single-chamber pulse generator with an RF pulse period of 1000 ms resulted in an altered pace to pace cycle length, while an RF pulse period of 200 ms produced results as seen in the Cordis 415A. The Cordis 402B was tested in both unipolar and bipolar configurations. When used as a unipolar stimulator, the Cordis 402B exhibited no adverse reaction. However, when the Cordis 402B was configured in the bipolar mode, the 200-ms period RF pulses produced an adverse reaction, as seen in the Cordis 415A and 334A. The large decrease in arterial pressure was also seen when the Cordis 233F was present in the pulsed RF field. Similar responses were noted in all Telectronics models tested. The authors attributed the adverse reactions to antenna interference with the RF field. Device heating was not reported in these experiments.[38]

Gleason et al.[39] examined the Avery Laboratory Model I 110A (Avery Laboratories, Farmingdale, NY) and the Medtronic 3360A, both of which are single-channel, monopolar, passive receivers, in a 0.35-T Diasonics MT/S MR system (Diasonics, San Francisco, CA) and two 1.5-T GE Signa IIs. The third device examined was a dual-channel monopolar receiver, the Medtronic 7560A, and the fourth was a four-contact receiver, the Medtronic SE-4 3464, both of which are implanted passive devices activated by an external RF instrument. The Cordis MK II 904A and the Medtronic Itrel I 7421 IPGs were also examined in this study. The authors did not report TE times, but they did report effective pulse durations of 1.5 and 0.8 ms for the 0.35- and 1.5-T MR systems, respectively.[39]

The findings reported were as follows. For passive receivers, the induced voltages were not large enough to damage the devices; however, for the Avery I 110A, the induced voltage was about 12 V at isocenter. Heating in the presence of the Medtronic Itrel I 7421 was reported to be about 4°C.[39]

Lauck et al.[6] evaluated pacemakers in a 0.5 T-Gyroscan MR system (Philips Medical Systems North America, Shelton, CT) study using a saline phantom. The pulsed RF field was at 21.3 MHz, and a maximum power of 150 W was applied. Single-chamber units examined were the Medtronic Minix 8341 and Telectronics Meta II 1204. Dual-chamber units examined were the Medtronic Synergist II 7071, Medtronic Elite 7077, Intermedics Cosmos II 283-01 and 284-05, Telectronics Meta 1250, Pacesetter Synchrony 2020, and Biotronik Ergos 03 (Biotronik,

Lake Oswego, OR). The stimulation rate was not altered in any device tested in the asynchronous mode with both the RF and gradient fields active. Also, single-chamber pacemakers were inhibited and dual-chamber pacemakers were triggered in synchronous mode during the MRI pre-scan and scan.[6]

In another study by Lauck et al.,[40] eight patients with implanted dual-chamber and single-chamber pacemakers were scanned in a 0.5-T MR system, and no adverse effects were found. Johnson[41] examined four patients with implanted pacemakers, the Siemens Pacesetter 2020T, 261, 285, and 2016T. One transient in pacing was noted, but all others continued to operate normally.

Achenbach et al.[18] examined the Telectronics Meta 1206, Telectronics Simplex, Biotronik Pikos, CPI Vigor 460, and CPI Vigor 1130 single-chamber pacemakers and the Telectronics Meta 1254, Biotronik Ergos 03, Biotronik Physios 01, CPI Delta T, Pacesetter Paragon II, and Pacesetter Synchrony III dual-chamber pacemakers. Tests were performed using a 1.5-T Siemens Magnetom MR system on various electrode and pacemaker combinations in air and a saline phantom of unspecified concentration. When all pacemakers were programmed in VVI mode and subjected to untriggered spin-echo sequences, inhibition of the devices occurred. In addition, when the pacemakers were set in DDD mode, inhibition of the atrial and ventricular leads was seen, as well as rapid ventricular pacing with atrial triggering. If the spin-echo sequences were ECG triggered, effects similar to the above were seen, but since the scanning sequence was interrupted after 700 ms to await the next ECG trigger, total inhibition was not observed.[18] This resulted in a reduced pacing frequency which was as low as 27 pulses per minute. Finally, if gradient-echo sequences were triggered from the ECG, all pacemakers tested were completely unaffected.[18]

Although there appears to be a trend toward safe imaging when cardiac pacemakers are set in asynchronous mode, the reader should be extremely cautious in interpreting these results and aware of the conditions under which the results were obtained. For instance, Erlebacher et al.[8] found a cardiac pacemaker to malfunction at $B_0 = 1.5$ T, whereas Fetter et al.[7] found no malfunction in the same pacemaker at $B_0 = 0.5$ T.

IV. MECHANISM OF RF HEATING IN THE VICINITY OF CONDUCTING IMPLANTS

In this section, electromagnetic field theory is used to provide an understanding of how additional heating can occur in the presence of a conductive implant. A model is developed to describe how an elongated implant can concentrate the induced electric field and is applied to a conductive wire. Heating of a conductive ring is also considered. Next, a method of calculating temperature rise from the local SAR is described, and finally, the effect of perfusion on the temperature rise is discussed.

A. CONCENTRATION OF ELECTRIC FIELDS BY AN ELONGATED IMPLANT

An electrically conductive, elongated implant will concentrate the induced RF currents, resulting in an increase in current density and increased SAR at some locations near an implant. This is different from the phenomenon reported by Ladd et al.[20] and Ladd and Quick,[21] where the heating is due to current flow in a coil connected to the end of a coaxial lead. A simplified model that provides a semiquantitative understanding of the heating mechanism due to currents flowing in tissues near an implant is shown in Figure 16.6.

The eddy currents induced in the body by the RF field are modeled by a uniform current density of J_0. The implant is modeled as a conducting wire, which could be a lead wire, of length l and with a hemispherical tip of radius R_i in a medium of much higher resistivity, ρ. The wire is covered by insulation along its length, with the insulation removed from both ends of the wire. The eddy currents flow into one end of the wire and out of the other end, resulting in an eddy current concentration at the ends.

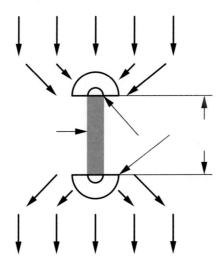

FIGURE 16.6 Model for calculation of enhanced SAR near the ends of a conductive wire.

The voltage drop in the phantom of resistivity ρ due to a uniform current density applied over its length is given by $\Delta V = \rho l J_0$. It is assumed that all the current passing through the tip of the wire also passes through a hemisphere of radius R_o, $R_o > R_i$, at either end of the wire. If the electrical impedance is neglected, there is no voltage drop across the wire. The potential drop ΔV across either of the hemispheres is assumed to be the voltage that would otherwise be dropped across a distance $l/2$ of the wire, $\Delta V = \rho l J_0/2$.

The radius R_o is found by evaluation of the voltage drop across the hemispherical shell between radii R_i and R_o. Considering that a current density, given by $J = J_0 R_o^2/r^2$, flows through a thin shell of radius r and thickness dr, the voltage drop across the hemisphere between radial distances R_o and R_i is calculated by

$$\Delta V = \rho J_0 R_o^2 \int_{R_i}^{R_o} \frac{dr}{r^2} = \rho J_0 R_o^2 \left[\frac{1}{R_i} - \frac{1}{R_o} \right] \tag{16.2}$$

The radius R_o is obtained by setting $\Delta V = \rho l J_0/2$ in Equation 16.2 and solving with the quadratic formula. The result is

$$R_o = \frac{R_i + \sqrt{R_i^2 + 2lR_i}}{2} \tag{16.3}$$

As a numerical example, consider an insulated wire of radius 1 mm and length of 5 cm. The radius R_o of the hemisphere with enhanced current density is calculated, using Equation 16.3, to be 5.5 mm. Using this value, the current density at the wire tip relative to background may be calculated to be

$$J(R_i)/J_0 = \frac{R_o^2}{R_i^2} = 30.5 \tag{16.4}$$

Because the current density is enhanced by a factor of 30.5, the SAR near the tip of the wire is a factor of 930 (30.5^2) greater than the average background level. It is important to note that the enhancement in the SAR increases with increasing wire length.

Bare wires, or wires with very thin insulation, are expected to exhibit a smaller temperature rise near the tip because the currents will be distributed over some distance near the ends of the wire. This spreading of the current occurs because a thin insulator has a small capacitive reactance at RF frequencies.

This calculation is clearly approximate, and more refined methods are needed to calculate the eddy current distribution accurately and hence the local SAR. For cases where the wire length exceeds a $1/4$ wavelength, $\lambda_{1/4}$, approximately, resonance effects will become important. It is important to note that for 64 MHz, $\lambda_{1/4}$ is about 1.2 m in air, but is only 0.13 m in muscle tissue. In this case, the most useful approximation may be a model where the electric field is considered to be scattered by the wire.[42]

B. Calculation of Power Deposition in a Conducting Ring

Another geometry of interest is a conducting ring or disk, which is illustrated in Figure 16.7. The conducting ring has a wire radius r_0, which is assumed to be small compared to the electrical skin depth, and a loop radius R_0, with the incident RF field being perpendicular to the loop. The RF field will induce a voltage in the loop according to Faraday's law of induction.

The resistance R_1 and inductive impedance per unit length ωL_1 are given by[43]

$$R_1 = \omega L_1 = \frac{R_s}{2\pi r_0} \qquad (16.5)$$

where $R_s = \sqrt{\rho \pi f \mu_0}$ is the surface resistivity, f is the frequency, and $\mu_0 = 4\pi \times 10^{-7}$ H/m is the permeability of free space. The equivalent circuit elements in Figure 16.8 are the self-inductance of the ring, L_{EXT}, the internal inductance of the wire, L_{WIRE}, and the internal resistance of the wire, R_{WIRE}. For a ring of radius R_0 and wire radius r_0,

$$R_{WIRE} = \omega L_{WIRE} = \frac{R_0 R_s}{r_0} \qquad (16.6)$$

where $\omega = 2\pi f$ is the angular frequency. The external inductance of the circular current loop is given by[43]

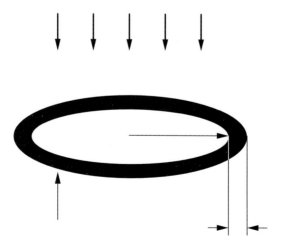

FIGURE 16.7 Conducting loop of radius R_0 and conductor radius r_0, with an RF field B_1 applied.

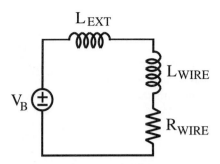

FIGURE 16.8 Equivalent circuit for the geometry shown in Figure 16.7.

$$L_{EXT} \approx R_0 \mu_0 \left[\ln \frac{8R_0}{r_0} - 2 \right] \tag{16.7}$$

The effective voltage V_B that is induced in the conducting loop by the RF field of amplitude B_1 and angular frequency ω is

$$V_B = \pi R_0^2 \omega B_1 \tag{16.8}$$

The current is the ring is

$$I_{WIRE} = \frac{V_B}{\sqrt{([\omega(L_{EXT} + L_{WIRE})]^2 + R_{WIRE}^2)}} \tag{16.9}$$

Using Equations 16.6 to 16.9, the average power dissipation in the wire is calculated by

$$P_{WIRE} = \frac{I_{WIRE}^2 R_{WIRE}}{2} \tag{16.10}$$

As a sample calculation, consider a wire radius of 1 mm, a loop radius of 2 cm, wire resistivity of 4×10^{-7} Ωm, and an RF field with amplitude 20 μT and frequency 64 MHz. The dissipated power calculated by Equation 16.10 is just 0.84 mW. Thus, the power dissipated in a closed conducting ring is quite small. Similarly, a disk-shaped device will also not produce significant inductive heating.

However, when an insulated wire is looped, a potentially hazardous situation arises. Almost all of the induced voltage will appear across the insulating gap where the wires cross. Resonance may result in a significant enhancement of the induced voltage.

V. CALCULATION OF TEMPERATURE RISE FROM LOCALIZED SAR

The estimation in Section IV.A indicates a potentially large SAR near the ends of an elongated implant. However, because of thermal diffusivity α, the heat will be dissipated in the tissue with no perfusion over a distance which is approximately given by

$$\Delta X_{TISSUE} \approx \sqrt{\alpha t} \tag{16.11}$$

where α is the thermal diffusivity and t is time. For tissue, α is about 1.45×10^{-7} m²/s. Assuming a 20-min scan, the distance of heat dissipation is calculated as $\Delta X_{TISSUE} \approx \sqrt{(1.45 \times 10^{-7})(1200s)} = 1.3$ cm. If the heat source is localized to a region much less than ΔX_{TISSUE} in size, the temperature rise will be much less than that predicted from the SAR alone.

For a more quantitative evaluation of temperature rise due to a localized heat source, it is necessary to solve the heat equation, Equation 16.12,

$$\nabla^2 T + \frac{q}{\kappa} - \frac{1}{\alpha}\frac{\partial T}{\partial t} = 0 \qquad (16.12)$$

where T is the temperature, q is the magnitude of the heat source, and κ is the thermal conductivity. Equation 16.12 is solved for a geometry with spherical symmetry and power deposition limited to a point centered at the origin, which models the intense heating that occurs near the tip of a wire. The solution of Equation 16.12 in response to a unit step of heat is

$$T(t, r) = \frac{1}{4\pi\kappa r} erfc\left(\frac{r}{2\sqrt{\alpha t}}\right) \qquad (16.13)$$

where r is the distance from the heat source and $erfc()$ is the complementary error function.[44]

The calculated temperature rise vs. time, at distances of 1.5, 2, and 5 mm from the center of a 10-mW heat source, is shown in Figure 16.9. As with the experimental results in Figure 16.3, there is a rapid initial rise followed by a gradual rise at the tip of the wire. Computed results of the type presented in Figure 16.9 may be compared to measured temperature rise near implants, as shown in Figure 16.3, to estimate the intensity of a concentrated heat source.

A. PERFUSION EFFECTS

If RF heating occurs in a localized volume, one can estimate how perfusion would reduce the temperature rise. Athey[45] calculates the steady state temperature rise as a function of the perfusion rate, the SAR, and the time required for the tissue temperature to reach 63% of its maximum value. A minimal perfusion for tissue may be taken to be 10 ml/min/100 g.[46] For this value, Athey's

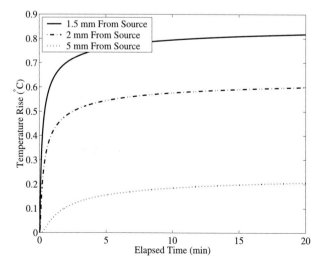

FIGURE 16.9 Calculated temperature rise in degrees Celsius as a function of time for distances of 1.5, 2, and 5 mm from the center of a 10-mW heat source.

method yields a steady state temperature rise of 0.14°C/(W/kg) and a time constant of 8 min. Thus, if the SAR is 4.0 W/kg, the steady state temperature rise is 0.56°C. If perfusion is neglected, an SAR of 4.0 W/kg applied for 20 min results in a temperature rise of 1.15°C, about a factor of 2.05 greater. This suggests that perfusion can significantly reduce RF-induced heating.

VI. CONCENTRATION OF GRADIENT-INDUCED CURRENTS BY METALLIC IMPLANTS

The pulsed gradient fields in MRI also induce currents in a subject, and these currents are in the range of audiofrequencies. One can envision that there would be a significant enhancement of the gradient-induced currents by a long wire as depicted in Figure 16.6. If there was indeed a significant electric field enhancement, it could result in nerve stimulation, which is the principal bioeffect of intense gradient fields. However, electric field enhancements less than a factor of three should not result in nerve stimulation because conductivity inhomogeneities within the body will provide a similar level of enhancement.[47] In addition, significant heating near implants by gradient-induced currents should not occur because the SAR from the gradient currents will be much smaller than that from the RF field.[48]

Previously, there was concern over retained cardiac pacing wires, which were considered to be a relative contraindication for MRI due to the possibility of arrhythmia instigated by induced currents.[49] Concern over the risk has been allayed in a study done by Hartnell et al.[50] in which patients with retained temporary epicardial pacing wires did not exhibit any changes in cardiac rhythm during MRI.

The model for electric field enhancement in Section IV.A does not consider the impedance between the tip of the implant and the surrounding tissue. Geddes and Baker[51] measured an impedance of 230 Ω at 1 kHz with a current density of 0.025 mA/cm^2 for a 0.157-cm^2 stainless steel electrode in 0.9% saline, and when measured at 10 kHz, the impedance was about 50 Ω. Given the smaller electrode area, the impedance is expected to be greater for the tip of a pacing wire and, thus, would significantly curtail concentration of eddy currents. Conversely, the impedance is expected to be small at the much higher RF frequencies.

There is a report of enhancement of the gradient-induced electric field by an implant in Reference 49. In phantom measurements using an electric field probe described by Tay et al.,[52] the presence of the Medtronic SynchroMed Infusion System resulted in up to a twofold increase in the electric field. This magnitude of enhancement is within expectations given the approximately cylindrical geometry of the device.[4] Presumably, the large surface area of the titanium case resulted in a small impedance.

Measuring the gradient-induced electric field near the tip of a long wire in a saline phantom would be interesting, but the electric field probe would need to be quite small. The noise voltage induced by the pulsed magnetic fields would likely overwhelm the signal of interest created by the induced currents.

VII. SUMMARY AND CONCLUSIONS

This chapter reviews interactions of medical implants with the RF and pulsed gradient fields in MRI. The RF field induces eddy current in patients, and these currents result in thermal energy deposition, which is quantified by the SAR. A metallic implant may result in concentration of RF-induced currents, producing an increased local SAR. Long wires especially may result in significant additional heating, particularly when the lengths approach resonant values, and they act as RF antennas. Perfusion and thermal heat flow can result in temperature rises much less than those calculated by solely considering the SAR.

The RF field has been found to interfere with the operation of a number of cardiac pacemakers, particularly when these devices utilize sensing leads. Furthermore, metallic implants may focus currents induced by the pulsed gradients, but few measurements are presently available. The impedance of the metal–electrolyte interface should serve to significantly reduce the concentration of gradient-induced currents.

The reader is encouraged to see other pertinent works, including the other chapters in this book, for a description of other relevant MR safety considerations.[49,53,54]

ACKNOWLEDGMENTS

The authors thank A. Ufuk Ağar, Joe D. Bourland, Kirk S. Foster, Leslie A. Geddes, and D. Joe Schaefer for their input, support, and invaluable assistance, both direct and indirect, in the creation of this chapter. The authors would also like to thank the Magnetic Health Science Foundation of Japan for their financial support.

REFERENCES

1. Stark, D. D. and Bradley, W. G., *Magnetic Resonance Imaging,* C.V. Mosby Company, St. Louis, 1988.
2. A primer on medical device interactions with magnetic resonance imaging systems, http://www.fda.gov/cdrh/ode/primerf6.html, February 1997.
3. Recommendations and report on petitions for magnetic resonance reclassification and codification, *Fed. Regist.,* 54(20), 5077–5088, 1989.
4. Smith, C. D., Kildishev, A. V., Nyenhuis, J. A., Foster, K. S., and Bourland, J. D., Interactions of magnetic resonance imaging radio frequency magnetic fields with elongated medical implants, *J. Appl. Phys.,* 87(9), 6188–6190, 2000.
5. Chou, C. K., McDougall, J. A., and Chan, K. W., RF heating of implanted spinal fusion stimulator during magnetic imaging, *IEEE Trans. Biomed. Eng.,* 44(5), 367–373, 1997.
6. Lauck, G., Von Smekal, A., Wolke, S., Seelos, K. C., Jung, W., Manz, M., and Luderitz, B., Effects of nuclear magnetic resonance imaging on cardiac pacemakers, *Pacing Clin. Electrophysiol.,* 18(8), 1549–1555, 1995.
7. Fetter, J., Aram, G., Holmes, D. R., Gray, J. E., and Hayes, D. L., The effects of nuclear magnetic resonance imagers on external and implantable pulse generators, *Pacing Clin. Electrophysiol.,* 7(4), 720–727, 1984.
8. Erlebacher, J. A., Cahill, P. T., Pannizzo, F., and Knowles, J. R., Effect of magnetic resonance imaging on DDD pacemakers, *Am. J. Cardiol.,* 57(6), 437–440, 1986.
9. Hartsgrove, G., Kraszewski, A., and Surowiec, A., Simulated biological materials for electromagnetic radiation absorption studies, *Bioelectromagnetics,* 8(1), 29–36, 1987.
10. Chou, C. K., Chen, G. W., Guy, A. W., and Luk, K. H., Formulas for preparing phantom muscle tissue at various radiofrequencies, *Bioelectromagnetics,* 5(4), 435–411, 1984.
11. Hagmann, M. J., Levin, R. L., Calloway, L., Osborn, A. J., and Foster, K. R., Muscle-equivalent phantom materials for 10–100 MHz, *IEEE Trans. Microwave Theory Tech.,* 40(4), 760–762, 1992.
12. Shellock, F. G. and Shellock, V. J., Cranial bone flap fixation clamps: compatibility at MR imaging, *Radiology,* 207(3), 822–825, 1998.
13. Gabriel, C. and Gabriel, S., Compilation of the dielectric properties of body tissues at RF and microwave frequencies, Technical Report AL/OE-TR-1996-0037, Physics Department King's College London and Armstrong Laboratory Radiofrequency Radiation Division Brooks Air Force Base, TX, 1996.
14. Durney, C. H., Massoudi, H., and Iskander, M. F., Radiofrequency radiation dosimetry handbook, Technical Report USAFSAM-TR-85-73, E.E. Department, the University of Utah, Salt Lake City, UT and Armstrong Laboratory Radiofrequency Radiation Division Brooks Air Force Base, TX, 1986.
15. Geddes, L. A. and Baker, L. E., The specific resistance of biological material — a compendium of data for the biomedical engineer and physiologist, *Med. Biol. Eng.,* 5(3), 271–293, 1967.

16. Burdette, E. C., Cain, F. L., and Seals, J., *In vivo* probe measurement technique for determining dielectric properties at vhf through microwave frequencies, *IEEE Trans. Microwave Theory Tech.,* MTT–28(4), 414–427, 1908.

17. Athey, T. W., Stuchly, M. A., and Stuchly, S. S., Measurement of radio frequency permittivity of biological tissues with an open-ended coaxial line: Part ii. Experimental results, *IEEE Trans. Microwave Theory Tech.,* MTT–30(1), 87–92, 1982.

18. Achenbach, S., Moshage, W., Diem, B., Schibgilla, V., and Bachmann, K., Effects of magnetic resonance imaging on cardiac pacemakers and electrodes, *Am. Heart J.,* 134(3), 467–474, 1997.

19. Chou, C. K., Bassen, H., Osepchuk, J., Balzano, Q., Petersen, R., Meltz, M., Cleveland, R., Lin, J. C., and Heynick, L., Radio frequency electromagnetic exposure: tutorial review on experimental dosimetry, *Bioelectromagnetics,* 17(3), 195–208, 1996.

20. Ladd, M. E., Quick, H. H., Boesinger, P., and McKinnon, G. C., RF heating of actively visualized catheters and guidewires, *Proc. Int. Soc. Magn. Reson. Med.,* 6, 473, 1998.

21. Ladd, M. E. and Quick, H. H., A 0.7 mm triaxial cable for significantly reducing RF heating in interventional MR, *Proc. Int. Soc. Magn. Reson. Med.,* 7, 104, 1999.

22. Chou, C. K., McDougall, J. A., and Chan, K. W., Absence of radiofrequency heating from auditory implants during magnetic resonance imaging, *Bioelectromagnetics,* 16(5), 307–316, 1995.

23. Nyenhuis, J. A., Bourland, J. D., Foster, K. S., Graber, G. P., Terry, R. S., and Adkins, R. A., Testing of MRI compatibility of the cyberonics model 100 NCP generator and model 300 series lead, Poster, American Epilepsy Society Meeting, December 1997.

24. Shellock, F. G., Nogueira, M., and Morisoli, S., MR imaging and vascular access ports: ex vivo evaluation of ferromagnetism, heating, and artifacts at 1.5-T, *J. Magn. Reson. Imaging,* 5(4), 481–484, 1995.

25. Shellock, F. G. and Morisoli, S. M., Ex vivo evaluation of ferromagnetism, heating, and artifacts produced by heart valve prostheses exposed to a 1.5-T MR system, *J. Magn. Reson. Imaging,* 4(5), 756–758, 1994.

26. Hartwell, R. C. and Shellock, F. G., MRI of cervical fixation devices: sensation of heating caused by vibration of metallic components, *J. Magn. Reson. Imaging,* 7(4), 771–772, 1997.

27. Fagan, L. L., Shellock, F. G., Brenner, R. J., and Rothman, B., Ex vivo evaluation of ferromagnetism, heating, and artifacts of breast tissue expanders exposed to a 1.5-T MR system, *J. Magn. Reson. Imaging,* 5(5), 614–616, 1995.

28. Shellock, F. G. and Shellock, V. J., Ceramic surgical instruments: ex vivo evaluation of compatibility with MR imaging at 1.5-T, *J. Magn. Reson. Imaging,* 6(6), 954–956, 1996.

29. Shellock, F. G. and Shellock, V. J., Cardiovascular catheters and accessories: ex vivo testing of ferromagnetism, heating, and artifacts associated with MRI, *J. Magn. Reson. Imaging,* 8(6), 1338–1342, 1998.

30. Shellock, F. G. and Shellock, V. J., Spetzler titanium aneurysm clips: compatibility at MR imaging, *Radiology,* 206(3), 838–841, 1998.

31. Shellock, F. G. and Slimp, G., Halo vest for cervical spine fixation during MR imaging, *Am. J. Roengtenol.,* 154(3), 631–632, 1990.

32. Shellock, F. G., Compatibility of an endoscope designed for use in interventional MR imaging procedures, *Am. J. Roentgenol.,* 171(5), 1297–1300, 1998.

33. Shellock, F. G., Detrick, M. S., and Brant-Zawadski, M. N., MR compatibility of Guglielmi detachable coils, *Radiology,* 203(2), 568–570, 1997.

34. Felmlee, J., Hokanson, D., Zink, F., and Perkins, W., Real time evaluation of EKG electrode heating during MRI at 1.5-T, *Proc. Int. Soc. Magn. Reson. Med.,* 3, 1226, 1995.

35. Nyenhuis, J. A., Kildishev, A. V., Bourland, J. D., Foster, K. S., Graber, G., and Athey, T. W., Heating near implanted medical devices by the MRI RF-magnetic field, *IEEE Trans. Magn.,* 35(5), 4133–4135, 1999.

36. Tronnier, V. M., Staubert, A., Hähnel, S., and Sarem-Aslani, A., Magnetic resonance imaging with implanted neurostimulators: an in vitro and in vivo study, *Neurosurgery,* 44(1), 118–125, 1999.

37. Pavlicek, W., Geisinger, M., Castle, L., Borkowski, G. P., Meaney, T. F., Bream, B. L., and Gallagher, J. H., The effects of nuclear magnetic resonance on patients with cardiac pacemakers, *Radiology,* 147(1), 149–153, 1983.

38. Hayes, D. L., Holmes, D. R., and Gray, J. E., Effect of 1.5 tesla nuclear magnetic resonance imaging scanner on implanted permanent pacemakers, *J. Am. Coll. Cardiol.,* 10(4), 782–786, 1987.
39. Gleason, C. A., Kaula, N. F., Hricak, H., Schmidt, R. A., and Tanagho, E. A., The effect of magnetic resonance imagers on implanted neurostimulators, *Pacing Clin. Electrophysiol.,* 15(1), 81–94, 1992.
40. Lauck, G., Sommer, T., Wolke, S., Luderitz, B., and Manz, M., Magnetic resonance imaging effects and considerations with permanent cardiac pacemakers, Euro–Pace Abstract, 7th European Symposium on Cardiac Pacing in Istanbul, Turkey, *Pacing Clin. Electrophysiol.,* May 1995.
41. Johnson, D., Magnetic resonance imaging effects and considerations with permanent cardiac pacemakers, NASPE Abstract, NASPE 15th Annual Scientific Sessions in Nashville, Tennessee, *Pacing Clin. Electrophysiol.,* April 1994.
42. Vitebskiy, S. and Carin, L., Moment-method modeling of short-pulse scattering from and the resonance of a wire buried inside a lossy, dispersive half-space, *IEEE Trans. Antennas Propag.,* 43(11), 1303–1312, 1995.
43. Ramo, S., Whinnery, J., and Van Duzer, T., *Fields and Waves in Communication Electronics,* John Wiley & Sons, New York, 1994.
44. Carslaw, H. S. and Jaeger, J. C., *Conduction of Heat in Solids,* Oxford University Press, New York, 1948.
45. Athey, T. W., A model of the temperature rise in the head due to magnetic resonance imaging procedures, *Magn. Reson. Med.,* 9(2), 177–184, 1989.
46. Report on the allerton workshop on the future of biothermal engineering, Technical Report, April 1997, Sponsored by the NSF, Grant No. NSF CTS 96-18518.
47. Nyenhuis, J. A., Mouchawar, G. A., Bourland, J. D., et al., A model for calculating the eddy currents induced by pulsed magnetic fields in the MRI environment, *Med. Biol. Eng. Comput.,* 29, 40, 1991.
48. Nyenhuis, J. A., Bourland, J. D., Kildishev, A. V., and Schafer, D. J., Bioeffects of intense MRI gradient fields, in *Magnetic Resonance Procedures: Health Effects and Safety,* Shellock, F. G., Ed., CRC Press, Boca Raton, FL, 2000, Chapter 2.
49. Shellock, F. G., *Pocket Guide to MR Procedures and Metallic Objects: Update 2000.* Lippincott, Williams & Wilkins, Philadelphia, 2000.
50. Hartnell, G. G., Spence, L., Hughes, L. A., Cohen, M. C., Saouaf, R., and Buff, B., Safety of MR imaging in patients who have retained metallic materials after cardiac surgery, *Am. J Roentgenol.,* 168(5), 1157–1159, 1997.
51. Geddes, L. A. and Baker, L. E., *Principles of Applied Biomedical Instrumentation,* John Wiley & Sons, New York, 1989, 333.
52. Tay, G. S., Chilbert, M. A., Battocletti, J. H., Sances, A., Jr., and Swiontek, T., Probe for measuring current density during magnetic stimulation, *Biomed. Instrum. Technol.,* 25(3), 220–228, 1991.
53. Shellock, F. G. and Kanal, E., *Magnetic Resonance: Bioeffects, Safety, and Patient Management,* Lippincott-Raven Publishers, New York, 1996.
54. Kanal, E., Shellock, F. G., and Talagala, L., Safety considerations in MR imaging, *Radiology,* 176(3), 593–606, 1990.

Appendix I

Medical Devices and Products Developed for Interventional, Intra-Operative, and Magnetic Resonance-Guided Procedures*

Various manufacturers and vendors of medical products, prompted by recommendations and requests from magnetic resonance (MR) healthcare workers, have recognized the need for developing specialized medical devices, equipment, instruments, and products for interventional, intra-operative, and MR-guided procedures. Similar to other devices and products utilized in the MR environment, *ex vivo* testing is required to demonstrate the safe use and operation before they are utilized for intra-operative or MR-guided procedures. The test procedures include an assessment of magnetic field interactions, heating, induced current (for certain devices), and artifacts using standardized techniques.

Thus, medical devices can then be characterized with respect to being "MR safe" or "MR compatible" with the MR environment. A device is considered MR safe if, when placed in the MR environment, it presents no additional risk to a patient, individual, or MR system operator from magnetic interactions, heating, or induced voltages, but it may affect the quality of the diagnostic information on MR scans. A device is considered MR compatible if it is MR safe, its use in the MR environment does not adversely impact the image quality, and it performs its intended function when used in the MR environment according to its specifications in a safe and effective manner.

This appendix provides a comprehensive listing of vendors that are a source for a variety of devices, instruments, and equipment that were designed for interventional, intra-operative, or MR-guided procedures.

---

* Note that some of the medical devices, equipment, and instruments may be pre-product prototypes that have completed evaluations by the U.S. Food and Drug Administration (FDA), European CE Mark, or other reviews for safety or effectiveness that may be necessary prior to commercial distribution of these devices. Some devices may not be available in all countries. No claims are made regarding patient/staff safety, MR compatibility, MR safety, or clinical capability of any of the medical devices included in this list. Before introduction of any medical device into the MR environment, the device should be inspected by qualified hospital personnel. The non-magnetic properties of the device and its clinical operation in the magnetic field should be verified before it is used for an MR procedure. Use of these medical devices for animal or human procedures must comply with any applicable government or local hospital safety and animal/human studies committee requirements. The MR facility should contact the vendor directly for technical specifications, pricing, and commercial availability of the medical product. Special thanks to Ms. Karen Streit of General Electric Medical Systems, Milwaukee, WI for providing the majority of the information on this compilation. Portions of this Appendix are reprinted with permission from Shellock, F. G., *Pocket Guide to MR Procedures and Metallic Objects: Update 2000*, Lippincott, Williams & Wilkins, Philadelphia, 2000.

Aesculap, Inc.
>1000 Gateway Blvd.
>So. San Francisco, CA 94080
>*Product(s)*
>General surgical instruments
>*Catalog or Special Items*
>MR-safe surgical instruments
>*Contact*
>Haio F. Fauser
>New Business Development Manager, U.S.
>Phone: 800-282-9000 or 415-876-7000
>*International Contact*
>Paul Wieneke (1st contact)
>Aesculap AG
>AM Aesculap-Platz
>P.O. Box 40
>78501 Tuttlingen/Germany
>Phone: 49-74-61-95-2801; Fax: 49-74-61-146-14

BIP
>AM Brand 1
>P.C. 0-82299 Tuerkenfeld, Germany
>*Product(s)*
>Core biopsy gun
>*Contact*
>Norbert Hece
>Phone: 49-81936026 or 49-81936548
>*International Contact*
>Same as above

Cogent Light
>26145 Technology Drive
>Santa Clarita, CA 91355-1137
>*Product(s)*
>Headlight/lightsource
>*Contact*
>Richard B. Davies
>Phone: 805-294-2989; Fax: 805-294-2904 (800–294-2989 #101)

Cook Medical
>P.O. Box 489
>Bloomington, IN 47402
>*Product(s)*
>Needles, biopsy guns, catheters
>*Contact*
>John DeFord, Ph.D.
>Product Development Manager
>Phone: 812-339-2235; Fax: 812-339-5369
>Toll-Free: 800-346-2686
>Customer Service: 800-457-4500

International Contact
   Same as above

Cryomedical Sciences
   1300 Piccard Drive, Suite 102
   Rockville, MD 20850
Product(s)
   Cryotherapy equipment
Contact
   John Baust
   Vice President of Research and Development
   Phone: 301-417-7070; Fax: 301-417-7077
International Contact
   German Distributor:
   Uwe Lindmfller
   B&K Medical
   Phone: 49-5143-93227; Fax: 49-5143-93228

Cuda Products
   600 Powers Avenue
   Jacksonville, FL 32217
Product(s)
   Light source adapters for endoscopes
Catalog or Special Items
   Olympus C-0200
   Wolff C-0201
   ACMI C-0202
Contact
   Phone: 904-737-7611; Fax: 904-733-4832

Daum Corporation
   Daum GmbH Deutschland
   Hagenower Strasse 73
   D-19061 Schwerin
   Phone: 49-385-6344-344; Fax: 49-385-6344-152
Product(s)
   Needles and various accessories
Contact
   Wolfgang Daum, President
   Phone: 410-455-5786; Fax: 410-455-5787
   E-mail: info@daum.de or medinfo@daum.de

Dornier Medizinlaser GMBH
   Industriestrasse 15
   82110 Germering, Germany
Product(s)
   MR-safe laser-delivery systems and
   various MR-safe applicators
   for laser-induced thermotherapy (LITT)

Contact
Wolfgang Illich
Development Engineer
Phone: 49-89-84108-133; Fax: 49-89-84108-745
E-mail: wolfgang.illich@domedtech.de
Dr. Werner Rother
Sales Manager
Phone: 49-89-84108-640; Fax: 49-89-84108-552
E-mail: werner.rother@domedtech.de

E-Z-EM, Inc.
717 Main Street
Westbury, NY 11590
Product(s)
Lufkin 22 gauge cytology biopsy needles
MRI histology biopsy needles
MRI core biopsy guns, 14 and 18 gauge
MRI lesion marking systems
Direct Sale or Distribution
Both, but primarily through distributors on six continents
Contact
Andy Zwarun, Vice President
Phone: 516-333-8230, ext. 304; Fax: 516-333-8278
E-mail: anzwar@worldnet.att.net
International Contact
Germany: Edwin Schneider (Guerbet)
Phone: 49-6196-7620; Fax: 49-6196-79934
Switzerland: Christopher Jackson
Manager, Medilink
Phone: 41-91-972-8417; Fax: 41-91-972-8568

Groupe Bruker Odam
34, Rue de l'Industrie
Wissembourg, France 67160
Product(s)
Patient monitoring equipment
Contact
Laurent Sigrist
Secretaire General
Phone: 33-88-63-36-06; Fax: 33-88-54-36-32
Sales Department:
Phone: 33-88-63-36-00; Fax: 33-88-94-12-82
International Contact
Same as above

In-Vivo Research
12601 Research Parkway
Orlando, FL 32826
Product(s)
Patient monitoring equipment

Direct Sale or Distribution
  Market through direct sales reps with some distributors
Contact
  Jerry O'Connor
  Product Manager
  Phone: 407-275-3220; Fax: 407-249-2022

J&J Ethicon, Inc.
  Route 22
  Somerville, NJ 08876
Product(s)
  Needles with sutures
Contact
  Bill McJames
  Phone: 908-218-2297; Fax: 908-218-2531

Johnson & Johnson Professional, Inc. (Codman Division)
  41 Pacella Park Drive
  Randolph, MA 02368
Product(s)
  CMC3 Irrigation Bi-Polar, Bookwalter Arm and
  Table Post, Rhoton
  Microsurgical, Hudson Twist Drill
Direct Sale or Distribution
  Direct sales through representatives
Contact
  Paula Papineau
  Associate Product Director
  Greg Auda
  Director of Instrumentation
  Phone: 508-828-3228; Fax: 508-828-3065
International Contact
  Blair Fraser
  Manager of new business development for
  European operation
  Phone: 44-13 44-86 40 30

Life Instruments
  14 Wood Road, Suite 002
  Braintree, MA 02184
Product(s)
  Penfields, curettes, mini cobbs, Hudson
  twist drill, drill bits, periosteal elevators
Contact
  Larry Foley
  Phone: 617-849-0209 or 800-925-2995; Fax: 617-849-0128
International Contact
  Same as above

Magnetic Resonance Equipment Corporation
P.O. Box 5489
5 Grant Avenue
Bay Shore, NY 11706
Product(s)
Patient monitors and patient communication and music systems
Catalog or Special Items
Catalog
Direct Sale or Distribution
Direct in the U.S. and Canada and through dealers in the rest of the world
Contact
John V. Plump
Phone: 516-243-3500; Fax: 516-243-3516

Magnetic VisiOn GMBH
Lochacher 6
CH-8630 Ruti, Switzerland
Product(s)
Neurosurgery drill, neurobiopsy needle guide, Dura hook, retractor
International Contact
Dr. Adriano Vigano
Phone: 41-55-260-1855; Fax: 41-55-260-1859
E-mail: avigano@swissonline.ch

Medrad
240 Alpha Drive
Pittsburgh, PA 15238-2870
Product(s)
Spectris MR Injector
(For injection of contrast media only, and explicitly not for drug or chemotherapy infusion.)
Contact
Phone: 800-633-7237 or 412-967-9700; Fax: 412-963-1964
International Contact
Medrad Europe
Postbus 3084
NL-6202 N.B. Maastricht, The Netherlands
Phone: 31-43-364-08-08; Fax: 31-43-365-00–20
Brigette Paltra (Meditron)
Phone: 41-55-4502121; Fax: 41-62-3900315

Midas Rex, L.P.
3001 Race Street
Ft. Worth, TX 76111
Product(s)
Pneumatic drill
Contact
Gary B. Gage
Director of R&D
Phone: 817-831-2604 or 800-433-7639; Fax: 817-834-4835

Möller Microsurgical
7 Industrial Park
Waldwick, NJ 07463
Product(s)
Microscope
Contact
Dick Montgomery
Vice President, Marketing & Sales
Phone: 201-251-9592; Fax: 201-251-9516
International Contact
Dr. Martin Schmidt, President
J.D. Möller Optische Werke GmbH
Rosengarten 10
D-22880 Wedel/Germany
Phone: 04103-70-93-33; Fax: 04103-70-93-50

MR Resources, Inc.
158R Main Street
P.O. Box 880
Gardner, MA 01440
Product(s)
MR parts and accessories
Contact
Ann Cochran, Catalog Manager
Phone: 800-443-5486 or 508-632-7000
International Contact
Same as above

North American Draeger
3136 Quarry Road
Telford, PA 18969
Product(s)
MRI anesthesia unit with electronic ventilator and monitoring system
Catalog or Special Items
Catalog
Direct Sale or Distribution
Direct
Contact
Greg Sutherland
Product Manager
Phone: 800-462-7566

Ohmeda Inc.
Ohmeda Drive
P.O. Box 7550
Madison, WI 53707-7550
Product(s)
Anesthesia machines, vaporizers, breathing circuit
Direct Sale or Distribution
Direct

Contact
Deb Schmaling
Marketing Product Manager for Excell
Phone: 800-345-2700, ext. 3357; Fax: 608-223-2476
E-mail: deb.schmaling@ohmeda.boc.com

Olympus America
4 Nevada Dr.
Lake Success, NY 11042-1179
Product(s)
Endoscopes, light sources, video systems
Contact
Gene Eldrige
Senior Design Engineer
Research & Development, Medical Instr. Div.
Phone: 516-844-5467; Fax: 516-326-9085

OMI Surgical Products
3924 Virginia Avenue
Cincinnati, OH 45227
Product(s)
Mayfield Skull Clamp
Catalog or Special Items
MR Safe Skull Pins
Contact
Chuck Dinkler
Research & Development
Phone: 800-755-6381 or 513-561-2705; Fax: 513-561-0195
International Contact
Same as above

Omnivent
Topeka, KS
Product(s)
Patient ventilation and ventilator monitors
Contact
Bill Gates, President
Phone: 800-933-7902 or 913-273-8924

Penlon
Abingdon,
Oxon, England OX14 3PH
Product(s)
MR Compatible Ventilator
Nuffield, Series 200
Contact
Craig Thompson
Marketing Manager
Phone: 44-1235-554-222; Fax: 44-1235-555-252
International Contact
Same as above

Pina-Vertriebs AG
Langrietstr. 17a
Neuhausen 2/Sh, Switzerland CH-8212
Product(s)
Surgical instruments, development of MR-safe custom devices, implants, scissors
International Contact
Axel Hoehn
Director of Sales and Marketing
Phone: 41-52-672-40-42; Fax: 41-52-672-40-48
Mobile: 49-171-349-41-19

Snowden Pencer
5175 S. Royal Atlanta Drive
Tucker, GA 30084
Product(s)
Titanium surgical instruments
Contact
Customer Service Department
Phone: 800-367-7874 or 770-934-4922
International Contact
Snowden-Pencer Customer Service Dept.
Phone: 770-496-0952

Studer Medical Engineering
Rundbuckstraße 2
CH-8212 Neuhausen am Reinfall, Switzerland
Product(s)
Moeller Microscopes and Stand
Contact
Rudolf Hensler
Phone: 41-52-674-0878; Fax: 41-52-674-0879
Karl Weissbach
Mobile: 49-171-210-6812

Synergetics, Inc.
17466 Chesterfield Airport Road
Chesterfield, MO 63005
Product(s)
Deep Neuro Dissection Set
Synerturn N000-160
Contact
Ed Tinn
Phone: 314-530-1440; Fax: 314-530-1143
To order: 800-600-0565

United Metal Fabricators
409 Eisenhauer Boulevard
Johnstown, PA 15904
Product(s)
Instrument tables, basin stands, OR furniture, case carts, etc.

Contact
Peter Terry
Phone: 800-638-5322 or 814-266-8726; Fax: 814-266-1870

United States Surgical
150 Glover Avenue
Norwalk, CT 06856
Product(s)
10 mm Surgiview Scope #176608, accessories
Contact
John Tovey
Phone: 617-533–1017

Valley Forge Scientific Corp.
136 Green Tree Road, Suite 100
Oaks, PA 19456
Product(s)
VFS-200 Bi-polar unit, electrocautery
Contact
Jerry Malis, Ph.D.
Bonnie Ritchie
Phone: 610-666-7500; Fax: 610-666-7565
International Contact
Same as above

Veenstra Instruments
Madame Curieweg 1
P.O. Box 115
N1-8500 Ac Joure, The Netherlands
Product(s)
Trolleys, case carts, OR furniture
Contact
Headquarters
Phone: 31-513-41-69-64; Fax: 31-513-41-69-19

Appendix II

Summary of Magnetic Resonance Safety Studies: 1985 to 1999

Frank G. Shellock

Study Description	Summary	Reference
1.5 T Simulated imaging conditions Human subjects Studied RF power levels equivalent to an SAR of 3 W/kg for 20 min	"Examinations on patients without thermoregulatory impairment can be carried out safely up to at least this SAR level (3 W/kg)."	Abart et al.[1]
Human subjects Clinical imaging conditions Study performed to assess the stimulation threshold for healthy adults using sinusoidally oscillating gradients	The greatest frequency of reported stimulations occurs when the y-gradient is used. This was confirmed by the results and supports the hypothesis that orthogonal to the y-axis the body has the largest conductive loop, resulting in the strongest peripheral simulation.	Abart et al.[2]
Mathematic modeling of thermoregulatory responses	"Assuming a criterion elevation in deep body temperature of 0.6 degrees C, Ta = 20 degrees C and v = 0.8 m/sec, a 70 kg patient could undergo an NMR exposure of infinite duration at SAR $\leq$ 5 W/kg."	Adair and Berglund[3]
Mathematic modeling of thermoregulatory responses with an emphasis on cardiovascular impairment	"Under conditions that are desirable in the clinic (Ta = 20 degrees C, 50% RH, still air), moderate restrictions (up to 67%) of SkBF yield tolerable increases in core temperature (TCO $\leq$ 1 degree C) during NMR exposures (SAR $\leq$ 4 W/kg of 40 minutes or less."	Adair and Berglund[4]
2.0 T Clinical imaging conditions Rats Studied effect of MRI on blood-brain barrier permeability	"No MRI-induced difference was detected"	Adzamli et al.[5]

Study Description	Summary	Reference
Mathematic modeling of thermoregulatory responses	"The model suggests that current practices in MR imaging will not cause a temperature rise in the center of small unperfused regions such as the eye of more than 1 degree C."	Athey[6]
1.5 T Exposure to RF radiation in excess of clinical imaging conditions Sheep Studied RF-radiation induced heating	"For exposure periods in excess of standard clinical imaging protocols the temperature increase was insufficient to cause adverse thermal effects."	Barber et al.[7]
0.5 and 1.5 T Clinical imaging conditions Human subjects Studied effect of MRI on the EEG and evaluated neuropsychological status	"No measurable influence of MRI on cognitive functions."	Bartels et al.[8]
0.04 T Clinical imaging conditions Human subjects Studied effects of MRI on cognition	"MRI did not cause any cognitive deterioration."	Besson et al.[9]
1.6 T Quenched magnet Pig Studied effect of quenching a magnet	"Our findings, which in the circumstances of this experiment, suggested that the risks are small."	Bore et al.[10]
MRI gradient-induced electric fields Dogs Studied bioeffects at high MRI gradient-induced fields	"As the strength of MRI gradient-induced fields increases, biological effects in order of increasing field and severity include stimulation of peripheral nerves, nerves of respiration and finally, the heart."	Bourland et al.[11]
1.5 T Simulated imaging conditions Human subjects	The dB/dt intensity to induce a sensation which the subject described as uncomfortable was about 50% above the sensation threshold. Experiments with dogs showed that cardiac stimulation by pulsed magnetic gradient fields is exceedingly unlikely.	Bourland et al.[12]
1.5 T Clinical imaging conditions Human subjects Studied memory loss	"No gross or subtle memory changes could be attributed to MR imaging, because control groups showed similar patterns of memory loss."	Brockway and Bream[13]
0.38 T Static magnetic field only Deoxygenated erythrocytes Studied orientation of sickle erythrocytes	"Further studies are needed to assess possible hazards of MRI on sickle cell disease."	Brody et al.[14]
0.35 and 1.5 T Clinical imaging conditions Human subjects with sickle cell disease Studied effects of MRI on patients with sickle cell disease	"No change in sickle cell blood flow during MR imaging in vivo.'	Brody et al.[15]

Study Description	Summary	Reference
0.35 T Clinical imaging conditions Human subjects Studied effects of noise during MRI on hearing	"Noise generated by MR imaging may cause temporary hearing loss, and earplugs can prevent this."	Brummet et al.[16]
Varying gradient fields Humans Studied neural stimulation threshold with varying oscillations and gradient field strength	"The threshold decreases with the number of oscillations and increases with frequency. The repeatable threshold of 63 T/s (1270 Hz) remains constant from 32 oscillations (25.6 msec) to 128 oscillations (102.4 msec)."	Budinger et al.[17]
60 T/s for 1.2-kHz sinusoids	"Assuming a 0.03-m radius current loop in the heart, 1,600 T/s corresponds to an induced electric field of 24 V/m. This field is approximately four times greater than that expected to cause perceptible sensation in the human torso."	Budinger et al.[18]
0.15 T Stimulated imaging conditions HL60 promyelocytic cells Studied effect of MRI on Ca^{2+}	"Results demonstrate that time varying magnetic fields associated with MRI procedures increase Ca^{2+}."	Carson et al.[19]
1.5 and 2.0 T Simulated imaging conditions Studied typical acoustic noise and analyzed the characteristics	"Through the analysis of acoustic noise, we find that the acoustic noise profiles and their frequency distributions are not only dependent on the pulse sequence employed but also greatly dependent on the types of scanners, especially the coil structures and their supports."	Cho et al.[20]
2.0 T Simulated imaging conditions Human volunteers Studied effects of acoustics, or sound noise arising in fMR imaging of the auditory, visual, and motor cortices	"…results show that the effects of acoustic noise on motor and visual responses are opposite…could have significant consequences in data observation and interpretation in future fMRI studies."	Cho et al.[21]
Gradient magnetic fields up to 66 T/s in dogs and 61 T/s in humans Dogs Human subjects studied physiologic responses to large amplitude time-varying magnetic fields	dogs — "No motion, twitch, or ECG abnormalities." Humans — "Brief minimal muscular twitches observed on various parts of the body due to magnetic stimulation."	Cohen et al.[22]
0.5 and 1.0 T Simulated imaging conditions Cultured human blood cells Studied effect of static magnetic fields and line scan imaging on human blood cells	"Neither treatment had any significant effect on any of the parameters measured"	Cooke and Morris[23]
4.7 T Exposures to static and RF electromagnetic fields only Isolated rabbit hearts Studied effects on cardiac excitability and vulnerability	No measurable effect on strength interval relationship or ventricular vulnerability.	Doherty et al.[24]

Study Description	Summary	Reference
1.5 T Human subjects Clinical imaging conditions Studied the incidence, type, and location of stimulation in a whole-body scanner	"Maximum stimulation typically occurred 30 to 40 cm from isocenter in the region of maximum dB/dt. Generally, y gradients produced truncal stimulation and x gradients produced stimulation in the head. ... Patients should be instructed to keep their hands apart."	Ehrhardt et al.[25]
Various MR systems and conditions This study assessed the safety, efficacy, and cost-effectiveness of the use of triple dose gadolinium-DTPA (Gd) in serial monthly brain MRI of patients with multiple sclerosis	No side effects were reported and no significant changes in blood test parameters were found throughout the study. This study shows that the serial use of triple dose Gd is safe, and that it increases the sensitivity of serial monthly enhanced MRI in detecting multiple sclerosis activity significantly.	Filippi et al.[26]
Gradient magnetic fields only Sinusoidal gradients at a frequency of 1.25 kHz with amplitudes up to 40 mT/min for a z-coil and 25 mT/min for an x-coil Human subjects studied physiologic effects, physiologic responses	Observed peripheral muscle stimulation, no extrasystoles or arrhythmias.	Fischer[27]
0.3, 0.5, 1.5 T Stimulated imaging conditions and static/RF and gradient fields separately Rats Studied blood-brain barrier permeability	"Increased brain mannitol associated with gradient fluid flux may reflect increased blood–brain barrier permeability or blood volume in brain."	Garber et al.[28]
2.2 to 2.7 T Simulated imaging conditions Mouse cells Studied oncogenic and genotoxic effects of MRI	"Data clearly mitigate against an association between exposure to MR imaging modalities and both carcinogenic and genotoxic effects."	Geard et al.[29]
60 T/s Gradient magnetic fields only Human subjects Studied effects of gradient magnetic fields on cardiac and respiratory function	"No changes were observed."	Gore et al.[30]
Mathematic modeling of rates of RF energy absorption	"Fair to good agreement was found between SAR and those predicted by simple phenomenological models."	Grandolfo et al.[31]
0.1 to 1.5 T Static magnetic field only Human subjects Studied effects of static magnetic fields on temperature	Temperatures increased or decreased depending on the field strength of the magnet.	Gremmel et al.[32]
2.11 T Static magnetic field only Isolated rat hearts Studied effect of static magnetic field on cardiac muscle contraction	"Static magnetic fields used in NMR imaging do not constitute any hazard in terms of cardiac contractility."	Gulch and Lutz[33]

Study Description	Summary	Reference
1.5 T Simulated imaging conditions Healthy volunteers Studied effects of high gradient amplitudes and switching rates	"…only for the imaging protocols characterized by the application of long bipolar repetitive gradient pulse trains, such as echo planar, peripheral nerve stimulation is reported at the threshold levels."	Ham et al.[34]
2.0 T RF at 90 MHz Simulated imaging conditions Phantom Caphuchin monkey Studied temperature changes in phantom and monkey brain during high RF power exposures	"Blood flowing through the brain used the body as a heat sink."	Hammer et al.[35]
0.35 T Simulated imaging conditions Mice Studied teratogenic effects of MRI	"Prolonged midgestional exposure failed to reveal any overt embryotoxicity or teratogenicity." "Slight but significant reduction in fetal crown–rump length after prolonged exposure justifies further study of higher MRI energy levels."	Heinrichs et al.[36]
1.5 T Static magnetic field only Human subjects Studied effect of static magnetic field on somatosensory evoked potentials	"Short-term exposure to 1.5 T static magnetic field does not affect SEPs in human subjects."	Hong and Shellock[37]
0.15 T Simulated imaging conditions Rats Studied effects on cognitive processes	"MRI procedure has no significant effect on spatial memory processes in rats."	Innis et al.[38]
2.0 T Static magnetic field only Human subjects Studied effect of static magnetic field on cardiac rhythm	Cardiac cycle length was significantly increased, but this is probably harmless in normal subjects. Safety in dysrrhythmic patients remains to be determined.	Jehenson et al.[39]
Survey of thermal injuries/incidents related to MR procedures	"The increasing incidence of such clinical MR-related reports of patient burns in conjunction with the ever-increasing number of MR sites, examinations, and applications (e.g., MRA) strongly indicate the need for increased physician awareness and education concerning this rare, but real, MR-related potential hazard."	Kanal and Applegate[40]
Various MR systems and conditions This study evaluated the safety and pharmacokinetics of gadolinium contrast agents in patients with hemodialysis; *in vitro* and clinical studies were performed	The results showed that all contrast agents and both dialysis membranes were suitable. Neither change in laboratory parameters nor side effects were observed. … consequently, there are no contraindications when using the ordinary dose of contrast agent even in patients with dialysis.	Katagiri et al.[41]

Study Description	Summary	Reference
1.5 T Simulated imaging conditions Frog embryo Studied effect of MRI on embryogenesis	"No adverse effects of MRI components on development of this vertebrate (*Xenopus laevis*)."	Kay et al.[42]
2.3, 4.7, and 10.0 T Static magnetic fields only Physiologic solutions (2.3 and 4.7 T) and mathematic modeling (10.0 T) Studied hydrostatic pressure and electrical potentials across vessels in presence of static magnetic fields	"A 10-T magnetic field changes vascular pressure in a model of the human vasculature by less than 0.2%."	Keltner et al.[43]
1.5 T Clinical imaging conditions Human subjects Studied physiologic changes during high-field-strength MRI	"Temperature changes and other physiologic changes were small and of no clinical concern."	Kido et al.[44]
1.5 T Simulated imaging conditions Rats Studied effects of MRI on receptor-mediated activation of pineal gland indole biosynthesis	"Strong magnetic fields and/or radiofrequency pulsing used in MRI inhibited beta-adrenergic activation of the gland."	LaPorte et al.[45]
1.0 and 1.5 T Clinical imaging conditions Human subjects Studied acoustic noise	"... many sequences produce noise levels above the safe levels defined by the Department of Health and the Health and Safety Executive."	McJury[46]
1.5 T Clinical imaging conditions Human subjects Studied acoustic noise	"...for certain protocols, the exposure to acoustic noise falls outside safety guidelines unless ear protection is used."	McJury et al.[47]
1.0 T Simulated imaging conditions Studied active noise control techniques that introduce antiphase noise to destructively interfere with MRI noise to produce a zone of quiet around the patient's ears	The results obtained show a useful attenuation of low-frequency periodic acoustic noise components. This suggests that MR-generated acoustic noise can be effectively attenuated at both low and high frequencies, leading to improved patient comfort.	McJury et al.[48]
3.5 to 12 T/s Gradient magnetic fields only Mice Studied effect of gradient magnetic fields on pregnancy and post-natal development	"No significant difference between the litter numbers and growth rates of the exposed litters compared with controls."	McRobbie and Foster[49]
Various strong magnetic field Gradient magnetic fields only Anesthetized rats Studied cardiac response to gradient magnetic fields	"The types of pulsed magnetic fields used in the present study did not affect the cardiac cycle of anesthetized rats."	McRobbie and Foster[50]

Study Description	Summary	Reference
1.89 T Simulated imaging sequence Rats Studied taste aversion in rats to evaluate possible toxic effects of MRI	"Rats exposed to MRI did not display any aversion to the saccharin solution."	Messmer et al.[51]
1.89 T Simulated imaging sequence Mouse spleen cells Studied possible interaction between ionizing radiation and MRI on damage to normal tissue	"For the normal tissues studied, MR imaging neither increases radiation damage nor inhibits repair."	Montour et al.[52]
0 to 2.0 T Clinical imaging conditions Human subjects Studied the extent of changes of the brainstem evoked potentials with MRI	"Routine MRI examinations do not produce pathological changes in auditory evoked potentials."	Muller and Hotz[53]
1.5 T Simulated imaging condition *In vitro* Studied the amalgamrelated mercury release for typical MRI conditions	"In vitro study demonstrated no evidence of an elevated mercury dissolution..."	Muller-Miny et al.[54]
0.75 T Static magnetic field only Hamster cells Studied effect of static magnetic field on DNA synthesis and survival of mammalian cells irradiated with fast neutrons	"Presence of the magnetic field either during or subsequent to fast-neutron irradiation does not effect the neutron-induced radiation damage or its repair."	Ngo et al.[55]
1.5 T Simulated imaging conditions Human subjects Studied effect of MRI on somatosensory and brainstem auditory evoked potentials	"It may be assumed that MRI causes no lasting changes."	Niemann et al.[56]
1.89 T Static magnetic field only Mice Studied effects of long-term exposure to a static magnetic field	"No consistent differences found in gross and microscopic morphology, hematocrit and WBCs, plasma creatine phosphokinase, lactic dehydrogenase, cholesterol, triglyceride, or protein concentrations in magnet groups compared to two control groups."	Osbakken et al.[57]
0.15 T Simulated imaging conditions Rats Studied effects of MRI on behavior of rats	"Results fail to provide any evidence for short or long term behavioral changes in animals exposed to MRI."	Ossenkopp et al.[58]
0.15 T Simulated imaging conditions Rats Studied effect of MRI on murine opiate analgesia levels	"NMRI procedures alter both day and night time responses to morphine."	Ossenkopp et al.[59]

Study Description	Summary	Reference
1.0 T Static magnetic field only Mice Studied effect of static magnetic field on *in vivo* bone growth	"Results suggest that exposure to intense magnetic fields does not alter physiological mechanisms of bone mineralization."	Papatheofanis and Papthefanis[60]
2.35 T Static and gradient magnetic fields only Nematodes Studied toxic effects of static and gradient magnetic fields	"Static magnetic fields have no effect on fitness of test animals." "Time-varying magnetic fields cause inhibition of growth and maturation." "Combination of pulsed magnetic field gradients in a static uniform magnetic field also has a detrimental effect on the fitness of the test animals."	Peeling et al.[61]
0.7 T Simulated imaging conditions Frog spermatazoa, fertilized eggs, and embryos Studied effects of MRI on development	"NMR exposure, at the dose used, does not cause detectable adverse effects in this amphibian."	Prasad et al.[62]
0.7 T Simulated imaging conditions Mouse bone marrow cells Studied the cytogenic effects of MRI	"NMR exposure causes no adverse cytogenic effects."	Prasad et al.[63]
2.35 T Simulated imaging conditions Mice Studied the effect of MRI on tumor development	"Immune response may be enhanced following MRI exposure, as indicated by the longer latency and smaller sizes of tumors in animals receiving MRI exposure."	Prasad et al.[64]
4.5 T Simulated imaging conditions Mice Studied the effects of high-field-strength MRI on mouse testes epididymes	"Little, if any, damage to male reproductive tissues from...high intensity MRI exposure."	Prasad et al.[65]
2.35 T Simulated imaging conditions Human peripheral blood mononuclear cells (PBMC) Studied effect of MRI on natural killer cell toxicity of PBMC with and without interleukin-2	"In neither case was cytotoxicity affected by prior exposure to MR imaging."	Prasad et al.[66]
0.15 T Simulated imaging conditions Mice Studied effects of MRI on immune system	"MR exposure has no adverse effect on the immune system, as evidenced by natural killer cell activity."	Prasad et al.[67]
0.15 and 4.0 T Simulated imaging conditions Fertilized frog eggs studied effect of MRI on developing embryos	"No adverse effect on early development."	Prasad et al.[68]

Study Description	Summary	Reference
0.15 T Exposed separately to static, gradient, and RF electromagnetic fields Mice Studied separate effects of static, gradient, and RF electromagnetic fields on morphine-induced analgesia in mice	"Time-varying, and to a lesser extent the RF, fields associated with the MRI procedure inhibit morphine-induced analgesia in mice."	Prato et al.[69]
4.7 T Clinical imaging conditions Human subjects Studied bioeffects of 4.7 T scanner	"Mild vertigo headaches, nausea magnetophosphenes metallic taste in mouth"	Redington et al.[70]
0.04 T Clinical imaging conditions Human subjects Follow-up study	"Average follow-up time was 6 months...none of the 35 deaths recorded was unexpected." "Using the magnetic field and radiofrequency levels currently in operation...we believe NMRI to be a safe, non-invasive method of whole-body imaging."	Reid et al. (71)
1.5 T Simulated imaging conditions Fetal mice Studied combined effect of exposure to gadopentetate dimeglumine and MRI on the developing embryo	"...MR exposure with and without gadopentetate dimeglumine had no adverse effect on the end points analyzed."	Rofsky et al.[72]
4.0 T RF at 8 to 170 MHz No gradient magnetic fields Human subjects Studied response of human auditory system to RF pulses	"In accordance with the used RF modulation envelope three distinct chirps per sequence could be resolved." "RF induced auditory noise is usually completely masked by noise from simultaneously switched gradient fields."	Roschmann[73]
Various MR systems and conditions 2,481 adult and pediatric subjects were studied with gadoteridol at doses from 0.025 to 0.3 mmol/kg in phase I-IIIb clinical trials in Europe and the U.S.	This report confirms the excellent safety profile of gadoteridol in healthy subjects and patients with a variety of known or suspected pathologies.	Runge and Parker[74]
2.7 T Simulated imaging conditions Rats Studied effects of MRI on ocular tissues	"There were no discernable effects on the rat eye.'	Sacks et al.[75]
0.5 T Static field only Wistar albino mice Studied possible alterations in enzyme activity of catalase and isoenzyme MB-creatine kinase induced by prolonged exposure of laboratory rodents to a static magnetic field	Results exclude any alteration in the activity of catalase and isoenzyme MB-creatine kinase caused by long-term exposure to a 0.5-T MR unit.	Salerno et al.[76]

Study Description	Summary	Reference
1.5 T Clinical imaging conditions Human subjects Studied effect of electromagnetic fields on melatonin levels	"MR imaging at high field strengths...did not suppress melatonin levels in human subjects.'	Schiffman et al.[77]
0.35 T Simulated imaging conditions Hamster ovary cells Studied effects of MRI on observable mutations and cytotoxicity	"NMR imaging caused no detectable genetic damage and does not affect cell viability."	Schwartz and Crooks[78]
1.5 T Static magnetic field only Human subjects Studied effect of static magnetic field on body temperature	"No effect on body temperature of normal human subjects."	Shellock et al.[79]
1.5 T Clinical imaging conditions Human subjects Studied thermal effects of MRI of the spine	"No surface 'hot spots.'" "Temperature effects were well-below known thresholds for adverse effects."	Shellock et al.[80]
1.5 T Clinical imaging conditions Human subjects Studied possible hypothalamic heating produced by MRI of the head	"There was probably no direct hypothalamic heating produced by clinical MRI of the head."	Shellock et al.[81]
1.5 T Clinical imaging conditions Human subjects Studied effect of MRI on corneal temperatures	"MR imaging...causes relatively minor increases in corneal temperature that do not appear to pose any thermal hazard to ocular tissue."	Shellock et al.[82]
1.5 T Clinical imaging conditions Human subjects Studied temperature, heart rate, and blood pressure changes associated with MRI	"MR imaging...not associated with any temperature or hemodynamic related deleterious effects."	Shellock and Crues[83]
1.5 T Clinical imaging conditions Human subjects Studied temperature changes associated with MRI of the brain	"No significant increases in average body temperature." "Observed elevations in skin temperatures were physiologically inconsequential."	Shellock and Crues[84]
1.5 T Static magnetic field only Human subjects Studied effects of static magnetic field on body and skin temperatures	"There were no statistically significant changes in body or any of the skin temperatures recorded."	Shellock et al.[85]
1.5 T Clinical imaging conditions Human subjects Studied effect of MRI performed at high SAR levels	"Recommended exposure to RF radiation during MR imaging of the body for patients with normal thermoregulatory function may be too conservative."	Shellock et al.[86]

Study Description	Summary	Reference
1.5 T Clinical imaging conditions Human subjects Studied effect of MRI on scrotal skin temperature	"Absolute temperature is below threshold known to affect testicular function."	Shellock et al.[87]
1.5 T Clinical imaging conditions Phantom Studied acoustic noise	"MR imaging performed with the worst-case pulse sequences did not produce noise levels that exceeded federal guidelines."	Shellock et al.[88]
1.5 T Simulated imaging conditions This study assessed gradient magnetic-field-induced acoustic noise levels associated with the use of echo planar imaging (EPI) and three-dimensional fast spin echo (3D-FSE) pulse sequences	"Gradient magnetic fields associated with the use of EPI and 3D-FSE techniques produced acoustic noise levels that were within the permissible levels recommended by federal guidelines."	Shellock et al.[89]
0.15 T Simulated imaging conditions Anesthetized rats Studied effect of MRI on blood-brain barrier permeability	"These findings raise the possibility that exposure to clinical MRI procedures may also temporarily alter the central blood-brain permeability in human subjects."	Shivers et al.[90]
1.5 T Simulated imaging conditions Anesthetized dogs Studied effect of MRI performed at high SAR levels	"These findings argue for continued caution in the design and operation of imagers capable of high specific absorption rates."	Shuman et al.[91]
0.4 to 8.0 T Static magnetic field only Mice Studied effect of static magnetic field on temperature	"Observed a field-induced increase in temperature."	Sperber et al.[92]
0.4 to 1.0 T Static magnetic field only Human subjects Studied the effects of static magnetic fields on tissue perfusion	"Neither at the skin of the thumb nor at the forearm were the changes in local blood flow attributable to the magnetic fields applied."	Stick et al.[93]
0.4 T Static magnetic field only Human subjects Studied magnetic field induced changes in auditory evoked potentials	"Strong steady magnetic fields induce changes in human auditory evoked potentials."	Stojan et al.[94]
0.15 T Clinical imaging conditions Human subjects Studied effect of MRI on cognitive functions	"No significant effect upon cognitive functions assessed."	Sweetland et al.[95]

Study Description	Summary	Reference
1.5 T Clinical imaging conditions Human subjects, neonates Studied heart rate (HR) and oxygen saturation before and during MR examinations of newborns	"Fluctuations in HR (but not oxygen saturation) that are temporally linked to the MR image acquisition occur in most neonates during routine clinical MR examinations."	Taber et al.[96]
0.6 T/s Gradient magnetic field only Mice Studied effect of gradient magnetic fields on the analgesic properties of specific opiate antagonists	"Results indicate that the time-varying fields associated with MRI have significant inhibitory effects on analgesic effects of specific myopiate-directed ligands."	Teskey et al.[97]
0.15 T Simulated imaging conditions Rats Studied effects of MRI on survivability and long-term stress reactivity levels	"Results fail to provide any evidence for changes in survivability and long-term reactivity levels in rats exposed to MRI."	Teskey et al.[98]
0.01 and 1.0 T Simulated imaging conditions and static magnetic field only *Echerichia coli* Studied effect of MRI and static magnetic field on various properties of *E. coli*	"No mutations or lethal effects observed."	Thomas and Morris[99]
1.5 T Simulated imaging conditions Mice Studied the potential effects of MRI fields on eye development	"These data suggest a potential for MRI teratogenicity in a strain of mouse predisposed to eye malformations.'"	Tyndall and Sulik[100]
1.5 T Simulated imaging conditions -C57BL/6J mouse Studied combined effects of MRI and X-irradiation on the developing eye of the mouse	"Results...suggested that the MRI techniques employed for this investigation did not enhance teratogenicity of X-irradiation on eye malformations produced in the 657BL/6J mouse."	Tyndall [101]
0.35 and 1.5 T Clinical imaging conditions Human subjects Studied effects of MRI on temperature	"No significant changes in central or peripheral temperatures resulting from the application of static or dynamic or radiofrequency."	Vogl et al.[102]
0.35 T Static magnetic field only Human subjects Studied effect of static magnetic field on auditory evoked potentials	"Magnetically induced shift may be explained by changes in electric capacities of the magnetically exposed biological system."	Von Klitzing[103]
0.2 T Static magnetic field only Human subjects Studied effect of static magnetic field on power intensity of EEG	"The increased control values following on inverted magnetic flux vector point to a reversible alteration of brain function induced by a static magnetic field."	Von Klitzing[104]

Study Description	Summary	Reference
0.2 T Static magnetic field only Human subjects studied Studied encephalomagnetic fields during exposure to static magnetic field	"Exposure to static magnetic fields as used in NMR-equipment generates a new encephalomagnetic field in human brain."	Von Klitzing[105]
1.5 and 4.0 T Static magnetic fields only Rats Studied effect of magnetic field on behavior	"At 4 T...in 97% of the trials the rats would not enter the magnet."	Weiss et al.[106]
0.16 T Static and gradient magnetic fields only Anesthetized rats and guinea pigs Studied effects of static and gradient magnetic fields on cardiac function of rats and guinea pigs	"No change in blood pressure, heart rate, or ECG."	Willis and Brooks[107]
1.5 T Simulated imaging conditions Human fetal lung (HFL) fibroblast cells Studied the effects of repetitive exposures to static magnetic field on cell proliferation	"The data do not provide evidence that repetitive exposures to a static magnetic field (1.5 T) exert effects on HFL proliferation."	Wiskerchen et al.[108]
0.3 T Static magnetic field only Mouse sperm cell Studied effect of static magnetic field on spermatogenesis	"Acute and subacute exposure to static magnetic fields associated with diagnostic MR imaging devices is unlikely to have any significant adverse effect on spermatogesis."	Withers et al.[109]
0.35 T Simulated imaging conditions Hamster ovary cells Studied effect of MRI on DNA and chromosomes	"The conditions used for NMR imaging do not cause genetic damage which is detectable by any of these methods."	Wolff et al.[110]
Varying gradient fields Human subjects Studied the effects of time-varying gradient fields on peripheral nerve stimulation using trapezoidal and sinusoidal pulse trains	"The thresholds of trapezoidal pulses were higher than those of sinusoidal pulses by 11% and 30%, respectively, at an equivalent power level."	Yamagata et al.[111]
1.5 T Simulated imaging conditions Chick embryos Studied teratogenicity of magnetic resonance field exposure	"...exposed embryos...showed a trend toward higher abnormality and mortality rates than their controls."	Yip et al.[112]
1.5 T Simulated imaging conditions Chick embryos Studied effect of of magnetic resonance exposure on proliferation and migration of motoneurons	"...birth rates, migration, and proliferation of lateral motoneurons were unaffected compared to their controls."	Yip et al.[113]

Study Description	Summary	Reference
1.5 T Simulated imaging conditions Chick embryos Studied effects of magnetic resonance exposure on the rate and specificity of sympathetic preganglionic axonal outgrowth	"...MR exposure conditions used in this study do not affect axonal growth in the sympathetic nervous system of the chick."	Yip et al.[114]
Various MR systems Clinical conditions The safety profile of ProHance® in special populations was evaluated by analyzing data extracted from the database of phase I-III studies Pediatric, elderly, and patients with renal disease studied	ProHance was administered at doses ranging from 0.1 to 0.3 mmol/kg and was found to be safe in all patient populations irrespective of age and pre-existing renal impairment. There appeared to be no correlation between incidence of adverse events and dose level in these special populations, and the higher dose level of 0.3 mmol/kg could be safely administered also to patients with end stage renal disease requiring hemodialysis, from whom the contrast medium was rapidly and efficiently dialyzed.	Yoshikawa and Davies[115]
0.5 and 1.5 T Static and gradient magnetic field Human subject Studied magnetic field effects on phantom limb pain	"The painful symptoms mimicked those experienced in the presence of the imagers."	Yuh et al.[116]

Note: Abbreviations used are radiofrequency (RF), specific absorption rate (SAR), nuclear magnetic resonance (NMR), magnetic resonance imaging (MRI), and electrocardiogram (ECG).

REFERENCES

1. Abart, J., Brinker, G., Irlbacher, W., and Grebmeier, J., Temperature and heart rate changes in MRI at SAR levels of up to 3 W/kg, in *Book of Abstracts*, Society of Magnetic Resonance in Medicine, Berkeley, CA, 2:683, 1991.
2. Abart, J., et al., Peripheral nerve stimulation by time-varying magnetic fields, *J. Comput. Assist. Tomogr.*, 21:532-538, 1997.
3. Adair, E.R. and Berglund, L.G., On the thermoregulatory consequences of NMR imaging, *Magn. Reson. Imaging*, 4:321-333, 1986.
4. Adair, E.R. and Berglund, L.G., Thermoregulatory consequences of cardiovascular impairment during NMR imaging in warm/humid environments, *Magn. Reson. Imaging*, 7:25-37, 1989.
5. Adzamli, I.K., Jolesz, F.A., and Blau, M., An assessment of blood-brain barrier integrity under MRI conditions: brain uptake of radiolabeled Gd-DTPA and In-DTPA-IgG, *J. Nucl. Med.*, 30:839, 1989.
6. Athey, T.W., A model of the temperature rise in the head due to magnetic resonance imaging procedures, *Magn. Reson. Med.*, 9:177-184, 1989.
7. Barber, B.J., Schaefer, D.J., Gordon, C.J., et al., Thermal effects of MR imaging: worst-case studies in sheep, *Am. J. Roentgenol.*, 155:1105-1110, 1990.
8. Bartels, M.V., Mann, K., Matejcek, M., et al., Magnetresonanztomographie und Sicherheit: Elektro-enzephalographische und neuropsychologische Befunde vor und nach MR-Untersuchungen des Gehirns, *Fortschr. Geb. Roentgenstr.*, 145:383-385, 1986.
9. Besson, J., Foreman, E.I., Eastwood, L.M., et al. Cognitive evaluation following NMR imaging of the brain, *J. Neurol. Neurosurg. Psychiatry*, 47:314-316, 1984.

10. Bore, P.J., Galloway, G.J., Styles, P., et al., Are quenches dangerous?, *Magn. Reson. Imaging*, 3:112-117, 1986.

11. Bourland, J.D., Nyenhuis, J.A., Mouchawar, G.A., et al., Physiologic indicators of high MRI gradient-induced fields, in *Book of Abstracts*, Society of Magnetic Resonance in Medicine, 3:1276, 1990.

12. Bourland, J.D., Nyenhuis, J.A., and Schaefer, D.J., Physiologic effects of intense MR imaging gradient fields, *Neuroimaging Clin. North Am.*, 9:363-367, 1999.

13. Brockway, J.P. and Bream, P.R., Does memory loss occur after MR imaging?, *J. Magn. Reson. Imaging*, 2:721-728, 1992.

14. Brody, A.S., Sorette, M.P., Gooding, C.A., et al., Induced alignment of flowing sickle erythrocytes in a magnetic field. A preliminary report, *Invest. Radiol.*, 20:560-566, 1985.

15. Brody, A.S., Embury, S.H., Mentzer, W.C., et al., Preservation of sickle cell blood flow patterns during MR imaging. An in vivo study, *Am. J. Roentgenol.*, 151:139-141, 1988.

16. Brummett, R.E., Talbot, J.M., and Charuhas, P., Potential hearing loss resulting from MR imaging, *Radiology*, 169:539-540, 1988.

17. Budinger, T.F., Fischer, H., Hentschel, D., et al., Physiological effects of fast oscillating magnetic field gradients, *J. Comput. Assist. Tomogr.*, 15:909-914, 1991.

18. Budinger, T.F., Brennan, K.N., Gilbert, J.C., et al., Excitation of the heart by rapidly oscillating magnetic fields, *Radiology*, 181(P):191, 1991.

19. Carson, J.J.L., Prato, F.S., Drost, D.J., et al., Time-varying fields increase cytosolic free Ca2+ in HL-60 cells, *Am. J. Physiol.*, 259:C687-C692, 1990.

20. Cho, Z.H., et al., Analysis of acoustic noise in MRI, *Magn. Reson. Imaging*, 15:815-822, 1997.

21. Cho, Z.H., et al., Effects of acoustic noise of the gradient systems on fMRI: a study on auditory, motor, and visual cortices, *Magn. Reson. Med.*, 39:331-336, 1998.

22. Cohen, M.S., Weisskoff, R., Rzedzian, R., et al., Sensory stimulation by time-varying magnetic fields, *Magn. Reson. Med.*, 14:409-414, 1990.

23. Cooke, P. and Morris, P.G., The effects of NMR exposure on living organisms. II. A genetic study of human lymphocytes, *Br. J. Radiol.*, 54:622-625, 1981.

24. Doherty, J.U., Whitman, G.J.R., Robinson, M.D., et al., Changes in cardiac excitability and vulnerability in NMR fields, *Invest. Radiol.*, 20:129-135, 1985.

25. Ehrhardt, J.C., et al., Peripheral nerve stimulation in a whole-body echo-planar imaging system, *J. Magn. Reson. Imaging*, 7:405-409, 1997.

26. Filippi, M., et al., A multi-centre longitudinal study comparing the sensitivity of monthly MRI after standard and triple dose gadolinium-DTPA for monitoring disease activity in multiple sclerosis. Implications for phase II clinical trials, *Brain*, 121(Pt. 10):2011-2020, 1998.

27. Fischer, H., Physiological effects of fast oscillating magnetic field gradients, *Radiology*, 173:(P)382, 1989.

28. Garber, H.J., Oldendorf, W.H., Braun, L.D., et al., MRI gradient fields increase brain mannitol space, *Magn. Reson. Imaging*, 7:605-610, 1989.

29. Geard, C.R., Osmak, R.S., Hall, E.J., et al., Magnetic resonance and ionizing radiation: A comparative evaluation in vitro of oncongenic and genotoxic potential, *Radiology*, 152:199-202, 1984.

30. Gore, J.C., McDonnell, M.J., Pennock, J.M., et al., An assessment of the safety of rapidly changing magnetic fields in the rabbit: implications for NMR imaging, *Magn. Reson. Imaging*, 1:191-195, 1982.

31. Grandolfo, M., Vecchia, P., and Gandhi, O.P., Magnetic resonance imaging: calculation of rates of energy absorption by a human-torso model, *Bioelectromagnetics*, 11:117-128, 1990.

32. Gremmel, H., Wendhausen, H., and Wunsch, F., Biologische Effekte statischef Magnetfelder bei NMR-Tomographie am Menschen. Wiss, Radiologische, Klinik, Christian-Albrechts-Universitat zu Kiel, 1983.

33. Gulch, R.W. and Lutz, O., Influence of strong static magnetic fields on heart muscle contraction, *Phys. Med. Biol.*, 31:763-769, 1986.

34. Ham, C.L.G., Engels, J.M.L., van de Wiel, G.T., and Machielsen, A., Peripheral nerve stimulation during MRI: effects of high gradient amplitudes and switching rates, *J. Magn. Reson. Imaging*, 7:933-937, 1997.

35. Hammer, B.E., Wadon, S., Mirer, S.D., et al., In vivo measurement of RF heating in Capuchin monkey brain, in *Book of Abstracts*, Society of Magnetic Resonance in Medicine, 3:1278, 1991.

36. Heinrichs, W.L., Fong, P., Flannery, M., et al., Midgestational exposure of pregnant balb/c mice to magnetic resonance imaging, *Magn. Reson. Imaging*, 6:305-313, 1988.

37. Hong, C.Z. and Shellock, F.G., Short-term exposure to a 1.5 Tesla static magnetic field does not effect somato-sensory evoked potentials in man, *Magn. Reson. Imaging*, 8:65-69, 1989.

38. Innis, N.K., Ossenkopp, K.P., Prato, F.S., et al., Behavioral effects of exposure to nuclear magnetic resonance imaging. II. Spatial memory tests, *Magn. Reson. Imaging*, 4:281-284, 1986.

39. Jehenson, P., Duboc, D., Lavergne, T., et al., Change in human cardiac rhythm by a 2 Tesla static magnetic field, *Radiology*, 166:227-230, 1988.

40. Kanal, E. and Applegate, G.R., Thermal injuries/incidents associated with MR imaging devices in the US: a compilation and review of the presently available data, in Society of Magnetic Resonance in Medicine, *Book of Abstracts*, Berkeley, CA, 1:274, 1990.

41. Katagiri, K., et al., Clearance of gadolinium contrast agent by hemodialysis: in vitro and clinical studies [Article in Japanese], *Nippon Igaku Hoshasen Gakkai Zasshi*, 58:739-744, 1998.

42. Kay, H.H., Herfkens, R.J., and Kay, B.K., Effect of magnetic resonance imaging on *Xenopus laevis* embryogenesis, *Magn. Reson. Imaging*, 6:501-506, 1988.

43. Keltner, J.R., Roos, M.S., Brakeman, P.R., et al., Magnetohydrodynamics of blood flow, *Magn. Reson. Med.*, 16:139-149, 1990.

44. Kido, D.K., Morris, T.W., Erickson, J.L., et al., Physiologic changes during high field strength MR imaging, *Am. J. Neuroradiol.*, 8:263-266, 1987.

45. LaPorte, R., Kus, L., Wisniewski, R.A., et al., Magnetic resonance imaging (MRI) effects on rat pineal neuroendocrine function, *Brain Res.*, 506:294-296, 1990.

46. McJury, M.J., Acoustic noise levels generated during high field MR imaging, *Clin. Radiol.*, 50:331-334, 1995.

47. McJury, M., Blug, A., Joerger, C., Condon, B., and Wyper, D., Acoustic noise levels during magnetic resonance imaging scanning at 1.5 T, *Br. J. Radiol.*, 64:413-415, 1994.

48. McJury, M., Stewart, R.W., Crawford, D., and Toma, E., The use of active noise control (ANC) to reduce acoustic noise generated during MRI scanning: some initial results, *Magn. Reson. Imaging*, 15:319-322, 1997.

49. McRobbie, D. and Foster, M.A., Cardiac response to pulsed magnetic fields with regard to safety in NMR imaging, *Phys. Med. Biol.*, 30:695-702, 1985.

50. McRobbie, D. and Foster, M.A., Pulsed magnetic field exposure during pregnancy and implications for NMR foetal imaging: a study with mice, *Magn. Reson. Imaging*, 3:231-234, 1985.

51. Messmer, J.M., Porter, J.H., Fatouros, P., et al., Exposure to magnetic resonance imaging does not produce taste aversion in rats, *Physiol. Behav.*, 40:259-261, 1987.

52. Montour, J.L., Fatouros, P.P., and Prasad, U.R., Effect of MR imaging on spleen colony formation following gamma radiation, *Radiology*, 168:259-260, 1988.

53. Muller, S. and Hotz, M., Human brainstem auditory evoked potentials (BAEP) before and after MR examinations, *Magn. Reson. Med.*, 16:476-480, 1990.

54. Muller-Miny, H., Erber, D., Moller, H., Muller-Miny, B., and Bongartz, G., Is there a hazard to health by mercury exposure from amalgam due to MRI?, *J. Magn. Reson. Imaging*, 1:258-260, 1996.

55. Ngo, F.Q.H., Blue, J.W., and Roberts, W.K., The effects of a static magnetic field on DNA synthesis and survival of mammalian cells irradiated with fast neutrons, *Magn. Reson. Med.*, 5:307-317, 1987.

56. Niemann, G., Schroth, G., Klose, U., et al., Influence of magnetic resonance imaging on somatosensory potential in man, *J. Neurol.*, 235:462-465, 1988.

57. Osbakken, M., Griffith, J., and Taczanowsky, P., A gross morphologic, histologic, hematologic, and blood chemistry study of adult and neonatal mice chronically exposed to high magnetic fields, *Magn. Reson. Med.*, 3:502-517, 1986.

58. Ossenkopp, K.P., Kavaliers, M., Prato, F.S., et al., Exposure to nuclear magnetic imaging procedure attenuates morphine-induced analgesia in mice, *Life Sci.*, 37:1507-1514, 1985.

59. Ossenkopp, K.P., Innis, N.K., Prato, F.S., et al., Behavioral effects of exposure to nuclear magnetic resonance imaging. I. Open-field behavior and passive avoidance learning in rats, *Magn. Reson. Imaging*, 4:275-280, 1986.

60. Papatheofanis, F.J. and Papthefanis, B.J., Short-term effect of exposure to intense magnetic fields on hematologic indices of bone metabolism, *Invest. Radiol.*, 24:221-223, 1989.

61. Peeling, J., Lewis, J.S., Samoiloff, M.R., et al., Biological effects of magnetic fields on the nemtode *Panagrellus redivivus*, *Magn. Reson. Imaging*, 6:655-660, 1988.
62. Prasad, N., Wright, D.A., Ford, J.J., and Thornby, J.I., Effect of nuclear magnetic resonance on early stages of amphibian development, *Magn. Reson. Imaging*, 1:35-38, 1982.
63. Prasad, N., Bushong, S.C., Thornby, J.I., et al., Effect of nuclear resonance on chromosomes of mouse bone marrow cells, *Magn. Reson. Imaging*, 2:37-39, 1984.
64. Prasad, N., Kosnik, L.T., Taber, K.H., et al., Delayed tumor onset following MR imaging exposure, in *Book of Abstracts*, Society of Magnetic Resonance in Medicine, Society of Magnetic Resonance in Medicine, Berkeley, CA, 1:275, 1990.
65. Prasad, N., Prasad, R., Bushong, S.C., et al., Effects of 4.5 T MRI exposure on mouse testes and epididymes, in *Book of Abstracts*, Society of Magnetic Resonance in Medicine, Society of Magnetic Resonance in Medicine, Berkeley, CA, 2:606, 1990.
66. Prasad, N., Lotzova, E., Thornby, J.I., et al., Effects of MR imaging on murine natural killer cell cytotoxicity, *Am. J. Roentgenol.*, 148:415-417, 1987.
67. Prasad, N., Lotzova, E., Thornby, J.I., et al., The effect of 2.35-T MR imaging on natural killer cell cytotoxicity with and without interleukin-2, *Radiology*, 175:251-263, 1990.
68. Prasad, N., Wright, D.A., Ford, J.J., et al., Safety of 4-T MR imaging: a study of effects of developing frog embryos, *Radiology*, 174:251-253, 1990.
69. Prato, F.S., Ossenkopp, K.P., Kavaliers, M., et al., Attenuation of morphine-induced analgesia in mice by exposure to magnetic resonance imaging: seperate effects of the static, radiofrequency and time-varying magnetic fields, *Magn. Reson. Imaging*, 5:9-14, 1987.
70. Redington, R.W., Dumoulin, C.L., Schenck, J.L., et al., MR imaging and bio-effects in a whole body 4.0 Tesla imaging system, in *Book of Abstracts*, Society of Magnetic Resonance Imaging, Berkeley, CA, 1:20, 1988.
71. Reid, A., Smith, F.W., and Hutchison, J.M.S., Nuclear magnetic resonance imaging and its safety implications: follow-up of 181 patients, *Br. J. Radiol.*, 55:784-786, 1982.
72. Rofsky, N.M., Pizzarello, D.J., Weinreb, J.C., Ambrosino, M.M., and Rosenberg, C., Effect on fetal mouse development of exposure to MR imaging and gadopentetate dimeglumine, *J. Magn. Reson. Imaging*, 4:805-807, 1994.
73. Roschmann, P., Human auditory system response to pulsed radiofrequency energy in RF coils for magnetic resonance at 2.4 to 170 MHz, *Magn. Reson. Med.*, 21:197-215, 1991.
74. Runge, V.M. and Parker, J.R., Worldwide clinical safety assessment of gadoteridol injection: an update, *Euro. Radiol.*, 7(Suppl. 5):243-245, 1997.
75. Sacks, E., Worgul, B.V., Merriam, G.R., et al., The effects of nuclear magnetic resonance imaging on ocular tissues, *Arch. Ophthalmol.*, 104:890-893, 1986.
76. Salerno, S., et al., Biologic effects of the static magnetic field generated by a 0.5 T magnetic resonance tomograph on the enzyme activity of catalase and creatine kinase in the rat, *Radiol. Med. (Torino)*, 97:174-178, 1999.
77. Schiffman, S.J., Lash, H.M., Rollag, M.D., Flanders, A.E., Brainard, G.C., and Burk, D.L., Effect of MR imaging on the normal human pineal body: measurement of plasma melatonin levels, *J. Magn. Reson. Imaging*, 4:7-11, 1994.
78. Schwartz, J.L. and Crooks, L.E., NMR imaging produces no observable mutations or cytotoxicity in mammalian cells, *Am. J. Roentgenol.*, 139:583-585, 1982.
79. Shellock, F.G., Schaefer, D.J., and Gordon, C.J., Effect of a 1.5 T static magnetic field on body temperature of man, *Magn. Reson. Med.*, 3:644-647, 1986.
80. Shellock, F.G. and Crues, J.V., Temperature, heart rate, and blood pressure changes associated with clinical MR imaging at 1.5 T, *Radiology*, 163:259-262, 1987.
81. Shellock, F.G., Schaefer, D.J., Grundfest, W., et al., Thermal effects of high-field (1.5 Tesla) magnetic resonance imaging of the spine: Clinical experience above a specific absorption rate of 0.4 W/kg, *Acta Radiol.*, 369(Suppl.): 514-516, 1986.
82. Shellock, F.G., Gordon, C.J., and Schaefer, D.J., Thermoregulatory responses to clinical magnetic resonance imaging of the head at 1.5 Tesla: Lack of evidence for direct effects on the hypothalamus, *Acta Radiol.*, 369(Suppl.):512-513, 1986.
83. Shellock, F.G. and Crues, J.V., Corneal temperature changes associated with high-field MR imaging using a head coil, *Radiology*, 167:809-811, 1986.

84. Shellock, F.G. and Crues, J.V., Temperature changes caused by clinical MR imaging of the brain at 1.5 Tesla using a head coil, *Am. J. Neuroradiol.*, 9:287-291, 1988.

85. Shellock, F.G., Schaefer, D.J., and Crues, J.V., Effect of a 1.5 Tesla static magnetic field on body and skin temperatures of man, *Magn. Reson. Med.*, 11:371-375, 1989.

86. Shellock, F.G., Schaefer, D.J., and Crues, J.V., Alterations in body and skin temperatures caused by MR imaging: Is the recommended exposure for radiofrequency radiation too conservative?, *Br. J. Radiol.*, 62:904-909, 1989.

87. Shellock, F.G., Rothman, B., and Sarti, D., Heating of the scrotum by high-field-strength MR imaging, *Am. J. Roentgenol.*, 154:1229-1232, 1990.

88. Shellock, F.G., Morisoli, S.M., and Ziarati, M., Measurement of acoustic noise during MR imaging: evaluation of six "worst-case" pulse sequences, *Radiology*, 191:91-93, 1994.

89. Shellock, F.G., Ziarati, M., Atkinson, D., and Chen, D.Y., Determination of gradient magnetic field-induced acoustic noise associated with the use of echo planar and three-dimensional, fast spin echo techniques, *J. Magn. Reson. Imaging*, 8:1154-1157, 1998.

90. Shivers, R.R., Kavaliers, M., Tesky, C.J., et al., Magnetic resonance imaging temporarily alters blood-brain barrier permeability in the rat, *Neurosci. Lett.*, 76:25-31, 1987.

91. Shuman, W.P., Haynor, D.R., Guy, A.W., et al., Superficial and deep-tissue increases in anesthetized dogs during exposure to high specific absorption rates in a 1.5-T MR imager, *Radiology*, 167:551-554, 1988.

92. Sperber, D., Oldenbourg, R., and Dransfeld, K., Magnetic field induced temperature change in mice, *Naturwissenschaften*, 71:100–101, 1984.

93. Stick, V.C., Hinkelmann, Z.K., Eggert, P., et al., Beeinflussen starke statische magnetfelder in der NMR-Tomographie die gewebedurchblutung? (Strong static magnetic fields of NMR: Do they affect tissue perfusion?), *Fortschr. Geh. Roentgenstr.*, 154(3):326-331, 1991.

94. Stojan, L., Sperber, D., and Dransfeld, K., Magnetic-field-induced changes in the human auditory evoked potentials, *Naturwissenschaften*, 75:622-623, 1988.

95. Sweetland, J., Kertesz, A., Prato, F.S., et al., The effect of magnetic resonance imaging on human congnition, *Magn. Reson. Imaging*, 5:129-135, 1987.

96. Taber, K., et al., Vital sign changes during infant magnetic resonance examinations, *J. Magn. Reson. Imaging*, 8:1252-1256, 1998.

97. Teskey, G.C., Prato, F.S., Ossenkopp, K.P., et al., Exposure to time varying magnetic fields associated with magnetic resonance imaging reduces fentanyl-induced analgesia in mice, *Bioelectromagnetics*, 9:167-174, 1988.

98. Tesky, G.C., Ossenkopp, K.P., Prato, F.S., et al., Survivability and long-term stress reactivity levels following repeated exposure to nuclear magnetic resonance imaging procedures in rats, *Physiol Chem. Phys. Med. NMR*, 19:43-49, 1987.

99. Thomas, A. and Morris, P.G., The effects of NMR exposure on living organisms. I. A microbial assay, *Br. J. Radiol.*, 54:615-621, 1981.

100. Tyndall, D.A. and Sulik, K.K., Effects of magnetic resonance imaging on eye development in the C57BL/6J mouse, *Teratology*, 43:263-275, 1991.

101. Tyndall, D.A., MRI effects on the tertogenicity of X-irradiation in the C57BL/6J mouse, *Magn. Reson. Imaging*, 8:423-433, 1990.

102. Vogl, T., Krimmel, K., Fuchs, A., et al., Influence of magnetic resonance imaging on human body core and intravascular temperature, *Med. Phys.*, 15:562-566, 1988.

103. Von Klitzing, L., Do static magnetic fields of NMR influence biological signals, *Clin. Phys. Physiol. Meas. (Bristol)*, 7(2):157-160, 1986.

104. Von Klitzing, L., Static magnetic fields increase the power intensity of EEG of man, *Brain Res.*, 483: 201-203, 1989.

105. Von Klitzing, L., A new encephalomagnetic effect in human brain generated by static magnetic fields, *Brain Res.*, 540:295-296, 1991.

106. Weiss, J., Herrick, R.C., Taber, K.H., et al., Bio-effects of high magnetic fields: a study using a simple animal model, *Magn. Reson. Imaging*, 8(S1):166, 1990.

107. Willis, R.J. and Brooks, W.M., Potential hazards of NMR imaging. No evidence of the possible effects of static and changing magnetic fields on cardiac function of the rat and guinea pig, *Magn. Reson. Imaging*, 2:89-95, 1984.

108. Wiskirchen, J., et al., Long-term effects of repetitive exposure to a static magnetic field (1.5 T) on proliferation of human fetal lung fibroblasts, *Magn. Reson. Med.*, 41:464-468, 1999.

109. Withers, H.R., Mason, K.A., and Davis, C.A., MR effect on murine spermatogenesis, *Radiology*, 156:741-742, 1985.

110. Wolff, S., Crooks, L.E., Brown, P., et al., Tests for DNA and chromosomal damage induced by nuclear magnetic resonance imaging, *Radiology*, 136:707-710, 1980.

111. Yamagata, H., Kuhara, S., Eso, Y., et al., Evaluation of dB/dt thresholds for nerve stimulation elicited by trapezoidal and sinusoidal gradient fields in echo-planar imaging, in *Book of Abstracts*, Society of Magnetic Resonance in Medicine, Berkeley, CA, 3:1277, 1991.

112. Yip, Y.P., Capriotti, C., Talagala, S.L., and Yip, J.W., Effects of MR exposure at 1.5 T on early embryonic development of the chick, *J. Magn. Reson. Imaging*, 4:742-748, 1994.

113. Yip, Y.P., Capriotti, C., Norbash, S.G., Talagala, S.L., and Yip, J.W., Effects of MR exposure on cell proliferation and migration of chick motoneurons, *J. Magn. Reson. Imaging*, 4:799-804, 1994.

114. Yip, Y.P., Capriotti, C., and Yip, J.W., Effects of MR exposure on axonal outgrowth in the sympathetic nervous system of the chick, *J. Magn. Reson. Imaging*, 4:457-462, 1995.

115. Yoshikawa, K. and Davies, A., Safety of ProHance in special populations, *Euro. Radiol.*, 7(Suppl. 5):246-250, 1997.

116. Yuh, W.T.C., Fisher, D.J., Shields, R.K., et al., Phantom limb pain induced in amputee by strong magnetic fields, *J. Magn. Reson. Imaging*, 2:221-223, 1992.

Appendix III

Web Site for MRI Safety
www.MRIsafety.com

The international information resource for MRI safety, bioeffects, and patient management.

PURPOSE

MRIsafety.com is a web site that provides up-to-date and crucial information to healthcare providers and patients seeking answers to questions on MRI safety-related topics. The latest information is also provided for screening patients with implants, materials, and medical devices. **MRIsafety.com** was developed and is maintained by Frank G. Shellock, Ph.D.

KEY FEATURES

- *The List.* A searchable database that contains over 700 implants and other objects tested for MRI Safety.
- *Safety Information.* Useful information that pertains to patient care and management in the MRI environment.
- *Research Summary.* A presentation and summary of over 100 peer-reviewed articles on MRI bioeffects and safety.
- *Pre-MRI Screening.* Important information pertaining to screening patients and individuals. In addition, a form for pre-MRI screening is available to download for use at your imaging facility.

E-MAIL ADDRESS

If you have a specific question about a bioimplant, material, or device or require testing of a medical product, please contact Dr. Shellock at: Frank.Shellock@gte.net.

Index

transmetallation considerations, 247–248
urticaria caused by, 248
viscosity of, 247
mangafodipir trisodium, 249–250
monitoring guidelines, 218
oral, 253–254
during pregnancy, 152–153
Cranial flap fixation clamps, 295–296, 402–403
Currents, induced
characteristics of, 272–273
flow-induced, 8
from intense gradient fields
finite element calculation of, 47–51
metallic implant effect on concentration of, 410
motion-induced, 8
Cutaneous blood flow monitoring, 230–232

D

Deflection angle test, for metallic implant assessments,
277–278
Demagnetizing factors, 14–15
Dental implants, 296–297, 303, 349–350
Devices, *see* Implants, devices, and materials
Diamagnetic repulsion, 12
Diaphragm, 296–298
Distress, *see also* Claustrophobia
adverse outcomes secondary to, 198
contributing factors, 199–207
definition of, 198
impact of, 198–199
incidence of, 197–198
motion artifacts caused by, 199
pre-existing psychiatric problems and, 206–207
severity of, 198
system design and, 199–207
systematic desensitization techniques, 213
techniques for minimizing, 207–213
Dotarem, *see* Gadoterate meglumine

E

Ear
anatomy of, 116
cochlear implants, 292–293, 310, 402
hearing sensitivity of, 116
Echo planar imaging
acoustic noise associated with, 119–120
monitoring guidelines during, 218
Electric fields
calculation of, 48–51
concentration of, by elongated implant, 405–407
radiofrequency coil induction of, 62
specific absorption ratio calculations, 57–58
Electrocardiogram
electrodes for, 298, 350–352, 403
monitoring uses of, 222–223
Emergency plan, 220
Endoscopy, 304–305

End-tidal carbon dioxide monitor, 226–227
Eyes, radiofrequency energy-induced heating effects, 90

F

Fatio eyelid wire, 309–310
Ferric ammonium citrate, 253–254
FerriSeltz, *see* Ferric ammonium citrate
Ferumoxides, 250–251
Fields, *see* Electric fields; Magnetic fields; Radiofrequency
field
Filters, 293, 295, 342–349
Finite-difference time-domain method, for assessing
specific absorption rate, 98–99
Fluoroptic thermometry system, 232
Food and Drug Administration
authority of, 184–185
description of, 183–184
functions of, 183–184
guidance by
devices compatibility, 192–193
materials biocompatibility, 189
1998 MRDD 510(k), 190–192
safety, 192, 194–195
significant risk criteria, 190
software, 189–190
IEC standard 60601-2-33
description of, 188–189
revision forthcoming, 193–194
insurance reimbursement secondary to approval by,
184–185
magnetic resonance regulatory activity
class III devices, 185–186
magnetic fields, 187–188
MR Diagnostic Device 510(k) guidance, 186–187
reclassifications, 186–187
regulatory powers of, 184–185
Food and Drug Administration Modernization Act, 185
Foreign bodies, metallic, *see also* Implants, devices, and
materials
description of, 266
in orbital region, 266–267, 303
screening guidelines for, 267
Fringe magnetic fields
description of, 144
missile effect hazards secondary to, 268–269

G

Gadodiamide, 242, 244–246, 252
Gadolinium chelates
adverse reactions caused by, 242, 248–249
anaphylactoid reactions caused by, 248–249
differentiation of, 245, 247–248
dosing of, 252
gadodiamide, *see* Gadodiamide
gadopentetate dimeglumine, *see* Gadopentetate
dimeglumine
gadoterate meglumine, *see* Gadoterate meglumine